Oral Health: Principles and Practice

Oral Health: Principles and Practice

Edited by Edward Thomas

hayle medical
New York

Hayle Medical,
750 Third Avenue, 9th Floor,
New York, NY 10017, USA

Visit us on the World Wide Web at:
www.haylemedical.com

ISBN: 978-1-63241-570-7

Cataloging-in-Publication Data

Oral health : principles and practice / edited by Edward Thomas.
p. cm.
Includes bibliographical references and index.
ISBN 978-1-63241-570-7
1. Mouth--Care and hygiene. 2. Oral medicine. 3. Dental care. 4. Dental public health.
5. Mouth--Diseases. 6. Dentistry. I. Thomas, Edward.
RK60.7 .O73 2019
617.601--dc23

Table of Contents

Preface

The world is advancing at a fast pace like never before. Therefore, the need is to keep up with the latest developments. This book was an idea that came to fruition when the specialists in the area realized the need to coordinate together and document essential themes in the subject. That's when I was requested to be the editor. Editing this book has been an honour as it brings together diverse authors researching on different streams of the field. The book collates essential materials contributed by veterans in the area which can be utilized by students and researchers alike.

The practice of maintaining cleanliness of one's mouth and keeping it germ-free is called oral hygiene. Dental and gum diseases which affect oral hygiene include dental caries, gingivitis and periodontitis. The common and effective methods to maintain oral hygiene and to prevent oral diseases include routine tooth brushing, flossing and the use of tongue scrapers. Regular brushing plays an important role in the reduction of dental plaque. This can be done using a brush with soft bristles as it causes little damage to the gums. Flossing is a technique used to remove plaque from the space between the teeth. Tongue scrapers are used to remove the debris built up on the tongue. This book elucidates the concepts and innovative models around prospective developments with respect to oral health. It traces the progress of this field and highlights some of its key concepts and applications. This book includes contributions of dentists and experts which will provide innovative insights into this field.

Each chapter is a sole-standing publication that reflects each author´s interpretation. Thus, the book displays a multi-facetted picture of our current understanding of application, resources and aspects of the field. I would like to thank the contributors of this book and my family for their endless support.

Editor

1

A structural equation model to test a conceptual framework of oral health in Japanese edentulous patients with an item weighting method using factor score weights

Eijiro Yamaga*, Yusuke Sato and Shunsuke Minakuchi

Abstract

Background: To investigate Locker's multidimensional model of oral health in Japanese edentulous patients with an item weighting method using factor score weights, which is more accurate than the sum scoring method. A previous study tested Locker's model in edentulous elders in the UK, using empirical evidence from the Short-Form Oral Health Impact Profile (OHIP-14). Investigating the model using the OHIP for edentulous subjects (OHIP-EDENT), which contains 19 items suitable for these patients, may complement that study. Testing Locker's model in Japanese patients may support generalization of the model.

Methods: A total of 394 patients who were edentulous in both arches and visited the Dental Hospital of Tokyo Medical and Dental University for new complete dentures were recruited. This cross-sectional study had a non-probabilistic sampling design and included the following: data collection; application of the new item weighting method that involves hierarchical confirmatory factor analysis (CFA) to derive factor score weights for each item, using the bootstrap method, to check the significance of the factor score weights; and empirical testing of Locker's conceptual model of oral health in Japanese edentulous patients, using structural equation modelling analysis with the bootstrap method for precise estimations and model generation.

Results: Factor score weights derived from CFA were significant. After item weighting, the initial model was analyzed and found to have an inconsistent direct path (functional limitation to disability). This path was eliminated from the model and the modified model was re-run. All effects were significant. The model showed acceptable fit on indices including the model chi-squared, standardized root-mean-square residual, root mean-square error of approximation, goodness-of-fit index, comparative fit index, and *P*-value.

Conclusions: Our findings showed an empirical fit to Locker's model in Japanese edentulous patients when using the item weighting method, which was more accurate than the sum scoring method. These results could contribute to the generalization of Locker's model.

Keywords: Oral health quality of life, Edentulous, Conceptual model, Structural equation model, Factor score weight, Generalization

* Correspondence: e.yamaga.gerd@tmd.ac.jp
Gerodontology and Oral Rehabilitation, Department of Gerontology and Gerodontology, Graduate School of Medical and Dental Sciences, Tokyo Medical and Dental University, Yushima Bunkyo-ku, Tokyo 113-8549, Japan

Background

Oral health-related quality of life (OHRQoL) is a multidimensional construct. OHRQoL has been researched mostly based on Locker's conceptual model of oral health [1]. Locker proposed a scientific model that aims to specify the complicated consequences of oral disease on quality of life. Nevertheless, no study, except for that by Baker [2], has investigated Locker's model explicitly using empirical evidence. In that study [2], data for three samples (general adults, edentulous elders, and patients with xerostomia) were analyzed and the short version of the Oral Health Impact Profile (OHIP-14) [3] was used as the measure.

The OHIP [4] is often used to evaluate the multidimensional construct of OHRQoL. However, the large number of items included makes it difficult for participants to complete the survey. Therefore, the OHIP-14 was designed and has been widely adopted to assess the association between OHRQoL and a clinical intervention [5]. However, because of a floor effect, the OHIP-14 cannot determine improvements in edentulous persons following clinical intervention [6]. The OHIP-EDENT is a shortened version of the OHIP, which includes 19 items suitable for edentulous persons. By including an item on chewing and eating difficulty, the OHIP-EDENT could detect OHRQoL changes in edentulous persons with new or different prostheses [6]. In the present study, the Japanese version of the Oral Health Impact Profile for edentulous subjects (OHIP-EDENT-J), a cross-culturally adapted scale, was used [7].

Historically, the numbers of edentulous persons in developed countries have been decreasing. However, given the present ageing of societies, the need for treatment of edentulous persons is not anticipated to decrease overall [8]. The World Health Organization recommends that socioepidemiological research focusing on high-risk groups, including edentulous patients, is needed in order to improve the health of older adults [9]. Further, Critchlow and Ellis [10] concluded that the evidence base in complete denture research suffers from an insufficient number of well-conducted studies. Using the OHIP-14, Baker [2] succeeded in indicating that Locker's conceptual model of oral health is supported by empirical evidence in edentulous elders as well as in the general adult population. An investigation applying the OHIP-EDENT to Locker's model in edentulous patients may complement Baker's study.

Item weighting is a process by which the relative weight of events can be expressed. Using a weighted scoring system, the discriminant validity of OHIP was improved to a small extent [11]; however, it does not have good cost-performance [12]. That is, item weighting is a time-consuming process that offers only slight improvement of discriminant validity. On the other hands, DiStefano et al. [13] reported that sum scoring was a non-refined method because its score does not necessarily indicate adequate contribution to the factor (e.g., negative factor loading). Zucoloto et al. [14] also regarded sum scoring as an inaccurate method, and proposed a second-order or third-order model for derivation of the scores on the subscales and an overall score for the measure that adequately improves the accuracy of estimation of the construct using the structural equation modelling (SEM) method. SEM is a powerful multivariable analytical method that can present direct and indirect effects separately and express complicated relationships in a path diagram [15].

The aim of this study was to investigate Locker's conceptual model of oral health in Japanese edentulous patients with the OHIP-EDENT-J using SEM with the item weighting method proposed by Zucoloto et al. in order to generalize Locker's model. The following hypotheses were tested: functional limitations would be related to disability, which would be related to handicap, which in turn would be related to pain and discomfort; both pain and discomfort would be associated with disability; and pain would be related to discomfort. These hypotheses were adopted as the conceptual model of oral health in a sample of edentulous elders in a previous study by Baker [2].

Methods

The study was conducted in three stages: 1) collection of data; 2) deriving weighting formulae from hierarchical confirmatory factor analysis (CFA) to improve the accuracy of the estimation [14]; and 3) empirical testing of Locker's conceptual model of oral health in Japanese edentulous patients with the OHIP-EDENT-J [7] using SEM analysis after item weighting derived from CFA. A cross-sectional design with non-probabilistic sampling was adopted.

Participants

The participants were systemically healthy persons who were edentulous in both arches and visited the Dental Hospital of Tokyo Medical and Dental University requesting new complete dentures during the period from January 2009 to April 2015. The exclusion criteria included no existing denture or dentures and non-attendance before measurements. Three hundred and ninety-four patients were recruited for the study. One patient was hospitalized, another one was withdrawn, 49 had missing data, leaving 343 patients (87.1%, mean age 76.3 ± 8.3 years) for analysis. The patient characteristics, oral condition, and quality of previous dentures were investigated by calibrated prosthodontists with more than 4 years of clinical experience, during the creation of the new complete dentures (Table 1). The method devised

Table 1 Patient characteristics, oral condition, and quality of previous dentures

Variable	Participants (N = 343), n (%)	
Sex		
Male	140 (40.8)	
Female	203 (59.2)	
Edentulous period (years)		
< 1	77 (22.4)	
1 to < 3	28 (8.2)	
3 to < 5	18 (5.3)	
5 to < 10	42 (12.2)	
10+	174 (50.7)	
Forgotten	4 (1.2)	
Age of present denture (years)		
< 5	127 (37.0)	
5 to < 10	132 (38.5)	
10+	81 (23.6)	
Forgotten	3 (0.9)	
Ridge form (Cawood & Howell classification)[a]		
	Maxilla	Mandible
Class II	6 (1.7)	18 (5.3)
Class III	249 (72.6)	103 (30.0)
Class IV	57 (16.6)	81(23.6)
Class V	28 (8.2)	106 (30.9)
Class VI	1 (0.3)	31 (9.0)
Others	2 (0.6)	4 (1.2)
Denture stability (Kapur method)[b]		
0	37 (10.8)	132 (38.5)
1	109 (31.7)	139 (40.5)
2	197 (57.4)	72 (21.0)
Denture retention (Kapur method)[c]		
0	24 (7.0)	134 (39.1)
1	62 (18.1)	105 (30.6)
2	85 (24.8)	57 (16.6)
3	172 (50.1)	47 (13.7)
Jaw relation		
Premature contact (−)	232 (67.6)	
Premature contact (+)	111 (32.4)	

[a]Class II, immediately post extraction; Class III, well-rounded ridge form, adequate in height and width; Class IV, knife-edge ridge form, adequate in height and inadequate in width; Class V, flat ridge form, inadequate in height and width; Class VI, depressed ridge form, with some basal loss evident. [b]Scoring system: 0, no stability, when a denture base demonstrates extreme rocking on its supporting structures under pressure; 1, some stability, when a denture base demonstrates moderate rocking on its supporting structures under pressure; 2, sufficient stability, when a denture base demonstrates slight or no rocking on its supporting structures under pressure. [c]Scoring system: 0, no retention, when a denture is seated in place, it displaces itself; 1, minimum retention, when a denture offers slight resistance to vertical pull and little or no resistance to lateral force; 2, moderate retention, when a denture offers moderate resistance to vertical pull and little or no resistance to lateral force; 3, good retention, when a denture offers maximum resistance to vertical pull and sufficient resistance to lateral force

by Cawood and Howell [16] was employed to assess the residual ridge forms. Denture stability and retention were estimated using the Kapur method [17]. Jaw relation was estimated by investigating whether premature contact was existing or not in centric relation. The assessments of patient characteristics, oral condition, and quality of previous dentures are part of the screening process for patients requesting new complete dentures, and thus were not purely for purpose of this study. All subjects provided written informed consent to participate in this study.

OHIP-EDENT-J

To investigate the multidimensional construct of OHRQoL, the OHIP was assessed using the OHIP-EDENT-J [7]. The OHIP-EDENT-J has 19 items and consists of seven subscales (functional limitation, pain, psychological discomfort, physical disability, psychological disability, social disability, and handicap) and is based on Locker's model [1]. Functional limitation is defined as the extent of depression of function of body parts or systems. The definition of discomfort is the self-assessment of physical and psychological distress, including pain and other feelings that are not directly observable. Disability is expressed as three dimensions of well-being (physical, psychological, and social). Handicap is concerned with the social effects of disease, which are broader than those of disability [1]. Participants were asked how many times they had experienced the impact of each item in the previous month using a scale ranging from 0 (never) to 4 (very often).

Factor score weights

To improve the accuracy of estimation of the construct, we employed hierarchical CFA using SEM analysis [14, 15]. The SEM analysis was conducted with AMOS (SPSS Statistics version 17.0, SPSS Inc., Chicago, IL). Given that many authors have indicated their calculation of the OHIP by summing all items, the existence of the third-order factor (OHIP) is presumably assured [14]. Therefore, we performed CFA using a third-order hierarchical CFA model and derived a formula whereby the third-order factor (OHIP) could be estimated. The third-order model has been described in the literature [14]. The scores derived from the formula can obtain a more accurate estimation than the simple summing method. In detail, the weighting formula derived from the third-order model included factor score weights for items 1–19. The product of the factor score weight and average deviation of item score for the raw data was adopted as the final item score to investigate the hypothesized model. Evaluation of the significance of factor score weights was conducted using bias-corrected bootstrapped 95% confidence intervals (CIs) [18] based on

1000 replications. The method used to assess the model fit of CFA is described in the following paragraph.

Testing the Locker model

Locker's conceptual model of oral health in edentulous patients was empirically investigated using SEM. The hypothesized model was that used in a previous study of edentulous patients by Baker [2]. The maximum likelihood method is adopted for estimation of free parameters and requires data that have a normal distribution. More than 1.0 of absolute value of kurtosis was regarded as non-normal distribution. The bootstrap method can also be used to determine parameter estimates in data that have a non-normal distribution [18]. Parameter estimates of the direct and indirect effects were determined using the bootstrapping method with 1000 iterations.

Estimation of model fit

We assessed model fit to the data using five indices commonly used in SEM analysis, i.e., the chi-squared test and *P*-value, the standardized root-mean-square residual (SRMR), the root mean-square error of approximation (RMSEA), the comparative fit index (CFI), and the goodness-of-fit index (GFI) [15]. As the chi-squared value increases and the *P*-value consequently decreases, the fit of the model becomes increasingly worse. A 'larger' *P*-value indicates a 'better' model fit. SRMR values less than 0.08 are generally considered to be favorable [19, 20]. In general, an RMSEA less than 0.05 indicates a close fit, values between 0.05 and 0.08 indicate a reasonable fit, and an RMSEA more than 0.1 indicates a poor fit [21]. A GFI and a CFI of 1.0 indicates a complete model fit. Generally, a GFI and a CFI greater than 0.95 indicates a good fit [19, 20].

Strategy in model specification

There are some strategies involved in specification and evaluation of the model. MacCallum and Austin [21] proposed three SEM analysis strategies: (a) a strictly confirmatory strategy, in which a single a priori model is investigated; (b) a model generation strategy, in which an initial model is fitted to the data and then modified as necessary until the fit is adequate; and (c) an alternative model strategy, in which various a priori models are studied. We employed (a) a strictly confirmatory strategy for CFA and (b) a model generation strategy for the Baker model.

Results

The means, medians, and standard deviations (SDs) of the observed variables before weighting and Pearson's correlations between observed variables after weighting are shown in Table 2. There were no correlations with high coefficients (> 0.85), indicating that multicollinearity did not occur in the SEM analysis.

Univariate kurtosis in items 2, 7, 10, 13, and 15–19 (CFA section), handicap (Baker model section after weighting), and multivariate kurtosis (CFA and Baker model section) indicated a non-normal distribution.

Factor score weights

We derived the weighting formula from hierarchical CFA in which the third-order model was employed using raw data (OHIP item score). The CFA model and the bootstrap standardized estimates of direct effect are shown in Fig. 1. The fit indices were as follows: chi-squared = 897.03 (146 degrees of freedom), $P < 0.001$, CFI = 0.83, GFI = 0.76, RMSEA = 0.12 (90% CI 0.11–0.13), and SRMR = 0.089. The fit of the model was poor. The bootstrap standardized estimates and the standard error and CI values for the factor score weights of each item (OHIP) are shown in Table 3. All factor score weights were significant. Based on the model, the item scores for the third-order factor (OHIP) can be estimated by the following formula [14]:

$$\begin{aligned}\text{OHIP}, y = {} & 0.025\text{it}1 + 0.035\text{it}2 + 0.045\text{it}3 + 0.037\text{it}4 + 0.019\text{it}5 \\ & +0.049\text{it}6 + 0.092\text{it}7 + 0.202\text{it}8 + 0.114\text{it}9 \\ & +0.019\text{it}10 + 0.050\text{it}11 + 0.032\text{it}12 + 0.101\text{it}13 \\ & +0.115\text{it}14 + 0.015\text{it}15 + 0.037\text{it}16 \\ & +0.029\text{it}17 + 0.100\text{it}18 + 0.022\text{it}19\end{aligned}$$

Table 2 Pearson's correlations after item weighting

	Pearson's correlations				Summary measures			
	Functional limitation	Physical pain	Psychological discomfort	Disability	Mean	Median	SD	Score range
Functional limitation	–	–	–	–	5.93	6	3.04	0–12
Physical pain	0.812***	–	–	–	6.54	6	3.91	0–16
Psychological discomfort	0.694***	0.812***	–	–	3.21	3	2.26	0–32
Disability	0.545***	0.676***	0.736***	–	7.47	7	5.97	0–8
Handicap	0.438***	0.544***	0.589***	0.756***	1.72	2	1.86	0–8

SD standard deviation, the means, SDs, and ranges indicate the scores for each variable before item weighting. ***$P < 0.001$

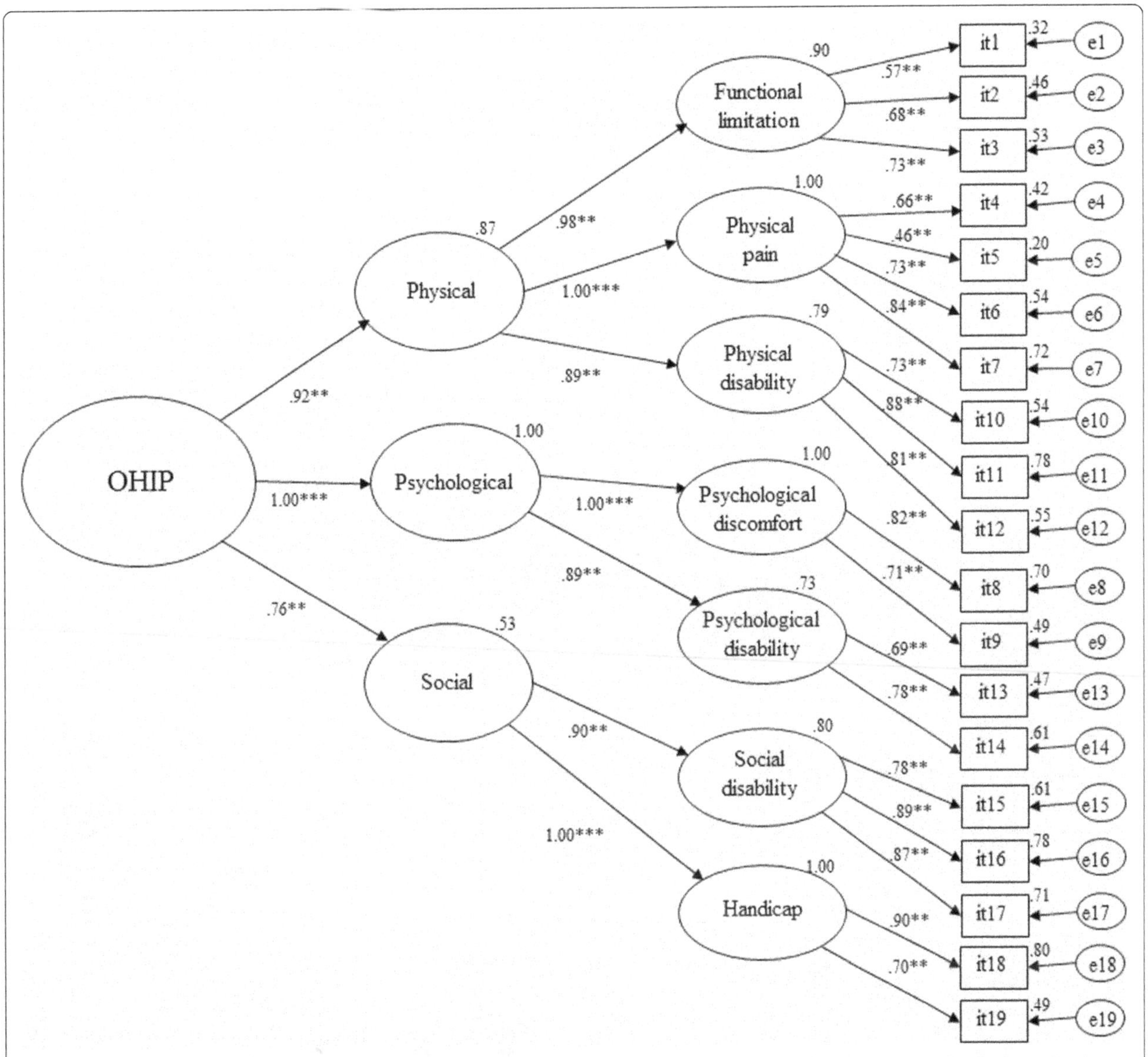

Fig. 1 The confirmatory factor analysis model to derive factor score weights. Bootstrap standardized direct effects for third-order hierarchical model of the Oral Health Impact Profile for edentulous subjects (OHIP-EDENT). Numbers on the upper right-hand side of the rectangles and ellipses represent the coefficient of determination associated with each structural equation. $^{**}P < 0.01$, $^{***}P < 0.001$

Testing the locker model

The main (Baker) model for the a priori hypotheses showed an acceptable fit on all indices: the GFI was 1.00, the CFI was 1.00, the RMSEA was 0.00 (90% CI 0.00–0.08), the SRMR was 0.013, the chi-squared value (3 degrees of freedom) was 2.139, and the *P*-value was 0.544 with weighted data. However, the direct effect of functional limitation on disability was a minus quantity, which was inadequate considering the consistency of association (worse functional limitation was associated with improving disability). Therefore, the path was deleted from the initial hypothesized (modified Baker) model. When the modified Baker model was re-run, the data supported Locker's conceptual model [1] in terms of the estimation of effects and fit indices. The fit indices of the modified Baker model were as follows: GFI = 1.00, CFI = 1.00, RMSEA = 0.00 (90% CI 0.00-0.08), SRMR = 0.013, chi squared value (4 degrees of freedom) = 3.431, and *P*-value = 0.488. Therefore, all five criteria were met. The modified Baker model accounted for 66% of the variance in pain, 66% in discomfort, 56% in disability, and 57% in handicap. The bootstrap standardized estimates, standard error values, and bias-corrected 95% CIs of direct effects and indirect effects are shown in Fig. 2.

Discussion

The present findings support Locker's conceptual model of oral health [1] and complement a previous well-

Table 3 Factor score weights for each item derived from the CFA model using the bootstrap method

Item	B	Bootstrap SE	Bias-corrected 95% CI
1	0.025**	0.008	0.012 / 0.044
2	0.035**	0.012	0.015 / 0.065
3	0.045**	0.014	0.022 / 0.079
4	0.037**	0.010	0.019 / 0.059
5	0.019***	0.006	0.009 / 0.035
6	0.049**	0.016	0.022 / 0.083
7	0.092**	0.034	0.039 / 0.166
8	0.202**	0.044	0.112 / 0.280
9	0.114**	0.033	0.054 / 0.180
10	0.019**	0.008	0.007 / 0.040
11	0.050**	0.016	0.022 / 0.086
12	0.032**	0.011	0.014 / 0.056
13	0.101**	0.056	0.041 / 0.261
14	0.115**	0.055	0.051 / 0.251
15	0.015**	0.008	0.005 / 0.040
16	0.037**	0.019	0.015 / 0.089
17	0.029**	0.016	0.010 / 0.074
18	0.100*	0.032	0.053 / 0.177
19	0.022*	0.013	0.007 / 0.060

OHIP Oral Health Impact Profile, *CFA* confirmatory factor analysis, *SE* standard error, *CI* confidence interval, $^{**}P < 0.01$, $^{***}P < 0.001$

designed study [2]. Both the study by Baker and the present study show that Locker's model can be generalized to various samples, including both edentulous patients and the general adult population, and that in both UK and Japanese edentulous sample, Locker's model can be applied.

By empirical analysis of the structure of a model, a theoretical model may be evaluated as highly sophisticated when compared with models that explain the nature of directional relationships between elements [22]. SEM is a powerful analytical method that is useful for investigating complex relationships like the structure of the elements of OHIP and presents the percentage of variance of the variables. In this study, the final (modified Baker) model explained 66% of the variance in pain, 66% in discomfort, 56% in disability, and 57% in handicap. That is, 34%–44% of the variance was not expressed in the model. Baker [2] referred to coping strategies, social support, sense of coherence, and negative affectivity as key contextual factors that may have improved interpretability. Moreover, we propose that elements of personality, such as neuroticism and life satisfaction, play an important role in oral health. Fenlon et al. [23] demonstrated that neuroticism had an influence on satisfaction with complete dentures and Yamaga et al. [24] indicated that satisfaction with complete dentures was associated with OHIP. Therefore, neuroticism may influence oral health. Locker et al. [25] showed a significant relationship between life satisfaction and oral health in older adults. Therefore, life satisfaction may be related

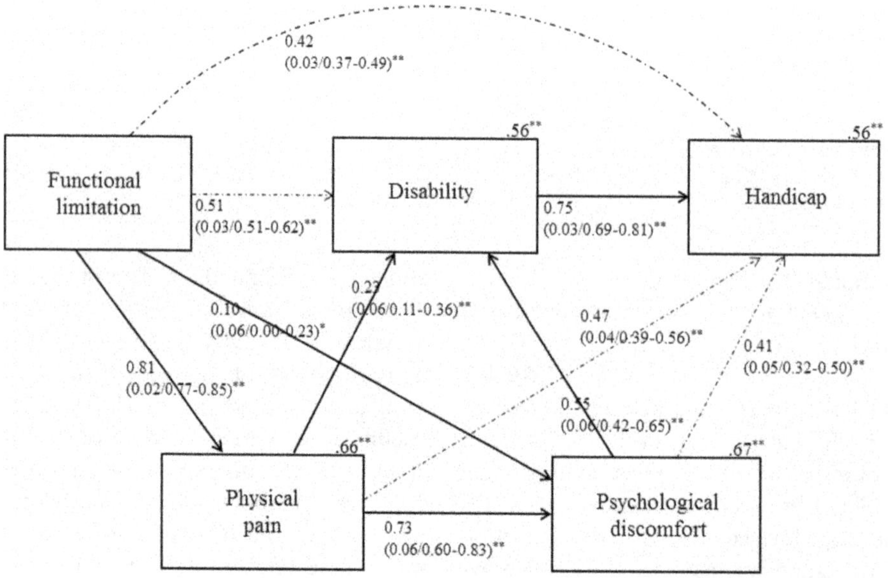

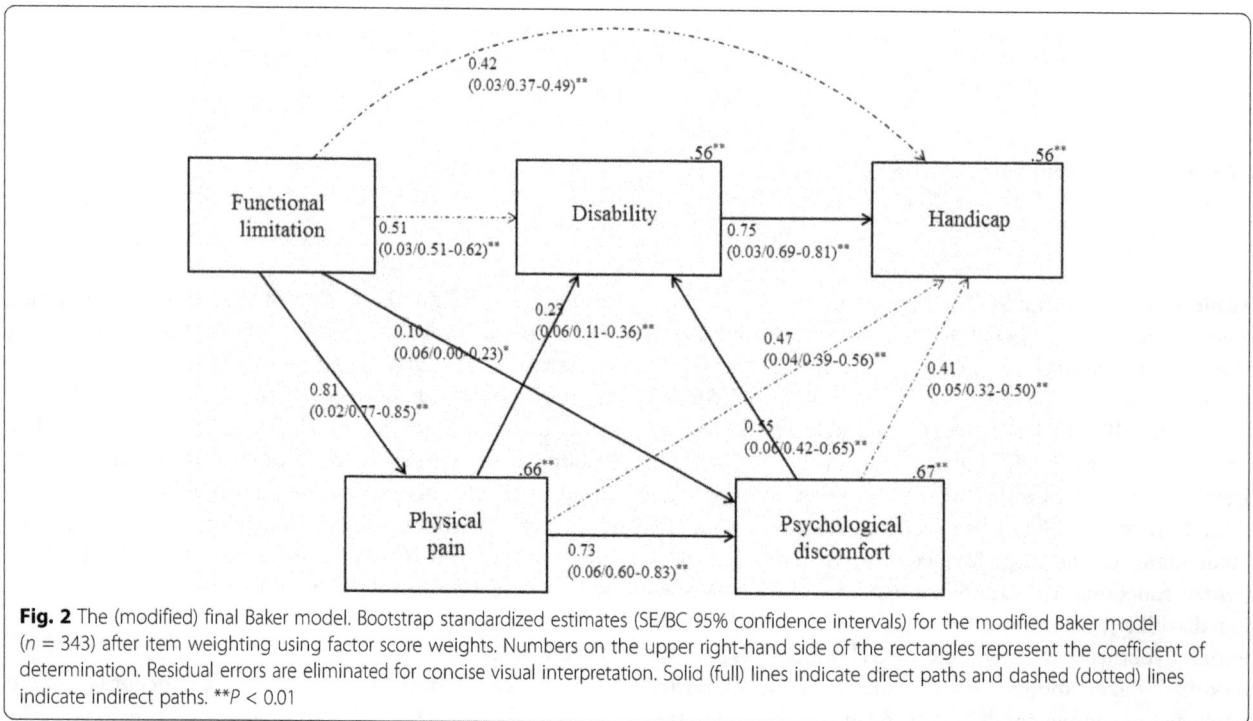

Fig. 2 The (modified) final Baker model. Bootstrap standardized estimates (SE/BC 95% confidence intervals) for the modified Baker model (n = 343) after item weighting using factor score weights. Numbers on the upper right-hand side of the rectangles represent the coefficient of determination. Residual errors are eliminated for concise visual interpretation. Solid (full) lines indicate direct paths and dashed (dotted) lines indicate indirect paths. $^{**}P < 0.01$

to oral health, especially in edentulous patients. If these variables had been included in this study model, more variation in OHIP elements may have been obtained.

In the present study, the final (modified Baker) model indicated higher fit indices than those indicated in the previous study [2] in edentulous patients. The *P*-value in the previous study was 0.350 and in the present study was 0.488. This may be because we used the OHIP-EDENT, which succeeded in eliminating the ceiling effect by including items relevant to chewing and eating difficulty [12], and not the sum scoring method but the item weighting method using hierarchical CFA with SEM analysis.

Jenkinson [26] indicated that the item weighting method is not so useful, whereas Zucoloto et al. [14] affirmed the correctness of item weighting. Jenkinson showed that measurements of health status are not significantly improved by weighting of items [26]. On the other hand, Zucoloto et al. [14] referred to the usefulness of the scoring method that adopted CFA with SEM. The theoretical concepts of physical, psychological, and social as second-order, or OHIP as third-order, have been discussed in the literature [27]. However, to date, its construct validity could not be tested by CFA analysis, which is important for accurate estimation. Therefore, further study is needed. The sum scoring method does not necessarily express the degree of effect of the score on the factor (OHIP). On the other hand, this weighting method can reflect how the score contributed to the factor (OHIP).

SEM analysis requires a large sample size (individuals) to obtain a precise estimation in free parameters. No absolute criteria for sample size exist in the literature. However, the complexity of the model is thought to be critical for sample size (individuals). A larger sample (individuals) was needed because the model was more complex and included more free parameters. In general, 20 individuals per free parameter is considered the desirable sample size [15]. Given that the hypothesized (Baker) model in the present study had 12 free parameters to be estimated, 240 individuals was considered the minimum adequate sample size. The third-order hierarchical (CFA) model had 44 free parameters to be estimated. Therefore, 880 individuals were needed. On the other hand, sample size (individuals) more than 200 was recommended in the field of social psychology for SEM analysis in the point of absolute criteria based on the general guide [15]. Both models met this recommendation.

In this study, the third-order model was used to interpret the multidimensional construct of OHRQoL and adjust item scores. It is possible to use various models, including CFA, to derive weight factor scores and understand the construct. For example, Baker [28] constructed a model for use in housebound edentulous elders in which functional (OHIP) was used as the latent variable (first order), physical, psychological, and social as indicator variables, and the covariance between the residual error of the psychological and social items was added. In the literature, the relevance of general health perception, functional (OHIP), and symptom status was investigated using a two-stage approach to SEM analysis [29]. Therefore, a more macroscopic view might be required to capture the multidimensional construct of OHRQoL rather than detailed elements, such as physical pain, as employed in this study. While a number of possible models exist, the third-order model was used to derive factor score weights because the third-order model covers all possible models and is not perfect but has been adequately tested in the literature [14]. A model fit was poor in the CFA model from which factor score weights were derived. However, bias-corrected bootstrapped 95% confidence intervals showed significance; the sample size recommendation in terms of absolute criteria was met. Moreover, the bootstrapping method had been recommended as the best approach for small-moderate sample sizes [18].

In the final (modified Baker) model, the direct effect of functional limitation on disability was not examined because of apparent inconsistency in the amount of direct effect. That is, it appears that more functional limitation decreases disability as derived from the initial hypothesized model, whereas functional limitation has a significant large indirect effect on disability. To wit, in edentulous patients, functional limitation influences disability indirectly rather than directly. This is because of the strong direct link between functional limitation and pain (0.81) and the indirect link between pain and discomfort (0.73). Clinically, it may be that functional limitation (e.g., dentures not fitting) has an indirect influence on disability (e.g., avoidance of eating) via pain or discomfort rather than a direct influence. In terms of general statistical principles, not all the potential direct relationships were incorporated (the parsimony principle) [15].

The main limitation of this study is its cross-sectional rather than longitudinal design. Thereby, a causal relationship could not be shown. Further studies including intervention would be required to determine the relationship between change in scores for before and after outcome variables. According to the theory of response shift [30], a follow-up response may be influenced by new information not available at the time of the initial response. On outcome evaluation, the response shift causes bias that confuses the meaning of the score. To eliminate this source of bias, future studies should include a longitudinal design.

Conclusions

The results of the present study show an empirical fit to Locker's model in Japanese edentulous patients by an item weighting method using factor score weights, which has more accuracy than the sum scoring method. This finding may contribute to the generalization of Locker's model.

Abbreviations

CFA: Confirmatory factor analysis; CFI: Comparative fit index; CI: Confidence interval; GFI: Goodness-of-fit index; OHIP-14: The Short-Form Oral Health Impact Profile,; OHIP-EDENT: OHIP for edentulous subjects; OHIP-EDENT-J: The Japanese version of the Oral Health Impact Profile for edentulous subjects; OHRQoL: Oral health-related quality of life; RMSEA: Root mean-square error of approximation; SD: Standard deviation; SEM: Structural equation modeling; SRMR: Standardized root-mean-square residual; UMIN: The University hospital Medical Information Network

Funding

This research was funded by a Grant-in-Aid for Scientific Research from the Japan Society for the Promotion of Science (Grant 26861628). The role of the funding agency was financial support, and it was not involved in the design of the study or collection, analysis, and interpretation of data or in writing the manuscript.

Authors' contributions

EY conceived and designed the study. EY also acquired and analyzed the data and drafted the manuscript. YS and SM coordinated and helped draft the manuscript and performed a critical review of the manuscript for important intellectual content. All authors read and approved the final version of the manuscript.

Competing interests

The authors declare that they have no competing interests.

References

1. Locker D. Measuring oral health: a conceptual framework. Community Dent Health. 1988;5:3–18.
2. Baker SR. Testing a conceptual model of oral-health: a structural equation modeling approach. J Dent Res. 2007;86:708–12.
3. Slade GD. Derivation and validation of a short form oral health impact profile. Community Dent Oral Epidemiol. 1997;25:284–90.
4. Slade GD, Spencer AJ. Development and evaluation of oral health impact profile. Community Dent Health. 1994;11:3–11.
5. Ikebe K, Watkins CA, Ettinger RL, Sajima H, Nokubi T. Application of short-form oral health impact profile on elderly Japanese. Gerodontology. 2004; 21:167–76.
6. Allen PF, Locker D. A modified short version of the oral health impact profile for assessing health-related quality of life in edentulous adults. Int J Prosthodont. 2002;15:446–50.
7. Sato Y, Kaiba Y, Yamaga E, Minakuchi S. Reliability and validity of a Japanese version of the oral health impact profile for edentulous subjects. Gerodontology. 2012;29:e1033–7.
8. Douglass CW, Shih A, Ostry L. Will there be a need for complete dentures in the United States in 2020? J Prosthet Dent. 2002;87:5–8.
9. Peterson PE, Yamamoto T. Improving the oral health of older people: the approach of the WHO global oral health Programme. Community Dent Oral Epidemiol. 2005;33:81–92.
10. Critchlow BC, Ellis JS. Prognostic indicators for conventional complete denture therapy: a review of the literature. J Dent. 2010;38:2–9.
11. Allen PF, Locker D. Do item weights matter? An assessment using the oral health impact profile. Community Dent Health. 1997;14:133–8.
12. Allen PF, Steele J. Data validity and quality. In: Lesaffre E, Feine J, Leroux B, Declerck D, editors. Statistical and methodological aspects of oral Health Research. Chichester: Wiley; 2009. p. 131–44.
13. DiStefano C, Zhu M, Mîndrilă D. Understanding and using factor scores: considerations for the applied researcher. Pract Assess Res Eval. 2009;14:1–11.
14. Zucoloto ML, Maroco J, Campos JADB. Psychometric properties of the oral health impact profile and new methodological approach. J Dent Res. 2014; 93:645–50.
15. Kline RB. Principles and practice of structural equation modeling. 3rd ed. New York: Guilford Press; 2011.
16. Cawood JI, Howell RA. A classification of the edentulous jaws. Int J Oral Maxillofac Surg. 1988;17:232–6.
17. Kapur KK. A clinical evaluation of denture adhesives. J Prosthet Dent. 1967; 18:550–8.
18. Efron B, Tibshirani R. Bootstrap methods for standard errors, confidence intervals, and other measures of statistical accuracy. Stat Sci. 1986;1:54–77.
19. Hu L, Bentler PM. Fit indices in covariance structure modeling: sensitivity to underparameterized model misspecification. Psychol Methods. 1998;3:424–53.
20. Hu L, Bentler PM. Cutoff criteria for fit indices in covariance structure analysis: conventional criteria versus new alternatives. Struct Equ Model. 1998;6:1–55.
21. MacCallum RC, Austin JT. Applications of structural equation modeling in psychological research. Ann Rev Psychol. 2000;51:201–26.
22. Taillefer MC, Dupuis G, Roberge MA, May SL. Health-related quality of life models: systematic review of the literature. Soc Indic Res. 2003;64:293–323.
23. Fenlon MR, Sherriff M, Newton JT. The influence of personality on patients' satisfaction with existing and new complete dentures. J Dent. 2007;35:744–8.
24. Yamaga E, Sato Y, Minakuchi S. A structural equation model relating oral condition, denture quality, chewing ability, satisfaction, and oral health-related quality of life in complete denture wearers. J Dent. 2013;41:710–7.
25. Locker D, Clarke M, Payne B. Self-perceived oral health status, psychological well-being, and life satisfaction in an older adult population. J Dent Res. 2000;79:970–5.
26. Jenkinson C. Why are we weighting? A critical examination of the use of item weights in a health status measure. Soc Sci Med. 1991;32:1413–6.
27. Slade GD. The oral health impact profile. In: Slade GD, editor. Measuring oral health and quality of life: Department of Dental Ecology, School of Dentistry, Chapel Hill: University of North Carolina; 1997. p. 93–104. https://www.adelaide.edu.au/arcpoh/downloads/publications/reports/miscellaneous/measuring-oral-health-and-quality-of-life.pdf. Accessed 24 Apr 2018.
28. Baker SR. Testing the applicability of a conceptual model of oral health in housebound edentulous older people. Community Dent Oral Epidemiol. 2008;36:237–48.
29. Anderson JC, Gerbing DW. Structural equation modelling in practice: a review and recommended two-step approach. Psychol Bull. 1988;103:411–23.
30. Schwartz CE, Sprangers MAG. Methodological approaches for assessing response shift in longitudinal health-related quality-of-life research. Soc Sci Med. 1999;48:1531–48.

2

Influence on interradicular bone volume of Invisalign treatment for adult crowding with interproximal enamel reduction: a retrospective three-dimensional cone-beam computed tomography study

Andreas Hellak[1,3*], Nicola Schmidt[1], Michael Schauseil[1], Steffen Stein[1], Thomas Drechsler[2] and Heike Maria Korbmacher-Steiner[1]

Abstract

Background: The aim of this study was to use three-dimensional datasets to identify associations between treatment for adult crowding, using Invisalign aligner and interproximal enamel reduction (IER), and changes in the volume of interradicular bone.

Methods: A total of 60 cone-beam computed tomography (CBCT) scans from 30 adult patients (28 women, two men; 30 CBCTs pre-treatment, 30 post-treatment) were examined retrospectively in order to measure bone volume three-dimensionally. The patients' average age was 36.03 ± 9.7 years. The interradicular bone volume was measured with OsiriX at four levels in the anterior tooth areas of the maxilla and mandible. Differences in bone between T0 and T1 were analyzed with IBM SPSS 21.0 using the Wilcoxon test for paired samples.

Results: Overall, a slight increase in the quantity of bone was found (0.12 ± 0.73 mm). There was a highly significant increase in bone in the mandible (0.40 ± 0.62 mm; $P < 0.001$), while in the maxilla there was a slight loss of bone, which was highly significant in the apical third (− 0.16 ± 0.77 mm; $P = 0.001$).

Conclusions: Overall, treatment for adult crowding using an aligner and IER appears to have a positive effect on interradicular bone volume, particularly in patients with severe grades of the condition (periodontally high-risk dentition). This effect is apparently independent of IER. This is extremely important with regard to the treatment outcome, since IER and root proximity have been matters of debate in the literature and teeth should remain firmly embedded in their alveolar sockets.

Keywords: Aligner, Adult crowding, Interradicular bone volume, IER, Bone quantity, CBCT

Background

Among adult patients there is growing interest in having a functionally healthy and aesthetically attractive dentition [1]. Patients often have adult crowding and wish to have malpositioning corrected as invisibly as possible [2, 3]. There are many treatment options e.g. using aligners and interproximal enamel reduction (IER).

One possible treatment for relieving crowding consists of expanding the dental arch in the labial direction in order to provide space for normal positioning of the affected teeth. Another method of creating space is IER. Potential periodontal changes in the anterior tooth area during orthodontic treatment with IER for adult crowding have been a topic of discussion in the literature [4–6]. In addition to the treatment of patients with periodontally healthy dentition, the question arises for the orthodontist

* Correspondence: hellak@med.uni-marburg.de
[1]Department of Orthodontics, University Hospital Giessen and Marburg, Campus Marburg, Georg-Voigt-Strasse 3, 35039 Marburg, Germany
[3]Abt. für Kieferorthopädie, UKGM Standort Marburg, Georg-Voigt-Strasse 3, 35039 Marburg, Germany
Full list of author information is available at the end of the article

of the way in which periodontally high-risk dentition is likely to behave during treatment. Vermylen et al. [7] defined an interradicular distance of 0.8 mm or less as root proximity and a risk marker for periodontal disease.

There have to date been no three-dimensional investigations of changes in interradicular bone volume in relation to treatment for adult crowding. The present study was carried out in order to investigate whether orthodontic treatment and resolution of crowding may even lead to an improvement in the bone situation. As a result of the use of conventional two-dimensional imaging to date, only limited quantification of the pre-therapeutic and post-therapeutic interradicular bone situation has been possible [8]. It is only modern three-dimensional cone-beam computed tomography (CBCT) scanning that has made it possible to carry out 3D analysis of the bone structures and the way in which they respond to tooth movements [9, 10, 11]. The aim of the present study was to investigate whether and to what extent orthodontic treatment with Invisalign aligners and IER leads to a change in the interradicular bone volume. Specifically, the following questions were addressed:

- How is the interradicular bone volume altered by aligner therapy?
- What effects on interradicular root distances are associated with interproximal enamel reduction (IER)?
- In what ways does the interradicular bone volume change after initial findings corresponding to a root proximity (=interradicular distance of ≤0.8 mm, a so called risk marker for periodontal disease [4])?

Methods

Changes in the interradicular distance were measured at a total of 720 measurement points in the present study. Pre-therapeutic and post-therapeutic cone-beam computed tomography (CBCT) scans from a total of 30 patients (28 women, two men) were examined retrospectively. In accordance with the SEDENTEXCT guidelines, the CBCT scans were taken for two reasons:

1. For periodontal assessment (a total of 26 cases). These patients had a fragile gingival type, with less bone in the anterior tooth area. Pre-treatment CBCT was therefore intended to visualize root proximity and resorption and help with therapeutic decision-making on whether to carry out IER or extraction of one anterior tooth. The following CBCT was intended to visualize root proximity and resorption after the completion of possible treatment, to check whether IER was still appropriate for creating space, since the teeth need to be covered by bone in order to avoid recession.
2. For temporomandibular joint assessment (a total of four cases). Some patients had craniomandibular disorders (CMD) with rheumatoid arthritis. In this small number of selected cases, pre-treatment CBCT was used to identify bone degenerative deformity, condylar positions, and bony structures in the temporomandibular joint. After successful CMD therapy and orthodontic treatment, CBCT scans were taken again to view the condylar positions and bony structures in the temporomandibular joint due to recurrent CMD problems and in order to adjust anti-inflammatory therapy.

The patients' average age was 36.03 ± 9.7 years. The use of the data was approved by the ethics committee of Marburg University Hospital (ref. no. 34/15).

The following inclusion and exclusion criteria were applied. Inclusion criteria:

- Presence of adult crowding capable of being adjusted using conservative orthodontic space-gaining measures such as protrusion, proclination, expansion and IER
- Permanent dentition
- Successfully completed treatment with Invisalign aligners
- Availability of one CBCT each from before and after treatment

The following parameters represented exclusion criteria:

- Extraction of anterior teeth during the course of treatment
- macrodontia/ hypoplasia
- abnormal change in tooth morphology
- Prosthetic treatment
- Skeletal anomalies
- General medical findings relevant to bone metabolism (e.g., osteoporosis, dysostosis, etc.)
- Periodontal disease and previous periodontal surgery procedures

All of the images were taken with a KaVo 3D eXam DVT system (KaVo Dental Ltd., Biberach an der Riss, Germany) using a scan with 360° revolution, a duration of 26.9 s (X-ray source voltage: 120 kVp; X-ray source current: 5 mA) and a voxel size of 0.25 mm. The datasets were collected and evaluated using OsiriX (Pixmeo, Bernex, Switzerland) with an Apple OS X operating system.

All of the patients had provided written consent to the use of their data in the study (in accordance with the Helsinki Declaration). The data were all analyzed on a semi-blinded basis.

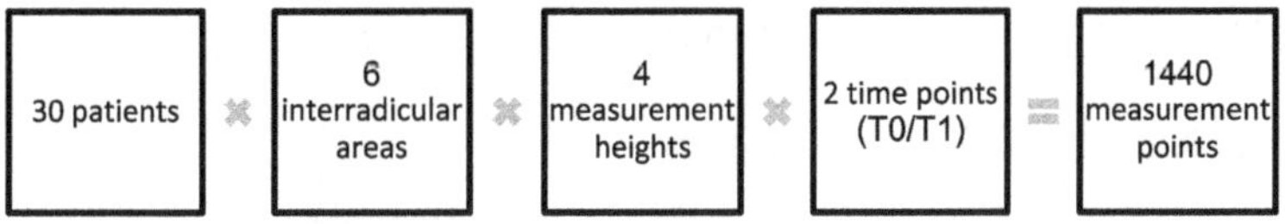
30 patients
6 interradicular areas
4 measurement heights
2 time points (T0/T1)
1440 measurement points

Fig. 1 Total measurement data

Measurement of interradicular bone volume

Measurements of the mesiodistal interradicular distance (Fig. 1) were modified in the OsiriX DICOM viewer using the method described by Sawada et al. [7]. The six interradicular areas between the lateral incisors in the maxilla and mandible were measured (Figs. 2 and 3).

The shorter of the roots in the two teeth adjoining the interradicular space was set as the reference tooth. A connecting line was drawn in the sagittal view from the buccal enamel–cement boundary (ECB) to the palatal or lingual enamel–cement boundary (Fig. 4). From the intersection of that line with the center of the root canal, the length to the apex was measured parallel to the dental axis/coronal plane (the ECB–apex distance), and the tooth was divided into four equal-sized sections. This resulted in the four measurement levels (Fig. 3). The sagittal view was used to adjust the axial plane to the desired height (Fig. 4).

The interradicular distance was measured in the axial view. For this purpose, two auxiliary lines were drawn parallel to the sagittal plane and were shifted in parallel as far as the root surfaces of the neighboring teeth (Fig. 5). In the measurement levels set, the interradicular distance was thus measured as the shortest distance between the root surfaces.

Whether and to what extent IER or expanding the dental arch in the labial direction influenced the interradicular space was investigated using ClinCheck software with the exact IER protocol. For each interradicular space we analyzed the change of the distance between the roots in comparison to the amount of IER. The total amount of IER was between 0.0 mm and 0.5 mm. In our study crowding was defined as the difference in millimeter between the arch perimeter and the mesial to distal tooth size total form S1-S3 (upper anterior jaw) and S4-S6 (lower anterior jaw) (Fig. 2). Maxillary and mandibular arches were classified separately. Each case was classified as presenting mild discrepancy crowding between − 0.1 mm to − 5 mm according to Proffit. W. R. and H. W. Field. *Contemporary Orthodontics*. St Louis, Mo: Mosby; 2000:224.

All of the digital volume tomograms were analyzed a second time by the same investigator (N.S.) one month later, to allow assessment of the reproducibility of the measurements. The means of the two evaluations were used for statistical analysis. All patients were treated by one operator (T.D.) in the same office.

Statistical analyses were carried out using IBM SPSS for Mac, version 21.0 (IBM Corporation, Armonk, New York, USA). The intraoperator correlation for each examination was initially calculated. For further analysis, the normal distribution of the values was checked. The values were tested for significant differences using the Wilcoxon test. The significance level was set at $P = 0.05$.

Results

Kendall's tau-b test showed a highly significant ($P < 0.001$, two-sided) intraoperator correlation ($r = 0.837$) for the interradicular distance measurements.

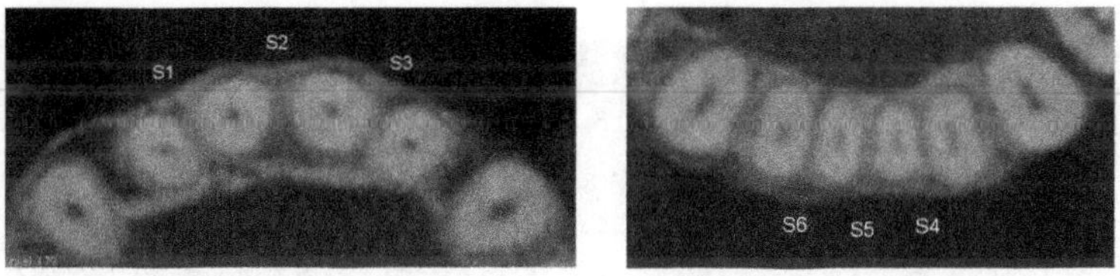

S1: space between 12 and 11
S4: space between 32 and 31

S2: space between 11 and 21
S5: space between 31 and 41

S3: space between 21 and 22
S6: space between 41 and 42

Fig. 2 Measurement points for interradicular distances

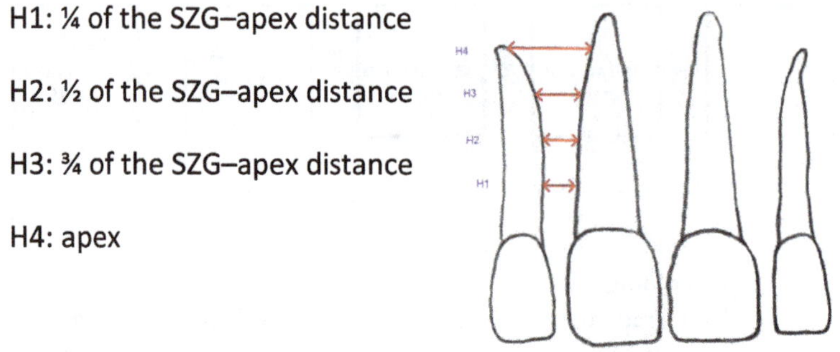

Fig. 3 Two-dimensional diagram showing the measurement distances used to determine interradicular distances

Increases in the interradicular distance were observed in the mandible, and decreases were observed in the maxilla (Table 1). The increase in interradicular space in the mandible was greater than the loss of space in the maxilla. The Wilcoxon test showed highly significant ($P \leq 0.001$) changes between T0 and T1 at all levels in the mandible, highly significant ($P \leq 0.01$) changes at the apex measurement level, and significant ($P \leq 0.05$) changes at the three-quarter level in the maxilla (Table 1).

Effects of IER

A positive effect was noted after treatment in 62.5% of all interdental spaces in which IER was carried out; however, the distance decreased in 37.5%. The effect was almost identical without IER (Table 2). Overall, it was found that IER did not have any statistically significant effects on the changing interradicular space conditions.

Periodontally critical situation (interradicular distance ≤0.8 mm)

In all, 17.2% of the pre-therapeutic interradicular measurement points had an interradicular distance ≤0.8 mm (Table 3), and the majority of these were in the mandible. As Table 3 shows, the treatment had a positive effect, since afterwards only 7.9% of the measurement points still had an interradicular distance ≤0.8 mm.

It was then investigated whether a periodontally high-risk dentition (≤ 0.8 mm) benefited more from aligner treatment than a periodontally healthy dentition (> 0.8 mm). Of the 124 measurement points that had a root distance ≤0.8 mm in the initial findings, 88.71% had increased space after treatment. An interradicular space increase of more than 0.8 mm was even observed in 71.77% (Table 4). An increase in space of more than 0.8 mm was observed in nine of 11 measurement points in the maxilla (81.82%), and in 80 of 113 measurement points in the mandible (70.8%).

By comparison, periodontally high-risk dentitions showed much larger increases in the interradicular bone volume (Table 5). As Table 5 shows, the result was highly significant statistically ($P \leq 0.001$).

Discussion

In the group of patients investigated in the present study, treatment for adult crowding was associated with an overall increase in interradicular space. The increased space was gained particularly in the mandible, as the increase was larger than the slight loss of space in the maxilla. One possible explanation for this might be the

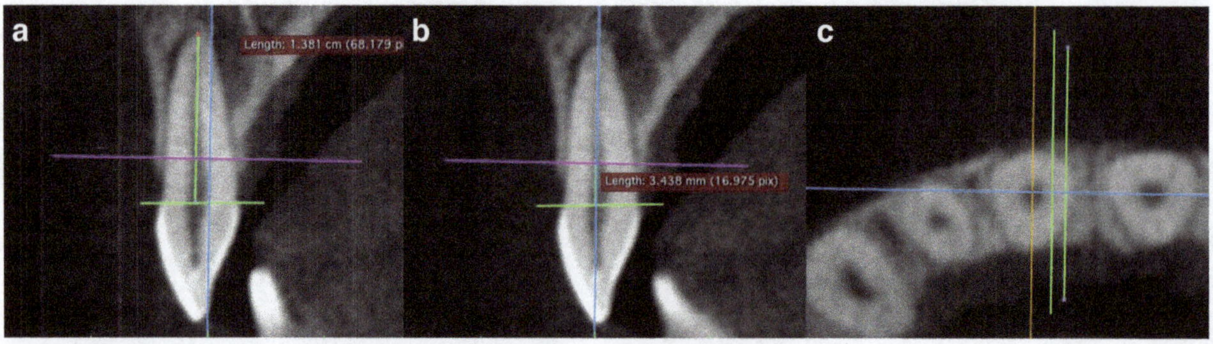

Fig. 4 Sagittal plane. **a** Measurement of the length of the apex to enamel–cement boundary (ECB) distance. **b** Setting the first measurement level, H1, at one-quarter of the ECB–apex distance. **c** Creating the auxiliary lines parallel to the sagittal axis in the axial view

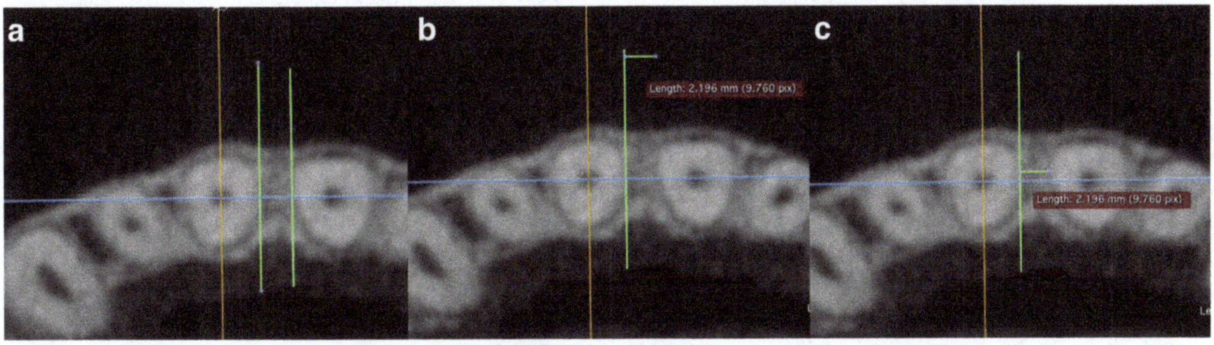

Fig. 5 Measurement of mesiodistal interradicular distance S1 at the H1 level on the axial plane. **a** Shifting of the auxiliary lines to the root surfaces. **b** Measuring the shortest interradicular distance by shifting an auxiliary line. **c** Display of the measurement distance

varying severity of the crowding. In this group of patients, adult crowding usually appeared earlier and with greater severity in the mandible than in the maxilla. More extensive measures to create space were therefore needed with a smaller bone volume. Another explanation might be the different methods used to create space.

One possible treatment for relieving crowding consists of expanding the dental arch in the labial direction in order to allow space for normal positioning of these teeth [12]. This method of space creation was used much more often in the mandible. The positive effect of reshaping the dental arch thus appears to have a strong influence on increases in interradicular space.

Another method of creating space is IER [13]. Although the roots ought to move closer to each other after the removal of enamel during IER, the positive effect of reshaping the dental arch appears to outweigh this, at least in the mandible. This increase in space despite IER has

Table 1 Descriptive comparison of differences in the interradicular distance measurements between T1 and T0, using the Wilcoxon test[a] for statistical analysis

Measurement level		n	Minimum	Maximum	Mean	SD	Wilcoxon test[a]	T1–T0
Maxilla								
¼	T1–T0	90	−1.75	1.27	−0.07	0.52	Z	−1.189 [b]
							A. significance (two-sided)	0.234
½	T1–T0	90	−2.40	1.33	−0.03	0.66	Z	−0.127 [b]
							A. significance (two-sided)	0.899
¾	T1–T0	90	−2.45	1.67	−0.22	0.75	Z	−2.505 [b]
							A. significance (two-sided)	0.012
Apex	T1–T0	90	−3.02	1.94	−0.32	1.03	Z	−2.565 [b]
							A. significance (two-sided)	0.01
Mandible								
¼	T1–T0	90	−0.68	1.35	0.30	0.46	Z	−5.237 [c]
							A. significance (two-sided)	< 0.001
½	T1–T0	90	−0.87	1.71	0.42	0.52	Z	−6.113 [c]
							A. significance (two-sided)	< 0.001
¾	T1–T0	90	−1.33	2.49	0.45	0.62	Z	−6.051 [c]
							A. significance (two-sided)	< 0.001
Apex	T1–T0	90	−1.86	2.60	0.40	0.84	Z	−4.048 [c]
							A. significance (two-sided)	< 0.001

SD standard deviation
[a]Wilcoxon signed rank test
[b]Based on positive ranks
[c]Based on negative ranks

Table 2 Effects of interproximal enamel reduction on the interradicular distance in 180 interproximal spaces

	With IER (*n* = 104)	Without IER (*n* = 76)
Interradicular distance increased	62.50%	63.16%
Interradicular distance decreased	37.50%	36.84%

IER interproximal enamel reduction

Table 4 Increase in the interradicular distance between T0 and T1 of periodontally high-risk dentition, including interradicular space increases to > 0.8 mm

n = 124 (≤ 0.8 mm)	Increases in space	Increases in space > 0.8 mm
Maxilla	90.91%	81.82%
Mandible	88.5%	70.80%
Total	88.71%	71.77%

also been confirmed in other studies. In two-dimensional studies, Zachrisson et al. [4] found that due to crowding, the roots have to be closer together than in correctly aligned teeth.

During treatment for adult crowding, interproximal enamel reduction (IER) was only carried out supportively in a few interdental spaces. When only the subtopic of IER is considered, it is notable that IER did not have any significant effect on the bone volume between the anterior dental roots. The distribution pattern of changes in the interradicular distance was almost identical with and without IER.

In general, the advantage of interproximal enamel reduction is that the extent of the expansion in the labial direction can be reduced, thereby reducing the risk of bone dehiscence occurring. In addition, the widened approximal contacts stabilize the treatment result [14]. These findings are also consistent with those reported in the clinical studies by Zachrisson et al. [4], in which no deterioration was observed on dental film more than 10 years later after approximal enamel reduction. However, precise three-dimensional measurement of interradicular spatial conditions was not possible due to the use of two-dimensional radiographic diagnosis in the study. An improvement in the aesthetic appearance can also be expected as a result of relieving anterior crowding, due to the avoidance of what are known as "black triangles." The creation of optimal apposition areas for the gingiva also reduces or prevents retrusion of the interdental papillae [15].

The most noticeable positive effect was seen when teeth with root proximity were treated. Vermylen et al. [7] defined 0.8 mm or less bone or interdental tissue as representing root proximity. Interdental spaces of this size are poorly accessible for periodontal treatment and are less able to resist periodontal disease [16]. Radicular distances with this potentially poor initial condition showed improvement in the spatial situation in approximately 89% of cases, and improvement beyond the critical range (> 0.8 mm after treatment) in approximately 72%. This means that a periodontally high-risk dentition benefited more from the aligner treatment than a periodontally healthy dentition. However, it must be mentioned here that root proximity is not the cause of periodontal disease, but only represents a risk factor [17–20]. Bacterial plaque is one of the main causes of periodontal inflammation [21].

Table 3 Interradicular distance ≤0.8 mm at time points T0 and T1 (*n* = 720)

	T0	T1
Maxilla	1.53%	1.11%
Mandible	15.69%	6.81%
Total	17.22%	7.92%

Another advantage of the present study is the three-dimensional imaging of the interradicular spaces. Other studies on measurement of bone volume have only been carried out using two-dimensional images, and have always noted the difficulty of depicting the interradicular distance precisely [8]. Two-dimensional images are also known as cumulative images. As a result of the cumulation, superimposed roots in crowded conditions are difficult to distinguish and the spaces are difficult to measure, due to differing enlargement factors. This lost information can be displayed in three-dimensional images [22]. For CBCT analysis, the question arises of whether the image resolution is sufficient to allow precise analysis. Gribel et al. [23] compared CBCT measurements with direct measurements of dry skulls. They found that CBCT scanning with a slice thickness of 0.3 mm was extremely precise, with a mean deviation of the measurements from the direct measurements of 0.1 mm.

Unfortunaly this study has a retrospective design with a risk of bias. A prospective randomized controlled trial would be interesting, but could currently not be carried out because of the ALARA principle. In view of the principle that radiation exposure should be "as low as reasonably achievable" (ALARA), CBCT is not indicated as a routine method for the imaging of bone support [24, 25]. A CBCT may only be indicated in selected cases in which clinical and conventional examinations do not provide the information needed for treatment. The operator always needs to consider its use carefully. If a CBCT is needed the use of shorter scans and a reduced effective radiation dose is recommended [26, 27]. A study group with a more balanced sex ratio would be desirable, because most of the patients included in this study were women. This is due to the retrospective

Table 5 Descriptive statistics for interradicular changes, classified into groups with a root proximity (periodontally high-risk dentition - interradicular bone quantity at T0 ≤ 0.8 mm) or with a periodontally normal dentition (interradicular bone volume at T0 > 0.8 mm) with Wilcoxon signed rank test for statistical analysis

Distance		n	Min.	Max.	Mean	SD	Wilcoxon test (≤ 0.8 mm vs. > 0.8 mm)	
≤ 0.8 mm	T1–T0	124	−0.45	2.49	0.60	0.54	Z	−8.071
> 0.8 mm	T1–T0	596	−3.02	2.60	0.02	0.75	A. significance (two-sided)	< 0.001

SD standard deviation

character of our study. However, presenting these data from the context of aligner treatment for adult crowding and possible interradicular bone changes may be helpful. Further research and additional information on the topic would be desirable.

Conclusions

Overall, treatment of adult crowding using Invisalign and IER, particularly in patients with severe conditions (with periodontally high-risk dentition), appears to have a positive effect on the interradicular bone volume, at least in adult female patients. The effect is also apparently independent of IER.

Abbreviations

ALARA: As low as reasonably achievable; CBCT: Cone beam computed tomography scans; IER: Interproximal enamel reduction

Acknowledgments

The authors thank Mr. Robertson for editing the manuscript.

Funding

The present study was not funded, nor supported by any grant. Therefore, the authors report no conflict of interest related to the present work.

Authors' contributions

AH conceived the study together with NS and HMKS, and carried out all experiments and drafted the manuscript. AH and MS performed the statistical analysis. TD treated the patients and SS helped with the collection of the data and made substantial contributions to conception and design. HMKS conceived the study, participated in its design and coordination and helped to draft the manuscript. All authors read and approved the final manuscript.

Competing interests

The authors declare that they have no competing interests.

Author details

[1]Department of Orthodontics, University Hospital Giessen and Marburg, Campus Marburg, Georg-Voigt-Strasse 3, 35039 Marburg, Germany. [2]Private practice, Wiesbaden, Germany. [3]Abt. für Kieferorthopädie, UKGM Standort Marburg, Georg-Voigt-Strasse 3, 35039 Marburg, Germany.

References

1. Nedwed V, Miethke RR. Motivation, acceptance and problems of Invisalign patients. J Orofac Orthop. 2005;66(2):162–73.
2. Weir T. Clear aligners in orthodontic treatment. Aust Dent J. 2017;62(1):58–62.
3. Meier B, Wiemer KB, Miethke RR. Invisalign—patient profiling. Analysis of a prospective survey. J Orofac Orthop. 2003;64(5):352–8.
4. Zachrisson BU, Nyøygaard L, Mobarak K. Dental health assessed more than 10 years after interproximal enamel reduction of mandibular anterior teeth. Am J Orthod Dentofac Orthop. 2007;131(2):162–9.
5. Zachrisson BU, Minster L, Ogaard B, Birkhed D. Dental health assessed after interproximal enamel reduction: caries risk in posterior teeth. Am J Orthod Dentofac Orthop. 2011;139(1):90–8.
6. Renkema AM, Navratilova Z, Mazurova K, Katsaros C, Fudalej PS. Gingival labial recessions and the post-treatment proclination of mandibular incisors. Eur J Orthod. 2015;37(5):508–13.
7. Vermylen K, De Quincey GN, van 't Hof MA, Wolffe GN, Renggli HH. Classification, reproducibility and prevalence of root proximity in periodontal patients. J Clin Periodontol. 2005;32(3):254–9.
8. Zachrisson BU, Alnaes L. Periodontal condition in orthodontically treated and untreated individuals. II. Alveolar bone loss: radiographic findings. Angle Orthod. 1974;44(1):48–55.
9. Fuhrmann R. Three-dimensional interpretation of periodontal lesions and remodeling during orthodontic treatment. Part III. J Orofac Orthop. 1996; 57(4):224–37.
10. Lund H. Cone beam computed tomography in evaluations of some side effects of orthodontic treatment. Swed Dent J Suppl. 2011;219:4–78.
11. Sawada K, Nakahara K, Matsunaga S, Abe S, Ide Y. Evaluation of cortical bone thickness and root proximity at maxillary interradicular sites for mini-implant placement. Clin Oral Implants Res. 2013;24 Suppl A100:1–7.
12. Stroud JL, English J, Buschang PH. Enamel thickness of the posterior dentition: its implications for nonextraction treatment. Angle Orthod. 1998; 68(2):141–6.
13. Sheridan JJ. Air-rotor stripping. J Clin Orthod. 1985;19(1):43–59.
14. Allais D, Melsen B. Does labial movement of lower incisors influence the level of the gingival margin? A case-control study of adult orthodontic patients. Eur J Orthod. 2003;25(4):343–52.
15. Melsen B, Allais D. Factors of importance for the development of dehiscences during labial movement of mandibular incisors: a retrospective study of adult orthodontic patients. Am J Orthod Dentofac Orthop. 2005; 127(5):552–61. quiz 625
16. Kim T, Miyamoto T, Nunn ME, Garcia RI, Dietrich T. Root proximity as a risk factor for progression of alveolar bone loss: the veterans affairs dental longitudinal study. J Periodontol. 2008;79(4):654–9.
17. Bollen AM. Effects of malocclusions and orthodontics on periodontal health: evidence from a systematic review. J Dent Educ. 2008;72(8):912–8.
18. Uysal T, Yagci A, Ozer T, Veli I, Ozturk A. Mandibular anterior bony support and incisor crowding: is there a relationship? Am J Orthod Dentofac Orthop. 2012;142(5):645–53.
19. Alsulaiman AA, Kaye E, Jones J, Cabral H, Leone C, Will L, Garcia R. Incisor malalignment and the risk of periodontal disease progression. Am J Orthod Dentofac Orthop. 2018;153(4):512–22.
20. Diedrich P. Periodontal relevance of anterior crowding. J Orofac Orthop. 2000;61(2):69–79.

21. Corbet EF, Davies WI. The role of supragingival plaque in the control of progressive periodontal disease. A review. J Clin Periodontol. 1993;20(5): 307–13.
22. Schulze D, Fleiner J. Digitale dentale Volumentomografie. Zahnmed Up2date. 2008;2:247–59.
23. Gribel BF, Gribel MN, Frazäo DC, McNamara JA Jr, Manzi FR. Accuracy and reliability of craniometric measurements on lateral cephalometry and 3D measurements on CBCT scans. Angle Orthod. 2011;81(1):26–35.
24. Ludlow JB, Davies-Ludlow LE, Brooks SL, Howerton WB. Dosimetry of 3 CBCT devices for oral and maxillofacial radiology: CB Mercuray, NewTom 3G and i-CAT. Dentomaxillofac Radiol. 2006;35(4):219–26. Erratum in: Dentomaxillofac Radiol 2006;35(5):392
25. Silva MA, Wolf U, Heinicke F, Bumann A, Visser H, Hirsch E. Cone-beam computed tomography for routine orthodontic treatment planning: a radiation dose evaluation. Am J Orthod Dentofac Orthop. 2008;133(5):640. e1–5
26. Cook VC, Timock AM, Crowe JJ, Wang M, Covell DA Jr. Accuracy of alveolar bone measurements from cone beam computed tomography acquired using varying settings. Orthod Craniofac Res. 2015;18(Suppl 1):127–36.
27. Padala S, Tee BC, Beck FM, Elias K, Kim DG, Sun Z. The usefulness of cone-beam computed tomography gray values for alveolar bone linear measurements. Angle Orthod. 2018;88(2):227–32.

3

Postoperative dental morbidity in children following dental treatment under general anesthesia

Yu-Hsuan Hu[1,2], Aileen Tsai[1,2], Li-Wei Ou-Yang[1,2], Li-Chuan Chuang[1,2] and Pei-Ching Chang[1,2*]

Abstract

Background: General anesthesia has been widely used in pediatric dentistry in recent years. However, there remain concerns about potential postoperative dental morbidity. The goal of this study was to identify the frequency of postoperative dental morbidity and factors associated with such morbidity in children.

Methods: From March 2012 to February 2013, physically and mentally healthy children receiving dental treatment under general anesthesia at the Department of Pediatric Dentistry of the Chang Gung Memorial Hospital in Taiwan were recruited. This was a prospective and observational study with different time evaluations based on structured questionnaires and interviews. Information on the patient demographics, anesthesia and dental treatment performed, and postoperative dental morbidity was collected and analyzed. Correlations between the study variables and postoperative morbidity were analyzed based on the Pearson's chi-square test. Correlations between the study variables and the scale of postoperative dental pain were analyzed using the Mann-Whitney U test.

Results: Fifty-six pediatric patients participated in this study, with an average age of 3.34 ± 1.66 years (ranging from 1 to 8 years). Eighty-two percent of study participants reported postoperative dental pain, and 23% experienced postoperative dental bleeding. Both dental pain and bleeding subsided 3 days after the surgery. Dental pain was significantly associated with the total number of teeth treated, while dental bleeding, with the presence of teeth extracted. Patients' gender, age, preoperative dental pain, ASA classification, anesthesia time, and duration of the operation were not associated with postoperative dental morbidity.

Conclusion: Dental pain was a more common postoperative dental morbidity than bleeding. The periods when parents reported more pain in their children were the day of the operation (immediately after the procedure) followed by 1 day and 3 days after the treatment.

Keywords: General anesthesia, Morbidity, Pediatric dentistry

Background

In developing countries, dental caries remain one of the most prevalent health problems in children. In most cases, dental treatment can be completed once children's behaviors are properly managed. However, for very young children, medically compromised children, and those who suffer extreme anxiety, mental or physical disabilities, general anesthesia (GA) will be needed [1].

The public's perception of GA has evolved in recent years and the use of GA has become more widely accepted [2–4]. The advantages rendered by GA include safety, efficiency, convenience, and high-quality restorative and preventive dental care [2]. Dental treatment under GA can also be completed during one single visit and minimize distress to the patient, parent, and dentist. However, children undergoing dental rehabilitation under GA do commonly experience postoperative symptoms such as dental pain and bleeding. However, dental practitioners usually have limited contact with patients after such treatment. Some studies revealed mild-to-moderate dental pain (16 to 48%) after dental treatment

* Correspondence: pearl.pcchang@gmail.com
[1]Department of Pediatric Dentistry, Chang Gung Memorial Hospital, Linkou, Taiwan, Republic of China
[2]Department of Pediatric Dentistry, Chang Gung Memorial Hospital, No. 5 Fu-Hsing Street. Kuei Shan Hsiang, Taoyuan, Taiwan, Republic of China

under GA [5–7]. Other studies found severe dental pain (74 to 95%) was the most common complication [8, 9]. While some studies have shown the prevalence of post-operative dental morbidity to be significant [8, 10–12], others have found it to be minimal [5, 13]. It is difficult to compare these studies because of the different variables used, such as the medical and cognitive status of subjects, socioeconomic status of caregivers, pain scales, standardization of GA and dental procedures, the number and types of dental procedures and postoperative analgesic usage.

Pain is a subjective phenomenon that varies from person to person, and the gold standard for pain assessment is self-reported pain [14, 15]. In the present study, pain was assessed using the Wong-Baker FACES Pain Rating Scale (Fig. 1), a self-report rating system that is easy to use for assessing the intensity of children's pain [15]. The scale shows a series of faces ranging from a happy face at 0 which represents "no hurt" to a crying face at 10 which represents "hurts worst." This scale has been validated for pediatric patients between 2 and 12 years of age as well as parents who report the pain intensity on their child's behalf [16].

However, the majority of the studies were conducted among patient populations in Western countries. Our study reported data collected among Taiwanese patient populations with the goal of identifying (1) the frequency and duration of postoperative dental morbidity of dental pain and dental bleeding, and (2) the impact of selected variables (patient demographics, intraoperative data, and types of dental treatment) on postoperative dental morbidity in children.

Methods

This was an one-year prospective, descriptive, and comparative study among physically and mentally healthy children. All physically and mentally healthy children who were scheduled for dental treatment under GA at the Department of Pediatric Dentistry of the Chang Gung Memorial Hospital in Taiwan were included in our study. Physically and mentally compromised children were excluded from the study. A total of 56 children participated in the study from March 2012 to February 2013. Approval from the Institutional Review Board (100-2964B) for the study was also obtained by the Ethical Committee of the Chang Gung Memorial Hospital, Taoyuan, Taiwan. The study was explained to all participants in detail, including both the principle and germane risks involved. Written informed consent was obtained from participants' legal guardians in accordance with the ethical principles of the World Medical Association agreed upon in the Declaration of Helsinki (version 2002).

After patients arrived in the operating room, standard anesthetic procedures were applied by the anesthesiologist. Nasotracheal intubation was performed on all children. The induction and maintenance agents used were sevoflurane. Dental treatment was performed by four pediatric dentists in accordance with the Guidelines of the American Academy of Pediatric Dentistry [17], including composite resin restoration, pulp treatment, stainless steel crowns (SSCs) of posterior teeth, strip crowns (SCs) of anterior teeth, and extraction of carious teeth or supernumerary teeth. After the dental treatment, children were moved to the post-anesthesia recovery room and later discharged on the same day. No children took postoperative analgesic medications such as acetaminophen.

Preoperative, intraoperative, and postoperative data were recorded. Preoperative data included gender, age, chief complaint, and preoperative dental pain (if any). Intraoperative data included the American Society of Anesthesiologist (ASA) Classification, method of intubation, induction and maintenance agents used, the number of teeth treated, and the type of treatment. Postoperative dental morbidity data were collected through questionnaires in the post-anesthesia recovery room the day of the operation (usually 1 h postoperatively) as well as 1 day, 3 days, 7 days and 14 days postoperatively. Dental pain and dental bleeding were the postoperative dental morbidity that the current study focused on. The questionnaires covered the following items: (1) Did the children have dental pain? and (2) Did the children have dental bleeding? Due to the young age of the children in

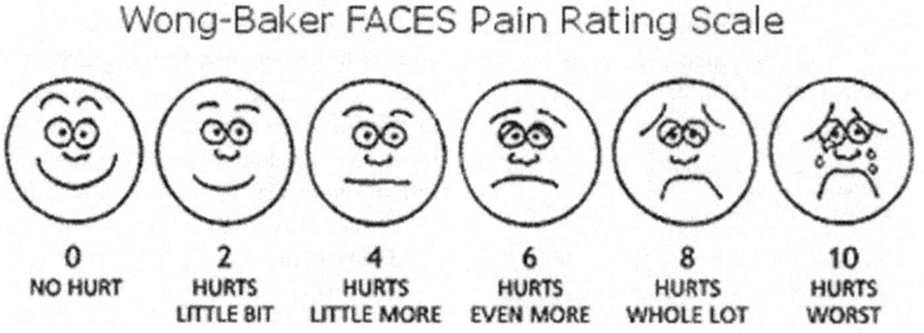

Fig. 1 Wong-Baker FACES Pain Rating Scale

the study (ranging from 1 to 8 years), the parents were the ones that reported children's pain intensity using the Wong-Baker FACES Pain Rating Scale. Before the dental treatment, parents were instructed on how to rate their children's postoperative pain. Postoperative dental pain was labeled as "yes" if the rating reported was equal to or greater than 2.

Statistical analysis of the data collected was performed using SPSS version 16.0 (SPSS, Inc., Chicago IL, USA). Descriptive data included the duration and frequency of postoperative morbidity. Correlations between the study variables and postoperative morbidity were analyzed based on the Pearson's chi-square test. Correlations between the study variables and the scale of postoperative dental pain were analyzed using the Mann-Whitney U test. A p-value less than 0.05 was considered statistically significant.

Results

The demographics and intraoperative data of the children are presented in Table 1. The mean age of the children was 3.34 ± 1.66 years, ranging from 1 to 8 years. Fifty-one children (91%) were brought by parents for caries treatment, and five (9%), for extraction of supernumerary teeth. The mean anesthesia time was 208.89 ± 67.27 min, and the mean duration of operation was 192. 70 ± 67.40 min. The type distribution of the teeth treated is reported in Table 2, and the frequency of postoperative dental pain and bleeding, in Table 3 and Fig. 2.

The associations between postoperative dental morbidity and children's gender, age, ASA classification, anesthesia time, duration of the operation, and the type of treatment are presented in Table 4. Postoperative dental pain did not vary with children's gender, age, ASA classification, anesthesia time, and duration of the operation in a statistically significant way. Postoperative dental pain did, however, vary significantly with the total number of teeth treated. A significantly higher frequency of dental pain was associated with the group where the total number of teeth treated was equal to or greater than 14, compared with the group where the total number was less than 14 ($p < 0.05$). Meanwhile, postoperative dental pain was not significantly related to the number of teeth restored with composite resin, the number of teeth with stainless steel crowns, the number of teeth with strip crowns, the number of pulp treatment received, or the number of teeth extracted, respectively.

The scale of postoperative dental pain as related to the total number of teeth treated was further analyzed and presented in Table 5. The highest pain rating was recorded in the post-anesthesia recovery room (1 h postoperatively). The ratings gradually dropped over 1 day, 3 days, 7 days, and 14 days postoperatively. The scale of postoperative dental pain was significantly related to the total number of teeth treated, in the recovery room as well as 1 day and 3 days postoperatively. This significance disappeared as more days passed. Although higher postoperative pain ratings during the first 3 days were seen with the group experiencing preoperative dental pain, this difference was not significant between the group that experienced preoperative dental pain and the group that did not.

The rating of postoperative dental pain as related to the dental procedure performed was further analyzed and presented in Table 6. The highest pain rating was associated with exodontia, followed by restoration with SSCs. The postoperative dental pain rating was significantly related to the number of teeth receiving pulp therapy 1 day postoperatively. The postoperative dental pain rating was also significantly related to the number of teeth restored with SSCs, in the recovery room as well as 1 day and 3 days postoperatively.

Postoperative dental bleeding did not vary significantly with children's gender, age, ASA classification, anesthesia time, and duration of the operation. The presence of teeth extracted was significantly related to postoperative dental bleeding. A significantly higher frequency of dental bleeding was found in the children with teeth extracted, compared with the children without teeth extracted ($p < 0.05$). Postoperative dental bleeding was not significantly related to the total number of teeth treated, the number of teeth restored (with composite resin, stainless steel crown, or strip crown), or the number of pulp treatment received.

Discussion

All physically and mentally healthy children receiving various dental treatments under general anesthesia in this study saw their treatment completed in one single visit to the Department of Pediatric Dentistry. The treatments performed included composite resin restoration, pulp therapy, stainless steel crowns (SSCs) of posterior teeth, strip crowns (SCs) of anterior teeth, and extraction of carious teeth or supernumerary teeth. Postoperative morbidity of dental pain and bleeding was observed.

Table 1 Demographics and intraoperative data of the children

Gender			Age (Year)		ASA Classification		Anesthesia Time (Hour)		Duration of Operation (Hour)	
Variable	Male	Female	< 3	≧3	I	II	< 3	≧3	< 3	≧3
Number (%)	31 (55)	25 (45)	20 (36)	36 (64)	18 (32)	38 (68)	18 (32)	38 (68)	22 (39)	34 (61)

Table 2 Type distribution of the teeth treated

	Total number of teeth treated		Teeth restored		Pulp treatment		Teeth extracted		SSC		SC	
Mean ± S.D.	13.79 ± 4.86.		7.16 ± 3.81		6.54 ± 4.23		0.64 ± 1.39		3.48 ± 2.77		2.32 ± 1.97	
Number of teeth	< 14	≧14	< 7	≧7	< 7	≧7	0	≧1	< 3	≧3	< 2	≧2
Number of children (%)	22 (39)	34 (61)	26 (46)	30 (54)	29 (52)	27 (48)	41 (73)	15 (27)	21 (38)	35 (62)	21 (38)	35 (62)

SC Strip Crown, *S.D.* Standard Deviations, *SSC* Stainless Steel Crown

Postoperative morbidity of dental pain and bleeding was observed in 46 and 13 children respectively among the 56 children evaluated in this study.

Earlier studies have found that the most common postoperative dental complication is toothache [8, 9, 16] and that the incidence of postoperative pain after dental rehabilitation under GA ranges from 36 to 93% [8, 10–12, 18]. Children in the present study thus appeared to experience a higher rate of dental pain (82%), which may be attributable to the higher number of dental procedures performed and longer duration of treatment. In addition, the induction and maintenance agent of anesthesia used in our study, sevoflurane, has been associated with more pain than halothane as reported by Ersin et al. [18].

In terms of the postoperative pain associated with particular dental treatments, the pain ratings were significantly related to pulp therapy and restoration with SSCs for teeth with pulp infection or inflammation. Gingivitis caused by poor oral hygiene among children receiving SSCs also induced more pain sensation after the treatment. On the other hand, a lower percentage (26%) of the children receiving tooth extraction experienced postoperative dental pain, which may be attributable to the local anesthesia administered before extraction. This echoes the finding by Atan et al. that the frequency of postoperative dental pain was lower in children who received local anesthesia [8]. Hence, when dental extractions are performed under general anesthesia, it is important to ensure that appropriate pain medication is provided.

Postoperative dental pain was found to correlate with the total number of teeth treated in our study. Children with 14 or more teeth treated experienced a significantly higher frequency of dental pain ($p < 0.05$) than those with a lower number of teeth treated. The current study also found that 82% of the children experienced dental pain both 1 h and 1 day after the operation, and 39% continued experiencing pain 3 days after the operation. Seven days after the operation, dental pain lingered among 5% of the children before completely stopping 14 days after the operation. These results are consistent with the findings reported by Needleman et al. and Atan et al. that postoperative dental pain occurred within 24 h and 1 day after the operation before subsiding 1 week after the operation [8, 9].

Table 3 Frequency of postoperative dental pain and bleeding

	Day 0	Day 1	Day 3	Day 7	Day 14
Dental pain N (%)	46 (82)	46 (82)	22 (39)	3 (5)	0 (0)
Dental bleeding N (%)	13 (23)	11 (20)	1 (2)	0 (0)	0 (0)

In this study, no pain killer or other medication for pain control was administrated to children. Since the highest pain rating (3.50 ± 2.59) was recorded in the postoperative recovery room, analgesics could be administered intravenously approximately 30 min before the termination of general anesthesia to reduce the pain that may occur during the first hour postoperatively. The higher pain rating was also associated with a higher number of teeth treated 1 day and 3 days

Table 4 Associations between postoperative dental morbidity and study variables

		Dental pain ($N = 50$)	Dental bleeding ($N = 15$)
Gender	Male	27(54)	10(66.7)
	Female	23(46)	5(33.3)
Age (Year)	< 3	18(36)	4(26.7)
	≧3	32(64)	11(73.3)
ASA Classification	I	17(34)	4(26.7)
	II	33(66)	11(73.3)
Anesthesia time (Hour)	< 3	14(28)	4(26.7)
	≧3	36(72)	11(73.3)
Duration of operation (Hour)	< 3	18(36)	5(33.3)
	≧3	32(64)	10(66.7)
Total number of teeth treated	< 14	17(34)	5(33.3)
	≧14	33(66)*	10(66.7)
Number of teeth restored	< 7	23(46)	8(53.3)
	≧7	27(54)	7(46.7)
Number of pulp treatment	< 7	24(48)	6(40)
	≧7	26(52)	9(60)
Number of teeth extracted	0	37(74)	8(53.3)
	≧1	13(26)	7(46.7)*
Number of teeth with SSC	< 3	17(34)	4(26.7)
	≧3	33(66)	11(73.3)
Number of teeth with SC	< 2	18(36)	7(46.7)
	≧2	32(64)	8(53.3)

*$p < 0.05$ (Pearson's chi-square test)

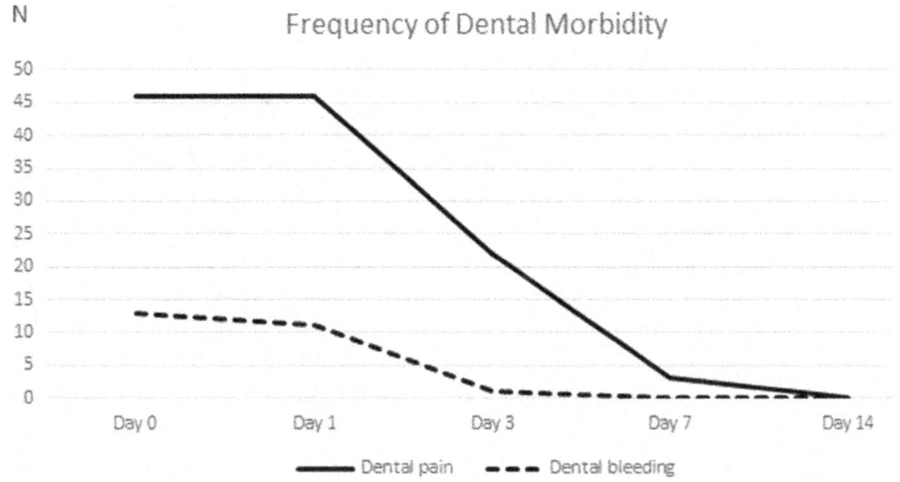

Fig. 2 Frequency of postoperative dental pain and dental bleeding

postoperatively. As the benefit of administering anti-inflammatory analgesics to control toothache in patients treated under GA has been documented [4, 5, 19], it is important to instruct parents to give analgesics regularly for the first few days postoperatively instead of waiting until the pain occurs [9]. According to the results of our study, in the case of comprehensive dental treatment, analgesic medication is recommended for at least 3 days postoperatively to prevent postoperative pain or lower the frequency and degree of the pain.

Postoperative bleeding was less frequent than postoperative dental pain in our study. Twenty-three per cent of the children experienced bleeding 1 h postoperatively, 20% experienced bleeding 1 day after the operation, and 3% experienced bleeding 3 days after the operation. No bleeding was found 7 and 14 days after the operation. The results of our study are consistent with the findings of Mayeda et al. that postoperative dental bleeding subsided within 24 h after the operation [7].

Given most Taiwanese parents' reticence toward tooth extraction, we endeavored to preserve the tooth treated even under general anesthesia in this study, which resulted in a lower extraction rate and in turn a lower rate of postoperative bleeding. The presence of extracted teeth was found to correlate with postoperative bleeding, as evidenced in the significantly higher frequency of dental bleeding ($p < 0.05$) in the group with teeth extracted. Blood clots formed over the extraction wound 1 day after the extraction, followed by epithelialization 3 to 7 days after the extraction. Bleeding usually occurred within 3 days after the extraction. There are different ways to control bleeding, such as using gauze packing, suture, and hemostasis agent. Using local anesthetic agents together with epinephrine can also reduce the incidence of bleeding during the early postoperative period. Well-controlled postoperative bleeding will reduce patients' and parents' anxiety.

Our study reports preliminary findings of postoperative dental morbidity after dental treatment under GA in Taiwan based on a prospective study conducted among a small sample of children. The key contribution of the study resides in the determination of the type and frequency of postoperative dental complaints among children. Future studies could exclude children under 2 or 3 and compare children's self-reported pain intensity with that based on parents' reporting. Given the high percentage of children who reported pain in our study, any correlation between the occurrence of pain and bleeding could be another potential topic for future studies. As the study participants were recruited only

Table 5 Mean ratings of postoperative dental pain related to preoperative pain and the total number of teeth treated

	Preoperative dental pain			Total number of teeth treated		
	No ($N = 31$)	Yes ($N = 25$)	p value	< 14 ($N = 22$)	≧14 ($N = 34$)	p value
Day 0	3.03 ± 2.36	4.08 ± 2.80	0.180	2.82 ± 2.52	3.94 ± 2.58	0.049*
Day 1	2.52 ± 1.93	3.28 ± 1.62	0.122	1.91 ± 1.80	3.47 ± 1.58	0.002*
Day 3	0.77 ± 1.33	1.20 ± 1.30	0.135	0.55 ± 1.10	1.24 ± 1.39	0.045*
Day 7	0.13 ± 0.50	0.08 ± 0.40	0.688	0.00 ± 0.00	0.18 ± 0.58	0.156
Day 14	0.00 ± 0.00	0.00 ± 0.00	1.000	0.00 ± 0.00	0.00 ± 0.00	1.000

*$p < 0.05$ (Mann-Whitney U test)

Table 6 Mean ratings of postoperative dental pain related to dental procedures

	Number of teeth restored with composite resin		Number of teeth treated with pulp therapy		Number of teeth extracted		Number of teeth restored with SSC		Number of teeth restored with SC	
	< 7 (*N* = 26)	≧7 (*N* = 30)	< 7 (*N* = 28)	≧7 (N = 28)	0 (*N* = 41)	≧1 (N = 15)	< 3 (*N* = 21)	≧3 (*N* = 35)	< 2 (N = 22)	≧2 (N = 34)
Day 0	3.15 ± 2.48	3.67 ± 2.78	3.07 ± 2.34	3.93 ± 2.80	3.12 ± 2.15	4.53 ± 3.42	2.38 ± 1.96*	4.17 ± 2.72*	3.18 ± 3.20	3.06 ± 2.04
Day 1	2.69 ± 1.78	3.00 ± 1.88	2.21 ± 1.75*	3.50 ± 1.69*	2.63 ± 1.76	3.47 ± 1.92	1.81 ± 1.54*	3.49 ± 1.70*	2.91 ± 1.93	2.82 ± 1.78
Day 3	0.77 ± 1.27	1.13 ± 1.36	0.64 ± 1.10	1.29 ± 1.46	0.83 ± 1.18	1.33 ± 1.63	0.38 ± 0.80*	1.31 ± 1.45*	1.00 ± 1.35	0.94 ± 1.32
Day 7	0.08 ± 0.39	1.13 ± 0.51	0.07 ± 0.38	0.14 ± 0.52	0.10 ± 0.44	0.13 ± 0.52	0.10 ± 0.44	0.11 ± 0.47	0.00 ± 0.00	0.18 ± 0.58
Day 14	0.00 ± 0.00	0.00 ± 0.00	0.00 ± 0.00	0.00 ± 0.00	0.00 ± 0.00	0.00 ± 0.00	0.00 ± 0.00	0.00 ± 0.00	0.00 ± 0.00	0.00 ± 0.00

*$p < 0.05$ (Mann-Whitney U test)

from the Taoyuan City, future studies could recruit children from other parts of Taiwan who receive dental treatment under GA. Furthermore, dental pain and bleeding were the two types of dental morbidity which the current study focused on. Similar studies could be initiated in the future among children receiving dental treatment under GA in other hospitals and with an expanded scope to include other types of postoperative morbidity.

Oral rehabilitation under general anesthesia can improve children's oral health as well as the quality of their physical, emotional, and social life [20]. However, to address parents' concern about the safety and postoperative morbidity related to general anesthesia, dentists should inform parents of the postoperative symptoms that may occur immediately and days after the operation under general anesthesia. Every effort must also be exerted to minimize the morbidity and ensure that both parents and children are comfortable with the procedures.

Conclusion

Our study showed that dental pain was a more common postoperative morbidity after dental treatment under general anesthesia than bleeding. Dental pain was related to the total number of teeth treated. The periods when parents reported more pain in their children were the day of operation (immediately after the procedure) followed by 1 day and 3 days after the treatment.

Abbreviations

ASA: American Society of Anesthesiologist; GA: General anesthesia; S.D.: Standard deviations; SC: Strip crown; SSC: Stainless steel crown

Authors' contributions

Y.H.H. was instrumental in the design and execution of the study and responsible for data analysis and manuscript preparation. A.T, L.W.O.Y. and L.C.C. contributed to the design and execution of the study as well as reviewing and revising the manuscript. P.C.C. contributed to the design and execution of the study as well as reviewing and revising the manuscript. She also served as the project advisor. All authors read and approved the final manuscript.

Competing interests

The authors declare that they have no competing interests.

References

1. American Academy of Pediatric D. Clinical guideline on the elective use of minimal, moderate, and deep sedation and general anesthesia for pediatric dental patients. Pediatr Dent. 2004;26:95–103.
2. Cantekin K, Yildirim MD, Cantekin I. Assessing change in quality of life and dental anxiety in young children following dental rehabilitation under general anesthesia. Pediatr Dent. 2014;36:12E–7E.
3. Salles PS, Tannure PN, Oliveira CA, Souza IP, Portela MB, Castro GF. Dental needs and management of children with special health care needs according to type of disability. J Dent Child (Chic). 2012;79:165–9.
4. Yildirim MD, Cantekin K. Effect of palonosetron on postoperative nausea and vomiting in children following dental rehabilitation under general anesthesia. Pediatr Dent. 2014;36:7E–11E.
5. Enever GR, Nunn JH, Sheehan JK. A comparison of post-operative morbidity following outpatient dental care under general anaesthesia in paediatric patients with and without disabilities. Int J Paediatr Dent. 2000;10:120–5.
6. Farsi N, Ba'akdah R, Boker A, Almushayt A. Postoperative complications of pediatric dental general anesthesia procedure provided in Jeddah hospitals, Saudi Arabia. BMC Oral Health. 2009;9:6.
7. Mayeda C, Wilson S. Complications within the first 24 hours after dental rehabilitation under general anesthesia. Pediatr Dent. 2009;31:513–9.
8. Atan S, Ashley P, Gilthorpe MS, Scheer B, Mason C, Roberts G. Morbidity following dental treatment of children under intubation general anaesthesia in a day-stay unit. Int J Paediatr Dent. 2004;14:9–16.
9. Needleman HL, Harpavat S, Wu S, Allred EN, Berde C. Postoperative pain and other sequelae of dental rehabilitations performed on children under general anesthesia. Pediatr Dent. 2008;30:111–21.
10. Fung DE, Cooper DJ, Barnard KM, Smith PB. Pain reported by children after dental extractions under general anaesthesia: a pilot study. Int J Paediatr Dent. 1993;3:23–8.
11. Holt RD, Chidiac RH, Rule DC. Dental treatment for children under general anaesthesia in day care facilities at a London dental hospital. Br Dent J. 1991;170:262–6.
12. Hosey MT, Macpherson LM, Adair P, Tochel C, Burnside G, Pine C. Dental anxiety, distress at induction and postoperative morbidity in children undergoing tooth extraction using general anaesthesia. Br Dent J. 2006;200: 39–43. discussion 27; quiz 50
13. Vinckier F, Gizani S, Declerck D. Comprehensive dental care for children with rampant caries under general anaesthesia. Int J Paediatr Dent. 2001;11:25–32.
14. Bieri D, Reeve RA, Champion GD, Addicoat L, Ziegler JB. The faces pain scale for the self-assessment of the severity of pain experienced by children: development, initial validation, and preliminary investigation for ratio scale properties. Pain. 1990;41:139–50.
15. Voepel-Lewis T, Merkel S, Tait AR, Trzcinka A, Malviya S. The reliability and validity of the face, legs, activity, cry, consolability observational tool as a measure of pain in children with cognitive impairment. Anesth Analg. 2002; 95:1224–9. table of contents
16. Escanilla-Casal A, Ausucua-Ibanez M, Aznar-Gomez M, Viano-Garcia JM, Sentis-Vilalta J, Rivera-Baro A. Comparative study of postoperative morbidity in dental treatment under general anesthesia in pediatric patients with and without an underlying disease. Int J Paediatr Dent. 2016;26:141–8.

4

Novel caries loci in children and adults implicated by genome-wide analysis of families

Manika Govil[1*†], Nandita Mukhopadhyay[1†], Daniel E. Weeks[2,3], Eleanor Feingold[1,2,3], John R. Shaffer[1,2], Steven M. Levy[4,5], Alexandre R. Vieira[1,2], Rebecca L. Slayton[6], Daniel W. McNeil[7,8], Robert J. Weyant[9], Richard J. Crout[10] and Mary L. Marazita[1,2,11]

Abstract

Background: Dental caries is a common chronic disease among children and adults alike, posing a substantial health burden. Caries is affected by multiple genetic and environmental factors, and prior studies have found that a substantial proportion of caries susceptibility is genetically inherited.

Methods: To identify such genetic factors, we conducted a genome-wide linkage scan in 464 extended families with 2616 individuals from Iowa, Pennsylvania and West Virginia for three dental caries phenotypes: (1) **PRIM**: dichotomized as zero versus one or more affected primary teeth, (2) **QTOT1**: age-adjusted quantitative caries measure for both primary and permanent dentitions including pre-cavitated lesions, and (3) **QTOT2**: age-adjusted quantitative caries excluding pre-cavitated lesions. Genotyping was conducted for approximately 600,000 SNPs on an Illumina platform, pruned to 127,511 uncorrelated SNPs for the analyses reported here.

Results: Multipoint non-parametric linkage analyses generated peak LOD scores exceeding 2.0 for eight genomic regions, but no LOD scores above 3.0 were observed. The maximum LOD score for each of the three traits was 2.90 at 1q25.3 for **PRIM**, 2.38 at 6q25.3 for **QTOT1**, and 2.76 at 5q23.3 for **QTOT2**. Some overlap in linkage regions was observed among the phenotypes. Genes with a potential role in dental caries in the eight chromosomal regions include *CACNA1E, LAMC2, ALMS1, STAMBP, GXYLT2, SLC12A2, MEGF10, TMEM181, ARID1B,* and, as well as genes in several immune gene families. Our results are also concordant with previous findings from association analyses on chromosomes 11 and 19.

Conclusions: These multipoint linkage results provide evidence in favor of novel chromosomal regions, while also supporting earlier association findings for these data. Understanding the genetic etiology of dental caries will allow designing personalized treatment plans based on an individual's genetic risk of disease.

Keywords: Dental genetics, Dental public health, Permanent dentition caries, Primary dentition caries, Non-parametric linkage, Genome-wide linkage study

Background

Dental caries is one of the most common chronic diseases among children and adults alike. Childhood caries is associated with failure to thrive, and it can affect self-esteem and school performance [1]. For both children and adults, caries is associated with pain and loss of teeth, and caries may adversely impact growth and weight gain in children, as well as nutrition among adults, thereby negatively affecting quality of life.

Caries is known to have a genetic component. Detection of genetic factors is complicated by the fact that numerous diverse environmental factors influence the incidence and severity of this disease, including the microbiome, dietary habits, fluoride exposure, salivary factors and tooth structure.

Prior studies have shown that caries experience in humans is determined by genetic causes with heritability

* Correspondence: manika.govil@gmail.com
†Manika Govil and Nandita Mukhopadhyay contributed equally to this work.
[1]Center for Craniofacial and Dental Genetics, Department of Oral Biology, School of Dental Medicine, University of Pittsburgh, Suite 500 Bridgeside Point, 100 Technology Drive, Pittsburgh, PA 15219, USA
Full list of author information is available at the end of the article

values between 20 and 60% [2–7]. To date, there have also been numerous studies investigating association of dental caries with candidate genes or with whole-genome Single Nucleotide Polymorphism (SNP) panels [8, 9]. The only previous genome-wide linkage study of caries was conducted using a panel of 392 microsatellite markers, on 46 extended Filipino families with 642 total individuals [10]. This study found suggestive linkage of low caries experience to chromosome regions 5q13.3, 14q11.2, and 13q27.1, and high caries experience to 13q31.1 and 14q24.3 However, results of previous studies have, in general, not been extensively replicated, possibly due to relatively small sample sizes [8, 9] and the enumeration of genetic factors is far from complete.

Our present study is the first to apply genome-wide multipoint linkage analysis to explore the genetic etiology of caries (whether in childhood or adulthood) using densely spaced SNPs on a population previously analyzed by genome-wide association. Genome-wide linkage analysis is a complementary strategy to genome-wide association analysis for gene-discovery. Whereas association identifies specific marker alleles correlated with the caries phenotype, linkage analysis strategies identify genomic regions shared between related individuals who show similar disease characteristics. The advantage of linkage analysis is that it makes full use of familial inheritance, is less sensitive to allelic heterogeneity, and, unlike association, can be used to detect rare disease-causing mutations. Furthermore, multipoint linkage utilizes genotypes from SNPs neighboring the test location, while association conducts tests at each location independently.

In this study, multipoint non-parametric linkage analysis was conducted, i.e., no assumptions were made with respect to the mode of inheritance of dental caries [11], and the analysis was, therefore, robust to uncertainty about the underlying genetic model. Empirical significance of the linkage signals was assessed across the genome by simulating multiple sets of genome-wide data such that the SNP genotypes were unlinked to caries status.

Methods

Study subjects and genotype data

The families and individuals included in this study are from western Pennsylvania, West Virginia, and Iowa. Subjects from Pennsylvania and West Virginia were ascertained through the Center for Oral Health Research in Appalachia (COHRA; [12]). Additional subjects from Pennsylvania were recruited under the University of Pittsburgh Dental Registry and DNA Repository (DRDR; [13]). Subjects from Iowa were recruited under two University of Iowa projects, the Iowa Fluoride Study (IFS; [14–17]) and Iowa Head Start (IHS; [18]). All subject recruitment and data collection was approved by site-specific Institutional Review Boards. Genotyping was conducted under the Gene Environment Association Studies Initiative (GENEVA) for approximately 600,000 SNPs on an Illumina platform (Human 610_Quadv1_B; Illumina, Inc., San Diego, CA, USA). All genotype and phenotype data is available on dbGaP (The database of Genotypes and Phenotypes; https://www.ncbi.nlm.nih.gov/gap; accession number phs000095.v3.p1). Details on genotyping and quality control protocols are also presented on dbGaP, or can be found in earlier studies [19, 20]. Table 1 summarizes the different subsets of data in terms of the sample available for this study. This study utilizes complete families, in other words, non-genotyped and non-phenotyped individuals also contribute to various aspects of the analysis. Prior studies primarily utilized unrelated individuals for conducting association analysis. The starting study sample comprised a total of 4727 self-reported non-Hispanic white individuals, of which 437 were unrelated, 1674 were in 558 two-parent and single offspring (trio) families, and 2616 were in 464 non-trio families. Approximately 76% of individuals were genotyped (Table 1).

Definition of dental caries phenotypes

Caries scores were assessed on the COHRA, IFC, and IHS subjects in accordance with the COHRA study protocol [12]. For subjects in the DRDR study, we used caries scores abstracted from clinical records by dental students trained by Dr. Alexandre R. Vieira, who is a co-author on this manuscript.

Table 1 Starting sample size

Site	Current study starting sample			
	Unrelated	Trios[a] (Individuals)	Non-trio pedigrees[b] (Individuals)	Genotyped/Total
COHRA	29	162 (486)	452 (2549)	2209/3064
IFS	–	394 (1182)	4 (32)	964/1214
IHS	169	1 (3)	7 (29)	183/201
DRDR	239	1 (3)	1 (6)	235/248
Total	437	558 (1674)	464 (2616)	3591/4727

Note: [a]Trios: Family structure of two parents and one child
[b]Non-trio pedigrees: Families with four or more members

We defined three dental caries phenotypes, one based on primary dentition (**PRIM**), and two that combine primary and permanent dentitions (**QTOT1**, **QTOT2**). **PRIM** was coded as a binary primary dentition caries phenotype based on the count of decayed and/or filled primary teeth (*dft*) score. An individual with a *dft* score of 1 or more was designated as being affected. The primary teeth from all subjects with primary or mixed dentition were assessed for **PRIM**. These individuals included adults with over retained primary teeth. **QTOT1**, an age-adjusted quantitative caries phenotype, is based on the sum of the *dft* score (primary teeth) and D_1MFT score (count of decayed, missing, and filled permanent teeth including white spot lesions). **QTOT1** scores were generated by adjusting this raw sum for age and age-squared effects using locally fitted splines. Scores for 113 individuals below 2 years of age and 5 individuals above 60 years, were excluded from linkage analysis due to a very low caries experience in the 0–2 years age group, and the presence of very few subjects above 60 years of age. Age-adjusted **QTOT2**, the second quantitative caries phenotype, is based on the sum of the *dft* score and the D_2MFT score (count of decayed, missing, and filled permanent teeth excluding white spot lesions). Age-adjustment was performed as for the **QTOT1** phenotype; and **QTOT2** scores for 115 individuals between 0 and 2 years of age and 44 individuals above 60 years were set to missing.

Data cleaning and preparation

Genetic map positions were generated for all SNPs. These genetic markers were filtered based on genotyping rates and Hardy-Weinberg proportions. The SNPs were then pruned for linkage disequilibrium (LD). SNPs with residual LD were clustered into super-markers. The procedures used for filtering SNPs, map creation, and LD-based SNP pruning and clustering are described below.

Genetic map creation

The Genetic Map Interpolator (GMI) program, [21] was used to calculate genetic map positions for all SNPs. Sex-averaged map positions were created for SNPs on chromosomes 1–22, and female map positions were created for SNPs on the X chromosome. In the GMI program, the physical basepair (bp) position of each SNP per March 2006 Build NCBI36/hg18 was transformed to the corresponding centiMorgan (cM) scale genetic map distance based on interpolation into the Rutgers Combined Linkage-Physical Map [22].

SNP filtering

In addition to the quality control and cleaning steps detailed on dbGap, we filtered SNPs on the basis of low genotyping success rate and deviation from Hardy-Weinberg equilibrium (HWE) proportions using the software PLINK [23]. SNPs with genotyping success rates below 95%, calculated using genotype data for all individuals, were excluded from analysis. Known genotypes of founders (i.e. those individuals in a family whose parents are not included in the study) and unrelated individuals were used to test SNPs for HWE proportions. The HWE proportions significance threshold was set at 10^{-5} for rejecting the null hypothesis of no deviation from HWE proportions.

Linkage disequilibrium-based SNP pruning and clustering

The genotyping panel available to this study was designed for genome-wide association analysis. When conducting linkage analysis on densely spaced SNP marker loci, the presence of substantial marker-to-marker LD is known to inflate linkage signals, especially if parental genotypes are missing [24]. In this study, LD was removed in two stages. First, the set of quality-filtered SNPs were pruned using PLINK such that the LD r^2 (a measure of LD based on the square of the correlation coefficient between loci) value among remaining SNPs fell below 20%. In PLINK, LD pruning consists of creating blocks of 50 consecutive SNPs followed by recursive removal of SNPs within blocks, until the LD r^2 value among the remaining SNPs is below the desired threshold (20% in our case). Only the unrelated genotyped individuals in our data – pedigree founders and unrelated cases/controls – were used to calculate LD in this step. Any remaining LD was then accounted for using LD-based clustering in Merlin [25]. In clustering, each block of consecutive SNPs that shows an r^2 value greater than a specified threshold (in our case 10%), is analyzed collectively as a super-marker.

Table 2 summarizes the data processing steps undertaken to select SNPs for linkage analysis, and the samples that contributed information to specific parts of this data cleaning. After HWE filtering and LD-based pruning, 127,511 SNPs in low LD (pairwise $r^2 \leq 20\%$) were retained. LD-based SNP clustering combined 92,495 SNPs into 20,634

Table 2 Sample for data cleaning

Procedure	Data
Low genotype rate filtering (PLINK)	3591 genotyped individuals
HWE testing (PLINK)	1839 genotyped (founders[a] + unrelated)[b]
LD-based pruning (PLINK)	1839 genotyped (founders[a] + unrelated)[b]
LD-based clustering and super-marker creation (Merlin)	1022 families (trios + non-trio pedigrees)[c]
Super-marker and SNP allele frequency estimation (Merlin)	1022 families (trios + non-trio pedigrees)[c]

Note: [a]Founders: Individuals in a pedigree or trio whose parents are not included in the study. For example, both parents in a trio are founders. Also note that some of the larger multigenerational pedigrees may have more than two founders
[b]The counts of individuals differs from totals provided in Table 1 since not all founders and unrelated individuals were genotyped for this study
[c]Trios: Family structure of two parents and one child; non-trio pedigrees: families with four or more members

super-markers, leaving 35,016 SNPs to be analyzed individually. The average genetic map distance between the final set of markers (super-marker index and singleton SNPs) is approximately 0.07 cM on the autosomes and 0.13 cM on the X-chromosome. Super-marker and singleton SNP allele frequencies were generated as maximum likelihood estimates using Merlin. The SNP clustering and allele frequency estimation steps utilized 1022 informative families.

Linkage analysis

Table 3 summarizes the sample of individuals used within the linkage analysis for the three traits. In the table are presented the number of informative pedigrees, individuals, and phenotyped relative pairs by relationship type that were included in NPL and QT linkage. A total of 160 relative pairs were informative for PRIM NPL. For QT linkage, the corresponding informative relative pair counts were 1026 and 1038 for QTOT1 and QTOT2.

Genome-wide linkage of PRIM

In non-parametric linkage (NPL) analysis, affected individuals within each pedigree are examined to detect whether affected relatives share genomic regions identical-by-descent (IBD) more often than expected due to their relatedness alone. This IBD sharing is tested at locations along each chromosome. Genome-wide NPL analysis was carried out for the **PRIM** phenotype using the S_{All} statistic [26] as implemented in Merlin [25].

Table 3 Linkage analysis final sample

	PRIM	QTOT1	QTOT2
Total Non-trio Pedigrees	108	376	385
COHRA	106	372	373
IFS	1	4	4
IHS	1	–	7
DRDR	–	–	1
Total Individuals	687	2200	2243
Phenotyped	243 affected	1738	1756
Genotyped	483	1582	1604
Total informative relative pairs[a]	160	1026	1038
Median [Min, Max] pairs/pedigree	1 [1–6]	1 [1–24]	1 [1–24]
Sibling-pairs	100	599	609
Half-sibling pairs	39	228	228
Cousin pairs	21	73	73
Grandparent-grandchild	0	28	28
Avuncular	0	98	100

Note: [a]PRIM: Affected relative pairs; QTOT1, QTOT2: phenotyped relative pairs

Genome-wide linkage of QTOT1 and QTOT2

The quantitative trait (QT) regression-based linkage method, Merlin-regress, [27] was utilized to carry out analyses of the two quantitative phenotypes across autosomes. The QT linkage method is based on regressing estimated IBD sharing between relative pairs on the squared sums and differences of their phenotypes. It does not handle X-linked SNPs, hence the X chromosome was not analyzed for the two quantitative traits. Merlin-regress analyses required specification of a heritability parameter (set at 50% based on published estimates for *DMFT*) and sample-based means and variances for **QTOT1** and **QTOT2.** All results, NPL and QT linkage, are reported as LOD (logarithm of the odds of linkage) scores.

Empirical significance of observed linkage signals

The most commonly used LOD score threshold of 3.0 used to test for significant linkage (Morton) was derived for parametric linkage analysis of a single locus on a binary trait phenotype. Subsequent research (e.g. those reviewed in [28]) that address newer linkage methods such as whole-genome analysis, affected-relative pairs and multipoint calculations are also based on assumptions on the study data, that are rarely true in real-life. Therefore, to correct for multiple testing, we carried out a simulation study to assess the genome-wide significance thresholds for the NPL and QT regression LOD scores. In general, for a null simulation, hundreds of simulated genetic data sets are generated and analyzed to produce an empirical distribution of LOD scores. Since this process would be prohibitively time consuming given the study data, we used an adaptive approach to generate null distributions. The replicate pool method, Pseudo [29] was used to derive the empirical null distribution of NPL scores for PRIM. An initial pool of 100 simulated genotype data sets was generated for this study using Merlin (simulate option) followed by the pseudo-simulation of 100,000 NPL genome-scans to create the empirical distribution of unlinked NPL LOD scores. Pseudo was not utilized for the quantitative data simulations since QT-regression does not produce pedigree-specific LOD scores. For QTOT1 and QTOT2, 5000 data sets each were simulated and analyzed using Merlin.

Selection of linkage peak regions and etiologic genes

For super-markers, the NPL and QT LOD scores correspond to the index (first) SNP of each cluster. In the linkage scan for each phenotype, maximizing markers in regions with LOD score ≥ 2.0 were identified as linkage peaks. A support interval of one LOD drop was used for exploring genes under selected linkage peaks. The one LOD drop support interval is the interval where the LOD score is within one unit of its maximum.

Regions with LOD scores ≥1.0 were identified for trait. Overlap of linkage signal among the three traits was determined based on overlap of peak support intervals or secondary peaks(s) of at least 1.0 LODs, lying within the primary peak support interval. In the event peaks for multiple phenotypes overlapped, the resulting support intervals were reduced to the region of overlap.

Genes within these support intervals were examined for a potential etiologic role in dental caries incidence. Genes identified as causal would include, for example, genes related to blood glucose levels, secretory function of the salivary glands, and host immune response. Proximity of genes to SNPs corresponding to linkage peaks was determined by physical map positions obtained from UCSC Genome Browser corresponding to the March 2006 (NCBI36/hg18) Assembly [30]. When no genes were identified as potentially contributing to caries risk, we instead listed the gene closest to the SNP with the maximum observed LOD.

Comparison with prior published findings

A systematic search of literature was conducted to compile caries risk-conferring genes and genomic regions from previous studies utilizing some portion of our data, as well as from studies of other populations. Physical positions for these genes and genomic regions were then mapped to our linkage scans. Linkage regions with a LOD score of 1.0 or greater have been reported as indicative of concordance or replication, as appropriate.

Sensitivity analysis

Effect of variation in parameter values on NPL statistics

For multifactorial diseases such as caries, the true underlying genetic model for disease is difficult to ascertain. In this study, model-free linkage methods were used to detect linkage. The QT methods are sensitive to the misspecification of the required programmatic input values. We conducted a sensitivity analysis for the heritability parameter (HP), since published literature provides a wide range of heritability values (40–60%), and our work utilized HP = 50%. In the sensitivity analysis, HP values were set at 40, and 60% for **QTOT1** and **QTOT2**.

Mega2 [31] was used to re-format and create input files for all the software used in data cleaning, LD-based pruning and clustering, genetic map creation, linkage analysis and data simulation.

Results

Study sample characteristics

Figure 1 provides detailed information on the distribution of the three phenotypes, **PRIM** (panels A and B), **QTOT1** (panels C, D, E and I), and **QTOT2** (panels F, G, H and I). There were 287 individuals with known **PRIM** phenotypes (panel A), of which 243 individuals were affected for PRIM. Of these 243 subjects, 242 were 18 years or younger in age (panel B). Subjects with primary or mixed dentition included in the **PRIM** NPL analysis ranged from 15 months to 22.5 years of age, with a mean of 7.4 years. These subjects with primary dentition caries constitute mainly the youngest generation. The distribution of the raw caries index by decade, age-adjusted index by decade, and age-adjusted caries index within all phenotyped individuals compared to those between 2 and 60 years of age are shown for **QTOT1** (panels C, D, and E) and **QTOT2** (panels F, G, and H). The number of phenotyped individuals, range, mean and standard deviation are presented in panel I for both quantitative traits. A larger number of individuals were phenotyped for D_2MFT as compared to D_1MFT in this study. For **QTOT1** and **QTOT2**, there were 2484, and 2868 phenotyped individuals in the 2–60 age range. Both of the age-adjusted phenotypes follow an approximately normal distribution, with a mean of zero. The **QTOT1** and **QTOT2** mean and standard deviations for the 2–60 age group were included as distribution parameters within quantitative trait linkage.

Linkage analysis

Figure 2 shows genome-wide LOD scores by SNP (or super-marker index SNP) for **PRIM**, **QTOT1**, and **QTOT2**. The empirical 5% genome-wide significance level, indicated as a solid horizontal line, was 3.48, 3.61, and 3.76 for **PRIM**, **QTOT1**, and **QTOT2**, respectively. Overlapping LOD score peaks for multiple phenotypes were observed in a few regions.

Highest LOD Score Regions

Table 4 presents peak LOD scores and 1-LOD support intervals. The SNP (or index SNP) with the maximum LOD value in each peak is identified along with its genomic location. Regions with maximum LOD ≥ 2.0 are shown ordered by chromosome, along with secondary peak(s) of at least 1.0 LODs, if observed for other traits. The highest LOD scores by trait were 2.90 for **PRIM**, 2.38 for **QTOT1**, and 2.76 for **QTOT2**. Detailed results for all SNPs that lie within the support region for peaks reported in Table 4 with a LOD score of 2.0 or more are provided in supplementary material [see Additional File 1].

For each linkage peak, the table also reports the closest gene, if found, with a potential role in caries incidence. For two of these peaks, one on chromosome 2 (**QTOT2**; LOD 2.30) and the other on chromosome 3 (**PRIM**; LOD 2.50), no such etiologic genes were identified within the support intervals. In these intervals, genes *BCL11A* (60.538–60.634 Mb) and *KAT2B* (20.056–20.171 Mb) were found to be closest to the respective LOD score peak SNPs. The genes within linkage peak

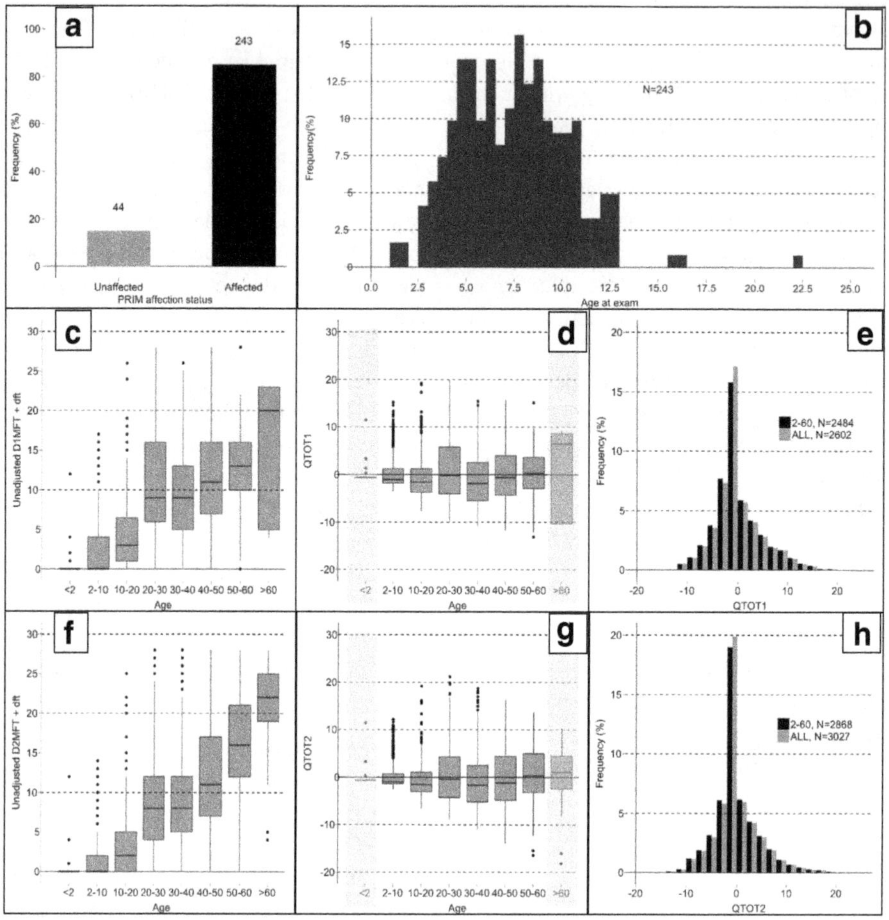

i **Distribution and sample size for new quantitative traits**

	QTOT1		QTOT2	
	0-60 years	2-60 years	0-60 years	2-60 years
Mean	0.00	-0.02	-0.04	-0.05
Standard Deviation	4.87	4.78	4.52	4.46
Minimum	-13.07	-13.07	-16.43	-18.17
Maximum	20.06	20.06	21.17	21.17
Number of Individuals	2,602	2,484	3,027	2,868

Fig. 1 Distribution of (**a**) **PRIM** by binary affection status, (**b**) age at exam of individuals categorized as **PRIM** affected, (**c**) raw $dft + D_1MFT$ (**d**) age-adjusted **QTOT1**, (**e**) age-adjusted **QTOT1** for the full sample compared to the distribution for the 2–60 age group, (**f**) raw $dft + D_2MFT$, (**g**) age-adjusted **QTOT2**, (**h**) age-adjusted QTOT2 for the full sample compared to the distribution for the 2–60 age group, and (**i**) mean, standard deviation, range and sample size for QTOT1 and QTOT2; shaded areas in panels D and G indicate individuals below the age of 2 and above 60 years with phenotypes excluded from quantitative trait linkage analysis

regions that may play an etiologic role in dental caries are described in the sections below.

Chromosome 1 The highest LOD 2.90 across all three traits was observed on chromosome 1 for PRIM (Table 4). Under this peak, the *CACNA1E* (179.719–180.037 Mb) gene has been shown to be involved in glucose-evoked insulin secretion in mice [32]. Poor glycemic control has potential implications for increased caries risk in humans. Mutations in the *LAMC2* (181.422–181.481 Mb) laminin gene are known to cause non-Herlitz form of junctional epidermolysis bullosa, which includes hypodontia and dental caries among its phenotypes [33].

Chromosome 2 The second **QTOT2** peak on chromosome 2 includes the *ALMS1* (73.466–73.691 Mb) gene. Mutations in this gene causes Alström syndrome, where gingivitis and discolored enamel are two clinical phenotypes [34]. Individuals with mutations in the *STAMBP* (73.910–73.944 Mb) gene have been reported to have cleft palate and facial dysmorphology [35].

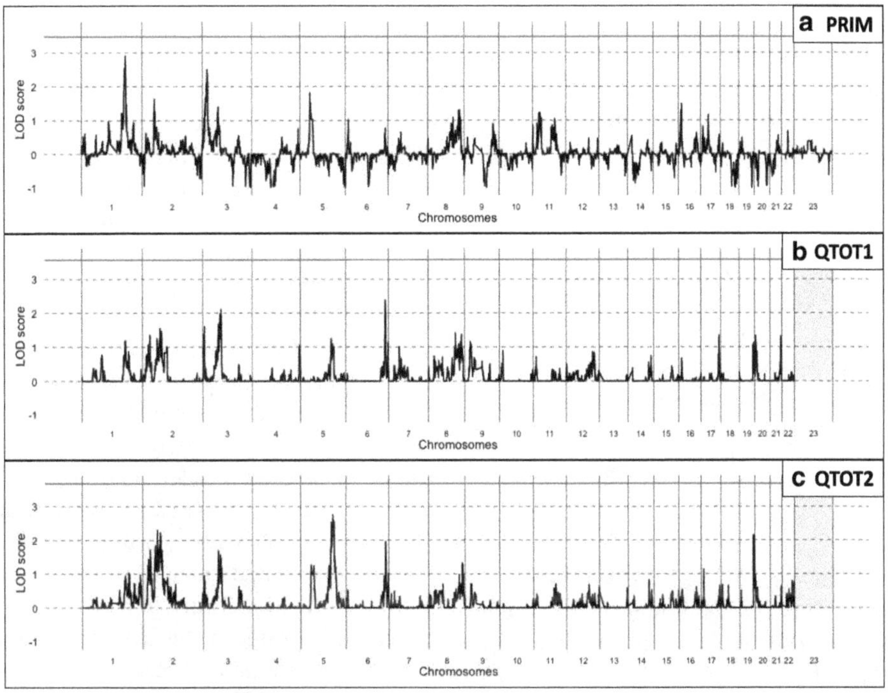

Fig. 2 Genome-wide LOD scores: (**a**) **PRIM**, (**b**) **QTOT1**, (**c**) **QTOT2**. **PRIM** results include the X chromosome. The empirical genome-wide 0.05 significance levels are indicated in each panel with a solid (red, online) horizontal line

Chromosome 3 The *GXYLT2* (73.020–73.107 Mb) gene is located within the chromosome 3 **QTOT1** peak. *GXYLT2* acts on epidermal growth factor, which is expressed in human submandibular and parotid glands, and important for the maintenance of oroesophageal and gastric tissue.

Chromosome 5 The highest genome-wide quantitative trait LOD was observed for **QTOT2**. This **QTOT2** peak contains the *SLC12A2* (127.447–127.553 Mb) gene, whose protein product helps the movement of chloride ions in saliva, thereby assisting in salivary function. Also

Table 4 Linkage peaks in highest LOD score regions

Chr	Trait	Peak[a]			Support Interval (Mb)[b] for Peak with LOD ≥ 2		Closest Genes within Support Interval[c]
		SNP	bp	LOD	Left	Right	
1	**QTOT1**	rs12096999	178,046,412	1.19			*CACNA1E*; *LAMC2*
1	**PRIM**	rs1281317	180,232,077	**2.90**	174.78	182.03	
2	**QTOT2**	rs7572396	59,893,993	**2.30**	58.63	64.29	*BCL11A*[d]
2	**QTOT1**	rs13420242	71,117,276	1.55			*ALMS1*; *STAMBP*
2	**QTOT2**	rs831535	73,976,537	**2.10**	65.23	79.72	
3	**PRIM**	rs9842115	20,378,197	**2.50**	15.06	22.19	*KAT2B*[d]
3	**QTOT1**	rs2044594	74,474,447	**2.12**	67.65	76.08	*GXYLT2*
5	**QTOT1**	rs11748635	123,232,224	1.24			*SLC12A2*; *MEGF10*; *IL* gene family
5	**QTOT2**	rs6866597	128,905,516	**2.76**	122.43	133.84	
6	**QTOT1**	rs240642	158,117,314	**2.38**	156.81	159.48	*TMEM181*; *ARID1B*
6	**QTOT2**	rs9295289	158,387,494	1.96			
19	**QTOT1**	rs11084325	59,424,868	1.12			*NLRP2*; *NLRP7*; *NLRP*, *KIR*, and *LILR* gene families
19	**QTOT2**	rs1671133	60,198,861	**2.15**	59.42	61.47	

Note: [a]Novel regions with LOD ≥ 2.00, and secondary peaks ≥1.0 observed for the other phenotypes; peak LOD ≥ 2.00 shown in bold
[b]Support interval for LOD ≥ 2.00; Mb: 10^6 (or 1 million) bp
[c]Genes with a potential role in caries incidence. If no such gene is identified, then the closest gene to the peak reported
[d]Unknown role in caries incidence; closest gene to the linkage peak SNP

within the support interval are genes from the *IL* family, which code for cytokines involved in blood production and immune system function. Defects in these genes result in autoimmune diseases and immune deficiency. A third gene, *MEGF10* (126.654–126.825 Mb) has been implicated in MARDD (Myopathy, areflexia, respiratory distress, and dysphagia), with cleft palate as an associated phenotype [36].

Chromosome 6 The *TMEM181* (158.877–158.976 Mb) gene under the **QTOT1** linkage peak codes for a putative G-coupled protein receptor which mediates reaction to cytolethal distending toxins secreted by many pathogenic bacteria. *ARID1B* (157.141–157.572 Mb) mutations result in mental retardation along with minor teeth anomalies [37].

Chromosome 19 This region harbors several genes from the *NLRP*, *KIR*, and *LILR* immune gene families that code for various receptors within immune cells. *NLRP2* (60.170–60.204 Mb), and *NLRP7* (60.127–60.151 Mb) were closest to the peak.

Comparison with previous relevant signals

Table 5 shows regions reported by previous studies, where our current LOD score is 1.0 or greater. Two regions were found to contain genes reported in prior studies.

Chromosome 11 A **PRIM** LOD of 1.23 was observed 8500 bp from the *MPPED2* (30.338–30.558 Mb) gene. A suggestive association of primary teeth caries was reported by a previous study on 1305 children aged 3–12, some of whom are also part of this analysis (Shaffer et al., 2011). The phenotype was defined similarly to our PRIM phenotype.

Chromosome 19 A gene-set enrichment analysis study [38] reported an association of primary teeth caries to *NLRP12* (58.989–59.019 Mb) in 1142 children aged 3–13, a subset of whom are also included in our study. **QTOT1** and **QTOT2** LOD scores ≥1.0 were observed 0.4–1.2 Mb from this gene.

Sensitivity analysis

For each of the two quantitative traits, **QTOT1** and **QTOT2**, Fig. 3, panels A, B, C, and D show the percentage deviation of LODs obtained using HPs of 40% or 60% from baseline LODs produced with an HP of 50%. These deviations are plotted on the y-axis against the corresponding baseline LOD (x-axis). The red points indicate SNPs for which baseline LODs of 2.0 or greater dropped below 2.0 when the HP value was changed. Conversely, the green points show SNP positions with baseline LODs below 2.0, which subsequently switched to a score of 2.0 or more with a change in HP. Percentage deviations where the baseline LODs were between 0 and 0.05 are not presented in panels A through D. Within this range, the change in LOD combined across HP = 40% and HP = 60% ranges from – 0.04 to 0.11 LOD for **QTOT1**. For **QTOT2**, the corresponding range is – 0.05 to 0.1 LOD. Although in percentage terms they represent exponential changes as compared to the baseline, none of the deviations in the 0 to 0.5 baseline LOD score range result in the LOD score approaching significance. Panels E and F break down for each trait, the percentage of all SNPs that drop below—or exceed—the 2.0 LOD score threshold with a change in HP. For both traits, a decrease in HP to 40% results in a minimal percentage of SNPs changing status (be it an increase or decrease in LOD score). In contrast, SNPs with LOD scores of 2.0 or greater at HP 50% are more likely to drop below the 2.0 LOD threshold when the HP is increased to 60%.

Table 6 presents the change in **QTOT1** and **QTOT2** LOD scores due to a change in HP for only the linkage peaks reported in Table 4. All LOD score peaks, except for one, remain above 2.0 despite changes in HP.

Discussion

To our knowledge, this study was the first to apply genome-wide multipoint linkage analysis to explore the genetic etiology of caries using densely spaced SNPs.

We defined two new quantitative phenotypes which combine childhood and adulthood caries indices while also accounting for variability by age. The linkage findings in this study nominated genes on six chromosomes (1, 2, 3, 5, 6, and 19) with potential involvement in caries

Table 5 Linkage signals with LOD ≥ 1 concordant with published findings

Study, Gene, phenotype	Highest observed LOD Score			
	SNP	bp	LOD	Trait
Genome-wide association, *MPPED2*, dichotomized d_1ft^a in US children aged 3–12 (Shaffer et al. 2011)	rs1447267	30,643,586	1.23	PRIM
Association with gene set enrichment, *NLRP12*, dichotomized d_1ft^1 in children aged 3–12 (Wang et al. [38])	rs11084325	59,424,868	1.12	QTOT1
	rs1671133	60,198,861	2.15	QTOT2

Note: [a]Dichotomized d_1ft as used in our study

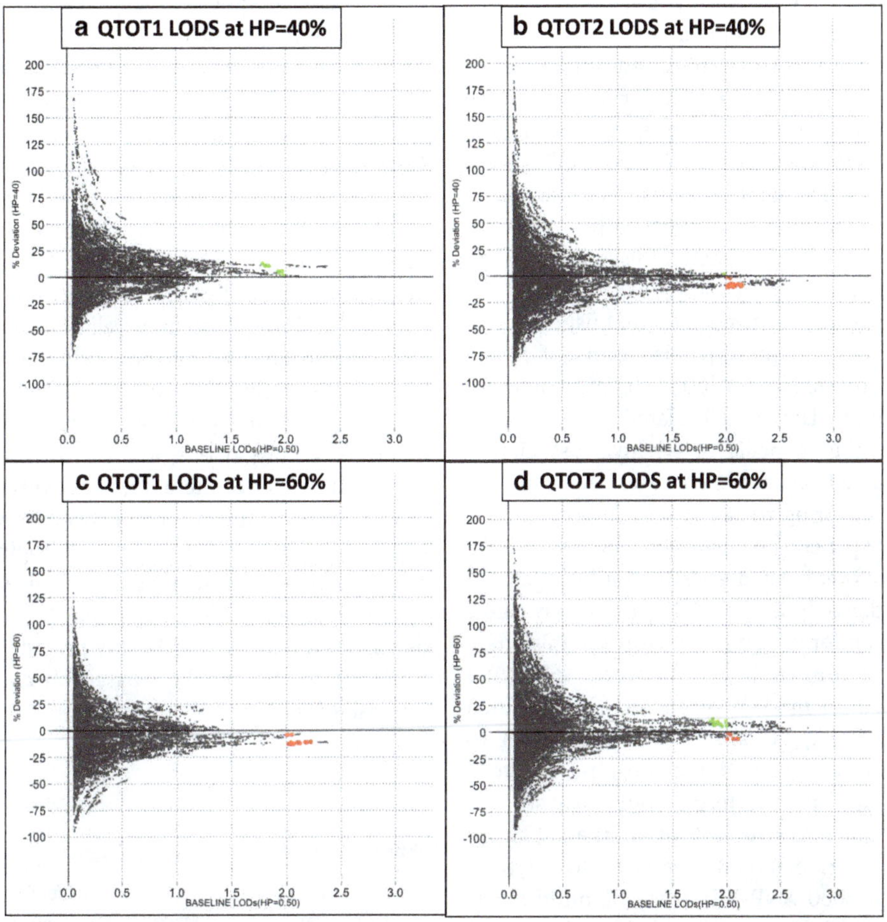

e QTOT1 SNPs Switching LOD Threshold

	HP=40%	HP=60%
HP=50% LOD < 2 switching ≥2	0.026%	0
HP=50% LOD ≥ 2 switching < 2	0	61.11%

f QTOT2 SNPs Switching LOD Threshold

	HP=40%	HP=60%
HP=50% LOD < 2 switching ≥2	0.002%	0.13%
HP=50% LOD ≥ 2 switching < 2	0.06%	5.39%

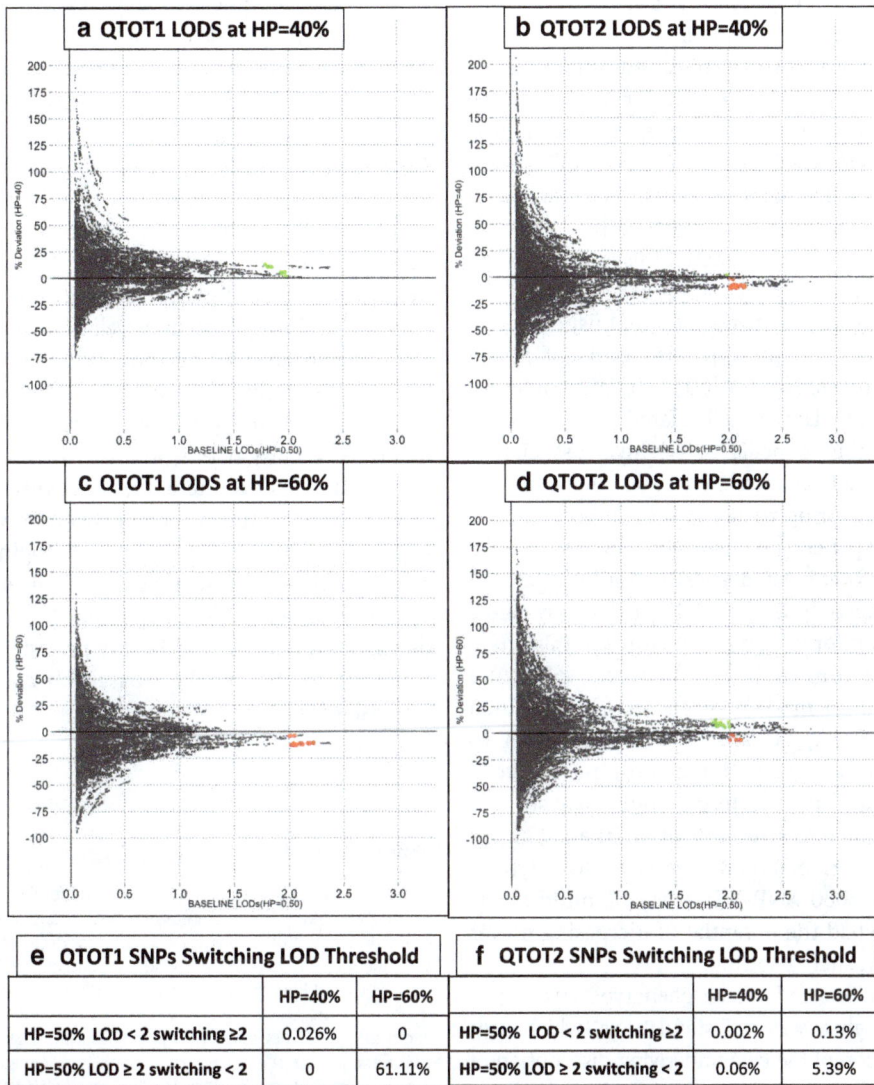

Fig. 3 Sensitivity of QT LOD score to changes in HP. Panels (**a**) and (**c**) are for **QTOT1**, and (**b**) and (**d**) are for **QTOT2**. In each scatterplot, the x-axis represents LOD scores reported in this paper, using HP = 50%. In panels (**a**) and (**b**), the y-axis represents LOD scores for HP = 40%. In panels (**c**) and (**d**), y-axis represents LOD scores calculated with HP = 60%. Panels E and F show the proportion (%) of SNPs switching from LOD ≤ 2.0 to LOD ≥ 2.0 for **QTOT1** and **QTOT2**

Table 6 Comparison of reported peaks in HP sensitivity analysis

Trait	Chr	SNP	A HP = 50%[a]	B HP = 40% [B-A]	C HP = 60% [C-A]
QTOT1	3	rs2044594	2.12	2.14 [0.02]	2.04 [−0.08]
	6	rs240642	2.38	2.62 [0.24]	2.10 [−0.28]
QTOT2	2	rs7572396	2.30	2.20 [−0.10]	2.36 [0.06]
	2	rs831535	2.10	2.16 [0.06]	2.00 [−0.10]
	5	rs6866597	2.76	2.64 [−0.12]	2.86 [0.10]
	19	rs1671133	2.15	1.95 [−0.20]	2.28 [0.13]

Note: [a]These values are the peak LOD score results reported in Table 4 for **QTOT1** and **QTOT2**

etiology. Some of the genes are known to cause syndromes with a dental or oral phenotype, while others have a role to play in human immune and host defense response, blood glucose levels, and secretory function of the salivary glands all of which may have a potential impact on incidence of dental caries (see, for example, Carneiro et al. (2015) for the relationship between diabetes and dental caries). After a comprehensive review of the literature, we also detected linkage to regions on chromosomes 11 and 19 previously reported as associated to caries.

As expected, we do not recapitulate all findings from all prior association studies published by our group although this linkage study and the previous association studies utilized data from the same sources (i.e.,

COHRA, IHS, DRDR, IFS). As mentioned previously, linkage and association are complementary strategies for gene-discovery. In linkage, similarities and differences in pairs of phenotypes are modeled in terms of genetic similarity over related pairs from families. In association, this modeling is performed at the level of individuals. Our linkage uses multi-point analysis, i.e., the LOD score at any specific location is influenced by linkage at neighboring loci. Association generally uses a set of independent one-locus tests. Finally, as described in methods, this study differs from prior published work, both in the number, and the type (in terms of family composition) of individuals included in the analysis. Linkage utilizes family data and all related pairs (affected or phenotyped) within a pedigree whereas association generally is conducted on unrelated cases and controls, or at most parent-offspring trios.

The genotyping panel was designed for association analyses, and therefore, is far denser than a linkage SNP panel. Although dense bi-allelic SNP panels may allow extraction of more information, a concern for this study was existing linkage disequilibrium between SNPs. We pruned SNPs based on marker-to-marker LD, and then exploited any remaining LD among the pruned set to create clusters which served as polymorphic markers. Despite the pruning and clustering, our analysis was conducted on a much denser set of markers (35,016 SNPs and 20,634 super-markers) compared to a typical linkage panel with 6000 SNPs. The use of multi-allelic super-markers also had the potential of increasing power of linkage studies in such a setting.

Genome-wide significance for each phenotype was empirically assessed through a series of simulations, which provides an approximation of the true underlying distribution of a statistic since not all features of the data can be completely replicated. In an exploratory study, adhering strictly to genome-wide significance thresholds may be overly conservative. Furthermore, of the 4727 subjects, only 2616 contributed to the linkage analysis, providing a comparatively small number of relative pairs given the large sample size.

The sensitivity analysis conducted for the parameter HP explores the impact of parameter value selection on a model-free QT method. The results from this analysis indicated that the non-parametric quantitative trait linkage method, as implemented in Merlin, was robust to variation in HP, and that changing the HP parameter had a minimal impact on LOD scores. Even more importantly, the linkage peaks were insensitive to parameter misspecification.

Environmental factors are not accounted for in this study due to unavailability of such data on many of our subjects, which would have drastically reduced the cohort size. We also did not attempt to analyze gene-by-gene interaction. The available methods for detection of gene-gene interaction that are applicable to our study design are computationally complex, thus making whole-genome interaction analysis beyond the scope of the current work (e.g. see the review of the various classes of interaction detection methods by Li [39]).

Conclusions

This study presents two new quantitative measures for dental caries which combine both the primary and permanent dentition, while adjusting for age effects. Genes identified in peak linkage regions underline the importance of exploring potential relationships between caries and other traits. We did not include environmental factors in this study. The interaction between putative caries risk conferring genes and factors including fluoride exposure, dietary habits, and the microbiome need to be investigated, as do interactions between the genes themselves. From a clinical perspective, individuals would be at an elevated lifetime risk of developing caries in both primary and permanent dentition, given increased genetic susceptibility. Understanding the genetic etiology of dental caries will allow health providers to design personalized treatment plans based on an individual's genetic risk of disease.

Abbreviations

bp: basepair; cM: centiMorgan; COHRA: Center for Oral Health Research in Appalachia; D_1MFT: Count of decayed, missing, and filled permanent teeth including white spot lesions; D_2MFT: Count of decayed, missing, and filled permanent teeth excluding white spot lesions; dbGaP: The database of Genotypes and Phenotypes; dft: Count of decayed and/or filled primary teeth (dft) score; DRDR: University of Pittsburgh Dental Registry and DNA Repository; GENEVA: Gene Environment Association Studies Initiative; GMI: Genetic Map Interpolator; HP: Heritability Parameter; HWE: Hardy-Weinberg Equilibrium; IBD: Identical-By-Descent; IFS: Iowa Fluoride Study; IHS: Iowa Head Start; LD: Linkage Disequilibrium; LOD: Logarithm of the odds of linkage; MARDD: Myopathy, areflexia, respiratory distress, and dysphagia; Mb: 10^6 (or 1 million) bp; NPL: Non-Parametric Linkage; PRIM: New binary dental caries phenotype based on dft; QT: Quantitative Trait; QTOT1: New age-adjusted quantitative caries phenotype based on the sum of the dft score and D_1MFT score; QTOT2: New age-adjusted quantitative caries phenotype based on the sum of the dft score and D_2MFT score; r^2: A measure of LD based on the square of the correlation coefficient between loci); SNP: Single Nucleotide Polymorphism

Acknowledgements

Many thanks are due to the study participants, and also to the dedicated research staff at all of the research sites, without whom these studies would be impossible.
Support for analyses was provided by the National Institute of Dental and Craniofacial Research (NIDCR) as a Pathway to Independence Award (R00-DE018085). Funding for genotyping was provided by NIDCR as part of the trans-NIH Genes, Environment and Health Initiative [GEI] (U01-DE018903). Genotyping was done by the Johns Hopkins University (JHU) Center for Inherited Disease Research (CIDR), with funding from the NIDCR, contract number HHSN268200782096C. Assistance with phenotype harmonization

and genotype cleaning, as well as with general study coordination, was provided by the GENEVA Coordinating Center (U01-HG004446) and by NCBI. Data and samples were provided by (1) the Center for Oral Health Research in Appalachia (a collaboration of the University of Pittsburgh and West Virginia University funded by NIDCR R01-DE 014899); (2) the Iowa Fluoride Study and the Iowa Bone Development Study, funded by NIDCR R01-DE09551and R01-DE12101, respectively); (3) the Iowa Comprehensive Program to Investigate Craniofacial and Dental Anomalies (funded by NIDCR, P60-DE-13076. The Dental Registry and DNA Repository project is supported by the University of Pittsburgh School of Dental Medicine. All analyses were conducted on the Centos 276-node cluster, Indy, also supported by the School of Dental Medicine at the University of Pittsburgh.

Funding
National Institute of Dental and Craniofacial Research (NIDCR), Award Numbers: R00-DE018085, U01-DE018903, HHSN268200782096C, R01-DE 014899, R01-DE09551, R01-DE12101, P60-DE-13076.
GENEVA Coordinating Center Award Number: U01-HG004446.
Neither NIDCR nor the GENEVA Coordinating Center played a role in the design of the study and collection, analysis, and interpretation of data and in writing the manuscript.

Authors' contributions
MG, NM, DEW, EF, MLM conceived and designed this study; NM and MG analyzed the data; MG and NM wrote the manuscript; SML, ARV, RLS, DWM, RJW, RJC, and MLM acquired the data; NM, MG, managed, cleaned and quality checked the data for linkage; MG, NM, DEW, EF, JRS, and MLM interpreted the results. All authors read and approved the final manuscript.

Competing interests
The authors declare that they have no competing interests.

Author details
[1]Center for Craniofacial and Dental Genetics, Department of Oral Biology, School of Dental Medicine, University of Pittsburgh, Suite 500 Bridgeside Point, 100 Technology Drive, Pittsburgh, PA 15219, USA. [2]Department of Human Genetics, Graduate School of Public Health, University of Pittsburgh, Pittsburgh, PA, USA. [3]Department of Biostatistics, Graduate School of Public Health, University of Pittsburgh, Pittsburgh, PA, USA. [4]Department of Preventive and Community Dentistry, University of Iowa College of Dentistry, Iowa City, IA, USA. [5]Department of Epidemiology, University of Iowa College of Public Health, Iowa City, IA, USA. [6]Department of Pediatric Dentistry, School of Dentistry, University of Washington, Seattle, WA, USA. [7]Dental Practice and Rural Health, West Virginia University School of Dentistry, Morgantown, WV, USA. [8]Department of Psychology, Eberly College of Arts and Sciences, West Virginia University, Morgantown, WV, USA. [9]Department of Dental Public Health and Information Management, School of Dental Medicine, University of Pittsburgh, Pittsburgh, PA, USA. [10]Department of Periodontics, West Virginia University School of Dentistry, Morgantown, WV, USA. [11]Clinical and Translational Science Institute, and Department of Psychiatry, School of Medicine, University of Pittsburgh, Pittsburgh, PA, USA.

References
1. Chou R, Cantor A, Zakher B, Mitchell JP, Pappas M: Prevention of Dental Caries in Children Younger Than 5 Years Old: Systematic Review to Update the U.S. Preventive Services Task Force Recommendation. Evidence Synthesis No. 104. ; 2014.
2. Boraas JC, Messer LB, Till MJ. A genetic contribution to dental caries, occlusion, and morphology as demonstrated by twins reared apart. J Dent Res. 1988;67(9):1150–5.
3. Bretz WA, Corby PM, Schork NJ, Robinson MT, Coelho M, Costa S, Melo Filho MR, Weyant RJ, Hart TC. Longitudinal analysis of heritability for dental caries traits. J Dent Res. 2005;84(11):1047–51.
4. Morrison J, Laurie CC, Marazita ML, Sanders AE, Offenbacher S, Salazar CR, Conomos MP, Thornton T, Jain D, Laurie CA, et al. Genome-wide association study of dental caries in the Hispanic communities health study/study of Latinos (HCHS/SOL). Hum Mol Genet. 2016;25(4):807–16.
5. Shaffer JR, Wang X, Desensi RS, Wendell S, Weyant RJ, Cuenco KT, Crout R, McNeil DW, Marazita ML. Genetic susceptibility to dental caries on pit and fissure and smooth surfaces. Caries Res. 2012;46(1):38–46.
6. Shaffer JR, Wang X, McNeil DW, Weyant RJ, Crout R, Marazita ML. Genetic susceptibility to dental caries differs between the sexes: a family-based study. Caries Res. 2015;49(2):133–40.
7. Wang X-J, Shaffer JR, Weyant RJ, Cuenco KT, DeSensi RH, Crout RJ, McNeil DW, Marazita ML. Genes and their effects on dental caries may differ between primary and permanent dentitions. Caries Res. 2010;44(3):277–84.
8. Vieira AR, Modesto A, Marazita ML. Caries: review of human genetics research. Caries Res. 2014;48(5):491–506.
9. Opal S, Garg S, Jain J, Walia I. Genetic factors affecting dental caries risk. Aust Dent J. 2015;60(1):2–11.
10. Vieira AR, Marazita ML, Goldstein-McHenry T. Genome-wide scan finds suggestive caries loci. J Dent Res. 2008;87(5):435–9.
11. Kruglyak L, Daly MJ, Reeve-Daly MP, Lander ES. Parametric and nonparametric linkage analysis: a unified multipoint approach. Am J Hum Genet. 1996;58(6):1347–63.
12. Polk DE, Weyant RJ, Crout RJ, McNeil DW, Tarter RE, Thomas JG, Marazita ML. Study protocol of the Center for Oral Health Research in Appalachia (COHRA) etiology study. BMC oral health. 2008;8:18.
13. Vieira AR, Hilands KM, Braun TW. Saving more teeth-a case for personalized care. J Pers Med. 2015;5(1):30–5.
14. Franzman MR, Levy SM, Warren JJ, Broffitt B: Tooth-brushing and dentifrice use among children ages 6 to 60 months. Pediatr Dent 2004, 26(1):87–92.
15. Levy SM, Warren JJ, Broffitt B, Hillis SL, Kanellis MJ. Fluoride, beverages and dental caries in the primary dentition. Caries Res. 2003;37(3):157–65.
16. Levy SM, Warren JJ, Davis CS, Kirchner HL, Kanellis MJ, Wefel JS. Patterns of fluoride intake from birth to 36 months. J Public Health Dent. 2001;61(2):70–7.
17. Marshall TA, Levy SM, Broffitt B, Warren JJ, Eichenberger-Gilmore JM, Burns TL, Stumbo PJ. Dental caries and beverage consumption in young children. Pediatrics. 2003;112(3 Pt 1):e184–91.
18. Slayton RL, Cooper ME, Marazita ML. Tuftelin, mutans streptococci, and dental caries susceptibility. J Dent Res. 2005;84(8):711–4.
19. Wang X, Shaffer JR, Zeng Z, Begum F, Vieira AR, Noel J, Anjomshoaa I, Cuenco KT, Lee MK, Beck J, et al. Genome-wide association scan of dental caries in the permanent dentition. BMC oral health. 2012;12:57.
20. Shaffer JR, Wang X, Feingold E, Lee M, Begum F, Weeks DE, Cuenco KT, Barmada MM, Wendell SK, Crosslin DR, et al. Genome-wide association scan for childhood caries implicates novel genes. J Dent Res. 2011;90(12):1457–62.
21. Genetic Map Interpolator [**https://watson.hgen.pitt.edu/register/**].
22. Matise TC, Chen F, Chen W, De La Vega FM, Hansen M, He C, Hyland FC, Kennedy GC, Kong X, Murray SS, et al. A second-generation combined linkage physical map of the human genome. Genome Res. 2007;17(12): 1783–6.
23. Purcell S, Neale B, Todd-Brown K, Thomas L, Ferreira MA, Bender D, Maller J, Sklar P, de Bakker PI, Daly MJ, et al. PLINK: a tool set for whole-genome association and population-based linkage analyses. Am J Hum Genet. 2007; 81(3):559–75.
24. Levinson DF, Holmans P. The effect of linkage disequilibrium on linkage analysis of incomplete pedigrees. BMC Genet. 2005;6(Suppl 1):S6.

25. Abecasis GR, Cherny SS, Cookson WO, Cardon LR. Merlin–rapid analysis of dense genetic maps using sparse gene flow trees. Nat Genet. 2002;30(1):97–101.
26. Whittemore AS, Halpern J. A class of tests for linkage using affected pedigree members. Biometrics. 1994;50(1):118–27.
27. Sham PC, Purcell S, Cherny SS, Abecasis GR. Powerful regression-based quantitative-trait linkage analysis of general pedigrees. Am J Hum Genet. 2002;71(2):238–53.
28. Nyholt DR. All LODs are not created equal. Am J Hum Genet. 2000;67(2): 282–8.
29. Wigginton JE, Abecasis GR. An evaluation of the replicate pool method: quick estimation of genome-wide linkage peak p-values. Genet Epidemiol. 2006;30(4):320–32.
30. UCSC Genome Browser [**http://genome.ucsc.edu**].
31. Baron RV, Kollar C, Mukhopadhyay N, Weeks DE. Mega2: validated data-reformatting for linkage and association analyses. Source Code Biol Med. 2014;9(1):26.
32. Jing X, Li DQ, Olofsson CS, Salehi A, Surve VV, Caballero J, Ivarsson R, Lundquist I, Pereverzev A, Schneider T, et al. CaV2.3 calcium channels control second-phase insulin release. J Clin Invest. 2005;115(1):146–54.
33. Bircher AJ, Lang-Muritano M, Pfaltz M, Bruckner-Tuderman L. Epidermolysis bullosa junctionalis progressiva in three siblings. Br J Dermatol. 1993;128(4): 429–35.
34. Ozgul RK, Satman I, Collin GB, Hinman EG, Marshall JD, Kocaman O, Tutuncu Y, Yilmaz T, Naggert JK. Molecular analysis and long-term clinical evaluation of three siblings with Alstrom syndrome. Clin Genet. 2007;72(4):351–6.
35. Carter MT, Geraghty MT, De La Cruz L, Reichard RR, Boccuto L, Schwartz CE, Clericuzio CL. A new syndrome with multiple capillary malformations, intractable seizures, and brain and limb anomalies. Am J Med Genet A. 2011;155a(2):301–6.
36. Hartley L, Kinali M, Knight R, Mercuri E, Hubner C, Bertini E, Manzur AY, Jimenez-Mallebrera C, Sewry CA, Muntoni F. A congenital myopathy with diaphragmatic weakness not linked to the SMARD1 locus. Neuromuscul Disord. 2007;17(2):174–9.
37. Hoyer J, Ekici AB, Endele S, Popp B, Zweier C, Wiesener A, Wohlleber E, Dufke A, Rossier E, Petsch C, et al. Haploinsufficiency of ARID1B, a member of the SWI/SNF-a chromatin-remodeling complex, is a frequent cause of intellectual disability. Am J Hum Genet. 2012;90(3):565–72.
38. Wang Q, Jia P, Cuenco KT, Zeng Z, Feingold E, Marazita ML, Wang L, Zhao Z. Association signals unveiled by a comprehensive gene set enrichment analysis of dental caries genome-wide association studies. PLoS One. 2013; 8(8):e72653.
39. Li C: Detecting gene-gene interaction in linkage analysis. Current protocols in human genetics 2005, Chapter 1:Unit 1.15.

5

Deciduous dental caries status and associated risk factors among preschool children

Hongru Su[1†], Renren Yang[2†], Qinglong Deng[2], Wenhao Qian[1*] and Jinming Yu[2*]

Abstract

Background: This study aims to understand the deciduous dental caries status of preschool children in Xuhui District of Shanghai, China and to analyze the associated risk factors.

Methods: In January of 2016, a cross-sectional investigation was conducted to examine the oral health of all the kindergarten children in Xuihui District of Shanghai, China. Meanwhile, a field questionnaire survey was conducted with the children's guardians to ascertain the potential risk factors associated with deciduous dental caries.

Results: Among 11,153 children, the prevalence of deciduous dental caries was 47.02%, and the mean dmft score was 2.21. The first three predilection sites were maxillary central primary incisors, mandible second primary molars, and mandible first primary molars. There were statistically significant differences in caries prevalence and dmft among different age groups and different household registration (Hukou) types ($P < 0.001$). Multivariate Logistic regression suggested that the possible risk factors for deciduous caries included: older age, drinking sweetened beverages frequently, often or usually eating sweets before sleep compared to rarely/never eat them at this time, exclusive or predominant breastfeeding compared to exclusive or predominant artificial feeding and latter introduction of toothbrushing. On the other hand, Shanghai Hukou families, high educational level of guardians (high school or college education), regular parental support for children's toothbrushing, guardians' oral health knowledge, and a good perception about children's oral health conditions were shown as potential protective factors for deciduous dental caries.

Conclusions: The deciduous dental caries status of preschool children in Xuhui District of Shanghai was still serious. The caries prevalence in Xuhui, China, is associated with children's age, household registration type, oral health habits, feeding habits, guardians' education level, parental perception about children's oral health and knowledge about oral health.

Keywords: Deciduous dental caries, Preschool children, Risk factors, Logistic models

* Correspondence: pingyanlaoto@163.com; jmy@fudan.edu.cn
†Hongru Su and Renren Yang contributed equally to this work.
[1]Xuhui District Dental Centre, Shanghai, China
[2]Collaborative Innovation Centre of Social Risks Governance in Health, School of Public Health, Fudan University, Shanghai, China

Background

Early childhood caries (ECC) is defined as the presence of one or more decayed, missing, or filled surfaces in any primary tooth in children younger than 6 years of age [1]. It is a serious public health problem that adversely affects children's physical and mental health, since dental decay can cause pain, reduced growth and development, speech disorders, and premature tooth loss that lead to chewing problems, loss of self-confidence, and harm to the permanent dentition [2]. The World Health Organization (WHO) lists dental caries as the third most common chronic, non-infectious disease after cancer and cardiovascular disease [3].

In recent years, the material living standard in China has increased a lot; however, oral health services have not improved accordingly, and many people lack oral health knowledge, resulting in a high prevalence of dental caries in China, especially among children. According to the 3rd National Oral Health Survey [4], the caries prevalence among 5-year-old children in 30 provinces of China was 66.0%. The prevalence among urban and rural children was 62 and 70.2%, respectively. The average caries was 3.50. This was an improvement over the results of the 2nd National Oral Health Survey, which was conducted in 1995 (caries prevalence: 76.6%, average caries: 4.5). However, there still exists a large gap between the current status and the WHO's goal-a 90% caries free population of 5-year-old children by 2010.

When compared to some developed countries, the caries prevalence among Chinese children was also at a very high level. For instance, the American National Health and Nutrition Examination Survey (NHANES 1999–2004) showed that the caries prevalence among 5-year-old children in America was 28% [5]. An oral health survey in England in 2003 revealed that the caries prevalence among British children was 43% [6]. In 2009, a study suggested that the caries prevalence was 37% among 4–5 years old children in Singapore [7]. From these results, we can conclude that greater prevention efforts targeting childhood caries are urgently needed in China, especially among preschool children. Since deciduous teeth are the major mastication organs of preschool children; if these teeth are carious, masticatory function is negatively affected, which not only blocks the intake of nutrients but also harms the growth of permanent teeth and even damages the oral mucosa. Hence, deciduous caries has a negative impact on children's growth and development.

Xuhui District is in the southwest of central Shanghai, China, which covers a majority of high-income residents. Meanwhile, there are also quite a number of migrant workers from other cities. Even though there have already been several studies regarding dental caries status of the Chinese population, a large sample survey, especially on preschool children in the area like Xuhui District, is still lacking. In this setting, the present study, which covered a large sample of preschool children, aims to understand the epidemiology of deciduous caries through a cross-sectional investigation of kindergarten children in Xuhui District of Shanghai. We hope the findings will be useful for future intervention.

Methods

Research design and participants

This present study was carried out together with the "Teeth Fluoridization Program for Children" which covered every kindergartener in Xuhui District and it also served as the baseline investigation of this program. This cross-sectional investigation was conducted in Xuhui District of Shanghai in January 2016. According to a survey in Xuhui District in 2009, the deciduous caries prevalence among 883 kindergarteners was 54.9% [8]. With the admissible error set at 10% of the prevalence, the significance level set at 0.05, and the design effect set at 3.0, the calculated sample size was 947. In view of no response and invalid questionnaires, we expanded the sample size by 10%. As a result, the required minimum sample size turned out to be 1042.

We selected all the community kindergartens in Xuhui District of Shanghai, China via cluster sampling. Every child studying at these kindergartens was included in this study. Those who were younger than 3-year-old or older than 6-year-old were excluded. In addition, the children's guardians (parents and grandparents) were also included for a questionnaire investigation. The study protocol was approved by the Ethics Committee of Xuhui District Dental Centre.

Oral health questionnaire

The distribution and collection of these questionnaires was conducted by teachers in each kindergarten who received unified training before the field investigation began. The parents or guardians were asked to complete the questionnaire on the spot the same day before the clinical examination of their children in January 2016. The questionnaire used in this study (refer to the Additional file 1) which was derived from the 4th National Oral Health Survey in China included the following aspects: the education level of guardians, feeding patterns, the daily eating habits and oral health habits of the children, parental perception about child's oral health, and guardians' oral health knowledge. Written informed consent was obtained from all guardians who agreed to participate in the study.

Clinical examination

The dental examinations were conducted in the community kindergartens by trained dentists using a 0.5 mm ball-ended CPI probe and a disposable dental mirror.

The results were recorded by another investigator. Dental caries assessments were based on the criteria recommended by the WHO [9], and the dmft index was used to record the caries experiences of the primary dentition. All the examination results were recorded on a caries specified checklist (refer to the Additional file 2) along with the child's gender, birthdate and household registration. This study involved 14 examiners and all the examiners were experienced dentists who received uniform specialized training before the beginning of the study. Meanwhile, to estimate the intra-examiner agreement on the assessment of caries status, we conducted a pilot survey after the training. The Kappa value was 0.89, which suggested high internal consistency in the dental examination.

Statistical analysis

Data were entered with Epidata 3.1, analyzed with R 3.4.1, and plotted with GraphPad Prism 6.01. The significance level was set at 0.05. The multiple imputation with MICE [10] in R was conducted for missing data. Observations that contained more than 15% missing values were directly removed from the original data. Statistical description was performed to calculate the prevalence of deciduous caries and the mean dmft score. For enumeration data, the Pearson Chi-square test (nominal data) and the Cochran-Armitage test for trend (ordinal data) were adopted. For continuous data, the following test methods were used, each for a specific situation: t test (two groups), Mann-Whitney test (two groups; and the data did not meet the requirements of parametric test), one-way ANOVA (more than two groups), and Kruskal-Wallis test (more than two groups; and the data did not meet the requirements of parametric test). A binary non-conditional Logistic model was applied to conduct multivariate regression analysis. The dependent variable was dental caries status (1 = carious, 0 = caries free). The independent variables were all the factors surveyed in this study. Some variables were recoded: the education level of guardians was recoded into 3 categories (below high school, high school, college and above), the feeding patterns was recoded into 3 categories (exclusive or predominant artificial feeding, exclusive or predominant breastfeeding, combination); age, the frequency of eating desserts and candies, the frequency of drinking sweetened beverages, the age of starting toothbrushing, parental perception about children's oral health and score of guardians' oral health knowledge were included in the model as continuous variables according to questionnaire. Based on the Logistic model, prevalence ratio was estimated using conditional method which was proposed by Wilcosky & Chambless [11].

Results

General conditions

Eleven thousand three hundred thirty-five caries checklists and 10,211 questionnaires were obtained during the present investigation. After removing invalid checklists, 11,153 remained; the validity rate was 98.39%. Then, we merged the caries checklists with the questionnaires by ID, removing the invalid ones. There were 9804 remaining after this step.

Among 11,153 children, 5972 (53.55%) were boys and 5181 (46.45%) were girls. The age ranged from 3 to 6 years old and the average was (4.87 ± 0.89) years old. Among these children, 10,700 (95.94%) held a Shanghai Hukou, while 453 (4.06%) did not. In total, 91.82% of the children had biological parents as guardians. As for the guardians, 5.86% reported below high school education levels, 12.00% reported high school education levels and 82.14% reported college and above education levels.

Deciduous dental caries status

The prevalence of deciduous dental caries was 47.02%. The mean dmft score of the total population was 2.21 and of patients was 4.70. The predilection sites of caries were, in order, maxillary primary central incisors (5684), mandible second primary molars (4566), mandible first primary molars (4383), maxillary second primary molars (2977), maxillary first primary molars (2550), maxillary primary lateral incisors (2342), maxillary primary canines (975), mandible primary canines (470), mandible primary central incisors (324), and mandible primary lateral incisors (271). The deciduous caries status among different age groups, genders and household registration types was shown in Table 1. From the results, we can find that there were significant differences in caries prevalence and dmft between different age groups and different household registration types ($P < 0.001$). However, there were no significant differences in caries prevalence and dmft between genders ($P = 0.702$; $P = 0.574$). The frequency distribution of dmft was as shown in Fig. 1 (the bar for "dmft = 0" was removed). Children with 2 decayed teeth were the most frequent (11.08%), followed by those with 1 decayed tooth (7.04%) and 4 decayed teeth (5.87%).

Deciduous caries prevalence of the surveyed children categorized by different factors of the questionnaire was as shown in Table 2. Except for guardians ($P = 0.076$) and the frequency of toothbrushing ($P = 0.063$), every other factor revealed a significant difference in caries prevalence.

Table 1 Deciduous caries status of different age groups, genders and household registration types (n = 11,153)

Variables	Categories	Caries prevalence			dmft	
		No. of surveyed (No. of cases with dental caries)	Caries prevalence (%)	P-value (statistics[1])	Mean ± SD	P-value (statistics[2])
Age (years old)	3	531 (156)	29.38	< 0.001** (−15.992[a])	1.09 ± 2.45	< 0.001** (304.022[b])
	4	3626 (1141)	38.91		1.68 ± 3.08	
	5	3798 (1908)	50.24		2.45 ± 3.57	
	6	3198 (1769)	55.31		2.71 ± 3.69	
Gender	Boys	5972 (2818)	47.19	0.702 (0.146)	2.23 ± 3.43	0.574 (0.562[c])
	Girls	5181 (2426)	46.82		2.19 ± 3.45	
Household registration	Shanghai	10,700 (4959)	46.35	< 0.001** (47.890)	2.14 ± 3.38	< 0.001** (−8.806[d])
	Non-Shanghai	453 (285)	62.91		3.76 ± 4.43	
Total	–	11,153 (5244)	47.02	–	2.21 ± 3.44	–

**P < 0.01. SD = standard deviation
[1]a: Cochran-Armitage test for trend (the statistics is Z-value); the others were Pearson Chi-square test (the statistics is χ^2-value)
[2]b: Kruskal-Wallis test (the statistics is χ^2-value); c: t test (the statistics is t-value); d: Mann-Whitney test (the statistics is Z-value)

Univariate analysis of risk factors associated with deciduous caries prevalence

Univariate analysis indicated that the possible risk factors of deciduous caries included: older age, non-Shanghai Hukou, low education level of guardians, unhealthy eating habits, latter introduction of toothbrushing, a bad perception about children's oral health conditions and low scores of guardians' oral health knowledge. The cPRs and 95% CIs of these factors were listed in Table 3.

Multivariate Logistic regression analysis of risk factors associated with deciduous caries prevalence

Higher prevalence of dental caries had been associated with older age, non-Shanghai Hukou, low education level of guardians, rare or inexistent parental support for children toothbrushing, a bad perception of children's oral health, low scores of guardians' oral health knowledge and unhealthy eating habits, as frequent ingestion of sweetened beverages or regular consumption of sweets at night or before sleeping. Meanwhile, children who started toothbrushing at earlier age and brushed their teeth more than once daily were with less caries experience. In addition, children who were exclusively or predominantly formula-fed had significantly lower caries prevalence than those exclusively or predominantly breastfed. The aPRs and 95% CIs of these factors were listed in Table 4.

Discussion

This cross-sectional study described deciduous dental caries status quo and tried to assess factors affecting on

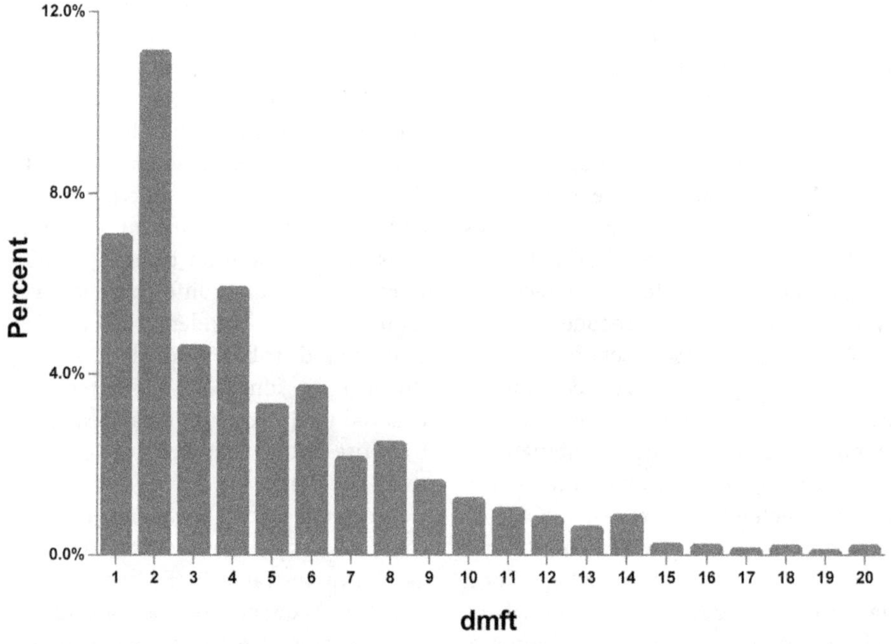

Fig. 1 The frequency distribution of dmft

Table 2 Deciduous caries prevalence of the surveyed children categorized by different factors of the questionnaire ($n = 9804$)

Variables	Categories	No. of surveyed (No. of cases with dental caries)	Caries prevalence (%)	*P*-value (statistics[1])
Guardians	Parents	9002 (4196)	46.61	0.076 (3.149[a])
	Grandparents	802 (400)	49.88	
Education level of guardians	Illiteracy	26 (19)	73.08	< 0.001** (13.436)
	Primary school	52 (36)	69.23	
	Middle school	497 (310)	62.37	
	High school	704 (403)	57.24	
	Technical secondary school	472 (270)	57.20	
	Junior college	2065 (1033)	50.02	
	Undergraduate	4532 (1958)	43.20	
	Graduate and above	1456 (567)	38.94	
Feeding patterns	Exclusive breastfeeding	3162 (1570)	49.65	< 0.001** (20.015[a])
	Predominant breastfeeding	2057 (934)	45.41	
	Exclusive artificial feeding	1133 (550)	48.54	
	Predominant artificial feeding	919 (402)	43.74	
	Combination feeding	2533 (1140)	45.01	
Eating desserts and candies (times per week)	< 1	503 (216)	42.94	< 0.001** (−4.432)
	1–2	908 (401)	44.16	
	3–4	1272 (595)	46.78	
	5–6	3217 (1427)	44.36	
	7–8	2824 (1403)	49.68	
	> 8	1080 (554)	51.30	
Drinking sweetened beverages (times per week)	< 1	3544 (1465)	41.34	< 0.001** (−8.810)
	1–2	2548 (1219)	47.84	
	3–4	1806 (890)	49.28	
	5–6	1259 (672)	53.38	
	7–8	506 (265)	52.37	
	> 8	141 (85)	60.28	
Eating sweets before sleep (days per week)	Rarely/never (< 1)	4079 (1563)	38.32	< 0.001** (13.962)
	Sometimes (1–3)	5132 (2696)	52.53	
	Often (> = 4)	593 (337)	56.83	
The age of starting tooth-brushing (years old)	< 1	540 (183)	33.89	< 0.001** (−8.635)
	1	1424 (598)	41.99	
	2	3304 (1503)	45.49	
	3	2915 (1483)	50.87	
	> = 4	1621 (829)	51.14	
Toothbrush (times per day)	< 1	5096 (2414)	47.37	0.063 (1.860)
	1	3562 (1683)	47.25	
	> = 2	1146 (499)	43.54	
Helping children brush teeth (days per week)	Rarely/never (< 1)	1984 (984)	49.60	0.001** (−3.332)
	Sometimes (1–3)	4480 (2115)	47.21	
	Often (4–6)	276 (124)	44.93	
	Everyday (7)	3064 (1373)	44.81	
Parental perception about children's oral health (score)	Poor (1–2)	800 (701)	87.63	< 0.001** (36.423)

Table 2 Deciduous caries prevalence of the surveyed children categorized by different factors of the questionnaire ($n = 9804$) *(Continued)*

Variables	Categories	No. of surveyed (No. of cases with dental caries)	Caries prevalence (%)	*P*-value (statistics[1])
	Fair (3)	2759 (1794)	65.02	
	Good (4–5)	6245 (2101)	33.64	
Score of guardians' oral health knowledge	0–4	385 (182)	47.27	< 0.001** (3.516)
	5–9	1506 (791)	52.52	
	10–14	7913 (3623)	45.79	
Total	–	9804 (4596)	46.88	–

**$P < 0.01$

[1]a: Pearson Chi-square test (the statistics is χ^2-value); the others were Cochran-Armitage test for trend (the statistics is Z-value)

Table 3 Univariate analysis of risk factors associated with deciduous caries prevalence (n = 9804)

Variables	Categories	β	Z-value	*P*-value	cPR	cPR 95% CI
Age	–	0.371	−15.710	< 0.001**	1.370	1.305–1.439
Gender	Boys					
	Girls	−0.033	− 0.817	0.414	0.983	0.942–1.025
Household registration	Non-Shanghai					
	Shanghai	−0.716	−6.766	< 0.001**	0.722	0.668–0.780
Guardians	Parents					
	Grandparents	0.131	1.774	0.076	1.070	0.995–1.151
Education level of guardians	Below high school	Ref	Ref	Ref		
	High school	−0.262	−2.497	0.013*	0.865	0.768–0.974
	College and above	−0.787	−8.791	< 0.001**	0.692	0.644–0.743
Feeding patterns	exclusive or predominant artificial feeding	Ref	Ref	Ref		
	exclusive or predominant breastfeeding	0.064	1.218	0.223	1.034	0.980–1.092
	Combination feeding	−0.056	− 0.938	0.348	0.971	0.911–1.033
Frequency of eating desserts and candies	–	0.069	4.427	< 0.001**	1.042	1.021–1.063
Frequency of drinking sweetened beverages	–	0.138	8.778	< 0.001**	1.085	1.064–1.108
Eating sweets before sleep (days per week)	Rarely/never (< 1)	Ref	Ref	Ref		
	Sometimes (1–3)	0.577	13.541	< 0.001**	1.362	1.302–1.426
	Often (> = 4)	0.751	8.443	< 0.001**	1.402	1.314–1.497
The age of starting tooth-brushing	–	0.162	8.607	< 0.001**	1.110	1.079–1.141
Toothbrush (times per day)	< 1	Ref	Ref	Ref		
	1	−0.005	−0.112	0.911	0.997	0.953–1.044
	> = 2	− 0.154	−2.346	0.019	0.919	0.855–0.988
Helping children brush teeth (days per week)	Rarely/never (< 1)	Ref	Ref	Ref		
	Sometimes (1–3)	−0.096	−1.772	0.076	0.950	0.898–1.006
	Often (4–6)	−0.187	− 1.452	0.146	0.901	0.779–1.043
	Everyday (7)	−0.192	−3.328	0.001	0.901	0.847–0.959
Parental perception about children's oral health	–	−0.957	−33.800	< 0.001**	0.952	0.947–0.958
Score of guardians' oral health knowledge	–	−0.030	−4.186	< 0.001**	0.987	0.981–0.992

cPR crude Prevalence Ratio, *CI* Confidence Interval, *Ref* Reference group
* $P < 0.05$; ** $P < 0.01$

Table 4 Association between caries and independent variables in Xuhui, China ($n = 9804$)

Variables	Categories	β	Z-value	*P*-value	aPR	aPR 95% CI
Age	–	0.351	12.875	< 0.001**	1.342	1.269–1.419
Gender	Boys					
	Girls	−0.015	− 0.331	0.741	0.992	0.946–1.040
Household registration	Non-Shanghai					
	Shanghai	−0.347	−2.811	0.005**	0.843	0.756–0.941
Guardians	Parents					
	Grandparents	0.051	0.589	0.556	1.027	0.940–1.122
Education level of guardians	Below high school	Ref	Ref	Ref	Ref	
	High school	−0.219	−1.884	0.060	0.886	0.777–1.010
	College and above	−0.624	−5.900	< 0.001**	0.740	0.677–0.810
Feeding patterns	exclusive or predominant artificial feeding	Ref	Ref	Ref	Ref	
	exclusive or predominant breastfeeding	0.147	2.519	0.012*	1.081	1.017–1.150
	Combination feeding	0.001	0.019	0.985	1.001	0.934–1.072
Frequency of eating desserts and candies	–	0.004	0.200	0.842	1.002	0.982–1.022
Frequency of drinking sweetened beverages	–	0.062	3.289	0.001**	1.035	1.013–1.058
Eating sweets before sleep (days per week)	Rarely/never (< 1)	Ref	Ref	Ref	Ref	
	Sometimes (1–3)	0.367	7.502	< 0.001**	1.216	1.155–1.281
	Often (> = 4)	0.553	5.469	< 0.001**	1.298	1.196–1.409
The age of starting tooth-brushing	–	0.124	5.010	< 0.001**	1.079	1.043–1.117
Toothbrush (times per day)	< 1	Ref	Ref	Ref	Ref	
	1	−0.100	−1.979	0.048*	0.948	0.899–1.000
	> = 2	−0.516	−5.527	< 0.001**	0.741	0.661–0.831
Helping children brush teeth (days per week)	Rarely/never (< 1)	Ref	Ref	Ref	Ref	
	Sometimes (1–3)	−0.188	−2.732	0.007**	0.905	0.841–0.972
	Often (4–6)	−0.134	−0.910	0.362	0.929	0.790–1.093
	Everyday (7)	−0.031	−0.411	0.681	0.983	0.907–1.066
Parental perception about children's oral health	–	−0.939	−32.053	< 0.001**	0.951	0.945–0.956
Score of guardians' oral health knowledge	–	−0.017	−2.007	0.045*	0.992	0.985–0.999
Constant	–	2.045	7.140	< 0.001**	–	–

The *P* value of goodness of fit test was 0.062
aPR adjusted prevalence ratio, *CI* confidence interval, *Ref* reference group
*$P < 0.05$; **$P < 0.01$

preschool children's oral health in Xuhui District. In spite of recent improvement in awareness of oral health among public, dental caries remains a significant problem especially in developing countries. In this study, we discovered that 47.02% of involved preschool children had caries experience. This finding was similar to that of other developing countries such as India (53%) [12] and South Africa (49%) [13]. Caries prevalence found in this investigation was lower than those of an oral health survey conducted in Xuhui District in 2009 (54.9%) [8] as well as a survey among 5-year-olds in Shanghai (66.42%) [14]. Furthermore, this prevalence was below the national average and the average of Shanghai.

Although we can conclude that there was a decrease in caries prevalence among preschool children in Xuhui District from these comparisons, it still had a very high prevalence of dental caries compared with the developed countries mentioned above, which suggested that deciduous dental caries was a serious oral health threat for preschool children. Since dental caries may not be eliminated but can be prevented, the result will be fruitful when appropriate prevention programs are implemented. Accordingly, a coordinated effort among health care providers, policy makers, and health institutions is desperately in need to minimize the prevalence of the disease.

It has been identified previously that socioeconomic status, education level of guardians and oral hygiene and eating habits of children were associated with dental caries [15–17]. This was in agreement with the current study. In our study, a strong association between age and dental caries was found. It was observed the caries severity gradually increased with age in primary dentition, which was consistent with many previous studies [17–19]. This is because caries is a cumulative process. This indicates that health promotion for the caries of dental prevention should begin in the first year of life among children in case the decayed teeth become too advanced to prevent.

Although American Academy of Pediatric Dentistry recommended that toothbrushing should be performed for children twice daily and started as soon as the first primary tooth erupted [1], only 48.02% of those in our study had brushed their teeth once a day or more and most of them had started tooth brushing at 2 years old or older. The children's dental behaviors have a significant influence on their oral health related quality of life and are important predictors of dental caries. Therefore, on basis of our findings, parents or guardians should be aware of consequences that not toothbrushing could result in children's oral health and should help children with toothbrushing since early years.

Our study showed that children who held a Shanghai Hukou had a lower caries prevalence and mean dmft score compared to those who did not (46.35%, 2.14 vs 62.91%, 3.76; $P < 0.001$). This significant difference can be explained by the fact that the parents of children without Shanghai Hukou are mainly migrant workers who come from other relatively underdeveloped cities. Migrant children had less access to services about health and education compared to children with local urban Hukou in Shanghai. For example, these children could only temporarily enrol in public schools as transient students and were not entitled to oral-related public health services funded by the tax revenue such as dental caries filling [20]. These findings were in accordance with a number of earlier studies [20–22] which reported the migrant children had higher prevalence of caries and dmft scores.

In recent years, the number of migrant workers in Shanghai has increased year by year [23]. Generally speaking, the socioeconomic status of this population is low. Having settled down in cities, the migrant children might have more delicious foods, more choice for sweet snacks than before they lived in rural areas, so they had higher risk of dental caries [24, 25]. In addition, according to Liu Chengjun et al.'s [20] survey, some bad oral health-related habits of migrant children such as most of children brushing their teeth less than twice daily and had sweet snacks before sleep without toothbrushing could also contribute to higher prevalence of decayed teeth. Thus, it is necessary for local communities to take targeted prevention measures to promote oral health of migrant population in order to improve the child's caries status.

This study also attempted to assess the influence of feeding habits on dental caries. It was concluded that there was a significant difference in caries prevalence between different feeding patterns ($P < 0.001$) and the prevalence was highest in the group of exclusive breastfeeding. This was the most controversial finding of this study. As for feeding patterns, a recent longitudinal survey [26] in Japan found that infants who had been breastfed for 6–7 months, both exclusively and partially, were at higher risk of dental caries at 30 months than those who had been exclusively formula-fed. Moreover, a cross-sectional investigation [27] about association between early life factors and dental caries in 5-year-old children involving 31 provinces of Mainland China had similar results. They found that exclusively and predominantly formula-fed children had lower caries experience than exclusively breastfed children. However, several reviews [28–30], contrary to our studies, showed strong evidence that breastfeeding was beneficial for the prevention of dental caries.

The results obtained in the present study may be caused by the fact that the involved children had a prolonged breastfeeding. A study [31] in Brazil by Peres, K.G. et al. revealed that prolonged breastfeeding (when children were breastfed for≥24 months) increased the risk of having dental caries. According to this study [31], the mechanism underlying this process may link to following risk factors such as frequent nocturnal breastfeeding, genes and environmental components modifying the susceptibility to caries in children, cariogenic potential component of human milk. Apart from that, like in most low- and middle-income countries, artificial feeding in China is mostly available to richer families in view of the cost of infant formula, and as such, it may represent a very strong indicator of family socioeconomic position. Adjusting for indicators of household income which were not surveyed in the present study would shed some light on this association and more studies should be conducted in the future. Due to these limitations, further study about association between breastfeeding and deciduous dental caries should be carried out. Meanwhile, other preventive measures should be implemented.

Dental caries is a preventable disease, there are many measures that could be taken to reduce the prevalence of deciduous caries. Oral health knowledge should be disseminated to every family, especially those of migrant workers or those with low education levels. Families and nursery institutions should help children develop good oral hygiene and eating habits. Early intervention programs for preschool children's oral health behavior should be developed based on the risk factors identified in this study. Most importantly, policy makers should work hand in hand to improve the quality and accessibility of oral health services.

Several limitations could be found in this present study. Firstly, the surveyed population was comprised of the kindergarten students in Xuhui District of Shanghai; therefore, those who did not attend kindergartens (although this population was very small) were not included. Secondly, some potential factors that contributed to dental caries, such as dentist visit [32] and the use of fluoride toothpastes, were not included in this study. We did not survey the use of fluoride toothpaste because many parents expressed uncertainty about toothpaste types when we conducted the pilot investigation. Thirdly, there was an unavoidable self-reporting bias since the children's guardians completed the self-administered questionnaires. Finally, the present study was a cross-sectional investigation, so causal inference was limited.

Conclusions

This study found that deciduous caries among preschool children in Xuhui District of Shanghai was still a severe problem. Enhancement of preventive measure at early age should be emphasized by guardian and dental health professionals. Furthermore, the caries prevalence in Xuhui, China, is associated with children's age, household registration type, oral health habits, feeding habits, guardians' education level, parental perception about children's oral health and knowledge about oral health.

Abbreviations

aPR: Adjusted prevalence ratio; CI: Confidence interval; CPP-ACP: Casein phosphopeptide-amorphous calcium phosphate; cPR: Crude prevalence ratio; SD: Standard deviation; WHO: World Health Organization

Acknowledgements

We would like first to thank the children and their guardians for the participation in this study. We also appreciated the support of the participating teachers, leaders, and other staff from the community kindergartens. Last but not least, we would like to thank all the dentists and investigators who contributed to this study.

Authors' contributions

WQ and JY designed this study. HS conducted the survey and data collection. RY and QD performed data analysis. HS and RY wrote this manuscript. All the authors read, revised and approved the final manuscript.

Competing interests

The authors declare that they have no competing interests.

References

1. Dentistry AAOP, Pediatrics AAO. Policy on Early Childhood Caries (ECC): classifications, consequences, and preventive strategies. Pediatric Dentistry. 2011;30(7 Suppl):31–3.
2. Kagihara LE, Niederhauser VP, Stark M. Assessment, management, and prevention of early childhood caries. J Am Acad Nurse Pract. 2009;21(1):1.
3. Petersen PE, Bourgeois D, Ogawa H, Estupinan-Day S, Ndiaye C. The global burden of oral diseases and risks to oral health. Bull World Health Organ. 2005;83(9):661–9.
4. Qi XQ. Report of the third national oral health survey. Beijing: People's Medical Publishing House; 2008.
5. Dye BA, Tan S, Smith V, Lewis BG, Barker LK, Thornton-Evans G, Eke PI, Beltran-Aguilar ED, Horowitz AM, Li CH. Trends in oral health status: United States, 1988-1994 and 1999-2004. Vital Health Stat. 2007;11(248):1–92.
6. Office for National Statistics. Decline in obvious decay in children's permanent teeth: Children's Dental Health Survey 2003 preliminary findings. London: Office for National Statistics; 2003.
7. Gao XL, Hsu CY, Loh T, Koh D, Hwamg HB, Xu Y. Dental caries prevalence and distribution among preschoolers in Singapore. Community Dent Health. 2009;26(1):12–7.
8. Zhao YJ, Wang KL. The observation of Children's oral health in the kindergartens of Xuhui District. Chin Prim Health Care. 2009;02:40–2.
9. WHO. Oral Health Surveys – Basic Methods. 4th version. Geneva: WHO; 1997.
10. Buuren S, Groothuis Oudshoorn K. Mice : multivariate imputation by chained equations in R. J Stat Softw. 2015;45(3):1–67.
11. Wilcosky TC, Chambless LE. A comparison of direct adjustment and regression adjustment of epidemiologic measures. J Chronic Dis. 1985;38(10):849.
12. Prakasha SS, Vinit GB, Giri KY, Alam S. Feeding practices and early childhood caries: a cross-sectional study of preschool children in Kanpur District, India. ISRN Dentistry. 2015;2013:275193.
13. Thekiso M, Yengopal V, Rudolph MJ, Bhayat A. Caries status among children in the west Rand District of Gauteng Province, South Africa. SADJ. 2012;67(7):318–20.
14. Feng JQ, Shen QP, Mi JG. Analysis of deciduous dental caries and high risk factors for 5-year-olds in shanghai. Stomatology. 2009;12:652–5.
15. Almeedani LA, Aldlaigan YH. Prevalence of dental caries and associated social risk factors among preschool children in Riyadh, Saudi Arabia. Pak J Med Sci. 2016;32(2):452.
16. Harris R, Nicoll AD, Adair PM, Pine CM. Risk factors for dental caries in young children: a systematic review of the literature. Community Dent Health. 2004;21(1 Suppl):71–85.
17. Mitali J, Ritu N, Meenakshi B, Samir D, Parul S, Arun K. Social and behavioral determinants for early childhood caries among preschool children in India. J Dent Res Dent Clin Dent Prospects. 2015;9(2):115–20.
18. Naidu R, Nunn J, Donnellyswift E. Oral health-related quality of life and early childhood caries among preschool children in Trinidad. BMC Oral Health. 2016;16(1):128.
19. Retnakumari N, Cyriac G. Childhood caries as influenced by maternal and child characteristics in pre-school children of Kerala-an epidemiological study. Contemp Clin Dent. 2012;3(1):2–8.
20. C-j L, Zhou W, X-s F. Dental caries status of students from migrant primary schools in Shanghai Pudong New Area. BMC Oral Health. 2016;16(1):28.
21. Cvikl B, Haubenberger-Praml G, Drabo P, Hagmann M, Gruber R, Moritz A, Nell A. Migration background is associated with caries in Viennese school children, even if parents have received a higher education. Bmc Oral Health. 2014;14(1):51.
22. Kühnisch J, Senkel H, Heinrichweltzien R. Comparative study on the dental health of German and immigrant 8- to 10-years olds in the Westphalian Ennepe-Ruhr district. Gesundheitswesen. 2003;65(2):96–101.
23. Xu W. Risk Factors for Dental Caries in 3-year-old and 6-year-old Children in Shanghai with the Preventive Strategies Research. Shanghai: Fudan University; 2012.
24. Huew R, Waterhouse P, Moynihan P, Kometa S, Maguire A. Dental caries and its association with diet and dental erosion in Libyan schoolchildren. Int J Paediatr Dent. 2012;22(1):68–76.
25. Li Y, Zhang Y, Yang R, Zhang Q, Zou J, Kang D. Associations of social and behavioural factors with early childhood caries in Xiamen city in China. Int J Paediatr Dent. 2011;21(2):103–11.

26. Kato T, Yorifuji T, Yamakawa M, Inoue S, Saito K, Doi H, Kawachi I. Association of breast feeding with early childhood dental caries: Japanese population-based study. BMJ Open. 2015;5(3):e006982.
27. Sun X, Bernabé E, Liu X, Gallagher JE, Zheng S. Early life factors and dental caries in 5-year-old children in China. J Dent. 2017;64:73.
28. Ge XJ, Zhang BS, Li B, Zhao LJ, Zhao B, Ren XY, Sun KQ. The effects of feeding methods on deciduous caries. Shanghai J Stomatol. 2004;13(5):365–6.
29. Tham R, Bowatte G, Dharmage SC, Tan DJ, Lau M, Dai X, Allen KJ, Lodge CJ. Breastfeeding and the risk of dental caries: a systematic review and meta-analysis. Acta Paediatr. 2015;104 suppl(467):62.
30. Avila WM, Pordeus IA, Paiva SM, Martins CC. Breast and bottle feeding as risk factors for dental caries: a systematic review and meta-analysis. PLoS One. 2015;10(11):e0142922.
31. Peres KG, Nascimento GG, Peres MA, Mittinty MN, Demarco FF, Santos IS, Matijasevich A, Ajd B. Impact of prolonged breastfeeding on dental caries: a population-based birth cohort study. Pediatrics. 2017;140(1):e20162943.
32. Liu L, Zhang Y, Wu W, Cheng M, Li Y, Cheng R. Prevalence and correlates of dental caries in an elderly population in Northeast China. PLoS One. 2013; 8(11):e78723.

Complex patterns of response to oral hygiene instructions: longitudinal evaluation of periodontal patients

Felice Amoo-Achampong[1], David E. Vitunac[1], Kathleen Deeley[1], Adriana Modesto[1,2] and Alexandre R. Vieira[1,2*]

Abstract

Background: Oral hygiene instruction is an intervention widely practiced but increased knowledge about oral health does not necessarily dramatically impact oral disease prevalence in populations. We aimed to measure plaque and bleeding in periodontal patients over time to determine patterns of patient response to oral hygiene instructions.

Methods: Longitudinal plaque and bleeding index data were evaluated in 227 periodontal patients to determine the impact of oral hygiene instructions. Over multiple visits, we determined relative plaque accumulation and gingival bleeding for each patient. Subsequently, we grouped them in three types of oral hygiene status in response to initial instructions, using the longitudinal data over the period they were treated and followed for their periodontal needs. These patterns of oral hygiene based on the plaque and gingival bleeding indexes were evaluated based on age, sex, ethnic background, interleukin 1 alpha and beta genotypes, diabetes status, smoking habits, and other concomitant diseases. Chi-square and Fisher's exact tests were used to determine if any differences between these variables were statistically significant with alpha set at 0.05.

Results: Three patterns in response to oral hygiene instructions emerged. Plaque and gingival bleeding indexes improved, worsened, or fluctuated over time in the periodontal patients studied. Out of all the confounders considered, only ethnic background showed statistically significant differences. White individuals more often than other ethnic groups fluctuated in regards to oral hygiene quality after instructions.

Conclusions: There are different responses to professional oral hygiene instructions. These responses may be related to ethnicity.

Keywords: Periodontitis, Dental plaque, Oral biofilm, Oral hygiene

Background

The two most common oral diseases (dental caries and periodontitis) are bacteria-mediated and can be prevented by satisfactory dental biofilm control. Dental biofilm starts forming soon after its removal from the tooth surface meaning that effective dental biofilm control requires effectively disturbing biofilm formation on a daily basis.

* Correspondence: arv11@pitt.edu
[1]Departments of Oral Biology, University of Pittsburgh School of Dental Medicine, 412 Salk Pavilion, Pittsburgh, PA 15261, USA
[2]Pediatric Dentistry, University of Pittsburgh School of Dental Medicine, 412 Salk Pavilion, Pittsburgh, PA 15261, USA

Epidemiology of dental caries and periodontitis in many developed countries has changed in the last five decades due to improved oral health practices. These changes also emphasize disparities in oral health, with most oral disease burden affecting the socially disadvantaged individuals [1].

A paradigm shift has occurred in dentistry where the emphasis has changed from it being a 'repair service' to being a health care service that prevents disease prior to damage occurring. Since the 1990's, oral health promotion has been considered of high importance to the service that dentists provide to their patients [2].

The implementation of oral health promotion has two aspects: the provider and the individual benefiting from this practice. On one hand, the dentist is the agent providing the intervention, and on the other hand is the patient, who will benefit from effectively implementing daily good oral health practices. In the United States, the dentist can be reimbursed by performing professional dental prophylaxis, which includes scaling and polishing procedures to remove coronal plaque, calculus, and stains (dental code D1110-Prophylaxis-Adult). This code also implies the provision of oral hygiene instructions, since dental code D1330 can be used in cases where additional time and expertise is directed toward the client's care beyond that of the routine brushing and flossing instructions included in the prophylaxis procedure codes, such as D1110. Regarding the patient, it is suggested that the psychology of behavior change is key to successful oral health promotion [3].

The two simplest and most widely used ways to promote oral health is through verbal and written advice. These two approaches are effective for increasing patient knowledge regarding oral health (reviewed in [3]) but data suggest that this does not have an impact on oral disease presentation. In our study, we took advantage of longitudinal data to determine how oral health instructions provided by a dentist impact oral health practices as measured by presence of dental biofilm and gingival bleeding in follow up dental visits. These direct measurements of oral hygiene practices are better surrogates than the traditional self-reported data of the number of times and when tooth brushing and flossing are performed every day.

Methods

Sample population

The subjects of this study were patients with active periodontitis being treated at the Department of Periodontics and Preventive Dentistry at the University of Pittsburgh's School of Dental Medicine. All of them were being treated by scaling and root planning and being monitored regarding personal oral hygiene improvements. Individual samples and clinical information were obtained through the Dental Registry and DNA Repository project. Since 2006, this project seeks to provide all patients seeking treatment at the School of Dental Medicine with the opportunity to be a part of the registry. All subjects in this study were selected from this database with a focus on those who have received periodontal treatment through the School of Dental Medicine. The information consisted of diagnostics, treatment planning and treatments provided as stated in each subject's record. All participants signed a consent form that authorized the use of information from their dental records and provided a saliva sample as a source of genomic DNA (deoxyribonucleic acid). Extracted DNA was done in accordance with the protocol set by the manufacturer's instructions. This project was approved by the University of Pittsburgh Institutional Review Board (IRB # 060991).

From January 2015 to January 2016, data from 2164 periodontal patients were analyzed. Of this, 227 patients fit the initial criteria of having at least ten teeth and more than one periodontal evaluation. All these subjects had a diagnosis of moderate to severe periodontitis and a code D1110 in their records that confirmed oral hygiene instructions were provided. No individuals selected for our study had any indication that they had bleeding disorders, physical disabilities that would affect oral hygiene ability or were pregnant. The intervention of interest, oral hygiene instructions, is provided to patients by all students at the same time at the initial appointment. Students are trained to present patients with the same content. We used the record that oral hygiene instructions were done and that patients were charged as the confirmation the intervention was provided. The number of marked surfaces for each tooth was recorded for both plaque and bleeding indexes (Löe and Silness, [4]; Silness and Löe, [5]) of each eligible patient. We determined full mouth percentages for affected areas, as well as by quadrant, left/right side, maxillary/mandibular, anterior/posterior, and incisor, canine, premolar, and molar teeth locations. From this, we sought to identify patterns to ascertain changes of the indexes over time. Following the analysis of clinical information, participants were grouped based on the number of evaluations; 104 selected subjects received only two periodontal evaluations over time (one every 6 months to 1 year) and 123 subjects received multiple periodontal evaluations ranging from three to eight visits (one evaluation every 6 months to 1 year). Several subgroup categories (based on if oral hygiene improved) were utilized to further determine trends in the oral hygiene surrogates we analyzed (plaque and bleeding indexes) including age, ethnicity, sex, tobacco use, and other concomitant health concerns/medication use such as diabetes, cardiovascular diseases, cancer, and gastrointestinal conditions. Of the total study population, 54% were aged 50 and above, 71% identified as White, and 21% as Black. In addition, 52% of study subjects identified as being female, 69% were determined to be nonsmokers, and 46 out of 227 individuals were reported to have diabetes.

Full mouth plaque indexes ranged from only 9.4% of the mouth affected to 100% (mean 47%). This variation was not statistically significant when sex was considered. When Blacks and Whites were compared, Black individuals had more teeth bleeding than White individuals ($p < 0.05$) (Table 1). The caries experience of the cohort was very high, with mean DMFT (Decayed, Missing due to caries, Filled Teeth) 15.62 (ranging from 0 to 28) and mean DMFS (Decayed, Missing due to caries, Filled Surface) 52.55 (ranging from 0 to 128). Only six individuals were caries free and 14 total individuals had a DMFT score of 2 or lower.

Genotyping

Genomic DNA was isolated from saliva samples according to established protocol. Taqman chemistry was used to determine genotypes for interleukin-1 alpha (*IL-1α*) and interleukin-1 beta (*IL-1β*) markers. These interleukins act as pro-inflammatory cytokines in the immune response towards infections and have been suggested as markers for periodontitis risk (reviewed in [6]). Reaction mixes were performed in 4-μL volumes using the two markers rs1800587 for *IL-1 α* and rs1143634 for *IL-1 β*. A non-template control (using water instead of DNA) was used as a negative control to ensure quality control of genotyping reactions. Clinic, demographic, and genotyping raw data can be seen in the Additional file 1.

Statistical analysis

Following subject genotyping, chi-square or Fisher's exact tests were used to determine Hardy-Weinberg equilibrium and to assess the significance of the differences observed in patterns of oral hygiene identified as well as genotypic and allelic frequencies between oral hygiene patterns as implemented in the PLINK software [7]. The distributions of subjects for each interleukin genotype were compared based on four out of the initial seven aforementioned subgroups found to be statistically significance. These included sex, ethnicity, tobacco use, and diabetes status, and were ultimately used in the study as key variables in determining evaluation trends. Intervention outcomes (improvement and worsening for subjects with data from only two assessments; or improved, worse, or fluctuation of oral hygiene surrogates over time for subjects with multiple assessments) provided an additional layer of characterization for this study population. We used chi-square and Fisher's exact tests for all comparisons. When considering oral hygiene status after the intervention based on sex, ethnic background, tobacco use, diabetes status, and interleukin genotypes, we applied Cochran-Mantel-Haenszel and regression models as implemented in the PLINK software [7]. A *p*-value of 0.05 or less was considered to be of statistical significance.

Table 1 Full mouth plaque and bleeding indexes means based on sex and ethnic background

Indexes	Relative frequency of full mouth affection
Total sample ($N = 227$)	
Plaque: Mean (Minimum-Maximum)	49 (9.4–100)
Bleeding: Mean (Minimum-Maximum)	25.2 (0.6–95)
Males	
Plaque: Mean (Minimum-Maximum)	50.1 (11.2–100)
Bleeding: Mean (Minimum-Maximum)	25.6 (0.6–95)
Females	
Plaque: Mean (Minimum-Maximum)	47.9 (9.4–100)
Bleeding: Mean (Minimum-Maximum)	24.8 (1.5–90.5)
Black	
Plaque: Mean (Minimum-Maximum)	50.1 (9.4–99)
Bleeding: Mean (Minimum-Maximum)	34 (9.4–92.5)
White	
Plaque: Mean (Minimum-Maximum)	48 (10.7–100)
Bleeding: Mean (Minimum-Maximum)	19.7 (0.6–95)

Results

In the first phase of statistical analysis (data not shown), separation of study subjects by interleukin genotypes revealed that genotypic and allelic differences in four of the seven subgroups were in fact borderline significant or significant. These included sex ($p = 0.07$) and ethnicity ($p = 0.02$) for *IL-1 β*, and tobacco use ($p = 0.07$) and diabetes status ($p = 0.06$) for *IL-1 α*. In terms of allelic differences, females were more likely to have the A allele and males were more likely to have the G allele. Additionally, for *IL-1 β*, White individuals were more likely to have the G allele when compared to Black individuals and those of other ethnicities. Further exploration of these data confirmed that this statistically significant difference was the result of population substructure, with those originating from Africa to be more likely to have the G allele for this interleukin. For *IL-1 α*, diabetics tended to have the G allele more frequently than those without diabetes and the A allele tended to be more prevalent for smokers than non-smokers. These initial findings suggested that further analysis needed to be done within these subgroups in terms of intervention outcome. The assigning of intervention outcomes (improved, worsened, or fluctuated) was based on plaque and bleeding indexes calculated for each visit and compared over time. Those who fluctuated did not display any clear trend of overall improvement or overall worsening in oral hygiene indexes. Only seven subjects did not show any changes (they stayed the same) and were not included for further analysis. The variation in number of available oral hygiene assessments was due to recording the oral hygiene, extension of follow-ups, and patient compliance to follow-up visits.

Results from comparisons between intervention outcomes within subgroups and interleukin genotypes are summarized in Table 2. Ethnicity was found to be the only subanalysis with statistical significant difference in that individuals not defined as African Americans or Whites were more likely to be inconsistent and fluctuate during treatment ($p = 0.02$). Also, 99 out of 148 White individuals showed an inconsistent pattern of oral hygiene status in comparison to 19 out of 56 African Americans (67% vs 34%; $p = 0.0002$). Sex, tobacco use, and diabetes status differences were not found to be statistically significant different for intervention outcome, although we can see a trend for non-smokers to not improve and diabetics that fluctuated more often improving by the end of the observation period.

Of particular interest during the study was to better understand the trends present for study subjects whose progress fluctuated throughout treatment. Individuals in this subpopulation were further separated based on if their plaque/bleeding indexes improved or worsened overall from their first periodontal evaluation to their last evaluation. Data for each subject was charted and graphed and from this, three progress curve patterns were determined as depicted in Fig. 1. A U-curve trend line defined subjects with initially high plaque/bleeding indexes that decreased and improved over time but increased and returned to high-percentages nearing the end of recorded treatment. An inverted U-curve trend line was also seen, that displays initially lower plaque/bleeding indexes that increased and worsened over time but ultimately dropped again to lower levels towards the end of their last recorded evaluation. The third pattern had a wavy curve. This pattern encompasses study subjects with a combination of both U- and inverted U-curve trend lines. With these definitions in mind, these curve patterns were compared against the four significant subgroups and interleukin genotypes to identify statistically significant differences between each if in fact present (Table 3). Previous caries experience determined based on DMFT/DMFS scores did not show any differences in the distribution of the assigned patterns of improvement or worsening of the plaque/bleeding indexes (i.e. among the 14 individuals with DMFT scores up to 2, six got worse overtime and eight got better; this trend could be seen throughout in the data).

In the fluctuation subpopulation, sex, tobacco use, diabetes status, and interleukin genotype were found to be statistically significant different in this group although not initially observed in the total sample. In regards to sex, more females presented with evaluation percentages defined by the U-curve pattern ($p = 0.001$). In contrast, more males displayed trends representative of the inverted U-curve pattern. For tobacco use, non-smokers more frequently displayed an inverted U-curve pattern

Table 2 Frequencies and Statistical Analysis of Intervention Outcomes for Plaque and Bleeding Indexes

	Improved ($N = 109$)	Worsened ($N = 118$)	*p*-value*	Fluctuated ($N = 123$)	Fluctuated Improved ($N = 73$)	Fluctuated Worsened ($N = 50$)	*p*-value**
Males	54	50	0.27	62	38	24	0.66
Females	55	68		61	35	26	
White	74	74	0.66	99	61	38	0.02
Black	26	30		19	12	7	
Other	9	14		5	0	5	
Smoker	35	25	0.06	41	28	13	0.15
Non-Smoker	74	93		82	45	37	
Diabetes	10	11	1.0	15	12	3	0.08
No Diabetes	99	107		108	61	47	
Genotype							
IL-1 α							
AA	20	18	0.23	16	10	6	0.79
AG	18	27		26	14	12	
GG	14	10		11	7	4	
IL-1 β							
AA	3	6	0.55	4	3	1	0.78
GA	18	16		23	13	10	
GG	36	41		43	26	17	

*p-value calculated using Chi-square test compares individuals whose plaque and bleeding indexes improved or worsened over the course of treatment. **p-value calculated using Chi-square test compares individuals whose plaque and bleeding indexes fluctuated but improved or fluctuated but worsened over the course of treatment. $p \leq 0.05$ were considered to be statistically significant

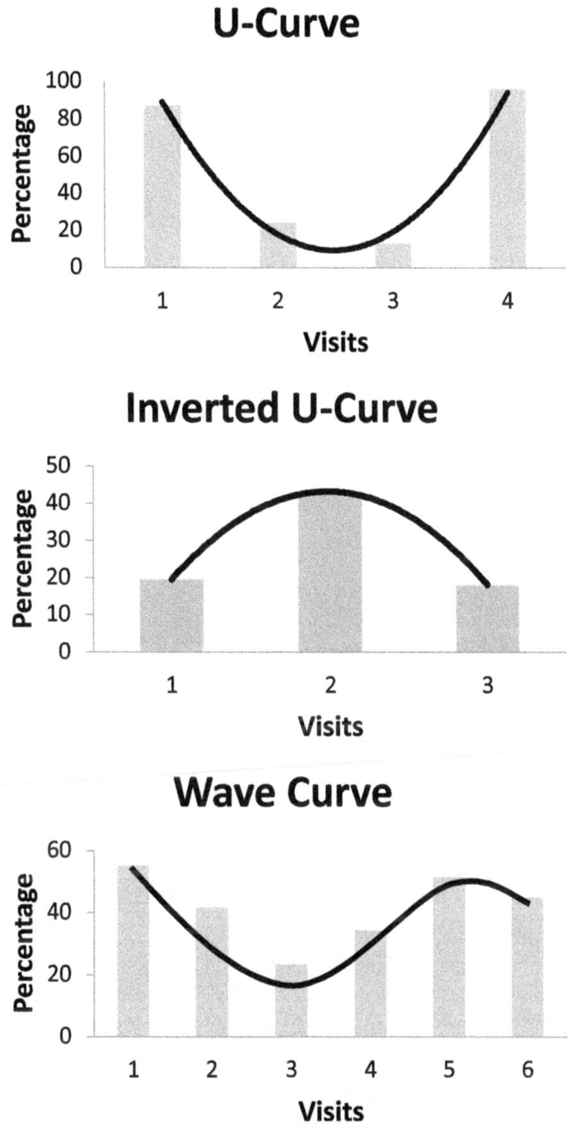

Fig. 1 Sample graphical representations of trend line patterns for individuals with more than two oral hygiene assessments ($N = 100$) whose plaque and bleeding index percentages fluctuated throughout periodontal treatment. Statistical results and number of subjects in each fluctuation subgroup are recorded in Table 2

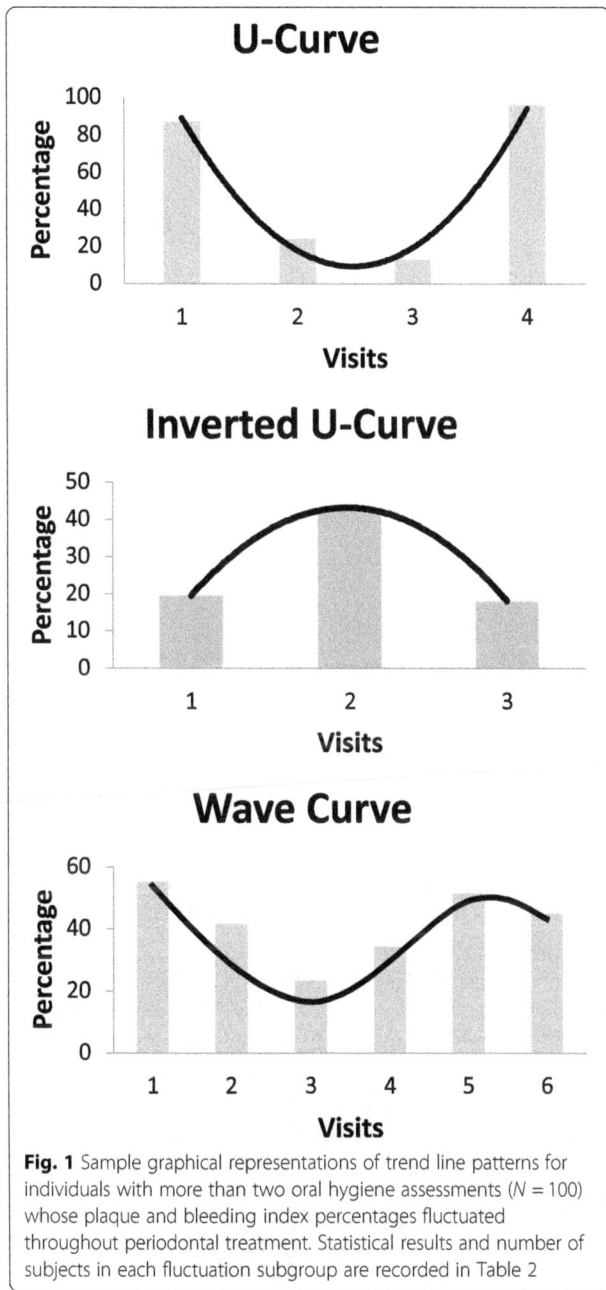

($p = 0.02$). Additionally, non-diabetics more frequently displayed a U- or inverted U-curve progression pattern whereas more diabetics were likely to follow a wavy curve pattern ($p = 0.03$).

Discussion

Oral hygiene instruction is an intervention that is provided essentially to every patient that visits a dental office, at least on the initial visit. There are thousands of scientific papers published on the topic of dental health education (reviewed in [3, 8, 9]) and the overall conclusion continues to be that there is weak evidence that improvements in knowledge lead to improved oral health behavior, at least in the short-term. The evidence is stronger for improving oral hygiene and gingival health by using psychological behavior change models [individually tailored oral health approaches, motivational interviews, autonomy-supportive interviews, counseling with six-step method, oral hygiene education based on social cognitive aid implementation theory, transtheoretical behavior change counseling [3]] but these models are not routinely used in a dental clinic such as the one we have in our school. Also, the dentists do not certify or assess if the patients understood the oral hygiene instructions received.

Since we have longitudinal data available, we decided to explore the presence of patterns that can be clinically useful. When the sample is analyzed as a whole, our data show no obvious changes in oral hygiene practices after treatment is initiated and an oral hygiene intervention is provided as measured by presence of dental biofilm and/or gingival bleeding. When these indexes were evaluated over time in patients receiving treatment for periodontitis, we noticed at least three clinical patterns: some patients obviously improved, some patients stayed the same or even got worse, and some patients fluctuated. Among the ones who fluctuated, some showed worsening that eventually returned to levels similar to baseline, some showed improvement that eventually returned to levels similar to baseline, and some continued to fluctuate. We believe these patterns need to be accounted for in future evaluations on the impact of any intervention (educational, clinical, or biological) aiming to improve oral health. Also, it is important to highlight that this study did not aim to compare subjects based on their periodontal disease classification, although most of the subjects had moderate to severe periodontitis, and we cannot draw any conclusions on the effects of these data on periodontal disease per se. Other limitations of our data are due to the inherited nature of our design. We relied on records that were filled by a number of different professionals in training. Although, we expect a good level of consistency, data are potentially affected by differences in how information is recorded or if information is missing. The evaluation of periodontal patients in particular and subjects in general with poorer oral health indicators may limit the potential of our results to be generalizable to other populations or geographic locations.

A randomized clinical trial is probably the ideal study design to demonstrate how effective is oral hygiene instructions provided at the dental office. However, due to its cost, this is an unlikely option for future studies. We approached the problem by using a pragmatic design, meaning that the data we studied came from a clinical setting where patients are treated routinely and

Table 3 Progress Curve Pattern Distributions and Statistical Analysis of Subjects with Fluctuating Intervention Outcomes

	U-Curve ($N = 16$)	Inverted U-Curve ($N = 19$)	Wavy Curve ($N = 13$)	*p*-value*
Males	4	14	7	0.0012
Females	12	5	6	
Caucasian	13	13	12	0.066
African American	3	4	1	
Other	0	2	0	
Smoker	7	4	6	0.018
Non-Smoker	9	15	7	
Diabetes	1	2	4	0.027
No Diabetes	15	17	9	
Genotype				
*IL-1 α***				Genotype
AA	4	5	6	$p = 0.3$
AG	10	10	3	Allele
GG	2	4	4	$p = 0.93$
*IL-1 β***				Genotype
AA	1	1	1	$p = 0.96$
GA	4	6	3	Allele
GG	11	12	9	$p = 1.0$

*p-value calculated using Fisher's exact test compares the progress curve patterns of subjects with fluctuating intervention outcomes
**p-values for genotypes were calculated for each interleukin based on genotype and allele ratios
$p \leq 0.05$ were considered to be statistically significant
Cochran-Mantel-Haenszel test or regression did not show different results and are not presented here for simplicity

not under controlled conditions. This approach brings the obvious challenges of understanding the multitude of influences that impact an individual response to oral hygiene instructions. Despite these characteristics, it is remarkable to see that oral hygiene quality, as measured by presence of plaque and gingival bleeding, have different patterns depending on the individual. One would assume that patients under dental treatment would be motivated to keep excellent oral hygiene levels but our data showed that individuals will not necessarily improve, which would suggest that professional oral hygiene interventions more often than twice a year might be warranted to certain individuals.

There is plenty of evidence that show that the success of oral health promotion interventions delivered in the dental office depends on the professional person's character, values, personality, and people skills. Data show that if professionals do not believe oral hygiene instructions will improve the health of their patient, then that professional will be less likely to practice an effective oral health promotion strategy [3]. In our sample, it was not possible to control for the professional delivering of oral hygiene instructions or the way that oral hygiene instructions were delivered (timing during consultation, length of time, how information was presented). Either a third or fourth year dental student provides oral hygiene instructions to our patients and in general they are very enthusiastic and passionate. But obviously, even among the students, there are more or less extraverted individuals, effective communicators, and proficient speakers. There was also no way to control for our patients' previous experiences. All of our patients have certainly gone to other dentists in the past and they received oral hygiene instructions before done by others, including exposure to oral health information in school and through television adds. The only assumption we can make is that despite these past experiences, the individuals that comprised our sample still needed periodontal treatment.

Genotypes for interleukin 1 have been suggested as potential markers that could help identify individuals that may have higher risk for tooth loss [10, 11]. By extension, this genomic assessment could help determine which individuals could visit the dentist less often since they would have decreased risk of tooth loss and would not benefit from additional preventive visits [10]. This suggestion, however, was refuted by later analyses [12]. We have suggested that looking at the combination of smoking, diabetes, cardiovascular diseases, and interleukin 1 genotypes may help determine who will benefit from coming more often to the dentist [11]. Our data showed that the interleukin 1 genotypes did not associate with the longitudinal patterns of oral hygiene practice surrogates that we studied. Interestingly, the "fluctuating" pattern was found more often in Whites comprising the studied sample. Specific associations with sex, diabetes status, and smoking were also found. We believe these results indicate the possibility that biological factors (i.e. genetic variants) related to behavior may be underlying these associations. Self-motivation to diet and exercise may be dictated by the same genetic variants influencing oral hygiene compliance. Similar arguments can be made for genetic variants that determine the will to quit smoking. The data also support differences between sexes.

Pittsburgh is the largest city adjacent to one of the poorest areas in the USA, Appalachia. This region is known for its predominantly settling of Anglo-Scottish people and poverty and subsistence living that has permeated the social and cultural structure of the region. Quantitative data clearly show socioeconomic indicators are much worse for the communities in the Appalachian region compared to those in the rest of the United States (reviewed in [13]). In regard to health indicators, Pittsburgh reflects what is found in the Appalachian region, and the population treated at the University of Pittsburgh Medical Center has some of the worst health indicators in the country, which makes Pittsburgh a perfect laboratory for studying disease risks. Despite these similar characteristics, our data showed that patients would respond differently to an intervention such as oral hygiene instructions. That makes us believe that the psychology of behavior change is potentially one of the key factors (if not the key factor) to oral health promotion. It is apparent that teaching health psychology to dentists would make oral health promotion more effective in dentistry [3].

Conclusions

Our data showed that response to interventions such as oral hygiene instructions have multiple identifiable patterns that may impact success and longevity of dental treatments.

Abbreviations

DMFS: Decayed, missing due to caries, filled surfaces; DMFT: Decayed, missing due to caries, filled teeth; DNA: Deoxyribonucleic acid; *IL-1 α*: Interleukin 1 alpha; *IL-1 β*: Interleukin 1 beta; IRB: Institutional Review Board

Acknowledgements

The authors thank Jacqueline Noel for administrative support.

Funding

The Dental Registry and DNA Repository project is supported by the University of Pittsburgh School of Dental Medicine.

Authors' contributions

Generated and analyzed clinical data: ARV, AM, FA-A, DEV, KD Generated and analyzed genotypes: ARV, AM, KD Statistical analyses: FA-A, ARV, Obtained funding: AM, ARV, Designed the study: ARV, AM, FAA, DEV, KD, Critically reviewed the manuscript: AM, FA-A, DEV, KD, Wrote the first draft: ARV. All authors read and approved the final manuscript.

Competing interests

The authors declare that they have no competing interests.

References

1. Yee R, Sheiham A. The burden of restorative dental treatment for children in third world countries. Int Dent J. 2002;52:1–9.
2. Pitts N. Are we ready to move to non-operative/ preventive treatment in dental caries in clinical practice? Caries Res. 2004;38:294–304.
3. Kay E, Vascott D, Hocking A, et al. A review of approaches for dental practice teams for promoting oral health. Community Dent Oral Epidemiol. 2016;44:313–30.
4. Löe H, Silness J. Periodontal disease in pregnancy. I. Prevalence and severity. Acta Odont Scand. 1963;21:533–51.
5. Silness P, Löe H. Periodontal disease in pregnancy II. Acta Odontol Scand. 1964;22(1):121–6.
6. Grigoriadou ME, Kputayas SO, Madianos PN, Strub JR. Interleukin-1 as a genetic marker for periodontitis: review of the literature. Quintessense Int. 2010;41:517–25.
7. Purcell S, Neale B, Todd-Brown K, Thomas L, Ferreira MA, Bender D, Maller J, Sklar P, de Bakker PI, Daly MJ, Sham PC. PLINK: a tool set for whole-genome association and population-based linkage analyses. Am J Hum Genet. 2007; 81:559–75.
8. Brown L. Research in dental health education and health promotion: a review of the literature. Health Educ Q. 1994;21:83–102.
9. Kay L, Locker D. Is dental health education effective? A systematic review of current evidence. Community Dent Oral Epidemiol. 1996;24:231–5.
10. Giannobile WV, Braun TM, Caplis AK, Doucette-Stamm L, Duff GW, Kornman KS. Patient stratification for preventive care in dentistry. J Dent Res. 2013;92:694–701.
11. Vieira AR, Hilands KM, Braun TW. Saving more teeth – a case for personalized care. J Pers Med. 2015;5:30–5.
12. Diehl SR, Kuo F, Hart TC. Interleukin 1 genetic tests provide no support for reduction of preventive dental care. J Am Dent Assoc. 2015;146:164–73.
13. McGarvey EL, Leon-Verdin M, Killos LF, et al. Health disparities between Appalachian and non-Appalachian counties in Virginia USA. J Community Health. 2011;36:348–56.

7

Comparative evaluation of the vertical fracture resistance of endodontically treated roots filled with Gutta-percha and Resilon: a meta-analysis of in vitro studies

Minmin Tan[1,2,3†], Zhaowu Chai[1,2,3†], Chengjun Sun[1,2,3], Bo Hu[1,2,3], Xiang Gao[1,2,3], Yunjia Chen[1,2,3] and Jinlin Song[1,2,3,4*]

Abstract

Background: Teeth treated endodontically are more susceptible to vertical root fracture (VRF). Some studies have suggested that obturating the root canals with Gutta-percha or Resilon can reinforce endodontically treated teeth, but a few others have presented conflicting results. These inconsistent results cannot guide clinicians in determining clinical approaches. The objective of this meta-analysis is to evaluate and compare the vertical fracture resistance of endodontically treated root canals obturated with Gutta-percha/AH plus and the Resilon system.

Methods: Comprehensive literature searches were performed in the PubMed, Cochrane Library, ScienceDirect, Web of Science and Embase databases. The titles and abstracts of all of the retrieved articles were independently assessed by two authors according to predefined selection criteria. Data in the included articles were independently extracted. Statistical analyses were conducted using Review Manager 5.3 and Stata 12.0 software. The pooled standardized mean differences (SMDs) with 95% confidence intervals (CIs) were calculated for the outcome indicators. The level of statistical significance was set at $p < 0.05$. The Cochran Q test (I^2 test) was used to test for heterogeneity among studies.

Results: Fourteen randomized controlled in vitro trials were included in the meta-analysis. The results demonstrated that the vertical root fracture resistance of unprepared and unfilled roots was significantly higher than that of roots obturated with Gutta-percha/AH plus (SMD = − 0.69, 95% CI = − 1.34 to − 0.04, $p = 0.04$) or the Resilon system (SMD = − 0.54, 95% CI = − 1.07 to − 0.00, $p = 0.05$). The differences in fracture resistance between the roots filled with Gutta-percha/AH plus and the prepared unfilled root canals was not significant (SMD = 0.59, 95% CI = − 0.02 to 1.21, $p = 0.06$). Roots obturated with Resilon had higher fracture resistance than instrumented unfilled roots (SMD = 0.83, 95% CI = 0.44 to 1.22, $p < 0.0001$) or roots filled with Gutta-percha/AH plus (SMD = 0.62, 95% CI = 0.01 to 1.23, $p = 0.05$).

Conclusions: The present study suggests that filling with Gutta-percha/AH plus dose not reinforce endodontically treated roots, whereas obturating with the Resilon system can increase vertical root fracture resistance of prepared roots. As this meta-analysis was based on in vitro studies, it should be careful to extrapolate its conclusion to the clinical context.

Keywords: Gutta-percha, Resilon sealer, Root canal obturation, Tooth fracture, Meta-analysis

* Correspondence: soongjl@163.com
†Minmin Tan and Zhaowu Chai contributed equally to this work.
[1]College of Stomatology, Chongqing Medical University, Chongqing, China
[2]Chongqing Key Laboratory of Oral Diseases and Biomedical Sciences, College of Stomatology, Chongqing Medical University, Chongqing, China
Full list of author information is available at the end of the article

Background

Endodontic therapy is a commonly used approach for the treatment of pulpitis and periapical periodontitis. Endodontically treated teeth have been demonstrated to be more prone to crown or root fracture than vital teeth [1, 2]. Vertical root fracture (VRF) is the most common and serious complication of the endodontically treated tooth, which typically leads to root resection and tooth extraction [3]. Therefore, the prevention of VRF is desirable. Many attempts have been made to increase the strength of endodontically treated roots, such as placing posts inside the roots [4, 5] and obturating dental materials in the root canals [6–8]. In recent years, the effects of different obturating materials on the strength of endodontically treated roots have received substantial attention.

Gutta-percha with the resin-based sealer AH plus is regarded as the gold standard in current obturation systems. Although Gutta-percha has many excellent properties, including good biocompatibility, low cytotoxicity [9], dimension stability and thermoplasticity, the ability of this material to strengthen roots that are treated endodontically remains unclear. Some studies [2, 10–12] reported that Gutta-percha/AH plus significantly increased the VRF resistance of instrumented roots, whereas other studies reported no significant effect [13–19]. Resilon, a root canal obturating material based on thermoplastic-filled polymer composites, has excellent sealing ability, antimicrobial activity, adhesive properties and retreatable properties [20, 21] when used in combination with one of the dual-cure resin-based root canal sealers Epiphany or Realseal. However, whether the fracture resistance of root canals can be increased by filling with Resilon and whether roots obturated with Resilon have higher fracture resistance than do those filled with Gutta-percha remain unclear. The inconsistent results cannot provide clear guidance to clinicians in making appropriate clinical choices.

Therefore, it is imperative to conduct a meta-analysis to investigate and compare the strengthening effects of Gutta-percha and Resilon on prepared roots. For the purposes of the meta-analysis performed here, data from randomized controlled in vitro trials were compiled to evaluate and compare the effects of these two root canal filling materials on the VRF resistance of teeth after root canal therapy.

Methods

Search strategies

Comprehensive searches of the relevant literature were performed in the PubMed, Cochrane Library, ScienceDirect, Web of Science and Embase databases from the earliest available date to November 21, 2017. The main keywords used were 'gutta-percha', 'resilon sealer' and 'tooth fracture'. For instance, the free search terms used in PubMed were as follows '(((gutta-percha) AND (AH plus)) OR (resilon)) AND ((tooth fracture) OR (fracture resistance))'. Specific searching strategies were developed for each database, as shown in Table 1. Additionally, the references in each retrieved articles were evaluated to avoid the omission of any relevant articles.

Literature selection criteria

The titles and abstracts of all of the retrieved articles were reviewed independently by two reviewers to determine their eligibility. If the information provided in the title and abstract was insufficient to determine the article's relevance to this study, the full text of the article was reviewed. When there was a disagreement between the two reviewers, a discussion was held in an attempt to reach a final decision. If a final agreement could not be reached by discussion, an experienced referee was consulted. The inclusion criteria and elimination criteria are shown in Table 2.

Table 1 Database search strategy

Pubmed	1. "Gutta-percha" [all fields] OR "Guttapercha" [all fields] 2. "AH-plus" [all fields] OR "Epoxy Resins" [all fields] OR "Resin Cements" [all fields] OR "epoxy resin-based root canal sealer" [all fields] 3. "Resilon" [all fields] 4. "tooth fracture" [all fields] OR "vertical fracture" [all fields] OR "fracture resistance" [all fields] 5. "english" [language] 6. (1 AND 2) OR 3 7. 4 AND 5 AND 6
Embase	#1. guttapercha OR 'gutta percha' #2. 'ah plus' OR (epoxy AND resins) OR (resin AND cements) OR (epoxy AND 'resin based' AND root AND canal AND sealer) #3. Resilon #4. (fracture AND resistance) OR (tooth AND fracture) #5. ((# 1 AND # 2) OR # 3) AND # 4
Cochrane Library	1. MeSH Terms: Root Canal Obturation 2. MeSH Terms: Root Canal Filling Materials 3. MeSH Terms: Gutta-Percha 4. MeSH Terms: resilon sealer 5. MeSH Terms: Tooth Fractures 6. MeSH Terms: Dental Stress Analysis 7. KEY WORD: fracture resistance 8. (# 1 OR # 2 OR (# 3 AND # 4)) AND (# 5 OR # 6 OR # 7)
Web of Science	#1. TOPIC: (gutta-percha) OR TOPIC: (guttapercha) #2. TOPIC: (AH-plus) OR TOPIC: (Epoxy Resins) OR TOPIC: (Resin Cements) OR TOPIC: (epoxy resin-based root canal sealer) #3. TOPIC: (resilon) #4. TOPIC: (tooth fracture) OR TOPIC: (vertical fracture) OR TOPIC: (fracture resistance) #5. ((# 1 AND # 2) OR # 3) AND # 4
ScienceDirect	(((gutta-percha or guttapercha) AND ((AH-plus) OR ((Epoxy Resins)) OR ((Resin Cements)) OR ((epoxy resin-based root canal sealer)))) OR (resilon)) AND (((tooth fracture)) OR ((vertical fracture)) OR ((fracture resistance)))

Table 2 Selection Criteria

Inclusion criteria	1. Participants: Freshly extracted single rooted human teeth with closed apices, and after standard root canal preparation, all specimens had regular space for obturation.
	2. Intervention: Root canals were obturated with Gutta-percha/AH plus and (or) the Resilon system.
	3. Control: Unprepared and unfilled roots (negative control roots) or prepared but unfilled roots (positive control roots).
	4. Outcomes: Vertical fracture resistance of roots.
	5. Study design: Randomized controlled in vitro trials.
Exclusion criteria	1. Studies that did not fulfill the inclusion criteria.
	2. .Studies that evaluated the influence of different factors on the resistance to fracture of endodontically treated roots obturated with Gutta-percha/AH plus or the Resilon system.
	3. Retreatment.

Data collection

Data in the included studies were extracted by two authors independently. These data included the first author, year of publication, sample size, tooth type, irrigation fluid, obturation technique, test machine loading rate, experimental groups and control groups.

Assessment of risk of bias

Risk of bias of each included study was assessed by two authors based on the article's descriptions of the following items: randomization of roots, roots free of caries or resorption, standardization of root dimensions, sample size calculation, endodontic treatment performed by a single operator, use of materials according to the instructions of the manufacturer, blinding of the examiner, and appropriateness of the statistical analyses. The category of the risk-of-bias was assessed according to the following criteria:

i. high risk of bias: one to three items were identified;
ii. medium risk of bias: four or five items were identified; and
iii. low risk of bias: six to eight items were identified.

Data analysis

To perform the meta-analysis, the standard deviation (SD) and mean force load to VRF (expressed in Newtons) values were selected and statistically pooled using RevMan 5.3 (Cochrane Collaboration). The pooled results were expressed as standardized mean differences (SMDs) along with the 95% confidence intervals (CIs) because the outcome variable of interest was continuous. The level of statistical significance was set as $p < 0.05$. The Cochran Q test (I^2 test) was adopted to test for heterogeneity among studies. If the heterogeneity was considerable ($I^2 > 50\%$), a random-effects model or subgroup analysis was used; otherwise, a fixed-effects model was employed. The reliability of the results was evaluated by performing a sensitivity analysis using Stata 12.0 software. Begg's rank correlation test was used to evaluate publication bias when there were a sufficient number of studies included in each forest plot.

Results

Study search

The initial search yielded 1706 articles. Among them, 241 were removed as duplicates, and 1441 were excluded after reviewing the titles and abstracts. Of the remaining 24 articles, ten were excluded after careful examination of the full text. Fourteen trials [11–16, 22–29] that met the inclusion criteria were finally included. The process of literature selection is shown in Fig. 1.

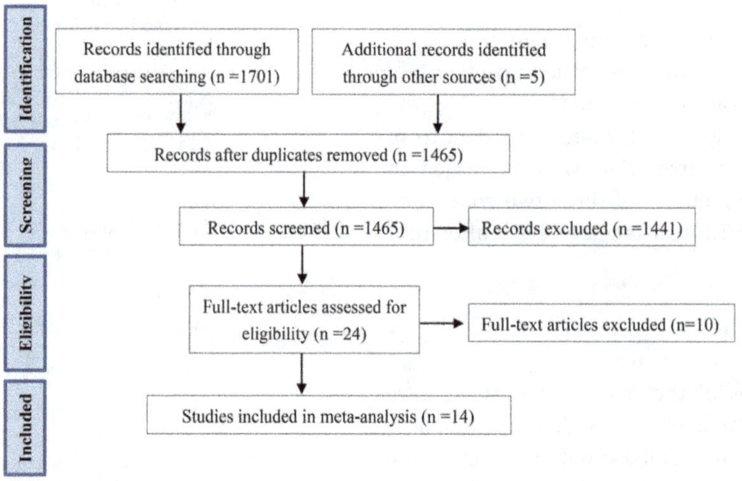

Fig. 1 PRISMA diagram of article retrieval

Description of studies

The studies included in this review were published from 2002 to 2017. All of the trials involved single rooted human teeth with closed apical foramen. A total of 659 roots were involved, including 92 unprepared and unfilled roots (negative control roots), 145 prepared and unfilled roots (positive control roots), 197 roots obturated with Gutta-percha/AH plus and 225 roots filled with the Resilon system. Regarding the type of tooth, human premolars were used as specimens in 10 studies [11–16, 22, 23, 25, 28], anterior teeth were used in 3 studies [26, 27, 29], and the type of tooth was not reported in 1 study [24]. Regarding the obturation techniques, a lateral condensation technique was utilized in 10 trials [13, 16, 22–29], a single-cone technique was used in 2 trials [11, 12], and no filling technique was reported in 2 trials [14, 15]. Vertical loading was applied to the teeth by the universal testing machine in all studies. The main features of the included studies are described in Table 3.

Assessment of risk of bias

Of the eligible studies, eight [11, 12, 16, 22, 23, 25, 26, 29] showed a low risk of bias and six [13–15, 24, 27, 28] presented a medium risk of bias (Table 4).

Meta-analysis

Gutta-percha/AH plus group verse negative control group

Differences between a Gutta-percha/AH plus group (roots filled with Gutta-percha/AH plus) and a negative control

Table 3 Main characteristics of included studies

Author	Year	Sample size/ Tooth type	Irrigants	Obturation technique	Test machine loading rate	Experimental group	Control group
Lertchirakarn et al. [27]	2002	20/Mandibular anterior teeth	EDTA and NaClO	Lateral condensation technique	0.5 mm/min	Gutta-percha/AH plus	Negative control
Hegde et al. [11]	2015	60/Mandibular premolars	EDTA and NaClO	Single-cone technique	1 mm/min	Gutta-percha/AH plus; Resilon/Epiphany	Negative control; Positive control
Topçuoğlu et al. [12]	2013	45/Mandibular premolars	EDTA and NaClO	Single-cone technique	1 mm/min	Gutta-percha/AH plus	Negative control; Positive control
Baba et al. [13]	2010	60/Mandibular premolars	EDTA and NaClO	Lateral condensation technique	1 mm/min	Gutta-percha/AH plus; Resilon/Epiphany	Positive control
Kumar et al. [15]	2014	60/Mandibular premolars	EDTA and NaClO	Not reported	1.25 mm/min	Gutta-percha/AH plus; Resilon/Realseal	Positive control
Jainaen et al. [14]	2008	40/Mandibular premolars	EDTA and NaClO	Not reported	1 mm/min	Gutta-percha/AH plus; Resilon/Realseal	Negative control; Positive control
Monteiro et al. [16]	2011	60/Mandibular premolars	EDTA and NaClO	Lateral condensation technique	1.25 mm/min	Gutta-percha/AH plus; Resilon/Realseal	Positive control
Elmakki et al. [23]	2014	60/Mandibular premolars	EDTA and NaClO	Lateral condensation technique	1 mm/min	Gutta-percha/AH plus; Resilon/Epiphany	Negative control; Positive control
Hammad et al. [24]	2007	23/Single rooted teeth	EDTA and NaClO	Lateral condensation technique	10 mm/min	Resilon/Realseal	Negative control
Nagpal et al. [28]	2012	40/Mandibular premolars	EDTA and NaClO	Lateral condensation technique	1 mm/min	Gutta-percha/AH plus; Resilon/Epiphany	Negative control
Langalia et al. [26]	2015	36/Maxillary anterior teeth	EDTA and NaClO	Lateral condensation technique	5 mm/min	Gutta-percha/AH plus; Resilon/Realseal	Negative control
Khan et al. [25]	2015	60/Mandibular premolars	EDTA and NaClO	Lateral condensation technique	1 mm/min	Resilon/Epiphany	Positive control
Dibajia et al. [22]	2017	35/Mandibular premolars	EDTA and NaClO	Lateral condensation technique	1 mm/min	Gutta-percha/AH plus; Resilon/Epiphany	Negative control
Sandikci et al. [29]	2014	60/Mandibular anterior teeth	EDTA and NaClO	Lateral condensation technique	1 mm/min	Gutta-percha/AH plus; Resilon/Epiphany	Negative control; Positive control

Table 4 Risk of bias considering parameters reported in the eligible studies

Study	Teeth randomization	Teeth free of caries or resorption	Standardization of root dimensions	Sample size calculation	Endodontic treatment performed by a single operator	Materials used according to the manufacturer's instructions	Blinding of the examiner	Appropriate of statistical analyses	Risk of bias
Lertchirakarn et al. [27]	Y	Y	N	N	Y	Y	N	Y	Medium
Hegde et al. [11]	Y	Y	Y	N	Y	Y	N	Y	Low
Topçuoğlu et al. [12]	Y	Y	Y	N	Y	Y	N	Y	Low
Baba et al. [13]	Y	N	N	N	Y	Y	N	Y	Medium
Kumar et al. [15]	Y	N	Y	N	Y	Y	N	Y	Medium
Jainaen et al. [14]	Y	Y	N	N	Y	Y	N	Y	Medium
Monteiro et al. [16]	Y	Y	Y	N	Y	Y	Y	Y	Low
Elmakki et al. [23]	Y	Y	Y	N	Y	Y	Y	Y	Low
Hammad et al. [24]	Y	Y	N	N	Y	Y	N	Y	Medium
Nagpal et al. [28]	Y	N	N	N	Y	Y	N	Y	Medium
Langalia et al. [26]	Y	Y	Y	N	Y	Y	N	Y	Low
Khan et al. [25]	Y	Y	Y	N	Y	Y	N	Y	Low
Dibaji et al. [22]	Y	Y	Y	N	Y	Y	N	Y	Low
Sandikci et al. [29]	Y	Y	Y	N	Y	Y	N	Y	Low

Y (Yes) indicates that the specific parameter was reported in the article
N (No) indicates that the specific parameter was not possible to be found in the article

group (unprepared and unfilled roots) were reported in nine studies [11, 12, 14, 22, 23, 26–29]. The results of the meta-analysis showed that the VRF resistance of negative control roots was significantly higher than that of roots in Gutta-percha/AH plus group (Fig. 2, SMD = – 0.69, 95% CI = – 1.34 to – 0.04, $p = 0.04$).

Resilon system group verse negative control group

Differences between a Resilon system group (roots filled with the Resion system) and a negative control group were investigated in eight studies [11, 14, 22–24, 26, 28, 29]. The results of the meta-analysis showed that the negative control roots had higher VRF resistance than roots

	Gutta-percha/AH plus			Negtive control				Std. Mean Difference
Study or Subgroup	Mean	SD	Total	Mean	SD	Total	Weight	IV, Random, 95% CI
Dibaji et al.2017	673.38	170.42	15	592.59	117.29	5	10.8%	0.48 [-0.54, 1.51]
Elmakki et al.2014	683.6	178.24	25	902.8	107.4	5	10.8%	-1.26 [-2.27, -0.24]
Hegde et al.2015	454	84.43	15	463	112.23	15	12.5%	-0.09 [-0.80, 0.63]
Jainaen et al. 2008	450.6	170.3	10	442.8	108.7	10	11.7%	0.05 [-0.82, 0.93]
Langalia et al.2015	200.2	21.96866	12	332.2	48.57022	12	9.2%	-3.38 [-4.70, -2.06]
Lertchirakarn et al.2002	246.9	23.6	10	324.2	35.3	5	8.1%	-2.62 [-4.16, -1.09]
Nagpal et al.2012	443.46	186.4223	15	466.9	96.7993	10	12.1%	-0.14 [-0.95, 0.66]
Sandikci et al.2014	424.02	108.18	20	464.36	134.6	10	12.3%	-0.33 [-1.10, 0.43]
Topçuoğlu et al.2013	452.97	95.65	15	470.68	110.89	15	12.5%	-0.17 [-0.88, 0.55]
Total (95% CI)			**137**			**87**	**100.0%**	**-0.69 [-1.34, -0.04]**

Heterogeneity: $Tau^2 = 0.73$; $Chi^2 = 35.82$, df = 8 ($P < 0.0001$); $I^2 = 78\%$
Test for overall effect: Z = 2.10 (P = 0.04)

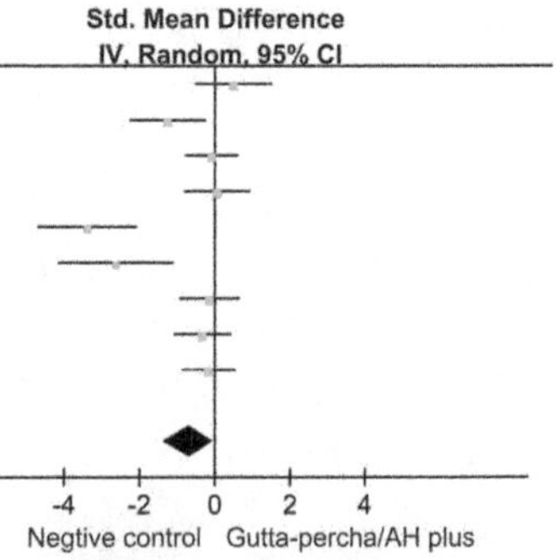

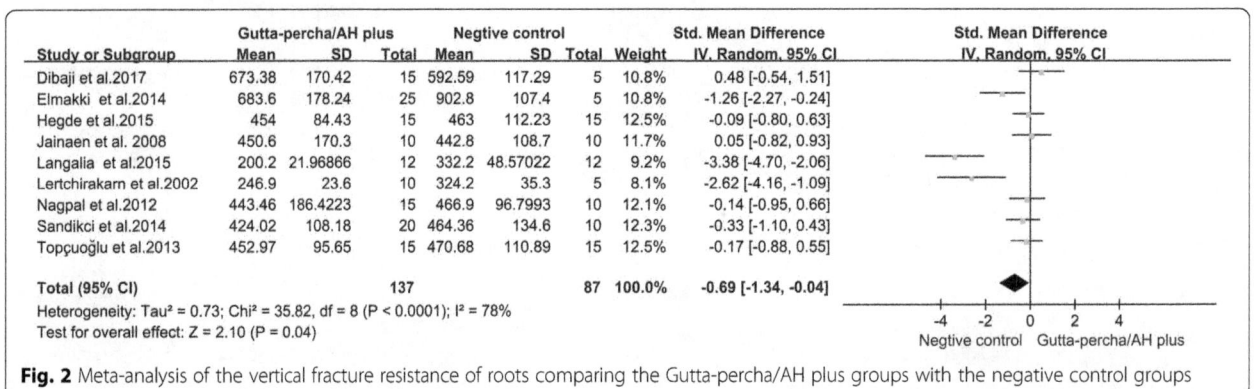

Fig. 2 Meta-analysis of the vertical fracture resistance of roots comparing the Gutta-percha/AH plus groups with the negative control groups

in Resilon system group (Fig. 3, SMD = – 0.54, 95% CI = – 1.07 to – 0.00, $p = 0.05$).

Gutta-percha/AH plus group verse positive control group

Eight studies [11–16, 23, 29] reported differences in VRF resistance between a positive control group (prepared but unfilled roots) and a Gutta-percha/AH plus group. The results of the meta-analysis showed no significant difference in VRF resistance between positive control roots and roots in Gutta-percha/AH plus group (Fig. 4, SMD = 0.59, 95% CI = – 0.02 to 1.21, $p = 0.06$).

Resilon system group verse positive control group

To investigate differences between a Resilon system group and a positive control group, the data from eight studies [11, 13–16, 23, 25, 29] were pooled. Analysis of the pooled data revealed that Resilon system filled roots were stronger than positive control roots (Fig. 5, SMD = 0.83, 95% CI = 0.44 to 1.22, $p < 0.0001$).

Gutta-percha/AH plus group verse Resilon system group

To investigate the differences between roots filled with Resilon and roots filled with Gutta-percha/AH plus, the data from ten studies [11, 13–16, 22, 23, 26, 28, 29] were pooled. The results of the meta-analysis showed that the Resilon-filled roots had higher VRF resistance than Gutta-percha/AH plus-filled roots (Fig. 6, SMD = 0.62, 95% CI = 0.01 to 1.23, $p = 0.05$).

Additional analysis

Substantial heterogeneity existed among several of the studies. Subgroup analysis was not performed due to a lack of related information in the included studies. Efforts were made to contact their corresponding authors, but no responses were received. We conducted a sensitivity analysis to investigate the influence of a single study on the overall effect size and thereby determine the stability of the results across studies. The results remain unchanged after we omitted any single study (Figs. 7, 8, 9, 10, 11), indicating that the results are statistically stable. Publication bias could not be evaluated because of the small number of trials included in the meta-analysis.

Discussion

VRF is often associated with the dehydration of dentin after endodontic therapy [30], removal of the root structure during root canal instrumentation [17, 19], loss of collagen cross-linking during root canal irrigation [31–34] or excessive pressure during root canal obturation [35]. At present, VRF has a high likelihood of occurring (up to 10.9%) after endodontic treatment [36]. Its occurrence typically leads to endodontic treatment failure and tooth extraction [37]. Therefore, it is important to seek an effective method to prevent VRF. Posts are typically used to reinforce endodontically treated roots [38–40]. However, their efficacy is very controversial, as it is associates with several factors which can influence the distribution of stress on the root canals and the amount of remaining dentin [41]. These factors include post type [42], length, diameter, material, and design [41], etc. If these factors are suitable, the posts might reinforce roots. If some of these factors are undesirable, the posts may play a negative role. Therefore, careful control of these factors must be taken when posts are used to reinforce endodontically treated teeth. Alternative methods to increase the VRF resistance of endodontically treated teeth have been investigated. Recently, obturating materials such as Gutta-percha and Resilon have been shown to influence the VRF resistance of root canals. However, there are different views in the literature with respect to whether these two materials can increase the postendodontic VRF resistance of roots and which one has a better reinforcement effect. These conflicting views make it difficult for clinicians to select the appropriate clinical approach. Therefore, a meta-analysis was performed to evaluate and compare the reinforcement efficacy of these two

	Resilon system			Negtive control				Std. Mean Difference
Study or Subgroup	Mean	SD	Total	Mean	SD	Total	Weight	IV, Random, 95% CI
Dibaji et al.2017	708.03	228.05	15	592.59	117.29	5	11.2%	0.53 [-0.50, 1.56]
Elmakki et al.2014	699.7	170.42	25	902.8	107.4	5	11.3%	-1.21 [-2.23, -0.20]
Hammad et al. 2007	146.31	49.64	13	245.26	41.29	10	11.0%	-2.06 [-3.12, -1.01]
Hegde et al.2015	470	107.54	15	463	112.23	15	14.2%	0.06 [-0.65, 0.78]
Jainaen et al. 2008	437.2	71.9	10	442.8	108.7	10	12.6%	-0.06 [-0.93, 0.82]
Langalia et al.2015	310	30.27283	12	332.2	48.57022	12	13.2%	-0.53 [-1.35, 0.29]
Nagpal et al.2012	453.8	119.5051	15	466.9	96.7993	10	13.4%	-0.11 [-0.91, 0.69]
Sandikci et al.2014	328	109.09	20	464.36	134.6	10	13.2%	-1.13 [-1.94, -0.31]
Total (95% CI)			**125**			**77**	**100.0%**	**-0.54 [-1.07, -0.00]**

Heterogeneity: $Tau^2 = 0.39$; $Chi^2 = 20.68$, df = 7 (P = 0.004); $I^2 = 66\%$
Test for overall effect: Z = 1.97 (P = 0.05)

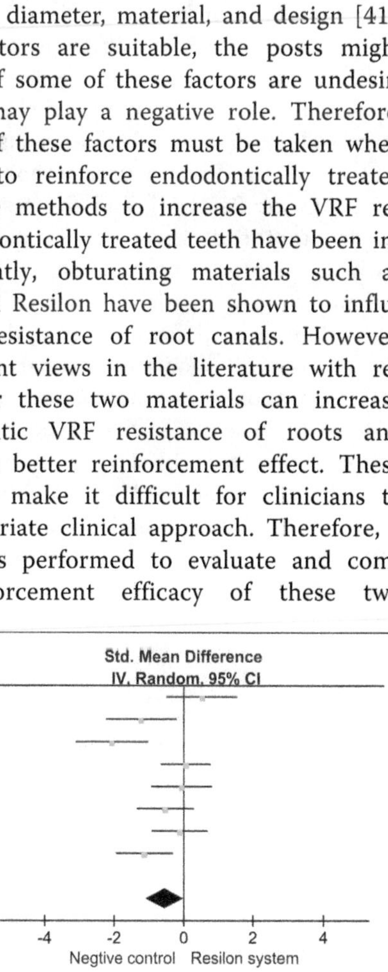

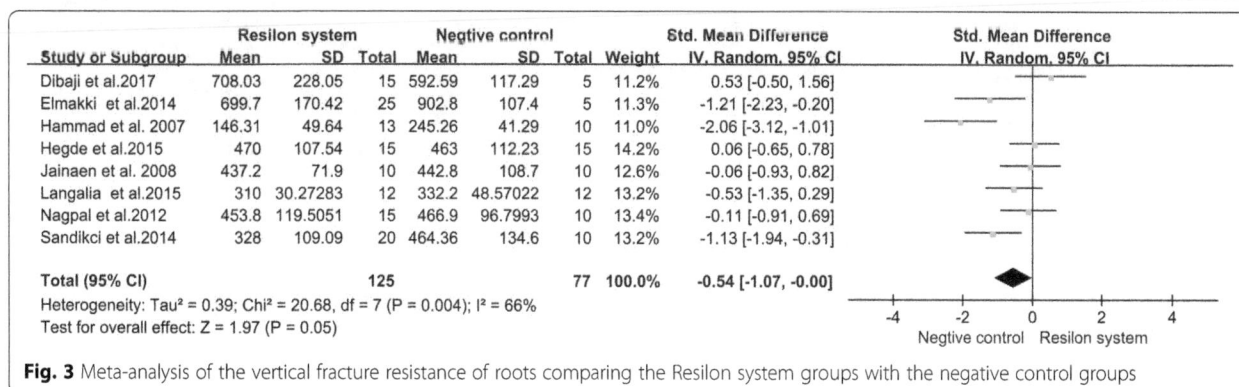

Fig. 3 Meta-analysis of the vertical fracture resistance of roots comparing the Resilon system groups with the negative control groups

Study or Subgroup	Gutta-percha/AH plus Mean	SD	Total	Positive control Mean	SD	Total	Weight	Std. Mean Difference IV, Random, 95% CI
Baba et al.2010	536.555	128.816	20	591.066	68.97	20	13.5%	-0.52 [-1.15, 0.11]
Elmakki et al.2014	683.6	178.24	25	547.2	63.7	5	11.2%	0.80 [-0.19, 1.78]
Hegde et al.2015	454	84.43	15	340	140.26	15	12.7%	0.96 [0.20, 1.72]
Jainaen et al. 2008	450.6	170.3	10	410.4	79.7	10	11.9%	0.29 [-0.59, 1.17]
Kumar et al. 2014	238.8	0.87	20	239.24	1.94	20	13.5%	-0.29 [-0.91, 0.34]
Monteiro et al.2011	414.72	111.86	20	395.79	171.41	20	13.6%	0.13 [-0.49, 0.75]
Sandikci et al.2014	424.02	108.18	20	206.01	94	10	11.5%	2.04 [1.10, 2.98]
Topçuoğlu et al.2013	452.97	95.65	15	320.19	49.45	15	12.1%	1.70 [0.85, 2.55]
Total (95% CI)			**145**			**115**	**100.0%**	**0.59 [-0.02, 1.21]**

Heterogeneity: Tau² = 0.64; Chi² = 36.90, df = 7 (P < 0.00001); I² = 81%
Test for overall effect: Z = 1.88 (P = 0.06)

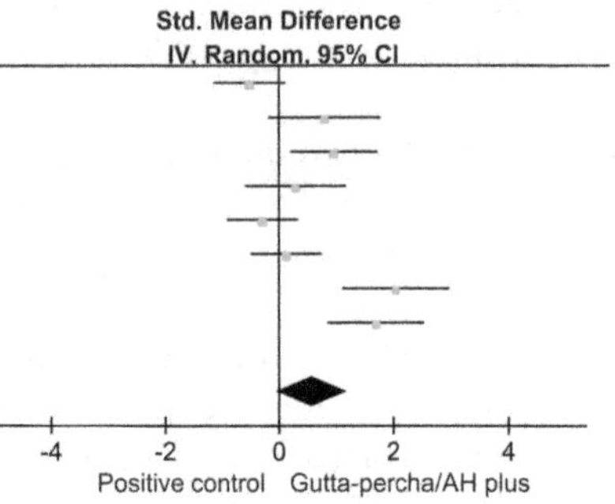

Fig. 4 Meta-analysis of the vertical fracture resistance of roots comparing the Gutta-percha/AH plus groups with the positive control groups

obturation systems on endodontically treated root canals. The results can offer guidance to clinicians in evidence-based decision making.

The results of this meta-analysis indicate that root canals filled with Resilon have higher fracture resistance than do prepared unfilled roots or roots filled with Gutta-percha/AH plus. These results can be attributed to the "monoblock" concept. According to Tay FR [43], a monoblock is a gap-free, solid and mechanically homogeneous mass in the root canal space that consists of different bondable materials and interfaces, which can facilitate favorable root canal sealing and simultaneously reinforce the filled canal [44, 45]. When Resilon is used to obturate a root canal, the Resilon core is bonded to the sealer (Epiphany or Realseal), and the resulting complex is bonded to the dentinal wall of the root canal [46], forming a monoblock system [47]. Resilon is a thermoplastic synthetic polymer composed of polyester with improved flexural strength. Compared with Gutta-percha, Resilon shows superior bonding potential when applied in combination with a resin-based sealer [15]. Therefore, the Resilon system has a superior ability to reinforce instrumented roots than dose the Gutta-percha/AH plus obturation system.

This meta-analysis found no significant difference in VRF resistance between prepared unfilled roots and Gutta-percha/AH plus obturated roots. Gutta-percha/AH plus has been accepted as the standard obturating system in root canal treatment. However, although the adhesive strength between the AH-plus sealer and the dentine wall is favorable [48], there is no chemical adhesion between Gutta-percha and AH-plus [8]; therefore, no monoblock system is formed, and no reinforcement is provided to the roots [49].

There was considerable heterogeneity among the included studies, which was primarily associated with methodological diversity. This diversity included differences in the type of tooth, root canal filling techniques and irrigation fluids, etc. The articles included in this meta-analysis involved different types of teeth, such as single-rooted straight maxillary anterior teeth, mandibular anterior teeth and mandibular premolars. Variation in root canal anatomies and root morphologies might affect fracture resistance of roots slightly [50]. In addition, the investigators in the eligible studies used different obturation techniques, including a lateral compaction technique and a single cone technique. The lateral compaction technique does not produce a homogeneous mass because the core material and accessory cones always remain separated, and the excessive wedge force while compacting may lead to initial root cracks [51], which might cause bias to the

Study or Subgroup	Resilon system Mean	SD	Total	Positive control Mean	SD	Total	Weight	Std. Mean Difference IV, Random, 95% CI
Baba et al.2010	885.943	194.41	20	591.066	68.97	20	12.1%	1.98 [1.21, 2.75]
Elmakki et al.2014	699.7	170.42	25	547.2	63.7	5	9.2%	0.93 [-0.06, 1.92]
Hegde et al.2015	470	107.54	15	340	140.26	15	12.1%	1.01 [0.25, 1.78]
Jainaen et al. 2008	437.2	71.9	10	410.4	79.7	10	10.5%	0.34 [-0.55, 1.22]
Khan et al. 2015	309.16	53.74	30	283.33	27.97	30	16.2%	0.60 [0.08, 1.11]
Kumar et al. 2014	239.42	0.001	20	239.24	1.94	20	14.4%	0.13 [-0.49, 0.75]
Monteiro et al.2011	510.11	143.38	20	395.79	171.41	20	14.1%	0.71 [0.07, 1.35]
Sandikci et al.2014	328.72	109.79	20	206.01	94	10	11.4%	1.14 [0.32, 1.96]
Total (95% CI)			**160**			**130**	**100.0%**	**0.83 [0.44, 1.22]**

Heterogeneity: Tau² = 0.18; Chi² = 16.25, df = 7 (P = 0.02); I² = 57%
Test for overall effect: Z = 4.14 (P < 0.0001)

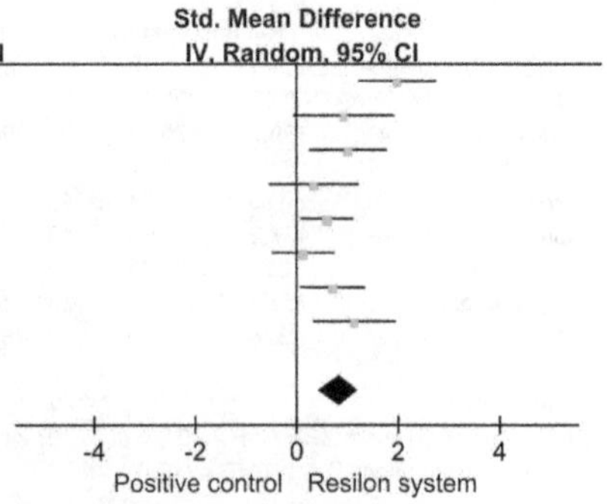

Fig. 5 Meta-analysis of the vertical fracture resistance of roots comparing the Resilon system groups with the positive control groups

Study or Subgroup	Resilon system Mean	SD	Total	Gutta-percha/AH plus Mean	SD	Total	Weight	Std. Mean Difference IV, Random, 95% CI
Baba et al.2010	885.943	194.41	20	536.555	128.816	20	10.0%	2.08 [1.29, 2.86]
Dibaji et al.2017	708.03	228.05	15	673.38	170.42	15	10.3%	0.17 [-0.55, 0.88]
Elmakki et al.2014	699.7	170.42	25	683.6	178.24	25	10.9%	0.09 [-0.46, 0.65]
Hegde et al.2015	470	107.54	15	454	84.43	15	10.3%	0.16 [-0.56, 0.88]
Jainaen et al. 2008	437.2	71.9	10	450.6	170.3	10	9.6%	-0.10 [-0.98, 0.78]
Kumar et al. 2014	239.42	0.001	20	238.8	0.87	20	10.5%	0.99 [0.33, 1.65]
Langalia et al.2015	310	30.27283	12	200.2	21.96866	12	7.0%	4.01 [2.53, 5.48]
Monteiro et al.2011	510.11	143.38	20	414.72	111.86	20	10.6%	0.73 [0.08, 1.37]
Nagpal et al.2012	453.8	119.5051	15	443.46	186.4223	15	10.3%	0.06 [-0.65, 0.78]
Sandikci et al.2014	328.72	109.09	20	424.02	108.18	20	10.5%	-0.86 [-1.51, -0.21]
Total (95% CI)			**172**			**172**	**100.0%**	**0.62 [0.01, 1.23]**

Heterogeneity: Tau² = 0.81; Chi² = 63.07, df = 9 (P < 0.00001); I² = 86%
Test for overall effect: Z = 1.99 (P = 0.05)

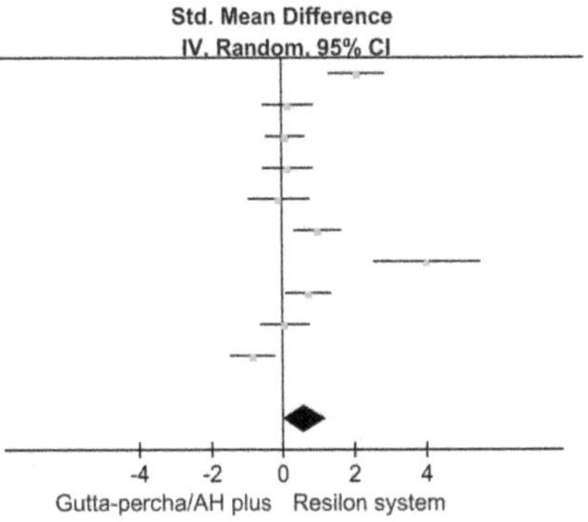

Fig. 6 Meta-analysis of the vertical fracture resistance of roots comparing the Resilon system groups with the Gutta-percha/AH plus groups

results of the studies with this technique and then affect the conclusion of our meta-analysis. Single cone techniques are often reliant upon sealers and may not densely obturate the canal in 3 dimensions [52], which may affect the efficacy of the obturating materials in reinforcing the roots. Furthermore, the irrigation step may influence the bonding of the obturating materials to the dentinal surface of the root. In all of the included studies, the investigators used ethylene diamine tetraacetic acid (EDTA) and sodium hypochlorite (NaClO) to remove the smear layer. However, the final irrigations differed among the studies. According to Lertchirakarn et al. [27], the high resistance of Resilon-obturated canals to fracture might be due to the clearance of the smear layer by EDTA after instrumentation which allowed the sealer to contact the canal wall and penetrate the dentinal tubules, resulting in increased root strength. In addition, it was reported that NaClO is not appropriate as the last irrigation to remove the smear layer because the residual solution may have adverse effects on the bonding strength of the primer to the dentine and may inhibit the curing of resin materials [53]. In contrast, Varela et al. [54] reported that the effect of NaClO on the polymerization of the sealer could be neglected. Due to these conflicting conclusions, the influence of final irrigation on the efficacy of the obturating materials in strengthening the roots remains unclear.

To our knowledge, this study presents the first meta-analysis performed to evaluate and compare the effects of Gutta-percha/AH plus and the Resilon system in reinforcing endodontically treated root canals. Strict inclusion and exclusion criteria were established. Only randomized controlled trials were included. Exhaustive searches of the relevant literature were performed. Fourteen studies were ultimately included. The risk of bias of these studies was strictly evaluated. Most of the included studies are well-designed research studies. A sensitivity analysis was used to explore the stability of results.

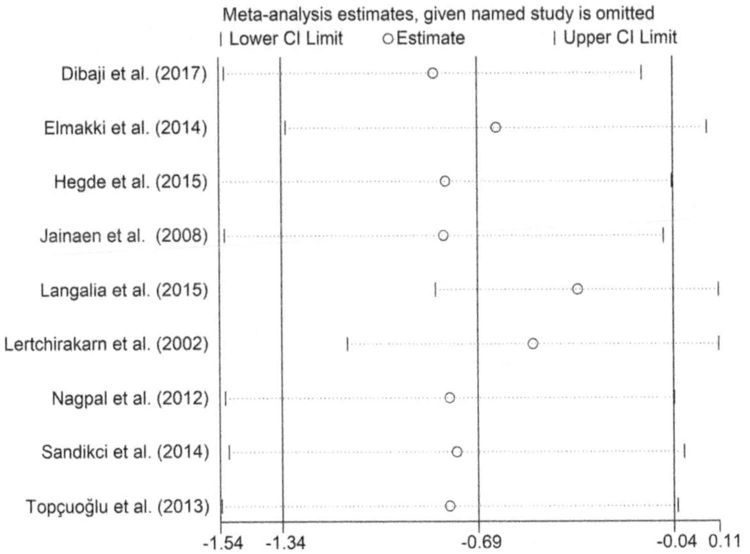

Fig. 7 Sensitive analysis of differences between the Gutta-percha/AH plus groups and the negative control groups

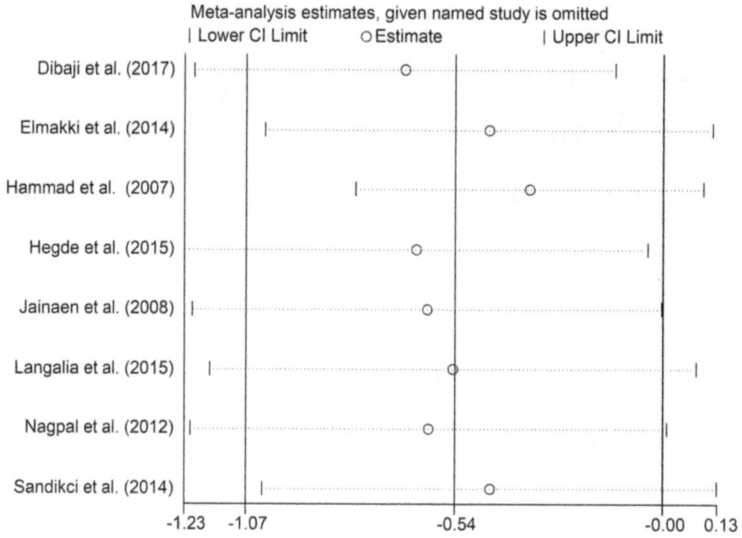

Fig. 8 Sensitive analysis of differences between the Resilon system groups and the negative control groups

The SMDs and 95% CIs did not change significantly when any one trial was removed. Therefore, our results are stable.

Although the meta-analysis was carefully conducted, some limitations remain. First, publication bias could not be evaluated because of the small number of trials included in the meta-analysis. Second, a medium risk of bias was found in some of the included studies. These studies scored especially poorly on the items including calculation of sample size and blinding of the examiner. Third, the meta-analysis is based on the findings of in vitro studies that were of low level of evidence. An in vitro approach is sometimes the only practical approach for medical or bio-medical research. However, in vitro studies have intrinsic limitations when attempting to accurately simulate biological, chemical or physical conditions in vivo [55, 56]. Although fracture resistance testing can be used to evaluate the fracture resistance of root canals filled with different materials, factors such as the temperature cycling, the wet environment, the direction of masticatory force, the frequency of loading and the presence of periodontal membrane need to be considered because they may affect the fracture resistance of roots in vivo. Therefore, the results of in vitro studies cannot be validly extrapolated to the clinical context. Even so, mechanical testing methods can offer useful

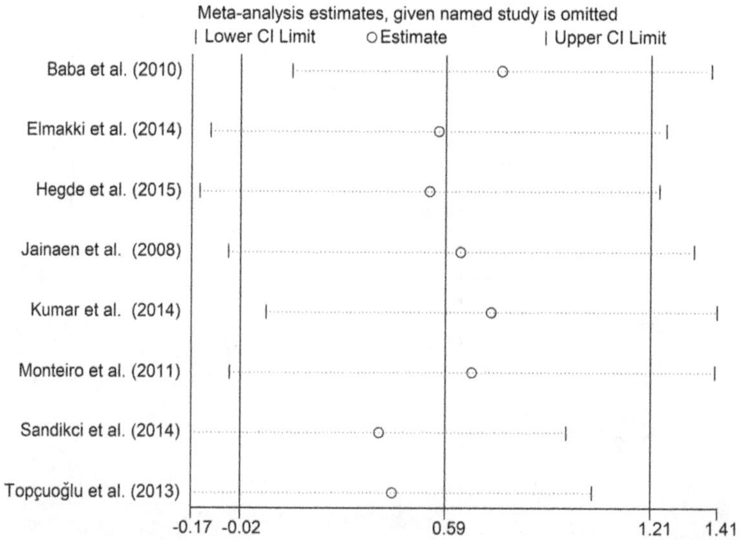

Fig. 9 Sensitive analysis of differences between the Gutta-percha/AH plus groups and the positive control groups

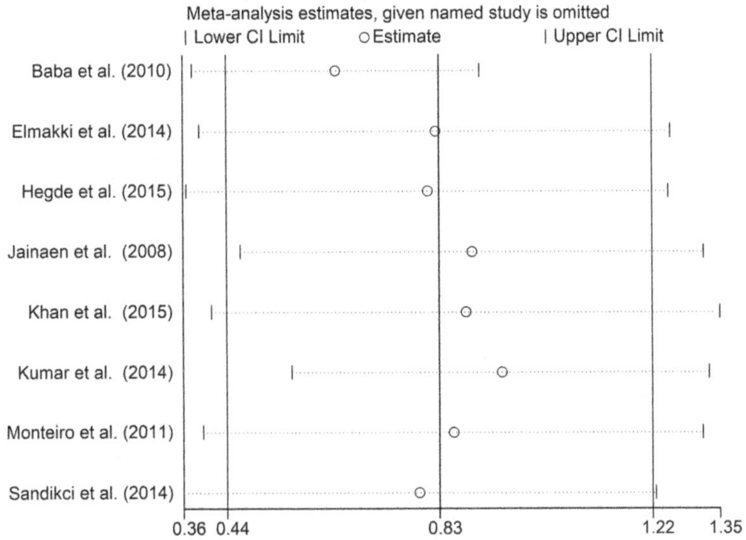

Fig. 10 Sensitive analysis of differences between the Resilon system groups and the positive control groups

information to identify substrate variables [57–60] and then provide guidance for application procedures [61, 62]. Thus, a meta-analysis based on in vitro studies is helpful to clinical practice, especially in the absence of evidence based on well-designed clinical trials [63–65]. Moreover, such a meta-analysis can suggest improvements and standardized methodologies for future studies [66, 67].

In consideration of the above results and limitations, we suggest that future randomized controlled studies perform appropriate sample size calculations, randomization and blinding, and control potentially confounding factors. Moreover, well-designed randomized controlled clinical trials are needed to evaluate the incidence of VRF of endodontically treated teeth while using these two obturating materials.

Conclusions

In conclusion, the present study suggests that filling the canals with Gutta-percha/AH plus fails to reinforce endodontically treated root canals, whereas the Resilon obturation system can increase the VRF resistance of prepared roots. It is to be noted that the conclusion should be interpreted cautiously because this meta-analysis was based on in vitro studies.

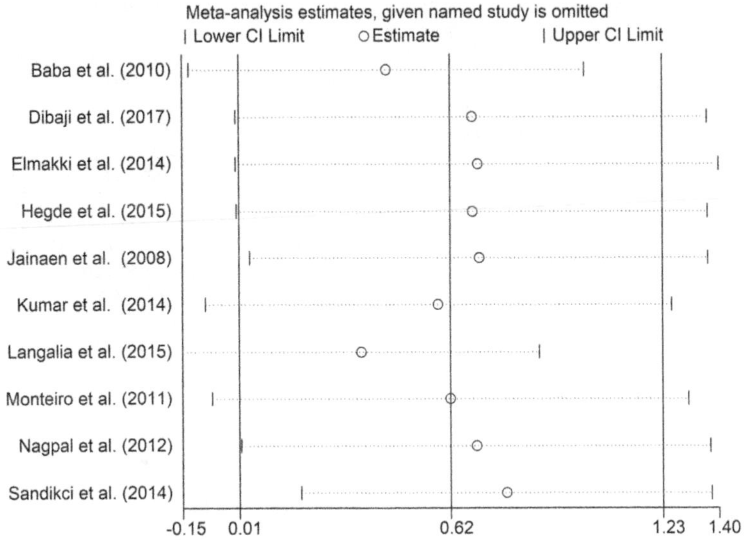

Fig. 11 Sensitive analysis of differences between the Resilon system groups and the Gutta-percha/AH plus groups

Abbreviations
CI: Confidence interval; EDTA: Ethylene diamine tetraacetic acid; NaClO: Sodium hypochlorite; SD: Standard deviation; SMD: Standardized mean difference; VRF: Vertical root fracture

Funding
This research was supported by the Project Supported by Program for Innovation Team Building at Institutions of Higher Education in Chongqing in 2016 (NO CXTDG201602006), the Project Supported by Chongqing Municipal Key Laboratory of Oral Biomedical Engineering of Higher Education, and the Medical Research Program of Chongqing Health and Family Planning Commission in 2015 (2015MSXM045). None of the funders played a role in the design of the study, data collection, analyses, and interpretation of the results or writing of the manuscript.

Authors' contributions
MMT and ZWC conceived the study. MMT and ZWC conducted the literature search. CJS and BH screened the results. YJC and XG performed the data extraction. MMT, ZWC, CJS, BH, YJC, XG and JLS contributed to the statistical analyses. MMT drafted the manuscript. BH and JLS contributed to the revision of the paper. All authors made substantial contribution to the drafting or revision of the manuscript for critically important intellectual content. All authors read and approved the final version to be published. Furthermore, all authors have agreed to be accountable for all aspects of the work in ensuring that questions related to the accuracy or integrity of any part of the work are appropriately investigated and solved.

Authors' information
Ms. MMT is a postgraduate student, College of Stomatology, Chongqing Medical University; a postgraduate student, Chongqing Key Laboratory of Oral Diseases and Biomedical Sciences; and a postgraduate student, Chongqing Municipal Key Laboratory of Oral Biomedical Engineering of Higher Education, Chongqing, China.
Dr. ZWC is a lecturer, College of Stomatology, Chongqing Medical University; a lecturer, Chongqing Key Laboratory of Oral Diseases and Biomedical Sciences; and a lecturer, Chongqing Municipal Key Laboratory of Oral Biomedical Engineering of Higher Education, Chongqing, China.
Ms. CJS is a postgraduate student, College of Stomatology, Chongqing Medical University; a postgraduate student, Chongqing Key Laboratory of Oral Diseases and Biomedical Sciences; and a postgraduate student, Chongqing Municipal Key Laboratory of Oral Biomedical Engineering of Higher Education, Chongqing, China.
Dr. BH is a lecturer, College of Stomatology, Chongqing Medical University; a lecturer, Chongqing Key Laboratory of Oral Diseases and Biomedical Sciences; and a lecturer, Chongqing Municipal Key Laboratory of Oral Biomedical Engineering of Higher Education, Chongqing, China.
Dr. XG is a lecturer, College of Stomatology, Chongqing Medical University; a lecturer, Chongqing Key Laboratory of Oral Diseases and Biomedical Sciences; and a lecturer, Chongqing Municipal Key Laboratory of Oral Biomedical Engineering of Higher Education, Chongqing, China.
Dr. YJC is a lecturer, College of Stomatology, Chongqing Medical University; a lecturer, Chongqing Key Laboratory of Oral Diseases and Biomedical Sciences; and a lecturer, Chongqing Municipal Key Laboratory of Oral Biomedical Engineering of Higher Education, Chongqing, China.
Dr. JLS is a professor, College of Stomatology, Chongqing Medical University; a professor, Chongqing Key Laboratory of Oral Diseases and Biomedical Sciences; and a professor, Chongqing Municipal Key Laboratory of Oral Biomedical Engineering of Higher Education, Chongqing, China.

Competing interests
The authors declare that they have no competing interests.

Author details
[1]College of Stomatology, Chongqing Medical University, Chongqing, China. [2]Chongqing Key Laboratory of Oral Diseases and Biomedical Sciences, College of Stomatology, Chongqing Medical University, Chongqing, China. [3]Chongqing Municipal Key Laboratory of Oral Biomedical Engineering of Higher Education, College of Stomatology, Chongqing Medical University, Chongqing, China. [4]Stomatological Hospital affiliated to Chongqing Medical University, No. 426, N. Songshi Rd, Chongqing 401147, China.

References
1. Çobankara FK, Üngör M, Belli S. The effect of two different root canal sealers and smear layer on resistance to root fracture. J Endod. 2002;28(8):606–9. https://doi.org/10.1097/00004770-200208000-00011.
2. Karapinar KM, Sunay H, Tanalp J, Bayirli G. Fracture resistance of roots using different canal filling systems. Int Endond J. 2009;42(8):705–10. https://doi.org/10.1111/j.1365-2591.2009.01571.x.
3. Lam PP, Palamara JE, Messer HH. Fracture strength of tooth roots following canal preparation by hand and rotary instrumentation. Aust Endod J. 2005; 31(2):529–32. https://doi.org/10.1097/01.don.0000150947.90682.a0.
4. D'Arcangelo C, De AF, Vadini M, D'Amario M, Caputi S. Fracture resistance and deflection of pulpless anterior teeth restored with composite or porcelain veneers. J Endod. 2010;36(1):153–6. https://doi.org/10.1016/j.joen.2009.09.036.
5. Ozcopur B, Akman S, Eskitascioglu G, Belli S. The effect of different posts on fracture strength of roots with vertical fracture and re-attached fragments. J Oral Rehabil. 2010;37(8):615–23. https://doi.org/10.1111/j.1365-2842.2010.02086.x.
6. Bortoluzzi EA, Souza EM, Reis JMSN, Esberard RM, Tanomaru-Filho M. Fracture strength of bovine incisors after intra-radicular treatment with MTA in an experimental immature model. Int Endod J. 2010;40(9):684–91. https://doi.org/10.1111/j.1365-2591.2007.01266.x.
7. Johnson ME, Stewart GP, Nielsen CJ, Hatton JF. Evaluation of root reinforcement of endodontically treated teeth. Oral Surg Oral Med Oral Pathol Oral Radiol Endod. 2000;90(3):360–4. https://doi.org/10.1067/moe.2000.108951.
8. Teixeira FB, Teixeira ECN, Thompson JY, Trope M. Fracture resistance of roots endodontically treated with a new resin filling material. J Am Dent Assoc. 2004;135(5):646–52. https://doi.org/10.14219/jada.archive.2004.0255.
9. Pascon EA, Spangberg LS. In vitro cytotoxicity of root canal filling materials: 1. Gutta-percha. J Endod. 1990;16(9):429–33. https://doi.org/10.1016/S0099-2399(06)81885-6.
10. Bhat SS, Hegde SK, Rao A, Shaji Mohammed AK. Evaluation of resistance of teeth subjected to fracture after endodontic treatment using different root canal sealers: an in vitro study. J Indian Soc Pedod Prev Dent. 2012;30(4): 305–9. https://doi.org/10.4103/0970-4388.108926.
11. Hegde V, Arora S. Fracture resistance of roots obturated with novel hydrophilic obturation systems. J Conserv Dent. 2015;18(3):261–4. https://doi.org/10.4103/0972-0707.154047.
12. Topçuoğlu HS, Tuncay Ö, Karataş E, Arslan H, Yeter K. In vitro fracture resistance of roots obturated with epoxy resin-based, mineral trioxide aggregate-based. and bioceramic root canal sealers J Endod. 2013;39(12): 1630–3. https://doi.org/10.1016/j.joen.2013.07.034.
13. Baba SM, Grover SI, Tyagi V. Fracture resistance of teeth obturated with Gutta percha and Resilon: an in vitro study. J Conserv Dent. 2010;13(2):61–4. https://doi.org/10.4103/0972-0707.66712.
14. Jainaen A, Palamara JE, Messer HH. The effect of resin-based sealers on fracture properties of dentine. Int Endod J. 2009;42(2):136–43. https://doi.org/10.1111/j.1365-2591.2008.01496.x.
15. Kumar P, Kaur NM, Arora S, Dixit S. Evaluation of fracture resistance of roots obturated with resilon and thermoplasticized gutta-percha: an in vitro study. J Conserv Dent. 2014;17(4):354–8. https://doi.org/10.4103/0972-0707.136510.
16. Monteiro J. de Noronha de Ataide I, Chalakkal P, Chandra PK. In vitro resistance to fracture of roots obturated with Resilon or Gutta-percha. J Endod. 2011;37(6):828–31. https://doi.org/10.1016/j.joen.2011.02.024.
17. Schäfer E, Zandbiglari T, Schäfer J. Influence of resin-based adhesive root canal fillings on the resistance to fracture of endodontically treated roots:

an in vitro preliminary study. Oral Surg Oral Med Oral Pathol Oral Radiol Endod. 2007;103(2):274–9. https://doi.org/10.1016/j.tripleo.2006.06.054.

18. Zamin C, Silva-Sousa YTC, Souza-Gabriel AE, Messias DF, Sousa-Neto MD. Fracture susceptibility of endodontically treated teeth. Dent Traumatol. 2012;28(4):282–6. https://doi.org/10.1111/j.1600-9657.2011.01087.x.
19. Zandbiglari T, Davids H, Schäfer E. Influence of instrument taper on the resistance to fracture of endodontically treated roots. Oral Surg Oral Med Oral Pathol Oral Radiol Endod. 2006;101(1):126–31. https://doi.org/10.1016/j.tripleo.2005.01.019.
20. Mohammadi Z, Jafarzadeh H, Shalavi S, Bhandi S, Kinoshita J. Resilon: review of a new material for obturation of the canal. J Contemp Dent Pract. 2015;16(5):407–14. https://doi.org/10.5005/jp-journals-10024-1698.
21. Soares C, Maia C, Vale F, Gadêneto C, Carvalho L, Oliveira H, et al. Comparison of endodontic retreatment in teeth obturated with Resilon or Gutta-Percha: a review of literature. Iran Endod J. 2015;10(4):221–5.
22. Dibaji F, Afkhami F, Bidkhori B, Kharazifard MJ. Fracture resistance of roots after application of different sealers. Iran Endod J. 2017;12(1):50–4.
23. Elmakki F, Abu-bakr N, Ibrahim Y. Fracture resistance of Resilon/epiphany and Gutta percha/AH plus. Indian J Dent. 2013;5(1):17–20. https://doi.org/10.1016/j.ijd.2013.11.002.
24. Hammad M, Qualtrough A, Silikas N. Effect of new obturating materials on vertical root fracture resistance of endodontically treated teeth. J Endod. 2007;33(6):732–6. https://doi.org/10.1016/j.joen.2007.02.004.
25. Khan S, Inamdar MN, Munaga S, Ali SA, Rawtiya M, Ahmad E. Evaluation of fracture resistance of endodontically treated teeth filled with Gutta-Percha and Resilon obturating material: an in vitro study. J Int Oral Health. 2015;7(Suppl 2):21–5.
26. Langalia AK, Dave B, Patel N, Thakkar V, Sheth S, Parekh V. Comparative evaluation of fracture resistance of endodontically treated teeth obturated with resin based adhesive sealers with conventional obturation technique: an in vitro study. J Int Oral Health. 2015;7(2):6–12.
27. Lertchirakarn V, Timyam A, Messer HH. Effects of root canal sealers on vertical root fracture resistance of endodontically treated teeth. J Endod. 2002;28(3):217–9. https://doi.org/10.1097/00004770-200203000-00018.
28. Nagpal A, Annapoorna BM, Prashanth MB, Prashanth NT, Singla M, Deepak BS, et al. A comparative evaluation of the vertical root fracture resistance of endodontically treated teeth using different root canal sealers: an in vitro study. J Contemp Dent Pract. 2012;13(3):351–5. https://doi.org/10.5005/jp-journals-10024-1150.
29. Sandikci T, Kaptan RF. Comparative evaluation of the fracture resistances of endodontically treated teeth filled using five different root canal filling systems. Niger J Clin Pract. 2014;17(6):667–72. https://doi.org/10.4103/1119-3077.144375.
30. Helfer AR, Melnick S, Schilder H. Determination of the moisture content of vital and pulpless teeth. Oral Surg Oral Med Oral Pathol Oral Radiol. 1972;34(4):661–70. https://doi.org/10.1016/0030-4220(72)90351-9.
31. Ari H, Erdemir A, Belli S. Evaluation of the effect of endodontic irrigation solutions on the microhardness and the roughness of root canal dentin. J Endod. 2004;30(11):792–5. https://doi.org/10.1097/01.DON.0000128747.89857.59.
32. Cruz-Filho AM, Sousa-Neto MD, Saquy PC, Pécora JD. Evaluation of the effect of EDTAC, CDTA, and EGTA on radicular dentin microhardness. J Endod. 2001;27(3):183–4. https://doi.org/10.1097/00004770-200103000-00011.
33. Rivera EM, Yamauchi M. Site comparisons of dentine collagen cross-links from extracted human teeth. Arch Oral Biol. 1993;38(7):541–6. https://doi.org/10.1016/0003-9969(93)90118-6.
34. Slutzkygoldberg I, Maree M, Liberman R, Heling I. Effect of sodium hypochlorite on dentin microhardness. J Endod. 2004;30(12):880–2. https://doi.org/10.1097/01.DON.0000128748.05148.1E.
35. Holcomb JQ, Pitts DL, Nicholls JI. Further investigation of spreader loads required to cause vertical root fracture during lateral condensation. J Endod. 1987;13(6):277–84. https://doi.org/10.1016/S0099-2399(87)80044-4.
36. Fuss Z, Lustig J, Tamse A. Prevalence of vertical root fractures in extracted endodontically treated teeth. Int Endod J. 1999;32(4):283–6. https://doi.org/10.1046/j.1365-2591.1999.00208.x.
37. Tsesis I, Rosen E, Tamse A, Taschieri S, Kfir A. Diagnosis of vertical root fractures in endodontically treated teeth based on clinical and radiographic indices: a systematic review. J Endod. 2010;36(9):1455–8. https://doi.org/10.1016/j.joen.2010.05.003.
38. Assif D, Gorfil C. Biomechanical considerations in restoring endodontically treated teeth. J Prosthet Dent. 1994;71(6):565–7. https://doi.org/10.1016/0022-3913(94)90438-3.
39. Cohen BI, Pagnillo M, Condos S, Deutsch AS. Comparison of the torsional forces at failure for seven endodontic post systems. J Prosthet Dent. 1995;74(4):350–7. https://doi.org/10.1016/S0022-3913(05)80373-7.
40. Gutmann JL. The dentin-root complex: anatomic and biologic considerations in restoring endodontically treated teeth. J Prosthet Dent. 1992;67(4):458. https://doi.org/10.1016/0022-3913(92)90073-J.
41. Fernandes AS, Dessai GS. Factors affecting the fracture resistance of post-core reconstructed teeth: a review. Int J Prosthodont. 2001;14(4):355–63.
42. Testori T, Badino M, Castagnola M. Vertical root fractures in endodontically treated teeth: a clinical survey of 36 cases. J Endod. 1993;19(2):87–91. https://doi.org/10.1016/S0099-2399(06)81202-1.
43. Tay FR, Pashley DH. Monoblocks in root canals: a hypothetical or a tangible goal. J Endod. 2007;33(4):391–8. https://doi.org/10.1016/j.joen.2006.10.009.
44. Schwartz RS. Adhesive dentistry and endodontics. Part 2: bonding in the root canal system-the promise and the problems: a review. J Endod. 2006;32(12):1125–34. https://doi.org/10.1016/j.joen.2006.08.003.
45. Teixeira FB, Teixeira EC, Thompson J, Leinfelder KF, Trope M. Dentinal bonding reaches the root canal system. J Esthet Restor Dent. 2004;16(6):348–54. https://doi.org/10.1111/j.1708-8240.2004.tb00066.x.
46. Shipper G, D Ø, Teixeira FB, Trope M. An evaluation of microbial leakage in roots filled with a thermoplastic synthetic polymer-based root canal filling material (Resilon). J Endod. 2004;30(5):342–7. https://doi.org/10.1097/00004770-200405000-00009.
47. Belli S, Eraslan O, Eskitascioglu G, Karbhari V. Monoblocks in root canals: a finite elemental stress analysis study. Int Endod J. 2011;44(9):817–26. https://doi.org/10.1111/j.1365-2591.2011.01885.x.
48. Sousa-Neto MD, Marchesan MA, Pécora JD, Junior AB, Silva-Sousa YT, Saquy PC. Effect of Er:YAG laser on adhesion of root canal sealers. J Endod. 2002;28(3):185. https://doi.org/10.1097/00004770-200203000-00010.
49. Aptekar A, Ginnan K. Comparative analysis of microleakage and seal for 2 obturation materials: Resilon/epiphany and gutta-percha. J Can Dent Assoc. 2006;72(3):245.
50. Obermayr G, Walton RE, Leary JM, Krell KV. Vertical root fracture and relative deformation during obturation and post cementation. J Prosthet Dent. 1991;66(2):181–7. https://doi.org/10.1016/S0022-3913(05)80045-9.
51. Meister F Jr, Lommel TJ, Gerstein H. Diagnosis and possible causes of vertical root fractures. Oral Surg Oral Med Oral Pathol. 1980;49(3):243–53. https://doi.org/10.1016/0030-4220(80)90056-0.
52. Whitworth J. Methods of filling root canals: principles and practices. Endod Top. 2005;12(1):2–24. https://doi.org/10.1111/j.1601-1546.2005.00198.x.
53. Darcey J, Roudsari RV, Jawad S, Taylor C, Hunter M. Modern endodontic principles. Part 5: obturation. Dent Update. 2016;43(2):114–6. 119–20, 123–6. doi: https://doi.org/10.12968/denu.2016.43.2.114
54. Varela SG, Rábade LB, Lombardero PR, Sixto JM, Bahillo JD, Park SA. In vitro study of endodontic post cementation protocols that use resin cements. J Prosthet Dent. 2003;89(2):146–53. https://doi.org/10.1067/mpr.2003.84.
55. Sarkisonofre R, Skupien JA, Cenci MS, Moraes RR, Pereiracenci T. The role of resin cement on bond strength of glass-fiber posts luted into root canals: a systematic review and meta-analysis of in vitro studies. Oper Dent. 2014;39(1):E31–44. https://doi.org/10.2341/13-070-LIT.
56. Masarwa N, Mohamed A, Abourabii I, Abu ZR, Steier L. Longevity of self-etch dentin bonding adhesives compared to etch-and-rinse dentin bonding adhesives: a systematic review. J Evid Based Dent Pract. 2016;16(2):96–106. https://doi.org/10.1016/j.jebdp.2016.03.003.
57. Frankenberger R, Krämer N, Lohbauer U, Nikolaenko SA, Reich SM. Marginal integrity: is the clinical performance of bonded restorations predictable in vitro? J Adhes Dent. 2007;9(Suppl 1):107–16. https://doi.org/10.3290/j.jad.a11974.
58. Hebling J, Castro FL, Costa CA. Adhesive performance of dentin bonding agents applied in vivo and in vitro. Effect of intrapulpal pressure and dentin depth. J Biomed Mater Res B Appl Biomater. 2007;83(2):295–303. https://doi.org/10.1002/jbm.b.30795.
59. Shono Y, Ogawa T, Terashita M, Carvalho RM, Pashley EL, Pashley DH. Regional measurement of resin-dentin bonding as an array. J Dent Res. 1999;78(2):699–705. https://doi.org/10.1177/00220345990780021001.
60. Shono Y, Terashita M, Pashley EL, Brewer PD, Pashley DH. Effects of cross-sectional area on resin-enamel tensile bond strength. Dent Mater. 1997;13(5):290–6. https://doi.org/10.1016/S0109-5641(97)80098-X.
61. Braga RR, Meira JBC, Boaro LCC, Xavier TA. Adhesion to tooth structure: a critical review of "macro" test methods. Dent Mater. 2010;26(2):e38–49. https://doi.org/10.1016/j.dental.2009.11.150.

62. Hashimoto M, Tay FR, Svizero NR, de Gee AJ, Feilzer AJ, Sano H, et al. The effects of common errors on sealing ability of total-etch adhesives. Dent Mater. 2007;97(2):560–8. https://doi.org/10.1016/j.dental.2005.06.004.
63. Nassar U, Aziz T, Flores-Mir C. Dimensional stability of irreversible hydrocolloid impression materials as a function of pouring time: a systematic review. J Prosthet Dent. 2011;106(2):126–33. https://doi.org/10.1016/S0022-3913(11)60108-X.
64. West NX, Davies M, Amaechi BT. In vitro and in situ Erosion models for evaluating tooth substance loss. Caries Res. 2011;45(Suppl 1):43–52. https://doi.org/10.1159/000325945.
65. Bayne SC. Correlation of clinical performance with 'in vitro tests' of restorative dental materials that use polymer-based matrices. Dent Mater. 2012;28(1):52–71. https://doi.org/10.1016/j.dental.2011.08.594.
66. Greenhalgh T. How to read a paper: papers that summarise other papers (systematic reviews and meta-analyses). BMJ. 1997;315(7109):672–5. https://doi.org/10.1136/bmj.315.7109.672.
67. Linde K, Willich SN. How objective are systematic reviews? Differences between reviews on complementary medicine. J R Soc Med. 2003;96(1):17–22. https://doi.org/10.1177/014107680309600105.

8

Oral health knowledge, behavior, and care seeking among pregnant and recently-delivered women

A. J. Lubon[1], D. J. Erchick[1], S. K. Khatry[2], S. C. LeClerq[1,2], N. K. Agrawal[3], M. A. Reynolds[4], J. Katz[1] and L. C. Mullany[1*]

Abstract

Background: Oral health behavior and attitudes of pregnant women in low-income countries are rarely examined, yet should be considered when designing preventative or therapeutic studies to reduce burden of oral diseases. We aimed to understand dental care-seeking behavior, as well as oral health knowledge and attitudes of oral health among pregnant women in rural Nepal.

Methods: Semi-structured in-depth interviews ($n = 16$) and focus group discussions (3 groups, $n = 23$) were conducted among pregnant and recently-delivered women in Sarlahi, Nepal. Transcripts were translated from the local language to English then analyzed using a hybrid approach to thematic coding with Atlas.ti version 7.

Results: Women felt confident describing the signs and symptoms of tooth decay and gum disease, but were not knowledgeable about where to receive care for tooth and/or gum pain and relied heavily on the knowledge of their community. Some women used a toothbrush and toothpaste at least once a day to clean their teeth, but many reported the traditional use of a branch of a local shrub or tree as their teeth cleaning instrument. Women suggested a willingness to consider using an oral rinse throughout pregnancy, perceiving that it might have a positive impact on infant health.

Conclusions: Future studies should focus on providing adequate and sustainable resources for pregnant women in Nepal and other low income settings to engage in good oral health behaviors (possibly supported through community-based workers), to maintain dental hygiene, and to access qualified dentists as a means of improving their oral health.

Keywords: Nepal, Periodontal disease, Oral health, Oral health behaviors, Dental care seeking behavior, Pregnancy

Background

In low resource settings, oral health services are frequently inadequate to meet the needs of the population [1]. Poor accessibility, low quality, and human resources gaps – all key challenges to improving health systems in such settings – are more acutely felt for oral health systems. The limited capacity and insufficient distribution of trained oral health providers leads to utilization patterns almost exclusively focused on pain management or emergency treatment responses, at the expense of prevention [1]. In addition to supply side approaches that call for substantive human, infrastructural, and financial resources, demand side approaches require understanding of community norms, attitudes, practices, and knowledge toward oral health hygiene behavior, preventative care, and care-seeking practices.

Nepal is one of many low- and middle-income countries where attention and resources applied to oral health have lagged behind other domains of public health. Most oral health studies conducted in Nepal have tended to focus on burden of disease among school-aged children [2–7] or descriptive characteristics of dental professionals [8–10]. One study used a more broadly focused cross-sectional population-representative survey to identify factors

* Correspondence: lmullany@jhu.edu
[1]Department of International Health, Johns Hopkins Bloomberg School of Public Health, 615 N. Wolfe Street W5009, Baltimore, MD 21205, USA
Full list of author information is available at the end of the article

associated with improved practices. Researchers found that odds of teeth cleaning/brushing were higher among participants living in the rural plains region (*terai*) bordering India, compared to those in the mid-hill regions, and higher among those with higher educational backgrounds [11]. Additionally, while women were more likely than men to report seeking dental care services, only 4.8% of these women had seen a dentist in the past 6 months [11].

Formative research studies from Nepal are necessary to inform the design of context-appropriate interventions and programmatic approaches. One study conducted in Newalparasi, Nepal used the Theory of Planned Behavior [12] model to better understand oral hygiene and perceptions, and decisions related to care seeking. The study found that perceived self-efficacy in relation to oral hygiene practices and expected social outcomes of having healthy teeth were important predictors for oral health behavior [13]. For example, researchers found that once-daily tooth brushing was associated with the bathing ritual, which has a symbolic meaning of creating purity [13]. There are few studies on the particular aspects of oral hygiene behavior, perceptions, and attitudes among pregnant women. This group is of particular interest given the often observed association in other settings between periodontal disease during pregnancy and perinatal outcomes [14–18]. Therefore, in Sarlahi District, Nepal, we aimed to characterize these issues through in-depth interviews (IDIs) and focus group discussions (FGDs) among pregnant and recently-delivered women. Specifically, we aimed to understand dental care-seeking patterns, practices of oral hygiene, attitudes, and knowledge relevant to oral health of pregnant and recently-delivered women.

Methods

Data collection

This project was conducted by the Nepal Nutrition Intervention Project – Sarlahi (NNIPS), a multi-institution research collaboration that has been conducting community-based studies in rural Sarlahi district over the past 28 years. Between August and December 2016, we conducted 16 IDIs and 3 FGDs among pregnant and recently-delivered women in this setting using purposive sampling to identify participants.

For IDIs, we selected pregnant women enrolled in an ongoing randomized pilot trial of the acceptability of oral rinses (clinicaltrials.gov: NCT02788786). Four IDI participants were selected from each of three oral rinse groups, and an additional four participants were selected from a group of women randomized to no rinse. The rinse group individuals were selected to reflect diverse levels of adherence and reactions to taste, based on preliminary data available from the trial.

The pilot trial was being conducted in communities representing only one of the two broad ethnic groups in the region. To address this, our selection of women for the FGD phase of the research leveraged a population-representative database of reproductive aged women who were current (i.e. pregnant) or previous (i.e. recently-delivered) participants in a large community-based randomized trial of topical emollient therapies and neonatal health outcomes (clinicaltrials.gov: NCT01177111). These women were purposively selected to broaden representation to both major ethnic groups within the community: Madhesi women ($n = 2$ FGDs, originally from the northern plains of India and southern Nepal) and Pahadi women ($n = 1$ FGD, originating from Nepal's hill regions). Women were excluded if they had already participated in the IDIs or the pilot trial of oral rinses.

Prospective participants were approached by field staff to assess interest in participation, and an individually signed consent was obtained prior to initiating interviews or discussion groups. All IDIs and FGDs followed similar semi-structured interview guides with primarily open-ended questions and recommended probes. The IDI guide focused on oral hygiene behaviors and dental health care seeking, whereas the FGD guide additionally included questions on the symptoms and causes of tooth decay and gum disease and perceptions of dental health. Interviewers took hand-written notes during interviews; all interviews and group discussions were audio recorded. Field researchers wrote expanded field notes within 24 to 48 h of completing the interview or discussion group. Audio recordings were transcribed verbatim from Maithili (the local language) into Nepali with the aid of expanded field notes. Completed Nepali transcripts were translated into English and reviewed for any apparent errors in translation.

Prior to initiating the field activities, the NNIPS qualitative research team, consisting of female staff members with prior formal training and experience in conducting qualitative studies of a range of public health domains, received a two-week refresher training conducted by the authors (AJL, DJE). An additional training session using illustrative examples from the first two interviews was subsequently conducted to strengthen interviewer technique by one of the authors (AJL). Interviews (avg. 43 min) took place in the informants' homes, while FGDs (avg. 74 mins) were conducted in field offices throughout the study area.

Data analysis

Demographic characteristics of IDI and FGD participants were available as participants were enrolled in one or both of the ongoing randomized control trials that collected quantitative data. Transcripts were analyzed using a hybrid approach combining deductive thematic analysis with inductive coding during analysis enabling themes to emerge from the data [19]. An initial deductive coding structure was created based on the anticipated themes and on the content of the IDI and FGD guides. The codebook was revised using inductive coding to reflect emerging themes from initially coded IDIs and FGDs. The list of codes was then narrowed down into categories to produce a final codebook used for coding of transcripts. After each field activity, the research team used reflective memoing and debriefing sessions to analyze data quality, scrutinize assumptions and approaches to the research, and develop the codebook. Data were compiled and coded using Atlas.ti, version 7 using memos to track the process. Data across IDIs and FGDs were analyzed to identify themes related to dental hygiene methods, community oral health knowledge, and dental care seeking behavior among pregnant women. This study closely approached thematic saturation indicated by the aforementioned repeating thematic categories and lack of new coding structures during these debriefing and memoing sessions [20].

Table 1 Demographic Characteristics of IDI and FGD Participants

	IDIs [n = 16]		FGDs [n = 23]	
Age (years)				
- Mean	20		21	
- Median	19		21	
- Range	16–29		15–33	
Previous live births	Frequency N (%)			
- 0	5	(31)	8	(35)
- 1	5	(31)	7	(30)
- 2	3	(19)	7	(30)
- 3	3	(19)	–	–
- 4	–	–	1	(4)
Gestational Age				
- 0-3 months	–	–	–	–
- 4-6 months	10	(63)	10	(43)
- 7-9 months	6	(38)	4	(17)
Women's Education				
- No Schooling	7	(44)	12	(52)
- Years 1–9	8	(50)	9	(39)
- 10-SLC Pass	1	(6)	3	(13)
Ethnicity				
- Madhesi	16	(100)	16	(70)
- Pahadi	–	–	7	(30)

Results

Characteristics of IDI and FGD participants

The average age of all IDI and FGD participants was 20 years (Table 1). Among the 16 IDI participants, all were Madhesi, were pregnant in either their second (n = 10) or third (n = 6) trimester at the time of the interview, and had 0 to 3 prior children. Almost half (n = 7) reported no formal education. The three FGDs included 23 participants, fourteen of whom were pregnant, whereas the remaining nine women were in various stages of the post-partum period. A majority of FGD participants had no formal education, and number of prior live births ranged evenly from 0 to 2 (where one participant had 4).

Oral hygiene

Madhesi participants (i.e. all IDI participants and those from the Madhesi-comprised FGDs) reported that their usual teeth cleaning practice was to use either a toothbrush and toothpaste or *datuwan*, a teeth cleaning twig that serves as both a toothbrush and toothpaste, once a day prior to their morning meal. In contrast, women in the Pahadi FGD stated that the norm in their communities was for women to brush their teeth twice a day if not more.

IDI participants reported using either a toothbrush with Colgate (a toothpaste brand commonly found throughout shops and markets in the area) or "Dabur Lal Danta Manjan", an ayurvedic toothpaste without fluoride, or using *datuwan*. IDI participants used the word "medicine" to describe the toothpaste used for their tooth cleaning routine, which upon further probing was revealed to be 'Colgate' characterized by the red color of the brand. Within the Madhesi community, women used any available *datuwan* when doing farm work, but the other types of *datuwan* used included bamboo, mango, neem, snake's tail or chaff flower and black honey shrub (*sikat*) for specific purposes. For example, bamboo *datuwan* was reported by the participants to help whiten teeth, whereas women stated that the bitter taste of the black honey shrub helped to kill germs within the teeth. Mango *datuwan* was deemed "holy" as it can be used to clean teeth during fasting ceremonies since it is a twig of a fruit tree. This contrasts with the use of toothbrushes, which might have been in contact with meat and fish during prior brushings, contact that would be perceived as breaking one's fast. Other dentifrices mentioned included sand, mud/dirt, wood ash, and charcoal. Among the Pahadi community, women said that they used charcoal to whiten their teeth, and the types of *datuwan* used differed from the Madhesi community and included kamala tree (*sindure*), Bombay rosewood (*sisoo*), *Jatropha curcas* (*bagandi*), and Sal tree (*sakhuwa*).

When asked regarding motivations for cleaning one's teeth twice per day, Madhesi and Pahadi community members had similar reasons including reducing the risk of caries, overall cleanliness, and preventing infections. By keeping the mouth clean, one also prevented the development of other diseases:

It is possible to prevent some diseases by brushing your teeth. If you don't brush your teeth, many different types of germs enter the mouth and spoil the teeth. It goes inside the stomach and [causes] diseases. It is because of the teeth that many diseases occur.

–6 months pregnant, Madhesi FGD participant.

Women predominately learned about and developed their teeth cleaning routines from their parents, but others reported learning by watching people in their community, through radio and television advertisements, or indicated they were self-taught. In terms of maintaining more frequent brushing (i.e. twice per day), IDI participants identified the most pertinent barrier to be accessibility to a toothbrush and toothpaste. Many indicated, however, a willingness to increase frequency if instructed by community-based workers, such as NNIPS staff. In both Madhesi and Pahadi communities, other commonly mentioned barriers were lack of time due to work obligations, laziness, sleepiness, forgetfulness, and lack of awareness. In addition, Madhesi women said that some community members justified brushing only once daily because a toothbrush could "ruin their gums"; it was also suggested that the rough feel of a toothbrush on teeth or swollen gums could lead to women preferring to use *datuwan*.

Symptoms, causes, and severity of tooth decay and gum disease

Women generally felt confident describing the symptoms and causes of tooth decay, and toothache and swelling in gums were commonly listed as key symptoms of tooth decay. Madhesi women additionally described a sensation of *saksakauncha* ("itching") within the teeth that was accompanied by tingling, "swelling in teeth", lack of appetite, and feelings of nausea or vomiting. Pahadi women additionally listed black patches on teeth, holes in teeth, bad smell, and sensitivity when drinking water as signs of tooth decay. Not rinsing the mouth after eating sweets or getting food stuck between teeth were reported as potential causes of tooth decay; some women in the Pahadi focus group also reported that decay had a familial basis, where mothers could pass the condition to their children. Madhesi women suggested other possible causes included leftover food causing "a wound in the gums or tooth creating a ground for germs to infect other teeth", not brushing teeth before eating, eating eggplant or fish while having a toothache, chewing tobacco, drinking alcohol, or misusing a "toothpick to create a hole in a tooth".

When discussing the symptoms and causes of gum disease, however, women were not as forthcoming as they were when talking about tooth decay. Swollen gums and pain in the gums were listed as symptoms. While Madhesi women added "swelling of the teeth", specifically in the wisdom teeth area, and toothache as signs of gum disease, Pahadi women described a throbbing pain due to pus collecting within the gums. Madhesi women suggested that gum disease could result from wounds inflicted by poking the gums with *datuwan,* swollen gums due to caries, not brush teething before eating, allowing impurities within the mouth to cause disease, or drinking sweet tea after brushing. When similarly queried regarding cause of gum disease, Pahadi women described not knowing about gums, and could not provide any specific causes.

Women in the Madhesi community reported that children, the elderly, tobacco users, and poor people were more likely to suffer from tooth decay or gum disease. Some of these women felt strongly that poor people were at a disadvantage because they lacked the resources to buy a toothbrush and thus were forced to use *datuwan.* When prompted about the importance of oral health relative to other types of health issues, Madhesi women deemed that tooth decay and gum disease were very serious health problems because toothaches are extremely painful, can cause other diseases to manifest, and if toothache is a continuous problem, one may need to have their teeth removed, thus losing their ability to eat. In contrast, women in the Pahadi focus group expressed doubt as to the seriousness of tooth decay and gum disease, given the ubiquitous nature of the issue within their community; these women did acknowledge that such opinions, however, differed among individual community members.

Dental healthcare seeking

When experiencing tooth and/or gum pain, participants frequently indicated that they would seek "English" or "modern" medicine either from a local shop or from an allopathic provider if brushing one's teeth with toothpaste did not resolve the problem. Ibuprofen and paracetamol were mentioned as treatments to reduce or remove tooth pain. Several participants in both IDIs and FGDs indicated they would also consider going to a clinic or hospital. Other participants described that to alleviate tooth pain they would first get *jhar fuk,* a traditional approach where a healer performs a spell to chase "worms" (germs) out of the teeth. If this effort was unsuccessful, they would then seek allopathic medicine and/or medical treatment from an allopathic doctor. Another common treatment option for tooth pain was application of clove oil or "*sancho,*" a blend of Himalayan essential oils, which is a multipurpose herbal medicine used for the common cold, cough, body aches, and other illnesses. Pahadi women mentioned that people get fillings out of cement or silver when they have tooth pain, and if the filling is of poor quality, people are forced to get their teeth extracted.

Upon further probing as to where one could find a dentist, most IDI participants could not say with certainty where to go because they had never experienced pain that would warrant such care-seeking. Women said they would seek the counsel of their neighbors and community members on where to purchase medicine for tooth and/or gum pain, where to find a good doctor, and where to find a dentist. Among all IDI and FGD participants, no women reported ever visiting a dentist; one FDG participant summarized as follows:

> *Some may have said [they didn't need a dentist] because of lack of money. Some might have ignored it [the pain]. Some might have taken care of it and might have become all right after using herbal medicine. Some might have extracted the tooth with the cavity and thrown it away after breaking it. Some may not have been able to go because of other compulsions/ problems. Some guardians do not take them. They might have brought some tablets and said that this would make it all right. Some might have been told about herbal medicine and they must have taken it and become all right.*
>
> **– 6 months pregnant, Madhesi FGD participant.**

Even though participants expressed interest in seeing a dentist or doctor regarding tooth and/or gum pain, only a minority said that they would seek care in the absence of pain. Many stated that it did not make sense for them to treat a problem such as black spots on their teeth or bleeding gums if there was no pain. Instead of seeking medical attention, most women said they would either brush their teeth with medicine (toothpaste) or take no action and wait for the problem to self-resolve. Madhesi FGD participants described that when gums are very red, swollen, and/or bleeding without pain, people rinsed their mouths with hot water, applied mud or clove oil, purchased oral medicine, and went to the hospital for treatment of teeth. Pahadi women indicated that some people attempted to reduce bleeding through brushing with cooking oil and/or salt, or using *datuwan* made of *J. curcas*.

Pregnancy and oral hygiene

Many IDI participants, as well as FGD participants from both as both ethnic groups, did not report changes in teeth cleaning routines during pregnancy. All women agreed that keeping the mouth clean was essential in preventing diseases, but there were mixed views on the association between good oral hygiene during pregnancy and healthy birth outcomes. In one of the Madhesi FGDs (but not the other FGDs), women stated that poor oral hygiene causes cavities that enter the abdomen and negatively affect the baby, and that toothaches are a serious health problem because one does not eat, which can cause the child to become "lean and thin."

Discussion

Findings from this qualitative study highlight important implications regarding pregnant women and oral hygiene within rural Nepal. First, while tooth brushing is commonly practiced, the normal practice was limited to once daily, and consistent use of toothbrushes and toothpaste was lacking. Knowledge of symptoms and causes of tooth decay and gum disease were limited and varied substantially across community members. This suggests that standardized, culturally-specific, and simple educational messaging need to be developed and delivered through appropriate behavioral change communication approaches. One such possibility includes training rural women in oral health promotion activities, an approach that has demonstrated improved oral health knowledge among female community members in Nepal [21].

Second, formal preventative maintenance remains a largely unknown concept in this sub-population, and dental care health seeking is almost entirely driven by a direct response to tooth and/or gum pain. In the absence of pain, a majority of women stated it was unnecessary to seek a dentist because teeth brushing would be sufficient to address bleeding gums or spots on their teeth in cases where the problem would not resolve itself. Delay in care-seeking among this population is not unique to oral health and pregnant women. For example, among the same community in Sarlahi district, delays in care-seeking for maternal and newborn complications have been attributed to low perceived severity of the illness even when symptoms were recognized early [22]. In these cases, care was initially sought from informal health providers including traditional birth attendants, traditional healers, and village doctors whereas barriers to seeking care from any health facility included transportation, finances, and distance to the facility [22]. These care-seeking findings for maternal and newborn complications suggest that it is norm for pregnant or recently delivered women in the Sarlahi district to delay care-seeking from formal providers and/or health facilities for many health problems including ones related to oral health. Moreover, care-seeking for maternal illness improves significantly in low and middle income countries when antenatal or postnatal counseling stresses illness recognition and referrals by community health workers [23]. By changing the way illness is perceived in these low income settings and building a solid referral foundation using community health workers, the norm of delaying care-seeking among pregnant and recently delivered women can be changed.

Third, limited access to qualified providers tends to delay treatment seeking until pain is severe and/or home or traditional remedies have failed. When more formal care is sought, women often expressed going to a "hospital for treatment of teeth," of which there were two in this area at the time of data collection. While one of these was staffed by a practitioner with a dental certificate, neither practitioner was a fully trained or qualified dentist. During the study period, the nearest qualified dentists were in the neighboring districts of Janakpur and Birgunj, located 80 km and 100 km to the east and west, respectively. Public transportation to and from one of these providers would require a full day (or more if the providers were not able to immediately see clients). Given these substantive distance barriers, women (and the broader community) would most benefit from the improvement of local facilities through formal dental training of local practitioners and from increasing the number of qualified dentists in the area.

A limitation of this study is that our interviewers found it challenging to effectively probe women in this community about oral health, in order to elicit richer responses. These challenges in engaging respondents in conversation may not be surprising given that young women in this community, especially among the Madhesi, are frequently reticent to share their opinion or be assertive. Interviewers frequently commented that IDI participants were reluctant to speak about their oral health for fear of saying something incorrect (social desirability bias) or because they claimed that they had no knowledge on the subject. This challenge may have resulted in interviewers resorting to more direct or leading questions. Interviewers were women of the community an in approximately similar age range as participants, but there other characteristics about the interviewers (for example, cultural deference towards "guests"; formal employment in non-agricultural or "skilled" work can confer an extra level of respect, etc) that might have inhibited more full sharing of information or opinions.. Facilitators of FGDs indicated that the group setting allowed women to feel more comfortable not only expressing their opinion, but contrasting their viewpoints with those of others in the group. In addition, as some IDI respondents had also participated in the ongoing oral rinse pilot trial, exposure to positive oral health behavior messages might have influenced their responses; it is possible that other IDI or FGD participants who had not participated in that trial might also have indirectly been exposed to similar content. The impact, however of such exposures is likely limited, as interviewers were instructed to parse out behavior changes related to involvement in the oral health trial through effective probing during each interview, and analysis of transcripts did not indicate substantively different knowledge or attitudes regarding, for example, oral hygiene practices between those who did or did not participate in the rinse trial In terms of generalizability, while the knowledge, attitudes, and practices related to oral hygiene and care-seeking are likely generalizable to broad population in this region, this specific population might be more amenable to behavior change communication approach, given that NNIPS has been working closely with these communities for 28 years. Specifically their future readiness to engage in and follow instructions related to improved oral health behaviors such as improved frequency of brushing may be overestimated relative to other populations.

Conclusions

We found that pregnant or recently-delivered women in the Sarlahi community either brushed their teeth with a toothbrush and toothpaste once daily or used a teeth cleaning twig, but were receptive to switching their routine to brushing twice daily with toothpaste when instructed by a health worker. Women in this community were unable to correctly identify the signs and causes of tooth decay and gum disease and lacked knowledge on where to find qualified dentists within the study area. Based on our findings, we suggest that future efforts involving oral health and pregnant women in low-income settings focus on providing tools and resources to maintain dental hygiene, promoting good oral health behaviors and knowledge (possibly through context-appropriate cadres of trained community-based workers), and increasing access to qualified and fully trained dentists to improve the overall oral health of pregnant women.

Abbreviations

FGD: Focus group discussion; IDI: In-depth interview; NNIPS: Nepali Nutrition Intervention Project Sarlahi

Funding

This study was funded by the Bill & Melinda Gates Foundation through grants OPP1131701 and OPP1084399.

Authors' contributions

AJL helped design the sampling framework jointly with other authors, oversaw implementation of data collection, ensured quality of the data, conducted the analysis, and wrote the manuscript. DJE helped conceptualize and design the study jointly with other authors, assisted with implementation in the field, aided with interpretation of the results, provided comments and edits to the manuscript. SKK helped conceptualize and design the study jointly with other authors, oversaw field implementation and ensured quality, provided comments on the manuscript. SCL contributed to the study design and overall implementation in the field, helped with interpretation of the results, and provided comments on the manuscript. NKA helped design the study, provided input on the data collection approach and content, provided comments on the manuscript. MAR conceptualized and designed the study jointly with other authors, gave comments on the manuscript. JK contributed to the study design, quality of data collected, and gave comments on the manuscript. LCM conceptualized and designed the study jointly with other authors, obtained funding the study, oversaw implementation approach, obtained ethical approvals, and edited the manuscript. All authors read and approved the final manuscript.

Competing interests
The authors declare that they have no competing interests.

Author details
[1]Department of International Health, Johns Hopkins Bloomberg School of Public Health, 615 N. Wolfe Street W5009, Baltimore, MD 21205, USA. [2]Nepal Nutrition Intervention Project – Sarlahi (NNIPS), Krishna Galli, Lalitpur, Kathmandu, Nepal. [3]Department of Dentistry, Institute of Medicine, Tribhuhvan University, Kathmandu, Nepal. [4]Department of Periodontics, University of Maryland School of Dentistry, Baltimore, MD, USA.

References
1. Petersen PE, Bourgeois D, Ogawa H, Estupinan-Day S, Ndiaye C. The global burden of oral diseases and risks to oral health. Bull World Health Organ. 2005;83(9):661–9. doi:/S0042-96862005000900011.
2. Prasai Dixit L, Shakya A, Shrestha M, Shrestha A. Dental caries prevalence, oral health knowledge and practice among indigenous Chepang school children of Nepal. BMC Oral Health. 2013;13:20. https://doi.org/10.1186/1472-6831-13-20.
3. Yee R, David J, Lama D. The periodontal health of Nepalese schoolchildren. *Community Dent Health*. 2009;26(4):250–6. https://doi.org/10.1922/CDH_2397Yee07.
4. Knevel RJ, Neupane S, Shressta B, de Mey L. Buddhi Bangara project on oral health promotion: a 3- to 5-year collaborative programme combining support, education and research in Nepal. Int J Dent Hyg. 2008;6(4):337–46. https://doi.org/10.1111/j.1601-5037.2008.00345.x.
5. Kanal S, Acharya J. Dental caries status and oral health practice among 12-15 year old children in Jorpati, Kathmandu. Nepal Med Coll J. 2014;16(1):84–7.
6. Thapa P, Aryal KK, Dhimal M, et al. Oral health condition of school children in Nawalparsai district, Nepal. J Nepal Health Counc. 2015;13(29):7–13.
7. Shrestha N, Acharya J, Sagtani AR, Shrestha R, Shrestha S. Occurrence of dental caries in primary and permanent dentition, oral health status and treatment needs among 12-15 year old school children of Jorpati VDC, Kathmandu. Nepal Med Coll J. 2014;16(2–4):109–14.
8. Knevel RJM, Gussy MG, Farmer J, Karimi L. Perception of Nepalese dental hygiene and dentistry students towards the dental hygienists profession. Int J Dent Hyg. 2016; https://doi.org/10.1111/idh.12192.
9. Wagle M, Trovik TA, Basnet P, Acharya G. Do dentists have better oral health compared to general population: a study on oral health status and oral health behavior in Kathmandu, Nepal. BMC Oral Health. 2014;14(23). http://www.biomedcentral.com/1472-6831/14/23. Accessed 19 Jan 2017
10. Knevel RJM, Luciak-Donsberger C. Dental hygiene education in Nepal. Int J Dent Hyg. 2009;7:3–9. https://doi.org/10.1111/j.1601-5037.2008.00338.x.
11. Thapa P, Aryal KK, Mehata S, et al. Oral hygiene practice and their socio-demographic correlates among Nepalese adult: evidence from non communicable disease risk factors STEPS survey Nepal 2013. BMC Oral Health. 2016;16(105) https://doi.org/10.1186/s12903-016-0294-9.
12. Ajzen I. The theory of planned behavior. Organ Behav Human Decis Process. 1991;50:179–211. https://doi.org/10.1016/0749-5978(91)90020-T.
13. Buunk-Werkhoven YAB, Dijkstra A, Bink P, van Zanten S, van der Schans CP. Determinants and promotion of oral hygiene behavior in the Caribbean and Nepal. Int Dent J. 2011;61:267–73. https://doi.org/10.1111/j.1875-595X.2011.00071.x.
14. Prathahini P, Mahendra J. Toll-like receptors: a key marker for periodontal diseases and preterm birth –a contemporary review. J Clin Diagn Res. 2015; 9(9):ZE14–7. https://doi.org/10.7860/JCDR/2015/14143.6526.
15. Lopez NJ, Uribe S, Martinez B. Effect of periodontal treatment on preterm birth rate: a systematic review of meta-analyses. Periodontol 2000. 2015;67: 87–130. https://doi.org/10.1111/prd.12073.
16. Kim AJ, Lo AJ, Pullin DA, Thornton-Johnson DS, Karimbux NY. Scaling and root planing treatment for periodontitis to reduce preterm birth and low birth weight: a systematic review and meta-analysis of randomized controlled trials. J Periodontol. 2012;83(12):1508–19. https://doi.org/10.1902/jop.2012.110636.
17. George A, Shamim S, Johnson M, et al. Periodontal treatment during pregnancy and birth outcomes: a meta-analysis of randomised trials. Int J Evid Based Healthc. 2011;9(2):122–47. https://doi.org/10.1111/j.1744-1609.2011.00210.x.
18. Boutin A, Demers S, Roberge S, Roy-Morency A, Chandad F, Bujold E. Treatment of periodontal disease and prevention of preterm birth: systematic review and meta-analysis. Am J Perinatol. 2013;30(7):537–44. https://doi.org/10.1055/s-0032-1329687.
19. Fereday J, Muir-Cochrane E. Demonstrating rigor using thematic analysis: a hybrid approach of inductive and deductive coding and theme development. Int J Qual Methods. 2006;5(1):80–92. https://doi.org/10.1177/160940690600500107.
20. Saunders B, Sim J, Kingstone T, et al. Saturation in qualitative research: exploring conceptualization and operationalization. Qual Quant. 2017; https://doi.org/10.1007/s11135-017-0574-8.
21. Knevel RJM. Training rural women to improve access to oral health awareness programmes in remote villages in Nepal. Int J Dent Hyg. 2010;8: 286–93. https://doi.org/10.1111/j.1601-5037.2010.00481.x.
22. Lama TP, Khatry SK, Katz J, LeClerq SC, Mullany LC. Illness recognition, decision-making, and care-seeking for maternal and newborn complications: a qualitative study in Sarlahi District, Nepal. J Health Popul Nutr. 2017;36(Suppl1):45. https://doi.org/10.1186/s41043-017-0123-z.
23. Lassi ZS, Middleton PF, Bhutta ZA, Crowther C. Strategies for improving health care seeking for maternal and newborn illnesses in low- and middle-income countries: a systematic review and meta-analysis. Glob Health Action. 2016;9:1–13. https://doi.org/10.3402/gha.v9.31408.

9

Preferences of dentists and endodontists, in Saudi Arabia, on management of necrotic pulp with acute apical abscess

Ahmad A. Madarati[1,2]

Abstract

Background: This study aimed at investigating dental clinicians' preferences on management of necrotic pulp with acute apical abscess (NPAAA) cases.

Methods: Following an ethical approval and two pilot studies, an electronic survey was emailed to 400 general dental practitioners (GDPs) and 56 endodontists. The email explained the study's methods and assured that participants' identities and information given would remain anonymous and confidential. A reminder email was sent after eight weeks. Responses were collected and data were analyzed using the Chi-square test at $p = 0.05$.

Results: The majority of respondents (86.3%) would deal with NPAAA cases *"differently"* from vital-pulp ones ($p < 0.001$). More endodontists (40%) used two or three irrgants than GDPs (29.5%). Whilst the highest proportion of endodontists (29.7%) *rarely* prescribed antibiotics, the highest proportion of GDPs (26%) *generally did so* ($p < 0.001$). Whilst the highest proportion of GDPs (26.9%) *over-instrumented the largest canal* in the first visit, most endodontists (56.8%) performed *complete cleaning & shaping* (C&S) ($p < 0.001$). In cases of non-stopped exudates, whilst the highest proportions of endodontists would either *let the patient wait till the exudates significantly reduce then continue their intended approach* (40.5%) or *insert ICMs and temporize the tooth* (40.5%), the highest proportion of GDPs (30.8%) would *insert only dry cotton pellet without temporizing the tooth* ($p = 0.002$). Of those who would *leave the tooth open* if non-stopped exudates presents in the first visit, the majority (81.9%) would temporize the tooth if *little exudates* present after C&S ($p < 0.001$).

Conclusions: Clinicians, especially GDPs, opted to treat teeth involved in NPAAA differently from those with vital-pulp, such as: were using different ICMs and irrigants, C&S to different apical size preparation. GDPs should improve their practice by implementing multi-irrigants protocol while C&S, limit prescribing antibiotics, perform complete debridement of the root canal system and not to leave the tooth open between visits. Clinicians, especially GDPs, relied on their own experiences in managing NPAA cases which necessitates scientific-based guidelines.

Keywords: Acute, Apical, Abscess, Endodontics, Emergencies, Pus, Questionnaire, Necrotic, Survey

Background

The main objectives of root canal treatments are: a- to remove the infection from the root canal system (elimination of microbes), b- to perfectly seal the root canal system to prevent re-infection, and c- to promote healing of the periapical tissues. Accomplishment of these objectives, however, in some cases is challenging. Diagnosis and management of necrotic dental pulp cases that are associated with apical pathosis possess difficulties. Misdiagnosis or improper treatment procedures, due to lack of knowledge or insufficient clinical skills, may result in serious consequences for the patient. Clinicians must identify the etiology and mechanism of the periapical tissues' pathosis and manage the case properly by providing the appropriate treatment measures. The role of bacteria and their toxic by-products in pathosis of the dental pulp and periradicular tissues is well established [1]. Therefore, after determining the corrected working length, complete

Correspondence: amadarati@taibahu.edu.sa; ahmad.madarati@hotmail.co.uk
[1]Restorative Dental Sciences Department, College of Dentistry, Taibah University, P.O Box 2898, Madina 43353, Saudi Arabia
[2]Faculty of Dentistry, Aleppo University, Aleppo, Syria

canal debridement, with / without obturation, is the treatment of choice [2]. However, if the time is limited in the first visit, partial debridement at the estimated working length can be a practical and accepted therapeutic procedure [2]. It is suggested that the root canal system of the offended tooth is dried and then filled with calcium hydroxide and the coronal access cavity is sealed with a temporary filling [2]. While different inter-appointment medications can be recommended, there is a general belief that such a tooth should not be generally left open till next visit [2]. Moreover, in acute apical abscess, the use of systemic antibiotics has not been proved beneficial if the infection is localized [3] However, unfortunately general dental practitioners (GDPs) seem not to follow these recommended procedures. For example, in cases of pulp necrosis associated with periapical pathosis (especially acute apical abscess), leaving the tooth open has been a controversial, but disappointedly is a common practice, to some extent [4]. Walton and Keiser stated that placing a cotton pellet lightly dampened with an intracanal chemical medication in the pulp chamber before placing temporary filling is a useless procedure [2], though it is well adopted by GDPs. These are some of other procedures that GDPs may still follow without scientific evidence. Unfortunately, there has been lack of information regarding clinicians' practices and preferences in this respect. Two previous surveys, conducted in the United States, showed how clinicians change their decision over period of time (5–7]. To this end, there is a need to explore management aspects and practitioners' preferences and practices when dealing with cases of necrotic pulp associated with acute apical abscess (NPAAA). In particular, to date there are no reports on the real-life practice of GDPs and endodontists, neither in Saudi Arabia nor in any other country, when a case of NPAAA is encountered.

Therefore, the aim of this questionnaire study was to investigate the preferences, practices and experience of GDPs and endodontists in the Western Province, Saudi Arabia towards management of NPAAA cases. The survey mainly aimed to answer the following questions:

❑ Would be there any significant difference between clinicians (GDPs and endodontists) who used to leave the tooth with NPAAA open after the first visit and those clinicians who do not?
❑ Would be any significant difference between GDPs and endodontists regarding procedures adopted in the first visit of dealing with a tooth associated with NPAAA?

Therefore, the following two null hypotheses were tested:

❑ H0 (1): There would be no significant differences between clinicians (GDPs and endodontists) who would leave a tooth associated with NPAAA open in the first visit and those who wouldn't.
❑ H0 (2): There would be no significant difference between GDPs and endodontists regarding some procedures followed in the first visit when dealing with a tooth associated with NPAAA open in the first visit.

Methods

This Internet-based questionnaire study was ethically approved by the Research Ethics Committee at Taibah University College of Dentistry (Saudi Arabia) without the need for participants' consent form. The study was accomplished in accordance to the World Medical Association's Helsinki Declaration between March and August 2016. A first pilot survey study was conducted on the academic staff at College of Dentistry, Taibah University to ensure that the questions were easily understood without personal interpretation. An initial questionnaire comprised both close-ended and partially close-ended questions in two main categories:

- Demographics (three non-numbered questions)
- Pattern of practice and experience of management of cases associated with NPAAA (14 main questions)

A second pilot survey was performed on a group of GDPs and endodontists to facilitate the sample size calculation. The latter was performed taking into consideration the following factors:

❑ 90% power to detect the difference between groups' proportions
❑ The expected (minimum desired) response rate (40–60%)
❑ The populations of the study target (number of GDPs and all endodontists in the Western Province, SA)
❑ Level of statistical significant difference (0.05)

It was decided that the survey would be sent to 400 GDPs and all endodontist registered in the Western Province, Saudi Arabia (56). The 400 GDPs were selected randomly using the systematic sampling method. The final questionnaire (Additional file 1) was constructed electronically using the Google Drive sheet. The electronic survey was emailed to the selected sample size (400 GDPs and 56 endodontists). The email explained the aims and methods of the study and assured that participants' identities would remain anonymous and all information given would remain confidential and would be used for the purpose of the research only. A further email was sent to all candidates after eight weeks to remind non-respondents to participate in the survey. Responses were collected using the Google Drive Excel document. Data were entered into SPSS 19 for Windows software (SPSS Inc., Chicago, IL,

USA) and they were analyzed using the Chi-square and Linear-by-Linear Association tests at $p = 0.05$. Statistical tests were performed to compare mainly among the proportions of each question responses and to compare between GDPs and endodontists regarding these responses.

Results

Classification of Respondents & Study's response rate

Of the 456 who were approached, 234 responded to this study as follows: 189 (80.6%) were *GDPs*, 32 (13.7%) *endodontists*, 6 (2.6%) *postgraduate students or residents* in endodontic specialty programmes, and 7 (3%) *others*.

Eighteen respondents (16 GDPs and 2 others) never performed RCTs. Therefore, they were categorized ineligible respondents. Accordingly, the overall and non-endodontists (GDPs & otters) sample sizes were:

456–18 = 438 and 400–18 = 382, respectively, resulting in the following response rates:

Overall response rate: 234 / 438 = 53.4%.
Non-endodontists (GDPs, Endodontic Postgraduate Programmes students, and others) final response: 202 / 382: 52.9%
Endodontists: 32 / 56 = 57.1%

This study involves mainly theoretical aspects of endodontics rather than attaining hand skills or mastering new techniques. Dealing with cases of NAPP is well established in the first year of the postgraduate studies programmes in Saudi Arabia. Therefore, participants who were enrolled in Endodontic Postgraduate Studies or Residency programmes, were categorized as endodontists. This also enabled better statistics for some variables.

Participants' experience & number of cases they perform per week

Overall, significantly the lowest proportion of respondents (8.8%) had *more than 20 years' experience* ($p < 0.001$) (Table 1). The highest proportion of endodontists (44.4%) had *10.1 to 20 years' experience* compared to 17.3% in GDPs group ($p = 0.005$).

There were significant differences between endodontists and GDPs regarding the number of RCTs performed per week ($p < 0.001$) (Table 1). Whilst the highest proportion of GDPs performed *1 to 5 cases* (52%), the highest proportion of endodontists (44.7%) performed *more than 15 cases*.

Overall there were no significant differences between endodontists and GDPs ($p = 0.176$) regarding the decision on *how to deal with case associated with NPAAA* (Table 1). The vast majority of respondents (93.4%) *would treat the tooth* ($p < 0.001$) and only 8.8% of GDPs would either *refer to endodontic specialist* (7%) or *extract the tooth* (1.3%) [$p < 0.001$].

Management's differences between vital and NPAAA cases & main Treatment's modalities adopted in NPAAA cases

Overall, the majority (86.3%) (Endodontists and GDPs) would deal with cases of NPAAA *"differently"* from that of vital ones ($p < 0.001$) (Table 2).

Table 1 Participants' experience, number of root canal treatments (RCTs) they perform per week and their approach for necrotic pulp associated with acute apical abscess (NPAAA) cases

Respondents' Classification	Experience of Respondents (Years)					
	Up to 2	2.1 to 5	5.1 to 10	10.1 to 20	More than 20	Total
GDP	25.5%	25.4%	25.4%	17.3%	9.2%	100% (173)
Endodontists	0%	21.1%	26.3%	44.4%	7.9%	100% (38)
Others	0%	40%	20%	40%	0%	100% (5)
Total	18.1%	25%	25.5%	22.7%	8.8%	100% (216)
Respondents' Classification	Number of RCT cases performed per week					
	1–5	6–10	11–15	More than 15	Total	
GDP	52%	28.3%	11.6%	8.1%	100% (173)	
Endodontists	10.5%	26.3%	18.4%	44.7%	100% (38)	
Other	80%	0%	20%	0%	100% (5)	
Total	45.4% (98)	27.3% (59)	13% (28)	14.4% (31)	100% (216)	
Respondents' Classification	Management of permanent teeth with NPAAA					Total
	Treat the tooth		Extract the tooth	Refer to an endodontist		
GDP	91.2%		1.8%	7%		100% (173)
Endodontists	100%		0%	0%		100% (37)
Other	100%		0%	0%		100% (5)
Total	93.6%		1.3%	5.1%		100% (215)

Table 2 Management's differences between vital and NPAAA cases & main treatment's modalities adopted by Participants in NPAA cases

Would you deal with NPAA differently		Respondents' Classification				Total	
		GDPs		Endodontists	Others		
Using of Rubber Dam		13.3%		9.7%	0%	11.9%	
Type of sealer		15.6%		6.5%	20%	13.5%	
Size of apical preparation		33.3%		32.3%	60%	34.1%	
Type of intra-canal medication		78.9%		16.1%	80%	63.5%	
Apical extension of preparation		17.8%		29%	20%	20.6%	
Methods for WL measurement		6.7%		3.2%	0%	5.6%	
Use of rotary instruments		8.9%		0%	20%	7.1%	
Technique of C&S		24.4%		22.6%	0%	23%	
Type of irrigants		62.2%		38.7%	100%	57.9%	
Obturation technique		17.8%		3.2%	0%	13.5%	
Overall Total		100% (90)		100% (31)	100% (5)	86.3% (126)	
Respondents' Classification	Instrumentation techniques					Total	
	Conventional	Step Back		Crown Down			
GDP	21.2%	45.2%		57.7%		173 (100%)	
Endodontists	0%	8.6%		97.1%		38 (100%)	
Other	20%	60%		100%		5 (100%)	
Total	16%	36.8%		68.8%		216 (100%)	
	Irrigants used in NPAAA cases						Total
Respondents' Classification	EDTA	NAOCL	CH	NAOCL + (EDTA or CH)[a]	NAOCL + (EDTA + CH)[a]	Other	
GDP	23.1%	92.3%	17.3%	29.5%	8.2%	3.8%	104 (100%)
Endodontists	21.6%	100%	10.8%	21.6%	10.8%	28%	37 (100%)
Other	40%	100%	20%	40%	20%	0%	5 (100%)
Total	23.3% (82.3%)	94.5%	15.8% (100%)	27.7%	9.1%	2.7%	141 (100%)
Respondents' Classification	Patterns of Antibiotics Usage						Total
	Never	Always	Generally	Frequently	Sometimes	Rarely	
GDP	5.8%	21.2	26%	11.5%	24%	11.5%	100% (104)
Endodontists	13.5%	10.8%	10.8%	16.2%	18.9%	29.7%	100% (37)
Other	20%	20%	0%	0%	40%	20%	100% (5)
Total	8.2%	18.5%	21.2%	12.3%	23.3%	16.4%	100% (146)

The values in brackets represent proportion of those who used the assigned irrigant with sodium hypochlorite irrigant. [a]Proportions were calculated out of sodium hypochlorite users

Size of apical preparation

34.1% would prepare root canals in cases with NPAAA to *different apical sizes* from those of vital pulps cases; without significant difference between endodontists and GDPs *($p = 0.913$)* (Table 2).

Type of intra-canal medications (ICMs)

Whist the majority of GDPs (78.9%) would use different ICMs when dealing with NPAAA cases compared to vital ones, only 16.1% of endodontists would do so *($p < 0.001$)* (Table 2).

Type of sealer

Only 13.5% reported the difference in the type of sealer used for RCT with significantly greater proportion of GDPs (15.6%) compared to that of endodontists (6.5%) *[$p < 0.001$]* (Table 2).

Technique of cleaning & shaping (C&S)

23% would use different techniques for C&S of the root canal system in cases of NPAAA. Significantly, Crown *Down* was the most common technique used for C&S cases with NPAAA (68.8%) *[$p < 0.001$]*; with the vast majority of endodontists (97.1%) using it compared to significantly less GDPs (57.7%) *[$p < 0.001$]* (Table 2).

Type of Irrigants

Whilst the highest proportion of GDPs (62.2%) would use *different irrigants* during instrumentation of cases associated with NPAAA, only 38.7% would do so *($p = 0.023$)* (Table 2). Significantly, the vast majority of respondents (94.5%) used sodium hypochlorite irrigant *($p < 0.001$).* The proportion of endodontists who used two or three irrigants (40%) was significantly greater than that of GDPs (29.5%) *[$p < 0.001$].*

Prescribing of antibiotics

Whilst the highest proportion of endodontists (29.7%) rarely prescribed antibiotics, only 11.5% of GDPs did so (*$p = 0.004$*). By contrast, the highest proportion of GDPs (26%) *generally prescribe antibiotics* (Table 2).

First Visit's management of NPAAA cases and its reasons

The most common management of NPAAA cases in the first visit were *complete C&S of the root canal system* and *over-instrumentation of the largest root canal* (*$p < 0.001$*). Overall there were significant differences between endodontists and GDPs (*$p < 0.001$*) (Table 3).

Whilst the highest proportion of GDPs (26.9%) used to over-instrument the largest canal, the highest proportion of endodontists (56.8%) used to perform complete C&S (*$p < 0.001$*). Also, while (21.2%) of GDPs used to *partially C&S the root canal system to the estimated working length,* none of endodontists (0%) did so (*$p < 0.001$*). On the other hand, 21.6% of endodontists used *to perform complete RCTs*; with only 3.8% of GDPs were doing so (*$p < 0.001$*). Overall, significantly the highest proportion (51.7%) reported their *own experience* as the reason for their first visit's approaches to NPAAA cases followed by those who did it because *they were taught to do so during undergraduate training* (37.4%) *[$p = 0.002$].* Forty percent of endodontists reported the *postgraduate studies* as the reason for doing so. By contrast, the highest proportion of GDPs (56.2%) reported their *own experience* as the reason for their first visit's approaches.

First Visit's management of NPAAA cases with non-stopped exudates

Overall, there was no significant difference between the highest proportion of participants (41.4%) who used to *leave the tooth open* (without temporary restoration) and the lower proportion 36.3% who used to *place temporary restoration* if there was non-stopped excaudate after the first visit management (*$p = 0.521$*) (Table 4). However, significantly the lowest proportion (22.6%) would *let the patient wait till the exudates stop or significantly reduce then continue their intended approach [$p = 0.018$]*; with

Table 3 First visit's management of NPAAA cases and the reasons participants report

Management of NPAAA in the first visit	Respondents' classification			Total
	GDPs	Endodontists	Others	
Access Cavity	3.8%	5.4%	0%	4.1%
Over-instrumentation the largest canal	26.9%	8.1%	40%	22.6%
WL measurement	1.9%	0%	0%	2%
WL and C&S of the largest canal	7.7%	0%	0%	5.5%
Partial C&S at estimated WL	21.2%	0%	20%	15.8%
Partial C&S at Corrected WL	15.4%	8.1%	0%	13%
Complete C&S	19.2%	56.8%	40%	29.5%
Complete RCT	3.8%	21.6%	0%	8.2%
Overall Total	100% (104)	100% (37)	100% (5)	100% (146)
Reasons for first visit approach of NPAAA	Respondents' classification			Total
	GDPs	Endodontists	Others	
Taught during undergraduate study	41.9%	27%	20%	37.4%
Lack of time	12.5%	2.7%	0%	9.6%
Learnt from own experience	56.2%	40.5%	40%	51.7%
Colleagues' recommendation	16.5%	2.7%	20%	13.1%
Taught during postgraduation	0%	40%	60%	12.3%
Taught in a scientific meeting	1%	0%	0%	0.7%
Dental Literature	23.1%	32.4%	40%	26%
Total	100%	100%	100%	100%

Table 4 First visit's management of NPAA cases with non-stopped exudates and the reasons participants report

First visit management of cases with non-stopped exudates		Respondents' classification			Total	
		GDPs	Endodontists	Others		
Waite till the exudates stop or significantly reduce then continue the intended approach		17.3%	40.5%	0%	22.6%	
No temporary restoration	No intra-canal dressing	3.8%	5.4%	0%	4.1%	41.1%
	With dry cotton pellet	30.8%	5.4%	20%	24%	
	Insert intra-canal medication	11.5%	0%	0%	8.2%	
Place temporary restoration	Insert dry cotton pellet	7.7%	8.1%	20%	8.2%	36.3%
	Insert intra-canal medication	28.8%	40.5%	60%	32.9%	
Total		100% (104)	100% (37)	100% (5)	100% (146)	
Reasons for This Approach		Respondents' classification			Total	
		GDPs	Endodontists	Others		
Taught during undergraduate study		22.3% (95.8)	0% (0)	20% (4.2)	16.6% (100)	
Lack of time		12.6% (100)	0% (0)	0% (0)	9% (100)	
Learnt from own experience		48.5% (78.1)	35.1% (20.3)	20% (1.6)	44.1% (100)	
Colleagues' recommendation		6.8% (100)	0% (0)	0% (0)	4.8% (100)	
Taught during postgraduation		0% (0)	43.2% (88.9)	40% (11.1)	12.4% (100)	
Dental Literature		9.7% (52.6)	21.6% (42.1)	20 (5.3)	13.1% (100)	
Total		100%	100%	100%	100%	

significantly more endodontists (40.5%) than GDPs (17.3%) *[p = 0.002]*. By contrast, the highest proportion of GDPs (30.8%) would *insert only dry cotton pellet without temporizing the tooth till next visit.* In addition, the proportion of endodontists who would insert ICMs and temporize the tooth (40.5%) was significantly greater than that of GDPs who would do the same (28.8%) *[p = 0.002]*. The proportion of endodontists who would temporize the tooth in the first visit (81.8%) was significantly greater than that of GDPs (44.2%).

While the most common reason for endodontists' approaches (43.2%) was *postgraduate studies' learning*, the most common reason for GDPs was *learning from their own experience (p < 0.001)* (Table 4).

Management of NPAAA cases with little exudates after complete C&S and its reasons

The majority of respondents (80.8%) used to insert temporary restoration, with (69.2%) or without intracanal medications (11.6%), if there had been little exudates after the first visit management (Table 5). The second most common management (12.6%) was to *let the patient wait till the exudates stop or significantly reduce then continue their intended.* Overall, there were significant differences between GDPs and endodontists *(p < 0.010).* Whilst the second common approach by endodontists (29.7%) was *let the patient wait till the exudates stop or significantly reduce then continue their intended, insert dry cotton pellet only without temporizing the tooth till next visit* was the second most common management adopted by *GDPs* (15.4%). However, there was no significant difference between the proportion of endodontists who used to *insert temporary restoration with intracanal medications* (62.2%) and those of GDPs who were doing (70.2%) *[p < 0.097].*

Overall, there were significant differences between endodontists and GDPs in reporting the reasons for their management of *little exudate after C&S (p > 0.05).* The first and second most common reasons for GDPs were that they *were taught to do so during undergraduate study* and their *own experience* (52 and 46.1%, respectively). However, the most common reason for endodontists was that they *were taught to do so during postgraduate studies* (61.1%).

Comparison between Management of First Visit Significant Exudates and Little Exudates after C&S

Of those who would *wait till the significant exudate stops then continue treatment in the first visit,* a significantly high proportion (54.5%, *p = 0.020)* would *temporize the tooth till next visit if little exudates still present after C&S of the root canal system in the first visit* (Table 6). Of those who would *leave the tooth open* if non-stopped exudates presents in the first visit, the majority (81.9%) would temporize the tooth if little exudates present after C&S *(p < 0.001).* Of those who used to *temporize the tooth* after the first visit associated with non-stopped exudates, 5% *would wait till exudate stop then continue treatment* in case of little exudates presented in the first visit.

Table 5 Management of NPAA cases with little exudates after complete cleaning and shaping (C&S) of the root canal system and the reasons participants report

First visit management of little exudates after complete C&S	Respondents' classification			Total	
	GDPs	Endodontists	Others		
Waite till the exudates stop or significantly reduce then continue your intended approach	6.7%	29.7%	0%	12.3% (18)	
Leave tooth open without neither dressing nor temporization till next visit	1.9%	0%	0%	1.4%	6.8% (10)
Insert dry cotton pellet only without temporization till next visit	1.9%	5.4%	0%	2.7%	
Insert intra-canal medication without temporization till next visit	3.8%	0%	0%	2.7%	
Insert dry cotton pellet only and temporization till next visit	15.4%	2.7%	0%	11.6%	80.8% (118)
Insert intra-canal medication and temporization till next visit	70.2%	62.2%	100%	69.2%	
Total	100% (104)	100% (37)	100% (5)	100% (146)	

Discussion

There has been need to explore the real-life practice of GDPs and endodontists when dealing with cases of NPAAA and to identify the reasons behind their approaches. Generally, more endodontists had *more than ten years' experience* than GDPs than GDPs. This might be explained by the fact that endodontists have to spend three to five years acquiring endodontic postgraduate training. As expected, there were significant differences between endodontists and GDPs regarding the *number of RCTs performed per week*; whilst most GDPs performed up to five cases per week, the highest proportion of endodontists performed more than 15 cases. While the full time of endodontists is devoted for endodontic treatment, GDPs usually perform other types of dental treatments. Another possible reason is that GDPs may refer complex cases or retreatment cases to endodontist [5]. The definition of complex cases from GDPs' prospective should be established; because the vast majority of GDPs in the current study used to treat cases with NPAAA. It could be assumed that complex or difficult cases, from GDPs' point of view, imply those cases with complex root canal anatomy or defective old root canal fillings. Nevertheless, these findings reflect participants' intention to preserve teeth involved in NPAAA. This is especially true with the fact that 6.1% would refer the cases to endodontists and only (1.8%) would extract teeth involved with such cases. In addition, few years ago more GDPs in Saudi dental practice (5%) used to extract such cases [5]. However, dealing with NPAAA cases may be challenging and possess some difficulties. Accordingly, clinicians may deal with them differently when compared with vital-pulp cases. The majority of the current study's respondents would do so. In the following we will try to discuss some of these different aspects, if any.

Almost 12% of respondents would use rubber dam (RD) isolation when dealing with NPAAA cases. This may explain the perception of these respondents towards the different pathological condition of NPAAA cases compared to vital-pulp cases. Different types of bacteria are associated or involved with different pathological endodontic conditions [6], hence these respondents were careful to prevent or reduce additional microbial invasion to the root canal system. RD isolation may also better control pus drainage. Nevertheless, it is well documented that RD is not commonly used by GDPs in many countries [7–10]. A recent study showed that only 21.6% of GDPs were using RD in Saudi Arabia [11]. While it is common, though disappointedly, for GDPs not to use RD, it is unaccepted that 9.7% of endodontists to use RD in NPAAA cases rather than vital-pulp cases. With the fact that RD isolation in endodontics is a standard of care [12].

Only 13.5% of participants (GDPs and endodontists) used to use different sealers when dealing with NPAAA

Table 6 Comparison between management of first visit significant exudates and little exudates after C&S

Management of First Visit Non-stopped Exudates	Management of First Visit Little Exudates after C&S			Total
	Wait till exudate stop then continue treatment	Leave tooth open till next visit	Temporize the tooth till next visit	
Wait till exudate stop then continue treatment	45.5%	0%	54.5%	100% (33)
Leave tooth without temporization till next visit	0%	18.9%	81.9%	100% (53)
Temporize the tooth till next visit	5%	0%	95%	100% (60)
Total	12.3%	6.8%	80.8%	100% (146)

cases. One assumption for such practice is that this group of clinicians' demand better antimicrobial effects. The antimicrobial effects of zinc oxide & eugenol-based sealers is well established [13]. It has been thought that calcium hydroxide-based sealers would have better biological and antibacterial properties which could contribute to better perapical tissues healing and repair. However, clinical and experimental studies have not shown such superiority [14, 15]. The MTA-based sealer has been recently introduced and has shown promising results [16]. Nevertheless, drawing conclusions on the impact of different sealers on treatments' long-term outcome should be based on clinical studies with sufficient follow-up periods. In addition, the current study did not ask the participants about the type of sealer they used in cases of NPAAA. This could be one limitation that necessitates further investigation.

There is a general belief that necrotic pulp cases, especially those associated with apical pathosis should be prepared to a larger apical size than vital-pulp cases. A previous clinical study found that enlarging the apical portion of root canals three sizes larger than the first file that bound at working length was sufficient [17]. Some authors have suggested creating a 'larger' apical preparation followed by a one-week dressing of calcium hydroxide [18–20]. Other authors have suggested enlarging the canal terminus to a pre-determined size beyond 35 or 40 [20–27]. However, it was suggested that larger tapers is more important than the final apical size; because a small taper size of 0.10 allowed minimum instrumentation of the apical part of the root canal systems [28]. One systematic review showed that canal enlargement reduces bioburden within the root canal system [29]. It revealed that in cases with necrotic pulps and periapical lesions, enlargement of the apical size would result in an increased healing outcome (clinically and radio-graphically) [29]. A very recent study revealed significant bacterial reduction when root canals of teeth involved with apical periodontitis were prepared to an S3 TFA file compared to S2 and S1 files [30]. The current study revealed that one third of participants were following this trend and they would prepare the root canals of NPAAA cases to different sizes of that in vital-pulp cases. Nevertheless, the influence of different apical enlargement on the treatment long-term outcome, especially in NPAAA cases, should be established systematically. This need was reflected on the current study; because two third of participants would not prepare the NPAAA cases to different apical size of that in vital-pulp cases. It is important to indicate that some studies proposed and investigated the interaction between the apical size preparation and other factors such as irrigation and obturation).

In addition to the antimicrobial and tissues- dissolving effects, irrigants are essentially used to remove and wash the debris out of the root canal system. Due to the extensive microbial invasion in NPAAA cases compared to those of vital-pulp ones, different irrigation protocols and stronger irrigants may be used [31]. Unlike endodontists, most GDPs in the current study used different irrigants when dealing with NPAAA cases. This again may reflect their perception to the pathological condition of the pulpal and periapical tissues in NPAAA cases when compared to vital-pulp cases. If this is the case, GDPs need to not underestimate the desired antimicrobial effects of irrigants in vital-pup cases as well. By contrast, the lowest proportion of endodontists used different irrigants. Endodontists are usually aware of the important of irrigation in elimination intracanal infection regardless of the pathological condition. There have been many solutions used as irrigants in endodontics; including sodium hypochlorite (NaOCl), chlorohexidine (CHX) and Ethylene diamine tetra acetic acid (EDTA). NaOCl has been the most commonly used irrigants [32]. The current study is not an exception and showed that the vast majority of clinicians were using it in NPAAA cases. It is an excellent antibacterial agent, capable of dissolving necrotic and vital tissues and the organic components of dentin and biofilms. Hence it has been the standard irrigant with which other and new irrigants are compared [33]. Chlorohexidine has been also known for its good antimicrobial effects, especially as adjunctive irrigant [34]. However, one limitation of both irrigants, is that their inferior ability in removing intracanal smear layer. Hence EDTA is strongly recommended for such a purpose [31]. An irrigation protocol that ensures elimination of microbs, dissolving pulp tissues and removing smear layer by combined use of selective irrigants in different sequences, is paramount. It is well established that such a protocol is key factor in better cleaning of the root canal system and contributes to better long-term treatment outcome [34]. Within this respect, the current study revealed the need to raise the awareness of GDPs for implementing multi-irrigants protocol as only one third of them use more than one irrigant.

The most common different practice of GDPs towards NPAAA cases from that in vital-pulp ones was using different type of ICMs; with only 16.1% of endodontists were doing so. This again, almost reflect GDPs perception of the significant microbial invasion and the essential need to eliminate intracranial infection. Also, it may mirror GDPs' understanding of using different ICMs according to different pulpal and periapical pathological conditions and the associated symptoms. Nevertheless, the current results are consistent with those obtained in a very recent study conducted in Saudi Arabia which showed general trend among GDPs to use different ICMs according to different pulpal and periapical diseases [35]. These findings validate the current study and confirm that it was conducted systematically. The previous study revealed that CH was the most common ICM used by Saudi dental clinicians;

GDPs and endodontists [35]. A previous study in the United States, also, found that CH was the most frequently used ICM all necrotic pulps cases [36]. The antimicrobial properties of CH dressing has been controversial [37], though it has been recommended for use in teeth with necrotic pulp tissue and bacterial contamination [2] because of its effectiveness in inhibiting microbial growth [38]. It probably has little benefit with vital pulps [2].

With NPAAA cases, extra caution and care should be exercised so the necrotic debris are not pushed apically, hence beyond the apex, during C&S to reduce post-treatment discomfort or pain. Crown-down instrumentation technique has been known as the least technique causing debris extrusion beyond the apex [39]. In addition, it enables removing the intracanal infection sequentially from the coronal portion down to the apical portion of the root canal system. The proportion of respondents, in the current study, who used this technique in cases with NPAAA was significantly greater than those who used Step-Back or Conventional ones. Unsurprisingly, the vast majority of endodontists used Crown-Down technique compared to lower proportion of GDPs. This indicates that GDPs need to update their knowledge and implement Crown-Down more as a technique of choice when dealing with NPAAA cases.

The results showed a clear trend among GDPs towards prescribing antibiotics when dealing with NPAAA cases. Whilst the highest proportion of endodontists (29.7%) rarely prescribed antibiotics, the highest proportion of GDPs (26%) generally prescribe. These findings are consistent with those obtained in a very recent systematic review [40]. However, the current results should be carefully interpreted because the current survey did not differentiate between presence and absence of swelling. This can be one limitation of the study which suggests further research to explore clinicians' preferences on prescribing antibiotics for different endodontic diseases as well as to explore the most common antibiotics used in individual diseases. Systemic antibiotics are better prescribed for the diffuse, rapidly spreading or persistent infections with systemic signs and symptoms such as cellulitis or persistent swelling. The antibiotic therapy in such cases, is an adjunct to debridement of the root canal system [2]. A recent systematic review concluded that the use of systemic antibiotics is not necessary and not recommended if the the infection is localized [3]. Improper use of antibiotics is one main factor that contributes to the emerging oral bacteria resistance to commonly used antibiotics [41]. Improper use of antibiotics includes: use in cases with no infection, erroneous choice of the agent, dosage or duration of therapy, and excessive use in prophylaxis [42]. Nevertheless, the results indicate that clinicians, especially GDPs, should exercise additional care when prescribing antibiotics.

Management of NPAAA cases has been controversial, especially in terms of leaving the tooth open. Unfortunately, there is little evidence and reports on the best management and treatment modalities. An old survey in the United States revealed that most endodontists would do complete canal debridement shorter than the working length (WL) in cases no swelling present [43, 44]. By contrast, they would over-instrument the canals and leave the tooth open if there is swelling [43, 44]. Leaving the tooth open is no longer accepted nowadays and is rarely considered in very limited cases, especially for endodontists. A recent study in the United States revealed that most Endodontic Diplomats would do complete C&S regardless of the swelling; with up to 38% who left the tooth open in case of swelling [36]. It is well accepted among endodontists that full debridement of the root canal system, if time permits, in the first visit, is the preferred therapeutic procedure of NPAAA cases [2]. However, drainage should be considered if time is limited and does not allow complete C&S [2]. As expected, endodontists in the current study showed awareness of such good practice as most of them would C&S root canals to the full working length. By contrast, a lower proportion of GDPs would do so; with the highest proportion of them would over-instrument the largest canal only. Lack of time could be one main reason for this policy. Another possibility is that GDPs aim only at reducing the pressure and relief patients' emergency situation. Interestingly, 21.6% of endodontists would perform complete RCT. The long-term treatment outcome and post-operative pain are the crucial debate in this respect. Reports indicated that there may be no difference in post-treatment pain if root canals are filled at the time of the emergency versus a later date [45] (Eleazer and Eleazer 1998). However, the long-term prognosis of such treatment is questionable [46, 47]. Nevertheless, a previous study showed no difference in treatment outcome between single-visit and two-visit treatments [48]. Overall, most clinician of the current study, especially GDPs, reported their *own experience* as the reason for their approaches to NPAAA cases in the first visit. This reflects the lack of scientific evidence that clinicians can rely on when dealing with such cases. This is especially true as most endodontist were equally relying on either their own experience or on what they were taught during postgraduate endodontic programmes.

Decision on NPAAA cases with significant exudates after first visit's procedures is one of the most crucial decision-making skills, especially with the lack of strong scientific evidence [49]. This reflected clearly on GDPs options as the highest proportion reported their *own experience* as the main reason for their decision. This was confirmed, somehow, by endodontists group as it was the second most common reason. The highest proportion of GDPs (30.8%) would *insert dry cotton pellet only without temporizing the tooth till next visit.* Moreover, the trend within the GDPs group was to *leave the tooth open till next visit.* These findings are consistent with those obtained in a previous study which revealed that leaving the tooth open for drainage is still present in the United Kingdom's dental practice [4]. With only 12% of GDPs, in the current study, reporting *lack of time* as a reason for their decision, it is clearly that they need to understanding that leaving the tooth open till next visit is inappropriate because it allows more microbial invasion to the root canal system and may cause more complications [49, 50]. Foreign objects may enter the root canal system or even to the periapical area [51]. With very little scientific evidence [49], the best action a clinician may take in case of significant exudates is that he/she steps away from the patient, or ask the patient to wait in the waiting area, for some time to allow the drainage to continue and hopefully resolve on the same treatment visit [2]. As expected, endodontic showed, to some extent, good practice as one of the highest proportions of them opted this good approach. Nevertheless, the trend of leaving the tooth open dramatically reduced in cases of little exudates after C&S. Of those who would leave the tooth open if non-stopped exudates presents in the first visit, the majority (81.9%) would temporize the tooth if little exudates present after C&S. It is clearly that the presence of the exudates impairs clinicians from taking the right decision. Clinicians need to understand that even with the presence of exudates, giving the tooth enough time in the first visit then C&S is usually the practice of choice that results in good drainage. More importantly, they need to improve their practice and do their best not to leave the tooth open regardless the tooth initial conditions.

Nevertheless, this study was conducted in Saudi dental practice, which can be considered as one limitation. Further studies in other countries with different dental practices environment, regulations and set-ups are paramount to conclude general recommendations.

Conclusions

Within the limitations of the current study, the following can be concluded:

- Clinicians showed clear trend towards preserving teeth involved in NPAAA, though they, especially GDPs, opted to treat them differently from those with vital-pulp cases. The main differences were using different ICMs and different irrigants, C&S to different apical size preparation.
- GDPs need to improve their practicing in specific aspects when dealing with NPAAA cases such as implementing Crown-Down technique and multi-irrigants protocol while C&S, limit prescribing antibiotics, perform complete debridement of the root canal system and not to leave the tooth open between visits.
- Though endodontists showed overall good practice, they need to completely adhere to the obligatory use of rubber dam.
- There is urgent need for clear guidelines that are based on scientific evidence because clinicians, especially GDPs, relied on their own experiences in managing NPAA cases.

Abbreviations

C&S: cleaning and shaping; CH: calcium hydroxide; CHX: chlorohexidine; EDTA: ethylene diamine tetra acetic acid; GDPs: general dental practitioners; NPAAA: necrotic pulp with acute apical abscess

Acknowledgements

The author would like to thanks all participants who responded to this survey study.

Authors' contributions

This study has been conduct by a single author (AAM) who is submitting for publication consideration. The author read and approved the final manuscript.

Competing interests

The author declares that he has no competing interests.

References

1. Kakehashi S, Stanley HR, Fitzgerald RJ. The effects of surgical exposures of dental pulps in germfree and conventional laboratory rats. J South Calif Dent Assoc. 1966;34:449–51.
2. Torabinejad M, Walton R. Endodontics: principles and practice. 4th ed. St. Louis: Saunders; 2009.
3. Aminoshariae A, Kulild JC. Evidence-based recommendations for antibiotic usage to treat endodontic infections and pain: A systematic review of randomized controlled trials. J Am Dent Assoc. 2016;147:186–91.
4. Eliyas S, Barber MW, Harris I. Do general dental practitioners leave teeth on 'open drainage'? Br Dent J. 2013;215:611–6.
5. Al-Fouzan KS. A survey of root canal treatment of molar teeth by general dental practitioners in private practice in Saudi Arabia. Saudi Dent J. 2010; 22:113–7.
6. Siqueira JF Jr, Rocas IN. Diversity of endodontic microbiota revisited. J Dent Res. 2009;88:969–81.
7. Going RE, Sawinski VJ. Parameters related to the use of the rubber dam. J Am Dent Assoc. 1968;77:598–601.
8. Joynt RB, Davis EL, Schreier PH. Rubber dam usage among practicing dentists. Oper Dent. 1989;14:176–81.
9. Marshall K, Page J. The use of rubber dam in the UK. A survey. Br Dent J. 1990;169:286–91.
10. Whitworth JM, Seccombe GV, Shoker K, Steele JG. Use of rubber dam and irrigant selection in UK general dental practice. Int Endod J. 2000;33:435–41.
11. Madarati AA. Why dentists don't use rubber dam during endodontics and how to promote its usage? BMC Oral Health. 2016;25(16):24.
12. European Endodontic Society. Quality guidelines for endodontic treatment: consensus report of the European Society of Endodontology. Int Endod J. 2006;39:921–30.
13. Mickel AK, Nguyen TH, Chogle S. Antimicrobial activity of endodontic sealers on Enterococus faecalis. J Endod. 2003;29:257–8.
14. Desai S, Chandler N. Calcium hydroxide-based root canal sealers: a review. J Endod. 2009;35:475–80.

15. Mohammadi Z, Dummer PM. Properties and applications of calcium hydroxide in endodontics and dental traumatology. Int Endod J. 2011;44: 697–730.
16. Mestieri LB, Gomes-Cornelio AL, Rodrigues EM, Salles LP, Bosso-Martelo R, Guerreiro-Tanomaru JM, Tanomaru-Filho M. Biocompatibility and bioactivity of calcium silicate-based endodontic sealers in human dental pulp cells. J Appl Oral Sci. 2015;23:467–71.
17. Saini HR, Tewari S, Sangwan P, Duhan J, Gupta A. Effect of different apical preparation sizes on outcome of primary endodontic treatment: a randomized controlled trial. J Endod. 2012;38:1309–15.
18. Orstavik D, Kerekes K, Molven O. Effects of extensive apical reaming and calcium hydroxide dressing on bacterial infection during treatment of apical periodontitis: a pilot study. Int Endod J. 1991;24:1–7.
19. McGurkin-Smith R, Trope M, Caplan D, Sigurdsson A. Reduction of intracanal bacteria using GT rotary instrumentation, 5.25% NaOCl, EDTA, and ca(OH)2. J Endod. 2005;31:359–63.
20. JFJr S, Rocas IN, Riche FN, Provenzano JC. Clinical outcome of the endodontic treatment of teeth with apical periodontitis using an antimicrobial protocol. Oral Surg Oral Med Oral Pathol Oral Radiol Endod. 2008;106:757–62.
21. Ram Z. Effectiveness of root canal irrigation. Oral Surg Oral Med Oral Pathol. 1977;44:306–12.
22. Salzgeber RM, Brilliant JD. An in vivo evaluation of the penetration of an irrigating solution in root canals. J Endod. 1977;3:394–8.
23. Chow TW. Mechanical effectiveness of root canal irrigation. J Endod. 1983;9: 475–9.
24. Card SJ, Sigurdsson A, Orstavik D, Trope M. The effectiveness of increased apical enlargement in reducing intracanal bacteria. J Endod. 2002;28:779–83.
25. Rollison S, Barnett F, Stevens RH. Efficacy of bacterial removal from instrumented root canals in vitro related to instrumentation technique and size. Oral Surg Oral Med Oral Pathol Oral Radiol Endod. 2002;94:366–71.
26. Usman N, Baumgartner JC, Marshall JG. Influence of instrument size on root canal debridement. J Endod. 2004;30:110–2.
27. Bierenkrant DE, Parashos P, Messer HH. The technical quality of nonsurgical root canal treatment performed by a selected cohort of Australian endodontists. Int Endod J. 2008;41:561–70.
28. Albrecht LJ, Baumgartner JC, Marshall JG. Evaluation of apical debris removal using various sizes and tapers of ProFile GT files. J Endod. 2004 Jun; 30(6):425–8.
29. Aminoshariae A, Kulild J. Master apical file size - smaller or larger: a systematic review of microbial reduction. Int Endod J. 2015;48:1007–22.
30. Rodrigues RCV, Zandi H, Kristoffersen AK, Enersen M, Mdala I, Ørstavik D, Rôças IN, Siqueira JF Jr. Influence of the apical preparation size and the Irrigant type on bacterial reduction in root canal-treated teeth with apical periodontitis. J Endod. 2017;43:1058–63.
31. Johnson W, Kulid JC, Tay F. Obturation of the cleaned and shaped root canal system. Chapter 7. In: Hargreaves KM, Berman LH, editors. Cohens' pathways of the pulp. 11th ed. St. Louis, Missouri: Elsevier Inc; 2016.
32. Willershausen I, Wolf TG, Schmidtmann I, Berger C, Ehlers V, Willershausen B, Briseño B. Survey of root canal irrigating solutions used in dental practices within Germany. Int Endod J. 2015;48:654–60.
33. Jose J, Krishnamma S, Peedikayil F, Aman S, Tomy N, Mariodan JP. Comparative Evaluation of Antimicrobial Activity of QMiX, 2.5% Sodium Hypochlorite, 2% Chlorhexidine, Guava Leaf Extract and Aloevera Extract Against Enterococcus faecalis and Candida albicans - An in-vitro Study. J Clin Diagn Res. 2016;10(5):ZC20–3.
34. Ng YL, Mann V, Gulabivala K. A prospective study of the factors affecting outcomes of nonsurgical root canal treatment: part 1: periapical health. Int Endod J. 2011;44:583–609.
35. Madarati AA, Zafar MS, Sammani AMN, Mandorah AO, Bani-Younes HA. Preference and usage of intracanal medications during endodontic treatment. Saudi Med J. 2017;38:755–63.
36. Lee MJ, Stewart WGHJ, Caine R. Current trends in endodontic practice: emergency treatments and technological armamentarium. J Endod. 2009;35:35–9.
37. Balto KA. Calcium hydroxide has limited effectiveness in eliminating bacteria from human root canal. Evid Based Dent. 2007;8:15–6.
38. Law A, Messer HH. An evidence-based analysis of the antibacterial effectiveness of intracanal medicaments. J Endod. 2004;30:689–94.
39. Sowmya HK, Subhash TS, Goel BR, Nandini TN, Bhandi BSH. Quantitative assessment of apical debris extrusion and intracanal debris in the apical third, using hand instrumentation and three rotary instrumentation systems. J Clin Diagn Res. 2014;8:206–10.
40. Segura-Egea JJ, Martín-González J, Jiménez-Sánchez MDC, Crespo-Gallardo I, Saúco-Márquez JJ, Velasco-Ortega E. Worldwide pattern of antibiotic prescription in endodontic infections. Int Dent J 2017; 67: 197–205.
41. Kuriyama T, Williams DW, Yanagisawa M, Iwahara K, Shimizu C, Nakagawa K, Yamamoto E, Karasawa T. Antimicrobial susceptibility of 800 anaerobic isolates from patients with dentoalveolar infection to 13 oral antibiotics. Oral Microbiol Immunol. 2007;22:285–8.
42. Pallasch TJ. Pharmacokinetic principles of antimicrobial therapy. Periodontol 2000. 1996;10:5–11.
43. Dorn SO, Moodnik RM, Feldman MJ, Borden BG. Treatment of the endodontic emergency: a report based on a questionnaire–part I. J Endod. 1977;3:94–100.
44. Dorn SO, Moodnik RM, Feldman MJ, Borden BG. Treatment of the endodontic emergency: a report based on a questionnaire–part II. J Endod. 1977;3:153–6.
45. Eleazer PD, Eleazer KR. Flare-up rate in pulpally necrotic molars in one-visit versus two-visit endodontic treatment. J Endod. 1998;24:614–6.
46. Sjogren U, Figdor D, Persson S, Sundqvist G. Influence of infection at the time of root filling on the outcome of endodontic treatment of teeth with apical periodontitis. Int Endod J. 1997;30:297–306.
47. Trope ME, Delano EO, Orstavik D. Endodontic treatment of teeth with apical periodontitis: single vs. multivisit treatment. J Endod. 1999;25:345–50.
48. Penesis VA, Fitzgerald PI, Fayad MI, Wenckus CS, BeGole EA, Johnson BR. Outcome of one-visit and two-visit endodontic treatment of necrotic teeth with apical periodontitis: a randomized controlled trial with one-year evaluation. J Endod. 2008;34:251–7.
49. Bence R, Meyers RD, Knoff RV. Evaluation of 5,000 endodontic treatments: incidence of the opened tooth. Oral Surg Oral Med Oral Pathol. 1980;49:82–4.
50. Wein F. Closing a tooth left open for drainage. Chronicle. 1975;38:406–7. 410
51. Simon JH, Chimenti RA, Mintz GA. Clinical significance of the pulse granuloma. J Endod. 1982;8:116–9.

10

Using community participation to assess demand and uptake of scaling and polishing in rural and urban environments

Ezi A. Akaji*, Nkolika P. Uguru, Sam N. Maduakor and Etisiobi M. Ndiokwelu

Abstract

Background: One of the control tools for periodontal disease besides individual home care is professional oral prophylaxis that is, Scaling and Polishing (S&P).The aim of this study is to assess the effect of oral health awareness on the demand and uptake of scaling and polishing among dwellers of rural and urban environments.

Methods: This interventional study was conducted in Enugu, Nigeria. A questionnaire was used to obtain data on demographic details, presenting complaints and requests, and prior dental visits from consenting attendees in 4 community outreaches. The number of those demanding for scaling of teeth at point of presentation was extracted from their requests. Oral health talk was then given as the intervention for the study. Periodontal assessment was done using Community Periodontal index (CPI) and participants who received scaling thereafter were recorded. Data were analyzed with SPSS [version 20] employing Chi square to compare categorical variables and p was significant at ≤0.05. Multiple regression analysis of factors affecting oral health awareness was done and outcome of intervention was determined by percentage difference in number of participants demanding and receiving S&P.

Results: A total of 454 participants enlisted for the study. The outreaches served as first point of contact with dental professionals for 383 (84.4%) participants. 60 (80%) and 15 (20%) participants demanded for scaling in the urban and rural locations respectively ($p = 0.00$). Out of 78 with CPI 3 score, only 8 (10.3%) demanded for S&P but uptake was by 73 (93.6%) [$p = 0.00$]. Outcome of oral health intervention was 80.6% difference among those with periodontitis. Multiple regression analysis of factors showed that participants' locations, that is, rural or urban, was the only factor that significantly affected oral health awareness ($C.I = 0.183–0.375$, $p = 0.000$).

Conclusion: Demand for scaling was sub-optimal but the uptake was satisfactory. Rural or urban location of the participants significantly influenced their oral health awareness. The keenness to take up scaling suggests benefits accruing from the oral health education. Appropriate health policies and planning could help bridge the gap between rural and urban areas and strengthen gains from this study.

Keywords: Periodontal disease, Community health education, Dental scaling, Utilization, Health services demand

Background

The term periodontal disease encompasses all pathological conditions of periodontal tissues categorized broadly as gingivitis and periodontitis [1].Gingivitis, an inflammatory lesion of marginal gingiva is highly prevalent in most populations and at most ages with global values ranging from 50 to 90% [2]. Gingivitis could resolve with improved oral hygiene, persist indefinitely or may result in attachment loss. [3] If loss or destruction of periodontal attachment or alveolar bone occurs, the condition is characterized as periodontitis [4]. Periodontitis is a major public health problem having met all the conditions for such, and the manifestations –bleeding, halitosis, gingival recession and tooth loss impact negatively on the affected individual [5, 6]. It is the most common chronic inflammatory disease seen in humans, affecting nearly half of adults in the United Kingdom and 60% of those over 65 years [7].Severe periodontitis, which may result in tooth loss, is found in most populations affecting both

* Correspondence: ezi.akaji@unn.edu.ng
Department of Preventive Dentistry, Faculty of Dentistry, College of Medicine, University of Nigeria, UNTH, Enugu, Nigeria

old and young age groups [8, 9]. A systematic analysis of global burden of oral conditions from 1990 to 2010 by Marcenes et al. (2013) showed that, severe periodontitis was the leading cause of Disability Adjusted Life Years (DALYs) in 9 regions of the world -Australia, Sub-Saharan Africa, East, Central, East, and Southeast Asia, and Southern, Central, Tropical, and Latin America [10]. A similar study specific for periodontitis found the disease had affected 743 million people worldwide with the age-standardized incidence rate of 701 cases per 100,000 person/years for severe periodontitis in 2010 [11].

The primary aetiological factor for periodontitis is dental plaque, which is a tenaciously adherent biofilm on teeth and gingival surfaces and is 70% bacteria while mineralized plaque deposits called calculus is one of the secondary factors [1]. Professional oral prophylaxis (that is scaling and polishing) performed by a dental care professional serves as one control measure for the disease [12]. Scaling is the removal of plaque, calculus, debris and staining from the crown and root surfaces of the teeth using specially designed sharp dental hand instruments or ultrasonic scalers. In order to smoothen teeth surfaces, a procedure called polishing is carried out. This involves removing any residual extrinsic stains and deposits using a rubber cup or bristle brush loaded with a prophylactic paste [12]. Scaling and polishing is nonsurgical procedure; intended to supplement the patient's home-care plaque control and is frequently provided as part of the dental recall appointment [13].With the removal of plaque and calculus, the clinical indicators of the active disease - bleeding and inflammation of the gums (gingivitis) – are also reduced and over time a reduction in gingivitis will reduce progression to periodontitis [12]. Individuals could benefit from this basic dental care every 6, 9 or 12 months depending on their peculiar needs [12, 13].Sadly, most do not access this basic dental care with negative implications to their periodontal health and this is often a function of level of awareness of oral diseases [14].

Access has being defined by several authors from different dimensions [15]. Utilization often used as a proxy of access, (that is, realised access) [16], is influenced by the supply as well as the demand for services, including individual attributes such as preferences, tastes and information [15].An individual or collective alertness to the existence and prevention of oral diseases and an equal alertness in taking necessary steps to obtain treatment for these diseases when they occur is referred to as oral health awareness [17]. According to some studies, poor oral health awareness among other factors is responsible for the occurrence of dental diseases [14, 18]. Other studies observed that when there is low oral health awareness, there is a direct effect on the illness seeking behaviour of the individual and population. The most common scenario is the underutilization of oral health facilities and/or late presentation at the clinic with resultant complications due to poor public enlightenment regarding prevention and treatment of these diseases [14].The concept of demand, utilization and awareness of dental services are all interrelated. Oral health utilization can be defined as the actual attendance by members of the public at oral health facilities to receive care. Demand on the other hand, 'which equates demand for uptake in our study' can be defined as a perception by the individual or community that a need exists. It can also be defined as the ability of the patient to seek dental health [19].

Observations from a study conducted in rural India show a significant association between dental awareness and demand for dental services [18]. Another study reported that awareness of individuals and communities need to be built in order to motivate the use of dental services. The same study also observed that imparting preventive dental education and strengthening of dental health facilities will increase utilization. It was also concluded that barriers to demand for dental care and utilization of dental services can be removed by motivating people and creating awareness about oral health problems prevention strategies and treatment in order to remove fear and anxiety [20]. Therefore, we hypothesize that if oral health education were provided to individuals to increase their oral health awareness, then, there will be increase in demand and uptake of oral health preventive services.

For a wider view on demand and uptake of scaling services, we conducted our study in rural and urban communities using outreach platforms. Community outreach programs offer opportunities for early diagnosis and treatment, dental health education, and institution of preventive measures so can spread awareness and disseminate treatment thereby enhancing access to care especially within the rural communities [21, 22].The aim of our study was to assess the effect of oral health awareness on the demand and uptake of scaling and polishing among dwellers of rural and urban environments.

Methods

Study area and design

This was an interventional study conducted in Enugu State Nigeria. The state is situated in inland south eastern Nigeria, and covers 7161 km^2 (Additional file 1). It is made up of 17 local government areas (LGAs) with at least one primary health care centre sited in each LGA [23]. From the list of LGAs obtained, we grouped them according to their geographic location (urban and rural). We selected two LGAs each from urban and rural areas by simple random sampling. This was done to ensure proper representation of both urban and rural communities. From each selected LGA, a community was selected by simple random method from the list of communities provided. Outreach was staged in each selected community and the Thailand's oral care model described by Professor P. Phantumvanit in the Peterson and Kwam's study (2004) was partly adopted here [24]. The model fosters community participation and capacity building for oral health promotion, hence, for our study, each selected community provided volunteers to help with the program.

Sample size and selection of participants

A minimum sample size of 453 was obtained using the formula $N = Z^2 P (1-P)/D^2$ with a consideration of the possibility of 20% non-response from participants (Araoye 2003) [25]. Our sample frame was drawn from households residing in the communities where outreach programs were held. Community heads and volunteers they endorsed facilitated the process by informing and inviting households and individuals to the outreach.

Inclusion and exclusion criteria

Consenting attendees who were willing to participate in study (see Additional file 2) were included while those who gave no consent were excluded.

Data collection

Phase 1

As attendees arrived at the outreach, a questionnaire (Additional file 2) was administered to the consenting ones by the researchers to obtain data on demographic details, frequency of tooth brushing and number of visits to an oral health care professional prior to the outreach and present dental concern/need if any. One of the options for dental concern /need stem question was "cleaning of teeth". Response to this question was used to measure demand for S&P. Thereafter, an oral health educational talk highlighting the need and methods for good oral care with tooth brushing demonstrations and the attendant implications were done. Volunteers translated the talk in the native dialect of the community. The oral health education (OHE) served as the intervention in this study. All attendees (study participants and others) were given tooth cleaning materials. Phase 1 ended with periodontal assessment of consenting participants. This was done by 3 examiners employing the modified Community Periodontal Index (CPI) [26] with a sterilized CPI probe and mouth mirror under artificial illumination provided by fluorescent light and head banded torch, in a temporarily created screened corner at the outreach venue. Face mask and examination gloves were worn by the examiner to prevent cross infection. Calibration of examiners was done by training them on the specific instruments to use. There was pre-assessment on 10 patients before the outreach in order to determine the uniformity of instruments of measure (CPI probe) and the grading system used by all examiners. The examiners were asked to measure and chart findings during the training and were assessed to ensure reliability and validity of measurement. Probing depth was used as the unit of measure among the three examiners.

Phase 2

Here, uptake of scaling and polishing (S&P) was recorded capturing those that requested for dental scaling when the questionnaire was administered initially and those who decided for it after the oral health intervention. The uptake was measured by the number of participants receiving S&P at the outreach or 6 months after in designated oral health care centres. S&P was carried out by dentists, dental therapists and final year dental students using disposable materials and instruments in separate packs for each participant in accordance with universal infection control standards prescribed by the World Health Organization [27]. The scaling procedure was done with the participants seated on a mobile dental chair which had a detachable sputum bowl. To ensure privacy, a collapsible standing shield was used to secure the place. Hand instruments such as jacquette scalers, and universal scalers were used to remove dental plaque and calculus from tooth surfaces; the recipients rinsed their mouth with water from disposable cups intermittently. Those who opted to have their scaling done later were given identifiers in form of tally numbers and sent to designated dental centres.

Our primary outcome was determined by percentage difference in demand and uptake of scaling services amongst those with scaling treatment need after delivery of the oral health education. For the purpose of this study, awareness was measured using number of dental visits as proxy for it. We did that because evidence from studies carried out in similar context show that the number of dental visits made by respondents for routine check up or otherwise was based on their level of awareness [14, 20, 28].

Data analysis

Data collected were analysed using the Statistical Package for Social Sciences software for windows (version 20 SPSS Inc. Chicago IL), describing categorical variables using frequencies and percentages. Statistical significant differences among groups were determined by the Chi-square test and Confidence intervals; the level of significance was set at $P \leq 0.05$. Percentage difference in demand and uptake of scaling of teeth was calculated.

Results

Four hundred and fifty four participants aged 2 to 86 years (mean: 38.5 ± 14.8 years) were included in the study. 245 (54.0%) participants enlisted in the rural outreaches and 209 (46.0%) in the urban centres; 219 (48. 2%) were males and 235 (51.8%) were females. The outreaches served as first point of contact with dental professionals for 383 (84.4%) participants and as second for 56 (12.3%). Other demographic details are in Table 1.

On the overall, 60 (28.7%) participants demanded for scaling of their teeth in the urban outreaches and 15(6. 1%) did in the rural communities ($p = 0.00$). Also, 50 (66. 7%) males and 25 (33.7%) females demanded for scaling at the outreaches (p = 0.00). A total of 364(80.2%) participants had scaling and polishing during the program and/or within 6 months after in designated dental facilities; 160 (44.0%) in the urban and 204 (56.0%) in the rural communities ($p = 0.04$).These are shown in Table 2.

We also considered the association between periodontal status with demand and uptake of scaling as presented in Table 3 and found 42 (26.8%) of those with mild gingivitis [CPI score1] demanded for S&P. However, even with CPI scores 3 and 4, 70 (89.7%) and 15 (93.8%) respectively did not indicate interest in S&P ($p = 0.00$). However, 73 (93.6%) of those with CPI 3 received scaling post intervention. From the Table 3, we extracted data for percentage difference in demand and uptake of scaling amongst those with the periodontal treatment needs and obtained an 80.8% difference; details of the calculation are in Table 4.

Table 1 Socio-demographic details of the participants

Participants' characteristics	Number ($N = 454$)	Percentage
Age group		
0–29 yrs	152	33.5%
30–59 yrs	255	56.2%
≥ 60 yrs. (Mean: 38.5 ± 14.8 yrs)	47	10.3%
Gender		
Male	219	48.2
Female	235	51.8
Location		
Urban	209	46.0
Rural	245	54.0
No of previous visit(s) for dental care		
1st visit	383	84.4
2nd visit	56	12.3
> 2 visits	15	3.3
Demand for dental scaling		
Yes	75	16.5
No	379	83.5
Uptake of dental scaling		
Yes	364	80.2
No	90	19.8

The outreach served as first contact with dental professionals for 84.4% of the participants

Table 2 Level of demand and uptake of dental scaling according to location and gender

Variable	Demand		Uptake	
	Yes	No	Yes	No
Urban	60 (80%)	149 (39.3%)	160 (44%)	49 (54.4%)
Rural	15 (20%)	230 (60.7%)	204 (56%)	41 (45.6%)
Total	75 (100%)	379 (100)	364 (100)	90 (100)
p-value	$p = 0.00$*		$p = 0.07$	
Male	50 (66.7%)	169 (44.6%)	175 (48.1%)	44 (48.9%)
Female	25 (33.3%)	210 (55.4%)	189 (51.9%)	46 (51.1%)
Total	75 (100)	379 (100)	364 (100)	90 (100)
	$p = 0.00$*		$p = 0.89$	

*Statistically significant

Using the number of dental visits prior to outreach as a proxy for awareness in our study, a multiple regression analysis of factors affecting oral health awareness was done. Analysis showed that there was 0.279 increase in awareness depending on the place of abode of the respondents ($p = 0.00$), so we can predict that the geographic location (urban or rural) of a person affects the oral health awareness. Our table also showed that for every unit increase in age there was a 0.004 reduction in number of dental visits ($p = 0.853$) and a 0.024 increase in uptake of S&P is predicted ($p = 0.652$) (Table 5).

Discussion

The ultimate aim of periodontal treatment is to control disease progression or achieve a rate of progression which is compatible with a functional dentition for the lifetime of the individual [2, 4]. Our study created an opportunity for such through oral health education as intervention and platform for interaction between populace and the dental professionals in the communities. It also served as an opportunity to introduce basic dental scaling to the people who though needed the service were yet to attend dental clinic.

From our study we observed that more females than males enlisted in the study. However, this higher attendance of women than men does not necessarily translate to increased awareness because the effect of gender on awareness was found not to be significant in this study. This could mean that females were probably more readily available at the time of our visit or that given the fact that women are the primary care givers in the home, and tend to visit health facilities more than males, either for themselves or their children; they had better opportunity to

Table 3 Demand and uptake of dental scaling according to periodontal status

Variable	Periodontal status of participants					
Demand for S&P	Healthy Periodontium	Mild gingivitis	Moderate Gingivitis	Periodontitis		Total
	CPI 0	CPI 1	CPI 2	CPI 3	CPI 4	
	n (%)	*n* (%)	*n* (%)	*n* (%)	*n* (%)	*N*
Yes	1 (7.7))	42 (26.8)	23(12.1)	8 (10.3)	1 (6.3)	75
No	12 (92.3)	115 (73.2)	167 (87.9)	70 (89.7)	15 (93.8)	379
Total	13 (100)	157 (100)	190 (100)	78 (100)	16 (100)	454
$X^2 = 18.8$ $p = 0.01$ Significant						
Uptake	CPI 0	CPI 1	CPI 2	CPI 3	CPI 4	
Yes	6 (46.2)	113 (72.0)	160 (84.2)	73 (93.6)	12 (75.0)	364
No	7 (53.8)	44 (28.0)	30 (15.8)	5 (6.4)	4 (25.0)	90
Total	13 (100)	157 (100)	190 (100)	78 (100)	16 (100)	454
$X^2 = 24.4$ $p = 0.00$ Significant						

CPI = Community Periodontal Index
CPI Score 0 = Healthy periodontium; CPI Scores 1 & 2 = Gingivitis; CPI Score 3 & 4 = Periodontitis

partake than the males. A previous study on gender influence on oral health proposed that females are more informed about oral health than men and take more interest in their oral health than men [29]. In as much as we do not disagree with this notion, most public or community dental practices are usually incorporated in a regular medical facility and as such women who visit for other purposes such as maternal and child health issues, are readily available for dental awareness creation programs. Therefore, they were in a better position to get more information about preventive oral health services.

We observed that only a minority of the participants with scaling treatment need (9.6%) demanded for scaling services at the outreaches, however post-intervention, we recorded an uptake of scaling by 90.4% of participants which most likely was spurred up by some factors (see Table 4). We attributed this mainly to the motivation and educational talks received during the program having positive effect on participants. This corroborates the statement by Nash and Brown (2012) that "Oral disease and the resulting need for information, therapy, and rehabilitation are the starting point for the demand for dental services" [30]. Our oral health intervention interlaced with the supply of the scaling services to the participants might have addressed the barriers posed by availability, and access to treatment similar to reports from other studies [31, 32]. Access can no longer be looked at from the patients' ability to obtain or utilize care alone but is now essentially a concept of supply - demand where both availability of dental care which can represent the supply side and individual factors related to patients need, cultural and community considerations relating to the demand side are both taken into consideration [33]. On the overall, with a recorded percentage difference of 80.8% in demand and uptake of scaling for those with scaling treatment need and 63.7% all participants (Table 4), we can infer that the intervention in this study positively influenced uptake of scaling. This is similar to the report of a study in school aged children that OHE is effective in increasing knowledge, attitude and practice of individuals [34].

Looking at gender influence on demand and uptake of scaling, males demanded for scaling of teeth more than women but more women took up the scaling treatment at the long run. This may be due to cultural and behavioural attributes of men where they are initially more decisive than women. However, the actual uptake of healthcare is subject to a myriad of factors such as their workplace demands, self- perceived oral health need, and their perception of the seriousness of the condition [32, 35, 36]. This is corroborated by a report that females had better oral healthcare habits than the males,

Table 4 Percentage difference in demand and uptake of dental scaling

Groups	% requesting or taking up scaling		Outcome
	Demand	Uptake	
For all participants	75/454 = 16.5%	364/454 = 80.2%	80.2–16.5 = 63.7% difference
For those with Scaling treatment need[a]	9/94 = 9.6%	85/94 = 90.4%	90.4–9.6 = 80.8% difference

[a]This group was made up of participants with CPI Scores of 3 and 4

Table 5 A multiple regression of factors affecting oral health awareness

Variables	Standardized coefficient	*P* value	Lower limit (Confidence Interval)	Upper limit (Confidence Interval)
Constant	.520	0.00	.252	.789
Uptake of S&P	0.024	.652	–.082	.131
No. of times brushed	0.047	.243	–.032	.125
Age category	–0.004	.853	–.049	.041
Demand for S&P	0.063	.293	–.055	.181
Gender	0.066	.140	–.022	.154
Location	.279	.0001	.183	.375

$R^2 = 0.116$
Dependent variable: Number of visit to dentist (as measure of awareness)
Predictors (constant), uptake of S&P, no. of times brushed, age category, demand for S&P, Gender and Location
Predictors coded as yes = 1; No = 2
Reference categories: No uptake of S&P, No brushing, Age category: 0 to 39 yrs., No demand for S&P, Gender- Male, For location- Rural, Unit of variables have been standardized

were more concerned about how their teeth looked than males, thus would be more inclined to get their teeth scaled and polished and retain their teeth in good health [37].

Furthermore, we observed that individuals with CPI scores 3 and 4, that is, more severe periodontal conditions, were not interested in S & P; we attributed this to lack of perceived need for it. In our environment, credible reports show perceived need of dental condition is a function of how aware the individuals are about oral health or health in general. [32, 35]. Awareness creation can motivate behavioural change in respondents and improve their dental health seeking pattern as reported in other studies. [14] It is our view that the oral health education created a platform to motivate those with severe periodontal condition who initially did not demand for scaling to take up.

Furthermore, a number of factors affected oral health awareness in the present study (Table 5). The location of the participants, that is rural or urban, affected awareness significantly. This observation also flows with our other finding stated above that more urban participants than rural demanded for scaling ($p = 0.00$). Rural dwellers have been known to face challenges of awareness and use of oral health facilities [14, 22]. By implication, low oral health awareness has a direct effect on the illness seeking behaviour of the individuals and population and need to be built up in order to motivate the use of dental services; our study was able to achieve this to a reasonable extent. Other factors such as age, gender and number of times brushed, illustrated a trend in influencing the outcome variable, but the results were not statistically significant.

The present study has limitations that must be taken into account to correctly interpret the findings. First, the use of prior dental visit alone as proxy for awareness may lead to partial assessment of oral health awareness as other facets exist but within the scope of our study, we were able to synergize the two. Secondly, using community outreach programs to recruit study participants could be a limitation for our study. However, this method has been known to aid recruitment of hard to reach populations or minority groups into studies. In the light of this, our approach was able to capture women, children as well as men who most often do not seek healthcare [38]. This approach has proved effective in other studies as a means of recruiting study participants. [21, 22]. Another limitation to our study could be the use of CPI to measure periodontal status of participants. CPI is saddled with the challenge of either underestimating or overestimating periodontal treatment needs as fake pockets resulting from gingival overgrowth without attachment loss could be mistaken for true periodontitis.

In terms of strengths, we were able to reach out to a good number of people especially the grassroots, hoist promotional activities like oral health education, and provide professional dental scaling of teeth to the individuals within the ambit of our study. These gains could be sustained by instituting appropriate health policies which will inform better planning and encourage the viability of oral health care activities in the communities possibly by incorporating them into existing primary health care centres.

Conclusions

The demand for scaling and polishing by the participants was sub-optimal; uptake during and after the outreaches was however satisfactory. The keenness to take up S&P suggests benefits accruing from the oral health education as intervention in our study. Only geographic location of the participants affected their oral health awareness significantly; other factors such as age and gender did not. Our findings could aid in appropriate policy making and planning for basic oral health services to reach the grassroots possibly using existing primary oral health care platforms.

Abbreviations

CPI: Community Periodontal Index; OHE: Oral health Education; S&P: Scaling and Polishing; WHO: World Health Organization

Acknowledgements

Our sincere gratitude goes to the community leaders, volunteers, resident doctors, dental therapists and the final year dental students for their assistance in carrying out this study. We also thank the dental clinics that helped with the post-outreach dental scaling services.

Funding

No internal or external funding was received from any individual or group.

Authors' contributions

EAA: Conceptualization, study design, data collection, data analysis, manuscript draft, critical editing of the manuscript for important intellectual content. NPU: Study design, data collection, data analysis and critical editing of the manuscript for important intellectual content. SNM: Data collection and critical editing of the manuscript for important intellectual content. EMN: Data collection and critical editing of the manuscript for important intellectual content. All authors read and approved the final draft.

Authors' information

EAA: Senior Lecturer/ Consultant in Community Dentistry, Department of Preventive Dentistry, College of Medicine, University of Nigeria /UNTH, Enugu State, Nigeria.
NPU: Senior Lecturer in Community Dentistry, Department of Preventive Dentistry, College of Medicine, University of Nigeria, Enugu State, Nigeria.
SNM: Lecturer /Consultant in Periodontology, Department of Preventive Dentistry, College of Medicine, University of Nigeria/UNTH, Enugu State, Nigeria.
EMN: Professor in Community Dentistry, Department of Preventive Dentistry, College of Medicine, University of Nigeria, Enugu State, Nigeria.

Competing interests

The authors declare that they have no competing interests.

References

1. Umeizudike KA, Ayanbadejo PO, Onojole AT, Umeizudike TI, Alade GO. Periodontal status and its association with self-reported hypertension in non-medical staff in a university teaching hospital in Nigeria. Odonto-Stomatol Trop. 2016;39:47–55.
2. Albandar JM. Global risk factors and risk indicators for periodontal diseases. Periodontol. 2000;2002(29):177–206.
3. Chestnut IG, Gibson J. Churchhill's pocketbook of clinical dentistry. 2nd edition, Churchill Livingstone, Glasgow 2002; pg 173–174.
4. Boehm TK, Scannapieco FA. The epidemiology, consequences and management of periodontal disease in older adults. J Am Dent Assoc. 2007; 138:26S–32S.
5. Batchelor P. Is periodontal disease a public health problem? British dental journal. 217: 405 – 409. Published online: 24 October 2014 | doi:101038/sjbdj2014.912.
6. Daly B, Batchelor PA, Treasure ET, Watt RG. Essential dental public health. 2nd ed. Oxford: Oxford University Press; 2013.
7. Chapple ILC. Time to take periodontitis seriously. Br Med J. 2014;348:2645.
8. Petersen PE. The world oral health report 2003: continuous improvement of oral health in the 21st century - the approach of the WHO global oral health Programme. Community Dent Oral Epidemiol. 2003;31(suppl. 1):3–24.
9. Petersen PE, Yamamoto T. Improving the oral health of older people: the approach of the WHO global oral health Programme. Community Dent Oral Epidemiol. 2005;33:81–92.
10. Marcenes W, Kassebaum NJ, Bernabé E, Flaxman A, Naghavi M, Lopez A, Murray CJL. Global burden of oral conditions in 1990-2010: a systematic analysis. J Dent Res. 2013 Jul;92(7):592–7.
11. Kassebaum NJ, Bernabé E, Dahiya M, Bhandari B, Murray CJL, Marcenes W. Global burden of severe periodontitis in 1990-2010: a systematic review and meta-regression. J Dent Res. 2014;93(11):1045–53.
12. Worthington HV, Clarkson JE, Bryan G, Beirne PV. Routine scale and polish for periodontal health in adults. *Cochrane Database of Systematic Reviews* 2013, Issue 11. Art. No: CD004625. DOI: https://doi.org/10.1002/14651858.CD004625.pub4 (accessed September 12, 2015).
13. Beirne P, Forgie A, Clarkson JE, Worthington HV. Recall intervals for oral health in primary care patients. *Cochrane Database of Systematic Reviews*, 2005; Issue 2 [DOI:https://doi.org/10.1002/14651858.CD004346.pub3] (Accessed September 12, 2015).
14. Sofola OO. Implications of low oral health awareness in Nigeria. Niger Med J. 2010;51:131–3.
15. Levesque J, Harris MF, Russel G. Patient-centred access to health care: conceptualising access at the interface of health systems and populations. Int J Equity Health. 2013;12:18.
16. Peters DH, Garg A, Bloom G, Walker DG, Brieger WR, Rahman MH. Poverty and access to health care in developing countries. Ann N Y. Acad Sci. 2007; 1136:161–71.
17. Jeboda SO. Implication of low dental awareness in Nigeria. Niger Dent J. 2008;16:43–5.
18. Preksha P, Bharath K, Rushabh D, Geetika A, Jitendra S. Utilization of dental services in public health center: dental attendance, awareness and felt needs. J Contemp Dent Pract. 2015;16:829–33.
19. Pradeep Y, Chakravarty KK, Simhadri K, Ghenam A, Naidu GM, Vundavalli S. Gaps in need, demand, and effective demand for dental care utilization among residents of Krishna district, Andhra Pradesh, India. J Int Soc Prev Community Dent. 2016;6(Suppl 2):S116–21. https://doi.org/10.4103/2231-0762.189737.
20. Gambhir RS, Brar P, Singh G, Sofat A, Kakar H. Utilization of dental care: an Indian outlook. J Nat Sci Biol Med. 2013;4(2):292–7. https://doi.org/10.4103/0976-9668.116972.
21. Kadaluru UG, Kempraj VM, Muddaiah P. Utilization of oral health care services among adults attending community outreach programs. Indian J Dent Res. 2012;23:841–2.
22. Asawa K, Bhanushali NV, Tak M, Kumar DRV, et al. Utilization of services and referrals through dental outreach programs in rural areas of India. A two year study. Rocz Panstw Zakl Hig. 2015;66(3):275–80.
23. Learn About Enugu State, Nigeria | People, Local ... - NgEX.com. Available at: *www.ngex.com/nigeria/places/states/enugu.htm*. (Accessed Jan 5, 2017).
24. Petersen PE, Kwan S. Evaluation of community-based oral health promotion and oral disease prevention – WHO recommendations for improved evidence in public health practice. Comm Dent Health. 2004;21(Suppl):319–29.
25. Araoye MO. Research methodology with statistics for health and social sciences. 1st ed. Ilorin: Nathadex; 2003. p. 117–21.
26. World Health Organization. Oral health surveys: basic methods. 4th ed. Geneva: World Health Organization; 1997.
27. World Health Organization: Infection control standard precaution in health care.2006 http://www.who.int/csr/resources/publications/4EPR_AM2.pdf. *(Accessed June 10, 2015).*
28. Denloye O, Ajayi D, Bankole O, Bamidele P. Dental service utilization among junior secondary school students in Ibadan, Nigeria. Pediatr Dent J. 2010; 20(2):177–81.
29. Azodo C, Unamatokp B. Gender difference in oral health perception and practices among medical house officers. Russian Open Med J. 2012;1(2)
30. Nash KD, Brown LJ. The market for dental services. J Dent Educ. 2012;76:973–86.
31. Croucher R, Sohanpal R. Improving access to dental care in East London's ethnic minority groups: community based qualitative study. Comm Dent Health. 2006;23:95–100.

32. Uguru NP, Akaji EA, Ndiokwelu E, Uguru CC. Assessing health workers knowledge on the determinants of health: a study in Enugu Nigeria. Niger. J Med. 2012;21(1):48–52.
33. Guay AH. Access to dental care, solving the problem of the underserved populations. J Am Dent Assoc. 2004;135:1599–605.
34. Haque SE, Rahman M, Itsuko K, Mutahara M, Kayako S, Tsutsumi A, Islam MJ, Mostofa MG. Effect of a school-based oral health education in preventing untreated dental caries and increasing knowledge, attitude, and practices among adolescents in Bangladesh. BMC Oral Health. 2016;16:44. https://doi.org/10.1186/s12903-016-0202-3.
35. Akaji EA, Jeboda SO, Oredugba FA. Comparison of normative and self-perceived dental needs among adolescents in Lagos-Nigeria. Niger Postgrad Med J. Dec 2010;17(4):283–6.
36. White BA. Factors influencing demand for dental services: population, demographics, disease, insurance. J Dent Educ. 2012;76:996–1007.
37. Kawamura M, Wright FAC, Sasahara H, Yamasaki Y, Suh S, Iwamoto Y. An analytical study on gender differences in self-reported oral health care and problems of Japanese employees. J Occup Health. 1999;41:104–11.
38. Wang Y, Hunt K, Nazareth I, Freemantle N, Petersen I. Do men consult less than women? An analysis of routinely collected UK general practice data. BMJ Open. 2013;3:e003320. https://doi.org/10.1136/ bmjopen-2013-003320.

11

Association between maternal acculturation and health beliefs related to oral health of Latino children

Tamanna Tiwari[1*], Matthew Mulvahill[2], Anne Wilson[1], Nayanjot Rai[3] and Judith Albino[4]

Abstract

Background: This report is presenting the association of maternal acculturation, measured by preferred language, and oral health-related psychosocial measures in an urban Latino population.

Methods: A cross-sectional survey was conducted with 100 mother-child dyads from the Dental Center at the Children's Hospital Colorado, the University of Colorado. A portion of Basic Research Factors Questionnaire capturing information about parental dental knowledge, attitudes, behavior and psychosocial measures was used to collect data from the participating mothers. Descriptive statistics were calculated for demographics and psychosocial measures by acculturation. A univariate linear regression model was performed for each measure by preferred language for primary analysis followed by adjusted model adjusting for parent's education.

Results: The mean age of the children was 3.99 years (SD = 1.11), and that of the mother was 29.54 years (SD = 9.62). Dental caries, measured as dmfs, was significantly higher in children of Spanish-speaking mothers compared to children of English-speaking mothers. English-speaking mothers had higher mean scores of oral health knowledge, oral health behaviors, knowledge on dental utilization, self-efficacy, and Oral Health Locus of Control as compared to Spanish-speaking mothers. Univariate analysis demonstrated significant association for preference for Spanish language with knowledge on dental utilization, maternal self-efficacy, perceived susceptibility and perceived barriers. The effect of language was attenuated, but significant, for each of these variables after adjusting for parent's education.

Conclusion: This study reported that higher acculturation measured by a preference for the English language had a positive association with oral health outcomes in children. Spanish-speaking mothers perceived that their children were less susceptible to caries. Additionally, they perceived barriers in visiting the dentist for preventive visits.

Keywords: Oral health knowledge, Acculturation, Health belief model

Background

Acculturation is defined as the process by which individuals from a community may adopt the values and behaviors from another culture, and this may, in turn, affect their beliefs [1]. According to recent literature, acculturation is considered a multidimensional process, in which sociocultural changes may occur throughout the person's life course and varying even for individuals living within the same community [1–3].

* Correspondence: Tamanna.tiwari@ucdenver.edu
[1]Department of Community Dentistry and Population Health, School of Dental Medicine, University of Colorado Anschutz Medical Campus, Aurora, Colorado, USA
Full list of author information is available at the end of the article

There are many potential frameworks to understand the acculturation process and how it impacts health in immigrant populations. According to one theoretical framework, migration may cause psychosocial distress or loss of social support, resulting in a new behavioral environment that could be associated with the level of acculturation for an individual [3]. The framework presented by Fox et al. describes how socioeconomic conditions of migrant families may influence higher assimilation into the host culture, thereby resulting in higher levels of acculturation [3]. Furthermore, length of stay, language spoken at home, and social networks may influence the level of acculturation for an individual or a family [4, 5]. For example, educational level, preferred language, and level of dental knowledge of the social networks are associated with a higher level of acculturation and, in turn, with the utilization of dental health services [6].

Another concept presented by Gao et al. discusses that the impact of acculturation on health can be mediated via a change in health behaviors and perceptions of one's ability to prevent disease or receive treatment [7]. In the context of health beliefs, acculturation can influence utilization of health services, doctor-patient communication, adopting new health behaviors, and treatment decisions [7, 8]. Furthermore, acculturation may have a positive or negative effect on the health outcome in question [1]. For example, acculturation can be a risk factor for adoption of behaviors such as increased alcohol consumption, smoking, and higher fast food consumption, and on the other hand, it may promote increased amount of time engaged in exercise and physical activity [2].

For oral health outcomes, acculturation has been seen to influence the oral health behaviors, access, and navigation of oral healthcare [9, 10]. A recent systematic review of the impact of acculturation on oral health concluded that though higher levels of acculturation had a positive effect on utilization of dental services, this did not necessarily lead to improving oral health outcomes [7]. The authors also concluded that lower levels of acculturation might increase the risk of uptake of some unhealthy oral health-related behaviors, such as consumption of high sugary foods and drinks, and increase the risk of poor oral health outcomes [7]. Although there is a growing recognition that acculturation is a complicated process and that it influences oral health by a complex interplay of psychosocial factors, there is a scarcity of dental research addressing these issues.

Latinos are the largest and fastest immigrant group in the US, with a growth of 39% in Latino children between 2000 to 2010 [8]. In addition, within the 21% US households that speak a language other than English, 62% of these households are Spanish speaking [11]. Thus this study aimed to examine the association of maternal acculturation, measured as preferred language, and oral health-related psychosocial measures in an urban Latino population.

Methods

A cross-sectional survey was conducted with 100 mother-child dyads. One hundred dyads consisting of Latina mothers who were at least 18 years of age with a child under the age of 6 years were enrolled at the Dental Center at Children's Hospital Colorado, the University of Colorado in Aurora, Colorado. Latino families make up about 50% of the patient population at the Dental Center. The study only enrolled mothers who are primary caregivers to maintain reliability in the same kind of caregivers they study. A convenience sample of Latina mothers was enrolled from the waiting room of the Dental Center at Children's Hospital. A co-investigator on the study prescreened the mothers, and because Latina mothers were eligible for the study, pre-screening enabled appropriate enrollment. Information about the study was provided in English and Spanish, with a consent form detailing the approach of the study. Participating mothers were given the option to hear about the study details, sign the consent form and complete the survey in English or Spanish. Certified translators provided study information to Spanish-speaking mothers. This study was approved by the Colorado Multiple Institutional Review Board (COMIRB).

Measures

A manuscript with the main outcomes and study methodology has been recently published and presents all the details of the study design and implementation [12]. The questionnaire used in this study is a portion of the Basic Research Factors Questionnaire (BRFQ) [13] (Table 1), which captures parental dental knowledge, attitudes, behaviors, and other psychosocial measures. The BRFQ was developed as a collaborative effort involving three Centers for Research to Reduce Oral Health Disparities: located at the University of Colorado Denver, Boston University, and the University of California San Francisco (UCSF), and funded by the National Institute of Dental and Craniofacial Research. The BRFQ is available in English and Spanish and is being used by all three centers in diverse populations.

All the children participating in the study received an oral examination by one of the co-investigators of the study. Decayed, missing, filled, surfaces (dmfs) were measured during this examination. Data was recorded using an electronic dental research recording instrument designated as CARIN (Caries Research Instrument), specifically designed for research documentation involving dmfs.

Table 1 provides the description of the measures and the subscales of the BRFQ used in this study. Psychosocial measures include oral health behavior, oral health knowledge, knowledge on dental utilization, self-efficacy, three subscales on Oral Health Locus of Control, and four subscales from the Health Belief Model (Table 1). Knowledge on dental care utilization is another variable that measures the mother's knowledge about when to take the child for dental care, preventive visits vs. visiting the dentist in response to pain and the impact of her friends and family on her dental care utilization for her child. Behavior and oral health knowledge scales range from 0 to 100 and were calculated as the percent of individual items marked correctly. The remaining measures utilized Likert-type scales, with scores on each item ranging from 1 to 5. The summary measures are the average of the values for answered questions, thus also ranging from 1 to 5.

Table 1 Description of Measures

Measure	Description
Oral Health Locus of Control (OHLOC) 3 subscales	OHLOC captures a person's attitudes about who or what has control over their child's oral health outcomes. There are 3 subscales, which represents the extent to which participants believe control of their child's oral health outcomes lies with the parent (internal LOC), the dentist (powerful other LOC), or chance factors (chance LOC).
Health Belief Model 4 subscales	The Health Belief Model is one of the major models that have been used to explain health behavior. The model predicts that behavior is a function of 4 subscales - Perceived susceptibility, Perceived severity, Perceived barriers, Perceived benefits.
Self-Efficacy	Self-efficacy represents a person's confidence that he/she can successfully engage in a specific health behavior. Self-efficacy score represents how sure participants are that they can engage in recommended behavior to take care of their children's teeth. Ten questions quantify this measure.
Oral Health Behavior	The overall behavior score represents the percentage of 13 oral health behavior items that were answered with an adherent response, where "adherent" means the participant engages in the recommended oral health behavior.
Oral Health Knowledge	The overall knowledge score represents the percentage of (how many) oral health knowledge items answered correctly. Nineteen questions quantify this measure.
Knowledge on dental utilization	Five items measured parental knowledge on utilization of oral health services for their children.

Language preference was used as a proxy for acculturation in this study. Several studies have used this proxy measure to capture acculturation, as use of non-native language has been associated with higher utilization of health services and better health in immigrant populations [5, 14]. Preference for English or Spanish was measured by asking the participating mothers if they wanted to complete the consent form and study survey in English or Spanish. Spanish-speaking mothers were considered to be less-acculturated

Table 2 Descriptive statistics for demographic variables by acculturation

	language: English ($N = 59$) mean (SD)	language: Spanish ($N = 40$) mean (SD)
Gender		
Male	32 (54.24%)	21 (52.50%)
Female	27 (45.76%)	19 (47.50%)
Child's Age	3.94 ± 1.09	4.05 ± 1.15
Mother's Age	28.20 ± 9.77	31.84 ± 9.05
Mother's Education		
Less than HS	17/56 (30.36%)	20/38 (52.63%)
HS or more	39/56 (69.64%)	18/38 (47.37%)
Mother's Employment		
Employed	23 (38.98%)	12 (30.00%)
Not employed	36 (61.02%)	28 (70.00%)
Household Size	4.66 ± 1.53	4.89 ± 1.23
Household Income		
\$10,830 - \$14,569	3/28 (10.71%)	1/13 (7.69%)
\$14,570 - \$18,309	3/28 (10.71%)	1/13 (7.69%)
\$18,310 - \$22,049	2/28 (7.14%)	3/13 (23.08%)
\$22,050 - \$25,789	3/28 (10.71%)	2/13 (15.38%)
\$25,790 - \$29,529	12/28 (42.86%)	3/13 (23.08%)
\$29,530 - \$33,269	0/28 (0.00%)	2/13 (15.38%)
\$33,270 - \$37,009	3/28 (10.71%)	1/13 (7.69%)
\$37,010	2/28 (7.14%)	0/13 (0.00%)
Household Minors	2.61 ± 1.42	2.72 ± 1.28
Household Years in Household	4.58 ± 3.67	3.79 ± 3.25
Dental Caries (dmfs)	7.56 ± 12.11	15.20 ± 21.48

or closer to the Latino culture, as compared to English- speaking.

Data analysis

Analyses for this study tested the effect of preferred language, which was considered a proxy for acculturation, on psychosocial measures of oral health. Descriptive statistics were calculated for demographics and psychosocial measures by acculturation. Descriptive statistics presented for continuous variables are both mean (SD) and median (IQR), where IQR is the 25% and 75% or inter-quartile interval. For categorical variables, count and percentages are presented. The primary analysis consists of univariate linear regression models for each measure by preferred language, as well as a model adjusting for parent's education. A significance level of 0.05 was used in all hypothesis testing and confidence intervals. Data cleaning and analysis were conducted using R version 3.3.2 (2016–10-31) (R Core Team 2013).

Results

Table 2 provides demographic characteristics of the study sample, presently separately by the preferred language of communication. Fifty-nine mothers were English speaking, and 40 were a Spanish speaker. The mean age of the children in the study was 3.99 years (SD = 1. 11), and that of the mother was 29.54 years (SD = 9.62). Dental caries, measured as dmfs, was significantly higher (15.20 ± 21.48) in children of Spanish-speaking mothers than for children of English-speaking mothers (7.56 ± 12. 11) ($p = 0.043$).

Table 3 provides the means of the psychosocial measures by preferred language. English-speaking mothers had higher mean scores of oral health knowledge (87.51 ± 7.65), behaviors (47.13 ± 14.98), knowledge of dental utilization (3.67 ± 0.51), and self-efficacy (4.34 ± 0.59), compared to Spanish-speaking mothers. English-speaking mothers had higher scores of Internal Oral Health Locus of Control (4.38 ± 0.68); Spanish-speaking mothers scored higher on one subscale of the Health Belief Model, Perceived Barriers (4.07 ± 1.25).

In the univariate models (Table 4), the preference for Spanish-language was significantly associated with knowledge of dental utilization (– 0.51, $P = 0.0006$), maternal self-efficacy (– 0.44, $P = 0.0024$). Preference for the Spanish language was also significantly associated with maternal Perceived Susceptibility (– 0.52, $P = 0.0046$) Perceived Barriers (0.53, $P = 0.0001$), and two subscales of Health Belief Model. After adjusting for parent's education, the effect of language was slightly attenuated, though still significant, for each of these variables, suggesting that parent's education was a significant confounder.

Table 3 Descriptive statistics for psychosocial measures by acculturation

	language: English ($N = 59$)	language: Spanish ($N = 40$)
Oral health Behavior ($P = 0.0988$)		
mean (SD)	47.13 ± 14.98	41.76 ± 16.18
median (IQR)	50.00 (34.85, 58.33)	41.67 (31.82, 50.00)
Oral health knowledge ($P = 0.3995$)		
mean (SD)	87.51 ± 7.65	85.67 ± 12.18
median (IQR)	88.89 (82.35, 93.54)	88.24 (82.35, 94.12)
Knowledge on dental utilization ($P = 0.0024$)		
mean (SD)	3.67 ± 0.51	3.15 ± 0.93
median (IQR)	3.60 (3.40, 4.00)	3.40 (2.45, 4.00)
Self-efficacy ($P = 0.0043$)		
mean (SD)	4.34 ± 0.59	3.91 ± 0.79
median (IQR)	4.50 (4.00, 4.80)	4.06 (3.60, 4.45)
Locus of control - Internal ($P = 0.1655$)		
mean (SD)	4.38 ± 0.68	4.07 ± 1.25
median (IQR)	4.67 (4.00, 5.00)	4.67 (3.67, 5.00)
Locus of control - External Others ($P = 0.6971$)		
mean (SD)	2.19 ± 1.01	2.27 ± 0.94
median (IQR)	2.00 (1.33, 2.67)	2.33 (1.67, 3.00)
Locus of control - External Chance ($P = 0.6227$)		
mean (SD)	2.10 ± 1.01	2.22 ± 1.19
median (IQR)	2.00 (1.33, 3.00)	2.00 (1.00, 3.00)
Health belief model - Severity ($P = 0.0574$)		
mean (SD)	4.29 ± 0.94	3.94 ± 0.82
median (IQR)	4.67 (3.67, 5.00)	3.67 (3.58, 5.00)
Health belief model - Barriers ($P = 0.0002$)		
mean (SD)	1.89 ± 0.61	2.42 ± 0.68
median (IQR)	1.80 (1.45, 2.20)	2.45 (1.80, 3.00)
Health belief model - Susceptibility ($P = 0.0080$)		
mean (SD)	3.34 ± 0.75	2.83 ± 1.03
median (IQR)	3.50 (3.00, 3.75)	3.00 (2.00, 3.50)
Health belief model - Benefits ($P = 0.1951$)		
mean (SD)	4.31 ± 0.67	4.03 ± 1.24
median (IQR)	4.40 (4.20, 4.80)	4.55 (3.70, 5.00)

Discussion

The impetus for acculturation research in health is to determine whether experiences of a particular group have effects on trends in health outcome [15]. In this study, higher acculturation, which was measured by a preference for the English language had a positive association with oral health outcomes, i.e., dental caries in children. Children of English-speaking mothers had significantly lower dmfs scores compared with children of Spanish-speaking mothers. Spanish-speaking mothers had low knowledge of dental care utilization, low self-

Table 4 Linear regression of each psychosocial variable on primary language (Spanish) on both a univariate basis and adjusted for parent's education

Outcome	estimate*	*p*.value	Edu Adj. estimate*	Edu Adj. *p*.value
Oral health Behavior	−5.37 (−11.66, 0.92)	P = 0.0932	−5.69 (−12.21, 0.84)	P = 0.0867
Oral health Knowledge	−1.84 (− 5.79, 2.11)	P = 0.3581	− 1.41 (− 5.45, 2.63)	P = 0.4894
Knowledge on dental service utilization	−0.51 (−0.80, −0.22)	P = 0.0006	−0.41 (− 0.71, − 0.11)	P = 0.0073
Self-efficacy	− 0.44 (− 0.71, − 0.16)	P = 0.0024	− 0.35 (− 0.62, − 0.09)	P = 0.0099
HBM - Severity	−0.34 (− 0.71, 0.02)	P = 0.0636	−0.26 (− 0.65, 0.12)	P = 0.1800
HBM - Barriers	0.53 (0.27, 0.79)	P = 0.0001	0.46 (0.20, 0.71)	P = 0.0006
HBM - Susceptibility	−0.52 (− 0.87, − 0.16)	P = 0.0046	−0.41 (− 0.78, − 0.05)	P = 0.0273
HBM - Benefits	−0.28 (− 0.66, 0.10)	P = 0.1477	−0.20 (− 0.57, 0.18)	P = 0.3045
LOC - Internal	−0.30 (− 0.69, 0.08)	P = 0.1213	−0.20 (− 0.57, 0.17)	P = 0.2867
LOC - External Others	0.08 (− 0.32, 0.48)	P = 0.7012	0.07 (− 0.36, 0.49)	P = 0.7600
LOC - External Chance	0.11 (− 0.33, 0.56)	P = 0.6114	0.10 (− 0.38, 0.58)	P = 0.6715

*Estimates are the difference in the psychosocial measure from primarily English-speaking and Spanish-speaking patients

efficacy; they perceived their children not susceptible to dental caries and perceived more barriers in visiting the dentist for prevention visits.

Our assumption was that recruiting a health center population should have neutralized any potential structural barriers related to utilization or access to care. However, Spanish-speaking mothers in this study perceived barriers in visiting the dentist for preventive visits and had poor oral health behaviors towards their children, when compared with English-speaking mothers. They also had perceptions that their children are less susceptible to developing dental caries, an attitude that may suggest why they did not do much about preventing dental caries. Spanish-speaking mothers had less knowledge related to dental care utilization, including timing and necessity of a dental visit, and they submitted to the notion that young children should only be taken for a dental visit if they were in pain. Furthermore, their social networks, including family and friends, supported not visiting the dentist unless there was an acute need, and they agreed that no one in their family told them the child should be taken for a preventive dental visit.

These perceptions could be related to cultural norms and beliefs, and because Spanish-speaking mothers were less acculturated compared with English-speaking mothers, their beliefs related to preventive dental visits would be inclined towards the Latino cultural norms [8], which in one study that was conducted with Mexican Americans has been described as a "reactive orientation" towards dental care [4]. Previous research also has shown that Latino parents can have fatalistic attitudes towards the oral health of their children and reduced utilization due to perceived barriers [16, 17]. Another study that collected qualitative data from Spanish-speaking Latina mothers at the same health center reported that they struggled to overcome the familial pressure against visiting the dentist for preventive appointments for their children and received suggestions that dental visits should be done in response to pain [18].

These differences in maternal oral health beliefs and behaviors can be embedded theoretically in the level of assimilation into the Anglo culture [2]. For example, partial acculturation of Latino families– that is, alienation from their traditional culture and incomplete integration into the new culture, may put them at greater risk for poor oral health related behaviors, which may also impact utilization and ultimately disease outcome [7, 8].

Although acculturation was measured by the proxy variable of preferred language use, it still shows an influence on maternal beliefs and perceptions related to caries prevention and dental care utilization – and ultimately the dental caries experience in children in this study. Lacking the ability to speak English can be seen as an external manifestation of "slow cultural transformation," which may influence access to care and navigation of the healthcare system, thus indirectly affecting health outcomes [19]. Within pediatric oral health research, lower dental care utilization, lower sealant applications and delayed first dental visits have been related to non-English speaking households [8]. For non-English speaking mothers, it may become difficult to follow the oral hygiene instructions and recommended behaviors given at the dental office, and because of the language barrier, their social networks might be limited to Spanish-speaking individuals. Recent studies have shown the complex role of social networks and acculturation in oral health [4]. Moreover, it has been reported that reduced English skills may cause significant difficulties for Latino families, making them less trusting towards dental care professionals and not establishing a dental home [10, 20].

The present study has some limitations. We drew our sample from a conveniently available urban health center population that may not be generalizable to the larger population. Acculturation was measured using the proxy variable of language preference, and we did not collect information on the birthplace of the mother if she was U.S. born or foreign born.

Conclusion

This study makes important contributions to understanding the underlying psychosocial and behavioral factors that predict how acculturation impacts oral health. Further longitudinal research is warranted in this direction, in using a multi-dimensional tool to measure acculturation rather than using a proxy variable. The author has secured funding to conduct a study that will use a multidimensional scale to measure acculturation.

Abbreviations

BRFQ: Basic Research Factors Questionnaire; IQR: Interquartile Range; SD: Standard Deviation; UCSF: University of California San Francisco

Acknowledgements

We would like to thank Dr. Sarah Horton and Dr. Sarah R. Baker for their comments on the draft. We would especially like to thank the children and their families who have participated in the study.

Funding

The grant support for this project is National Institute of Dental and Craniofacial Research award number K99DE024758 and R00DE024758.

Authors' contributions

TT designed the study, acquisition of the data, contributed to data analysis, data interpretation, manuscript writing and final approval of the manuscript. MM contributed to the analysis, interpretation, critically revised the manuscript and provided final approval of the manuscript. AW and JA contributed to the conception, design, critically revised the manuscript and provided final approval of the manuscript. NR contributed to the manuscript writing, acquisition of data and management of data, critically revised the manuscript and provided final approval of the manuscript. All authors read and approved the final manuscript. All authors agree to be accountable for all aspects of the work.

Competing interests

The authors declare that they have no competing interests with respect to the authorship and/or publication of this article.

Author details

[1]Department of Community Dentistry and Population Health, School of Dental Medicine, University of Colorado Anschutz Medical Campus, Aurora, Colorado, USA. [2]School of Medicine, University of Colorado Anschutz Medical Campus, Aurora, Colorado, USA. [3]Colorado School of Public Health, University of Colorado Anschutz Medical Campus, Aurora, Colorado, USA. [4]Center for Native Oral Health Research, University of Colorado Anschutz Medical Campus, Aurora, Colorado, USA.

References

1. Abraído-Lanza AF, Armbrister AN, Flórez KR, Aguirre AN. Toward a theory-driven model of acculturation in public Health Research. Am J Public Health. 2006;96:1342–6. https://doi.org/10.2105/AJPH.2005.064980.
2. Abraído-Lanza AF. Social support and psychological adjustment among Latinas with arthritis: a test of a theoretical model. Ann Behav Med. 2004;27: 162–71. https://doi.org/10.1207/s15324796abm2703_4.
3. Fox M, Entringer S, Buss C, DeHaene J, Wadhwa PD. Intergenerational transmission of the effects of acculturation on health in Hispanic Americans: a fetal programming perspective. Am J Public Health. 2015;105(Suppl 3): S409–23. https://doi.org/10.2105/AJPH.2015.302571.
4. Maupome G, McConnell WR, Perry BL, Marino R, Wright ER. Psychological and behavioral acculturation in a social network of Mexican Americans in the United States and use of dental services. Community Dent Oral Epidemiol. 2016;44:540–8. https://doi.org/10.1111/cdoe.12247.
5. Hunt LM, Schneider S, Comer B. Should "acculturation" be a variable in health research? A critical review of research on US Hispanics. Soc Sci Med. 2004;59:973–86. https://doi.org/10.1016/j.socscimed.2003.12.009.
6. Pullen E, Perry BL, Maupome G. "Does this look infected to you?" social network predictors of dental help-seeking among Mexican immigrants. J Immigr Minor Health. 2017:1–11. https://doi.org/10.1007/s10903-017-0572-x.
7. Gao X-L, McGrath C. A review on the oral health impacts of acculturation. J Immigr Minor Health. 2011;13:202–13. https://doi.org/10.1007/s10903-010-9414-9.
8. Tiwari T, Albino J. Acculturation and pediatric minority oral health interventions. Dental Clinics. 2017;61(95):35–42.
9. Farokhi MR, Cano SM, Bober-Moken IG, Bartoloni JA, Cunningham SE, Baez MX. Maternal acculturation could it impact oral health practices of Mexican-American mothers and their children? J Prim Care Community Health. 2011; 2:87–95. https://doi.org/10.1177/2150131910388942.
10. Patrick DL, Lee RSY, Nucci M, Grembowski D, Jolles CZ, Milgrom P. Reducing oral health disparities: a focus on social and cultural determinants. BMC Oral Health. 2006;6(Suppl 1):S4. https://doi.org/10.1186/1472-6831-6-S1-S4.
11. Zong J, Batalova J. Frequently requested statistics on immigrants and immigration in the United States. Washington, DC: Migration Policy Institute; 2016. http://www.migrationpolicy.org/article/frequently-requestedstatistics-immigrants-and-immigration-united-states#Top. Assessed Aug 24 2016.
12. Tiwari T, Wilson AR, Mulvahill M, Rai N, Albino J. Maternal Factors Associated with Early Childhood Caries in Urban Latino Children. JDR Clin Trans Res. 2017; https://doi.org/10.1177/2380084417718175.
13. Albino J, Tiwari T, Gansky SA, Barker JC, Brega AG, Gregorich S, et al. The basic research factors questionnaire for studying early childhood caries. BMC Oral Health. 2017;17:83. https://doi.org/10.1186/s12903-017-0374-5.
14. Abraído-Lanza AF, Chao MT, Florez KR. Do healthy behaviors decline with greater acculturation?: Implications for the Latino mortality paradox. Soc Sci Med. 2005;61(6):1243–55.
15. Fox M, Thayer Z, Wadhwa PD. Assessment of acculturation in minority health research. Soc Sci Med. 2017;176:123–32. https://doi.org/10.1016/j.socscimed.
16. Butani Y, Weintraub JA, Barker JC. Oral health-related cultural beliefs for four racial/ethnic groups: assessment of the literature. BMC Oral Health. 2008;8:26. https://doi.org/10.1186/1472-6831-8-26.
17. Hoeft KS, Barker JC, Masterson EE. Urban Mexican-American mothers' beliefs about caries etiology in children. Community Dent Oral Epidemiol. 2010;38: 244–55. https://doi.org/10.1111/j.1600-0528.2009.00528.x.
18. Tiwari T, Sharma T, Gutierrez K, Wilson A, Albino J. Learning about Oral Health Knowledge & Behavior in Latina Mothers. Boston: IADR/AADR/CADR General Session & Exhibition; 2015.
19. Flores G, Tomany-Korman SC. Racial and ethnic disparities in medical and dental health, access to care, and use of services in US children. Pediatrics. 2008;121:e286–98.
20. Graham MA, Tomar SL, Logan HL. Perceived social status, language and identified dental home among Hispanics in Florida. J Am Dent Assoc. 2005; 136:1572–82.

12

Assessment of prevalence of dental caries and the associated factors among patients attending dental clinic in Debre Tabor general hospital: a hospital-based cross-sectional study

Yilkal Tafere[1*], Selam Chanie[2], Tigabu Dessie[3] and Haileyesus Gedamu[4]

Abstract

Background: Dental caries is the most common dental health problem caused by the interaction of bacteria on tooth enamel. Risk factors for dental caries include salivary composition and inadequate fluoride. However, other factors, such as standard of living, behavior, hygiene, eating habits, social status and socio-demographic factors, also contribute to the evolution of caries. Therefore, this study aimed to determine the prevalence of dental caries and associated factors among patients attending the dental clinic in Debre Tabor General Hospital in North West Ethiopia.

Method: An institution based cross-sectional study was conducted among 280 systematically selected patients attending Debre Tabor General Hospital dental clinic from May 8–20, 2017. The data were collected using pre-tested questionnaire and oral examination by a qualified dental professional. Basic hygienic procedures were observed during an oral examination. The teeth were examined for dental caries by the presence of decay, missing and filled teeth. The data were entered into Epi-Info version 3.5 and cleaned and analyzed using SPSS version 20. Descriptive summary of the data and logistic regression were used to identify possible predictors using odds ratio with 95% confidence interval and *P*-value of 0.05.

Results: A total of 280 subjects participated in the study; among whom 129 (46.1%) were female and nearly two-thirds of the respondents 208 (74.3%) attended formal education. The study revealed k8that the overall prevalence of dental caries was 78.2%. Dental caries was lower among respondents who had good oral hygiene status (AOR = 0.05, 95% CI, 0.02, 0.81). Dental caries was higher among participants who earned less than 5000 Eth Birr per month (AOR = 8.43, 95% CI, 2.6, 27.2). Dental caries was lower among respondents who had good knowledge (AOR = 0.51, 95% CI, 0.03, 0.64).

Conclusions: Prevalence of dental caries was high and found public health problem. Socioeconomic status, educational level, and poor oral hygiene practices were associated factors for dental caries. Health promotion about oral hygiene and integration of services are supremely important for the prevention of the problem of dental caries.

Keywords: Dental caries, Associated factors Debre Tabor, Ethiopia

* Correspondence: yilkal2007@yahoo.com
[1]Department of Public health, College of Health Sciences, Debre Tabor University, Debre Tabor, Ethiopia
Full list of author information is available at the end of the article

Background

Dental caries is one of the oral health problems which cause the destruction of the hard parts of a tooth by the interaction of bacteria and fermentable carbohydrates [1, 2]. Now a day dental caries on the rise to become major public health problems worldwide, nearly 60–90% of children and about 100% of adults have dental cavities, often leading to pain and discomfort [3].

The problem related with dental caries leads to a decrease in the quality of life of the affected individuals and high economic costs for equally individuals and society, with disparities related to well-known issues of socioeconomics, immigration, lack of preventive efforts, and dietary changes [4]. The burden of dental caries in children is incredibly high. The Pain from dental caries can affect school attendance, eating and speaking, and, then impair growth and development [5, 6].

Even though the overall prevalence of dental caries decrease in developed countries, caries continues to be an important public health problem in most developing countries [7]. A study conducted in Lithuania showed that the overall prevalence of dental caries was 78.3%. [8]. Another study conducted in Brazil among adults aged 35 to 44 years showed that 82.0% consumed sugary foods up to four times a day. A study done in Brazil showed that 75% of the participants had enamel defects [9, 10]. Another study was done in Bulgaria also showed that Age, sex, and education were associated with tooth decay. Higher education was associated with a lower chance of having "missing" teeth. More frequent tooth brushing was associated with a lower chance of having decayed [11].

The prevalence of dental caries in Sudan was reported as 30.5% [12]. Another study done in Kenya revealed that the prevalence of dental caries was 37%. The main reason attributed was lack of knowledge on the causes and preventive methods of the disease [13].

An increasing utilization of sweet foods in the developing countries, poor tooth brushing habits, poor oral hygiene and low level of awareness are some of the factors that increased the levels of dental caries. In addition to this the way of life, eating habits, social status and socio-demographic factors also contribute to the development of caries. Caries can be prevented by decreasing sugar intake and brushing teeth after every meal using the appropriate techniques and regular check-ups [5–9, 14].

Although the trend is not clear in developing countries such as Ethiopia, Oral diseases have a growing impact on the health and well-being of people in the region and in particular on vulnerable and marginalized groups of the population. The burden of dental caries has been increasing due to the unlimited utilization of sugary foods, poor oral care practices and inadequate health service utilization [15, 16]. A study done in Finote Selam, Ethiopia showed that 48.5% of the students had dental caries. The prevalence was higher in female 54.6%. Lack of tooth brushing habit (AOR = 3.5, 95% CI: 1.9–6.4), frequent consumption of sugared foods (AOR = 3.4, 95% CI: 1.3–5.6) and residency (AOR = 1.8, 95% CI: 1.0–3.3) were found to have a significant association with dental caries [17]. Another study done Bahirdar city showed that the prevalence of dental caries was 21.8%, Poor habit of tooth cleaning was significantly associated with dental caries [18]. The study done in Gondar showed that there was a statistically significant association between dental caries and educational status (AOR = 0.37, 95% CI, 0.17, 0.80). Dental caries among children whose father were above grade 12 were 63% times at a lower risk compared to illiterates [19].

Untreated dental caries might lead to dental pain, which in turn results in impacts of affected play and sleep, avoidance of certain types of food and decreased performance [15]. In Ethiopia, existing dental health services are limited. Even though dental caries is high in the country, much is not known about the factors affecting it in the study area. Therefore this study was aimed to assess the prevalence of dental caries and its associated factors among patients attending Dental Clinic in Debre Tabor General Hospital.

Methods

Setting

This institution based cross-sectional study was conducted in Debre Tabor General Hospital Dental Clinic from May 8th and 20th 2017. Debre Tabor General Hospital that provides health service to over 1 million people and is located 654 Kms northwest of the capital city, Addis Ababa. Debre Tabor General Hospital is found in Debre Tabor town which is the capital of the South Gondar Zone. The hospital provides different inpatient and outpatient services including dental health services to the population in the surrounding area of Debre Tabor town and the nearby districts.

Participants

Source population

The source population was all patients who attending Debre Tabor Hospital, Dental clinic.

Study population

Systematically selected patients age 18 and above years old getting services from Debre Tabor hospital, dental clinic.

Exclusion criteria

Patients who were unable to communicate were excluded.

Sampling technique and procedure

A sample size of 288 was determined using single population proportion formula.

$$n = \frac{Z^2 p(p-1)}{d^2}$$

with the following assumptions: proportion (P) The prevalence of dental caries to be 21.8% as estimated from the study done in Bahir Dar, Ethiopia [19], a confidence level (CI) of 95%, and marginal error (d), 5 and 10% non-response rate.

Debre Tabor General Hospital was selected purposively. Daily patient flow to Debre Tabor general hospital dental clinic was calculated and. Finally, a systematic selection was done to identify study subjects.

Variables

The dependent variable was the prevalence of dental caries, and the independent variables were demographic, socioeconomic characteristics, information on dental caries, hygienic practice, and feeding habit and associated factors.

Operational definitions

Dental caries

The presence of tooth decay, missing and filled teeth at the time of the oral examination.

Good oral hygiene status

If no food particles and no accumulation of dental plaque and/or calculus is visible on the tooth surfaces at the time of the oral examination.

Poor oral hygiene status

If the presence of food particles in the mouth and there is a visible accumulation of dental plaque and/or calculus on the tooth surfaces at the time of oral examination.

Good knowledge

Those respondents who got a score greater than the mean (greater than five) from ten "yes/no" knowledge related questions about dental caries.

Poor knowledge

Those respondents who got a score less than or equal to the mean (got less or equal to five) from ten "yes/no" knowledge related questions about dental caries.

Data collection

Oral examination was done by a doctor of dental medicine. Hygienic statuses of the respondents were watched during an oral examination. A structured, pre-tested Amharic version questionnaire which was first drafted in English was used to collect data. The questionnaire was pre-tested and appropriate corrections were made for the main study. Data collectors were recruited in consultation with their immediate supervisors by considering their ability in establishing a good relationship with their clients, and their ability to record responses on questionnaire accurately. They were also trained by the principal investigators for two days on how to interview, handling, maintaining confidentiality and ethical issues. A day to day on site supervision was made during data collection by the investigators and one dentist professional.

Data analysis

Data were checked and entered using EPI-Info version 3.5.3 statistical software. Data were cleaned and edited accordingly and exported to SPSS version 20 for analysis. Descriptive analysis such as numerical summary measures, frequencies and proportions were computed. The association between the independent and outcome variables was first investigated using bivariate analysis. Those variables with p value ≤ 0.25 were included into multivariable analysis to determine the predictor variables for the outcome variables. Finally further analyses were carried out using multivariable analysis at significance level of p-value ≤ 0.05.

Ethical consideration

Ethical approval for this study was obtained from research evaluation and an ethical review committee of Debre Tabor University College of Health Sciences. Permission was obtained from Debre Tabor general Hospital. Verbal informed consent was obtained from each participant after providing complete information about the purpose and procedures of the study. At the end of the data collection session, all study participants were advised on how they can maintain their oral hygiene. The consent procedure was approved by the research evaluation and ethical review committee.

Results

Socio-demographic characteristics

A total of 280 subjects participated in the study; among whom129 (46.1%) were female andnearly two-thirds of the respondents 208 (74.3%) attended formal education. The mean age of the respondent was 33.23 with ±12.5 standard deviations (SD) and 103 (36.8%) of the respondents were in the age group of 20 to 29 years. Two hundred sixty-three (93.9%) were Orthodox Christian in religion, 271 (96.8%) were Amhara in ethnicity. One hundred ninety-three (69%) of the respondents were currently married. One hundred eighty-two (65.0%) of the respondents had a monthly income of less than 5000 Ethiopian birrs (Table 1).

Prevalence of dental caries, food consumption and practices related to oral hygiene

The results of this study revealed that the overall prevalence of dental caries was 219 (78.2%) among this the majority 80(36.6%) of the teeth affected by dental caries was molar. One hundred twelve (40%) of the study

Table 1 Socio-demographic characteristics of patients attending the dental clinic in DebreTabor General Hospital, Northwest Ethiopian, 2017

Variables	Frequency	Percent (%)
Age		
< 20	35	12.6
20–29	103	36.8
30–39	76	27
40–49	31	11
50–59	20	7.2
≥ 60	15	5.4
Sex		
Female	129	46.1
Male	151	53.9
Residence		
Urban	171	61.1
Rural	109	38.9
Religion		
Orthodox	263	93.9
Muslim	11	3.9
Protestant	6	2.2
Marital status		
Married	193	69
Single	76	27.1
Divorced	7	2.5
Widowed	4	1.4
Educational status		
Not attend formal education	72	9.7
Attend formal education	208	74.3
Occupation		
Farmer	96	34.3
Government employed	63	22.5
Merchant	80	28.6
Student	30	10.7
Other	11	3.9
Ethnicity		
Amhara	271	96.8
Tigray	6	2.2
Others	3	1
Monthly income in Eth.Birr		
< 5000	182	65.0
> 5000	98	35.0

Table 2 Prevalence of dental caries, food consumption and practices related to oral hygiene among patients attending the dental clinic in Debre Tabor General Hospital, Northwest Ethiopian, 2017

Variables	Frequency	Percent (%)
Knowledge about dental caries		
Good	104	38.2
Poor	176	62.8
Oral Hygiene status		
Good	112	40
Poor	168	60
Tooth brushing habit?		
Yes	70	24.9
No	210	75.1
The frequency of tooth brushing ($n = 70$)		
Once per day	20	28.6
Sometimes	50	71.4
Time of tooth brushing (n = 70)		
Morning	59	84.3
Mixed	5	7.1
Not fixed	6	8.6
Alcohol frequent consumption		
Yes	206	73.6
No	74	26.4
Sugared food consumption		
Yes	168	60
No	112	40
Frequency of consumption sugared foods ($n = 168$)		
Once per day	76	45.2
Twice per day	33	19.6
Sometimes	59	35.2
The family history of Dental Disease		
Yes	27	9.6
No	253	90.4
Dental caries (any type)		
Yes	219	78.2
No	61	21.8
Type of tooth decayed /missed ($n = 219$)		
Incisors	39	17.9
Canines	30	13.5
Premolars	70	32
Molar	80	36.6

subjects had good knowledge about causes and prevention of dental caries. Seventy (24.9%) of the respondents had tooth brushing of which 20(28.6) of the respondents brush their teeth once per day (Table 2).

Logistic regression analysis of factors associated with dental caries

The factors significantly associated with dental caries in bivariate analysis were entered into a multivariable logistic regression model as independent variables for the outcome of dental caries.

This finding demonstrated a significant association between respondent's level of education and dental caries (AOR = 0.24, 95% CI, 0.12, 0.49). Dental caries among respondents who had attended any formal education was 76% times lower risk of developing dental caries compared to those who were not attended formal education. Dental caries was lower among respondents who had good oral hygiene status as compared to those whose oral hygiene status was poor (AOR = 0.05, 95% CI, 0.02, 0.81).

A patient who lives in urban had 1.6 times (AOR = 1.6(1.2, 4.3)) chance of developing dental caries than those patients who were living in rural. Dental caries was higher among respondents who earned less than 5000 Eth Birr per month as compared to those earning greater than 5000 Eth Birr per month (AOR = 8.43, 95% CI, 2.6, 27.2). Dental caries was lower among respondents who had good knowledge about dental caries as compared to those patients who had poor knowledge about dental caries (AOR = 0.051, 95% CI, 0.03, 0.64) (Table 3).

Discussion

This study attempted to assess the prevalence and associated factors of dental caries amongpatients attending Debre Tabor General Hospital dental clinic. The overall prevalence of dental caries found in this study was 78.2%, which was consistent with study in Lithuania (78.3%), [8] and higher than the studies, (75%) in Brazil [9], 37% in Kenya, 30.5% in Sudan [12, 13], (48.5%) in Finote Selam, [17], Ethiopia, and 21.8% in Bahirdar city Ethiopia [18]. The high prevalence of dental caries in this study might be due to the fact that there were variations in study population, time and study setting, in this study since it is institutional based there might be high patient flow in health institutions compared to the community level; this indicates that there is a need to promote oral health. The difference with the Brazil, Kenya, and Sudan studies might be due study population variation and, the socio-demographic differences between those countries.

In the study, factors associated with dental caries were knowledge about prevention and causes of dental caries, oral hygiene status, monthly income, place of resident, educational status, and marital status.

The study found that dental caries was lower among respondents who had good oral hygiene status were 95% times less likely to be affected by dental caries as compared to those patients whose oral hygiene status was poor (AOR = 0.05, 95% CI, 0.02, 0.81). This finding is typically similar to the studies done in Finote Selam and Bahirdar [17, 18]. The study revealed that patients who did not attend any formal education were 76% times at a higher risk compared to those who attended formal education (AOR = 0.24, 95% CI, 0.12, 0.49) which is consistent with findings from a study conducted in Gondar [19].

Table 3 Bivariate and multivariate analyses of variables associated with dental caries among patients attending Debre Tabor General Hospital dental clinics, Debre Tabor, North West Ethiopia, 2017

Variables	Dental caries		COR (95%)	AOR (95%)	*p*-value
Monthly income	Yes	No			
< 5000 Eth birr	155	27	3.05, (CI, 1.7,5.5)	8.43(CI,2.61,27.20)	0.000*
> 5000 Eth birr	64	34	1.00	1.00	
Educational status					
Not Attend formal education	41	31	0.22(CI, 0.12,0.41)	0.24(CI,0.12,0.49)	
Attend formal education	178	30	1.00	1.00	0.000*
Resident					
Urban	141	30	1.95(CI 1.6,4.6)	1.6(CI,1.2,4.3)	0.01*
Rural	78	31	1.00	1.00	
Sex					
Female	108	21	3.98 (CI 1.85,6.73)	3.2 (CI,2.33,4.54)	0.001
Male	111	86	1.00	1.00	
Oral hygiene status					
Good	59	53	0.06(CI0.01,0.96)	0.05(CI,0.02,0.81)	0.001*
Poor	160	8	1.00	1.00	.
Knowledge about dental caries					
Good	86	18	0.7,(CI 0.40,.09)	0.51(CI,0.03,0.64)	0.001*
Poor	133	43	1.00	1.00	

*It means siginificantly associated

This study showed that Patient who lives in urban had 1.6 times (AOR = 1.6, 95% CI 1.2, 4.3) chance of developing dental caries than those patients who were living in rural. This could be that patients who live in urban settings could have access to consume commonly more sugary foods that cause dental caries.

There was also a significant difference between the monthly income of the households and dental caries. Dental caries was higher among respondents who earned less than 5000 Eth Birr per month as compared to those earning greater than 5000 Eth Birr per month (AOR = 8.43, 95% CI, 2.6, 27.2). This result is in line with the study done in Gondar town [19]. As the income of the families increasing, people are less likely to be affected by dental decays. This could be elaborated that those who have better monthly income can have potential to buy tooth cleaning materials. Dental caries was lower among respondents who had good knowledge about dental caries as compared to those patients who had poor knowledge about dental caries (AOR = 0.051, 95% CI, 0.03, 0.64). Having good knowledge about dental caries could help to have better health care seeking behavior of the community.

However, this study does have some inherent limitations. First, we did not use any of the recognized Oral Hygiene Index to assess oral hygiene status. Finally, though there are wide ranges of factors which affect the prevalence of dental caries among patients attending a dental clinic, only individual-level factors were addressed in this study. Hence, taking into consideration factors from the service providers' side and structural barriers would have been important.

Conclusions

In conclusion, this study showed, the prevalence of dental caries was high and found public, knowledge about dental caries, educational status, oral hygiene status, place of residence, and monthly income were important predictors of the prevalence of dental caries among patients attending Debre Tabor General Hospital Dental Clinic. Therefore, integrating oral health promotion service with other health services at the grass root levels could have a significant impact and are likely to benefit community's oral health problem at large. Health promotion about oral hygiene is supremely important for the prevention of the problem of dental caries.

Abbreviations

DMFT: Decayed, Missing, and Filled Teeth; OR: Odds ratios; SD: Standard deviation; SPSS: Statistical package for social sciences; WHO: World Health Organization

Acknowledgments

We are very grateful to the Debre Tabor University College of health science department of nursing for the approval of the Ethical Clearance. We express our heartfelt thanks to participants for their willingness to participate in the study, without whom this research would be impossible.

Funding

The authors have no support or funding to report.

Authors' contributions

YT Contributed in inception, design, analysis, interpretation, drafting the research, the manuscript and final approval of the revised manuscript for publication. SC Contributed in inception, design, analysis, interpretation, drafting of a research manuscript and final approval of the revised manuscript for publication. TD Contributed in inception, design, analysis, interpretation, drafting of a research manuscript and final approval of the revised manuscript for publication. HG. Contributed in inception, drafting of a research manuscript and final approval of the revised manuscript for publication. All authors read and approved the final version of the manuscript.

Authors' information

Yilkal Tafere, Lecturer of Epidemiology.
Selam Chanie: Professional nursing in Debre Tabor General Hospital.
Tigabu Dessie, Assistant Lecturer of Nursing.
Haileyesus Gedamu, Lecturer of Medical-surgical nursing.

Competing interests

The authors declare that they don't have competing interests.

Author details

[1]Department of Public health, College of Health Sciences, Debre Tabor University, Debre Tabor, Ethiopia. [2]Department of Nursing, Debre Tabor General hospital, Debre Tabor, Ethiopia. [3]Department of Nursing, College of Health Sciences, Debre Tabor University, Debre Tabor, Ethiopia. [4]Department of Nursing, College of Medicine and Health Sciences, Bahirdar University, Bahirdar, Ethiopia.

References

1. Ndiaye C. Oral health in the African region: progress and perspectives of the regional strategy. Afr J Oral Health. 2005;2:1–2.
2. WHO report 2015: http://www.who.int/mediacentre/factsheets/fs318/en/.
3. World Health Organization. Oral Health fact sheet April 2012. Available at. https://www.mah.se/CAPP/Oral-Health-Promotion/WHO-Oral-Health-Fact-Sheet1/.
4. Bagramian RA, Garcia-Godoy F, Volpe AR. The global increase in dental caries. A pending public health crisis. Am J Dent. 2009;22(1):3–8.
5. Yee R, Sheiham A. The burden of restorative dental treatment for children in third world countries. Int Dent J. 2002;52:1–9.
6. Petersen PE, Bourgeois D, Ogawa H, Estupinan-Day S, Ndiaye C. The global burden of oral diseases and risks to oral health. Bulletin of the WHO. 2005;83:661.
7. Namal N, Can G. Dental health status and risk factors for dental caries in adults in Istanbul, Turkey. East Mediterr Health J. 2008;14(1):110–8.

8. Miglė Ž, Rūta G, Ingrida V, Kristina S, Jaunė R, Eglė S. Prevalence and severity of dental caries among 18-year-old Lithuanian adolescents. Medicine. 2016; 52:54–60.
9. Vanessa R, Danuze B, Tatiana D, Ana C, Orlando A. Prevalence of dental caries and caries-related risk factors in premature and term children. Braz Oral Res. 2010;24(3):329-35.
10. Simone M, Mara V. High dental caries among adults aged 35 to 44 years: case-control study of distal and proximal factors. Int J Environ Res Public Health. 2013;10:2401-11.
11. Nikola D, Dick J, Ewald M, Nico H. Dental status and associated factors in a dentate adult population in Bulgaria: a cross-sectional survey. Int J Dent. 2011;2012(57840):11.
12. Nurelhuda NM, Trovik TA, Ali RW, Ahmed MF. Oral health status of 12-year-old school children in Khartoum state, Sudan; a school-based survey. BMC Oral Health. 2009;9:15.
13. Gathecha G, Makokha A. Dental caries and oral health practices among 12-year-old children in Nairobi west and Mathira west districts, Kenya. Pan Afr Med J. 2012;12:42.
14. Petersen EP. Oral health in the developing world, World Health Organization global oral health program chronic disease and health promotion. Geneva: Community Dentistry and Oral Epidemiology; 2009.
15. World Health Organization: Prevention methods and program for oral diseases WHO technical report series. Geneva: WHO; 2008.
16. Formulating Oral Health Strategy. Available at http://www.apps.searo.who.int/PDS_DOCS/B4433.pdf.
17. Amare T, Asmare Y, Muchye G. Prevalence of Dental Caries and Associated Factors Among Finote Selam Primary School Students Aged 12–20 years, Finote Selam Town, Ethiopia. OHDM. 2016;15(1).
18. Wondemagegn M, Tazebew D, Mulat Y, Kassaw M, Bayeh A. Dental caries and associated factors among primary school children in Bahir Dar city: a cross-sectional study. BMC Res Notes. 2014;7:949.
19. Fenta A, Belaynew W, Tadesse A, Kassahun A. Predictors of dental caries among children 7–14 years old in Northwest Ethiopia: a community based cross-sectional study. BMC Oral Health. 2013;13:7.

Knowledge of orthodontic tooth movement through the maxillary sinus

Wentian Sun[1], Kai Xia[1], Xinqi Huang[1], Xiao Cen[2], Qing Liu[1] and Jun Liu[1*]

Abstract

Background: To investigate the feasibility, safety and stability of current interventions for moving teeth through the maxillary sinus (MTTMS) by performing a systematic review of the literature.

Methods: The electronic databases PubMed, Embase, CENTRAL, Web of Science, CBM, CNKI and SIGLE were searched without a language restriction. The primary outcomes were parameters related to orthodontic treatment, including orthodontic protocols, magnitude of forces, type of tooth movement, duration and rate of tooth movement, and remolding of alveolar bone and the maxillary sinus floor. The secondary outcomes were safety and stability, including root resorption, perforation of the sinus floor, loss of pulp vitality and periodontal health and relapse.

Results: Nine case reports with 25 teeth were included and systematically analyzed. Fifty to two hundred g of force was applied to move teeth through the maxillary sinus. Bodily movement was accomplished, but initial tipping was observed in 7 cases. The rate was 0.6–0.7 mm/month for molar intrusion and 0.16–1.17 and 0.05–0.16 mm/month for mesial-distal movement of premolars and molars, respectively. Bone formation and remolding of the sinus floor occurred in 7 cases. Root resorption within 6 to 30 months was observed in 3 cases, while no cases of perforation of the sinus floor, loss of pulp vitality, periodontal health impairment or relapse were reported.

Conclusions: At the present stage, no evidence-based protocol could be recommended to guide MTTMS. The empirical application of constant and light to moderate forces (by TAD, segment and multibrackets) to slowly move teeth through or into the maxillary sinus in adults appears to be practical and secure. Bodily movement was accomplished, but teeth appear to be easily tipped initially, potentially resulting in root resorption. However, this conclusion should be interpreted with caution as the currently available evidence is based on only a few case reports or case series and longitudinal or controlled studies are lacking in this area.

Keywords: Intrusion, Maxillary sinus, Orthodontics, Root resorption, Systematic review, Tooth movement

Background

With the development of digitalization and material science in the past few decades, substantial progress has been achieved in orthodontic techniques for more efficient, precise, invisible, comfortable and rapid treatment [1–3]. However, orthodontists commonly encounter predicaments related to dental status, periodontal status, general health, orthodontic technique, anchorage, and other factors that may limit orthodontic treatment [4]. Among these challenges, movement of teeth against anatomic structures, such as the maxillary sinus (MS), appears to be non-evidence-based.

The MS is the largest paranasal sinus, located in the posterior maxilla, and has a close relationship with adjacent structures. It sprouts late in fetal life, existing at birth with a dimension of approximately 3*6*8 mm, and ends its growth in a pyramid shape in adults [5–7]. The MS floor (MSF) consists of a thin bony plate covered with a layer of mucosa. With pneumatization and aging, the floor extends into the posterior alveolar process and forms the alveolar recess, creating protrusions of root apices into the sinus [5]. Generally, the MSF is at the level of nasal floor at puberty

* Correspondence: junliu@scu.edu.cn
[1]State Key Laboratory of Oral Diseases, National Clinical Research Center for Oral Diseases, Department of Orthodontics, West China Hospital of Stomatology, Sichuan University, Chengdu 610041, China
Full list of author information is available at the end of the article

and reaches its lowest point with the eruption of the third molars [5, 6]. Morphologically, the sinus-root relationship (SRR) can fall into 5 categories: 0, the root is not in contact with the sinus floor; 1, the MSF curves inferiorly with the root in contact with the MSF; 2, the MSF curves inferiorly with the root projecting laterally on the sinus cavity but its apex is outside the sinus; 3, the MSF curves inferiorly with the root apex projecting on the sinus cavity; and 4, the MSF curves superiorly with part or all of the tooth root enveloped [8]. For individuals with excessive pneumatization, a type-1, 2, 3 or 4 relationship can be common.

The classic theory of orthodontic tooth movement stresses the dynamic balance of bone resorption on the pressure side and deposition on the tension side of the periodontal ligament (PDL) [9]. This theory has been successfully applied by orthodontists to move teeth in the alveolar bone. However, applying this concept to the MS, with potential tooth movement against cortex or soft tissue [10], is more difficult. Consequently, clinicians often fear the uncertainty of moving teeth through the maxillary sinus (MTTMS). However, recent experiments have revealed a particular biomechanical pattern regarding MTTMS. Mechanical stress could induce osteogenesis on the sinus side before bone resorption occurred on the PDL side, and the bone thickness of the sinus wall could be maintained [11–13], potentially indicating the feasibility of MTTMS. Furthermore, concurrent root resorption and higher efficiency of light forces were also observed in these experiments [11–13].

In orthodontic clinics, clinicians may encounter MTTMS. In some cases, planning the distalization of molars or the maxillary dentition to correct type-II occlusion or to achieve a better anterior profile is preferred because this technique has the benefit of avoiding extraction and is reported to be one of the advantages of clear aligners [1, 9, 14]. In other cases, when closure of posterior spaces [15–17], tooth intrusion to create spaces for opposing prosthetics [18, 19] or an alternative non-surgical sinus lift for implant sites [20–22] is required, orthodontists must implement MTTMS. MTTMS determines the feasibility, duration and quality of comprehensive treatment. No systematic reviews on MTTMS are currently available. The purpose of this research was to systematically review the literature and investigate the feasibility, safety and stability of current interventions for MTTMS.

Methods

This systematic review was conducted generally following the Preferred Reporting Items for Systematic Reviews and Meta-Analysis (PRISMA) checklist [23]. The literature search, data extraction and quality assessment were all performed independently by two reviewers. Any disagreement was resolved by discussion or by consultation with a third party.

Inclusion criteria

We set the following inclusion criteria to identify eligible studies: (1) Patients with at least one target tooth, defined as a tooth with at least one root protruding into the MS, were investigated. The morphological SRR (type-2, 3 or 4 for distal-mesial movement and type-1, 2, 3 or 4 for intrusion) must be confirmed by radiological diagnosis: periapical films, panoramics or cone-beam computed tomography (CBCT); (2) An orthodontic treatment to move target teeth through the MS was executed; (3) The primary outcomes were parameters related to orthodontic treatment, including orthodontic protocols, magnitude of orthodontic forces, tooth movement type, duration and rate of tooth movement, and remolding of the alveolar bone and MSF. The secondary outcomes were safety and stability, including orthodontically induced root resorption (OIRR), perforation of the sinus floor (Perforation of the sinus floor should be verified by occurrence of sinusitis or by radiological findings in sinus. The integrity of lamina dura should be assessed by radiography: periapical films, panoramics or CBCT, while the sinus membrane should be assessed with CT/CBCT, MRI or endoscopy [5, 18, 19, 24–28].), pulp vitality loss, and periodontal health impairment and relapse; and (4) The study was a clinical study, including randomized clinical trial, controlled clinical trial, cohort study, case-control study, cross-sectional study and case report.

Search strategy

Online searches were conducted in electronic databases, including PubMed, Embase, CENTRAL, Web of Science, Chinese Biomedical Literature Database (CBM), China National Knowledge Infrastructure (CNKI), without restriction of language. Grey literature was searched in the System for Information on Grey Literature in Europe (SIGLE). We used MeSH terms as well as free text words, and the key words were "maxillary sinus," "orthodontics," "orthodontic*," "tooth moving," and "tooth movement" for all databases. The reference lists of relevant articles were manually searched for additional studies. The searches were initially conducted in January 2017 and were updated on May 16, 2017.The search strategies are presented in Table 1.

Data extraction and analysis

Information regarding the characteristics and outcomes of the included studies was extracted. Specifically, the following characteristics were identified: country, age, sex, sample size, target teeth, SRR, source of active force and radiological method. The outcomes were those items defined in the inclusion criteria above.

Table 1 Search strategies for all databases (updated on May 16, 2017)

steps	PubMed	Embase	CENTRAL	Web of science	CNKI	CBM	SIGLE
1	"Maxillary Sinus" [Mesh] (9226)	Maxillary Sinus.mp. or Maxillary sinus/ (14263)	Maxillary Sinus.mp. or Maxillary Sinus/ (424)	Maxillary Sinus (21210)	Maxillary Sinus (8251)	"Maxillary Sinus" [Mesh] (3483)	Maxillary Sinus (26)
2	Maxillary Sinus (15823)	Orthodontics.mp. or Orthodontics/ (34932)	Orthodontics.mp. or Orthodontics/ (636)	Orthodontics (29732)	Orthodontics (12742)	Maxillary Sinus (7208)	Orthodontics (85)
3	"Orthodontics" [Mesh] (48362)	Orthodontic*.mp. (51672)	Orthodontic*.mp. (2402)	Orthodontic* (67283)	Tooth movement (1045)	"Orthodontics, Corrective" [Mesh] (11645)	Orthodontic* (235)
4	Orthodontics (63379)	Tooth moving.mp. (12)	Tooth movement.mp. or Tooth Movement/ (382)	Tooth moving (54506)	2 OR 3 (15616)	Orthodontics (16725)	Tooth movement (14)
5	Orthodontic* (62688)	Tooth movement.mp. (2970)	2 OR 3 OR 4 (2423)	Tooth movement (59130)	1 AND 4 (23)	"Tooth movement" [Mesh] (1104)	Tooth moving (3)
6	"Tooth Movement Techniques" [Mesh] (7834)	2 OR 3 OR 4 OR 5 (52143)	1 AND 5 (1)	2 OR 3 OR 4 OR 5 (157498)		Tooth movement (2280)	2 OR 3 OR 4 OR 5 (245)
7	Tooth movement (10981)	1 AND 6 (125)		1 AND 6 (305)		1 OR 2 (7208)	1 AND 6 (0)
8	Tooth moving (327)					3 OR 4 OR 5 OR 6 (18312)	
9	1 OR 2 (15823)					7 AND 8 (28)	
10	3 OR 4 OR 5 OR 6 OR 7 OR 8 (71532)						
11	9 AND 10 (195)						

CENTRAL Cochrane Central Register of Controlled Trials, *CNKI* China National Knowledge Infrastructure, *CBM* Chinese Biomedical Literature Database, *SIGLE* System for Information on Grey Literature in Europe

Results

Characteristics of the included studies

The online search yielded 677 articles. After excluding duplicate and irrelevant articles by reading titles and abstracts, 11 full texts remained. Then, the reference lists of these articles were read and one additional study was identified. No prospective or retrospective controlled clinical studies were found. Nine case reports meeting the inclusion criteria were included and systematically analyzed (Fig. 1). The characteristics of the 9 case reports are presented in Table 2.

Results of quality assessment

All included studies were case reports and consequently had a relatively high risk of bias.

Study outcomes analysis

In total, nine adult subjects with 25 target teeth were included. All target teeth had a type-2, 3 or 4 SRR (Table 3).

Protocol and magnitude of forces

Cacciafesta et al. [17] used segments to protract tooth numbers 27 and 28 mesially, and the force was 50 g by coil spring. Re et al. [22] used an endosseous implant in the retromolar area and a T-loop to move tooth number 25 distally, and the active load was 50 g/mm. In Kravitz et al.'s article [18], tooth number 16 was intruded using temporary anchorage devices (TADs), and the forces were 100 g by elastic power chain in the initial 2 months and 150 g by coil spring in the next 4 months. Yao et al. [19] also used TADs to intrude two adjacent molars (26 and 27), and the forces were 150–200 g by elastic power chain. Kuroda et al. [14] performed group distalization of the maxillary dentition using multibrackets and TADs, and 9 teeth were moved distally through the MS bilaterally with a load of 200 g by coil spring. Oh et al. [16], Park et al. [15], Saglam et al. [21] and Carvalho et al. [20] used multibrackets to move maxillary teeth mesially or distally through the MS (TADs were utilized in Park et al.'s article). In these reports, "light forces" or "mild to moderate forces" were used. Generally, light to moderate forces (50–200 g) were applied to accomplish MTTMS.

Tooth movement type

In general, 7 articles reported MTTMS in the sagittal direction [14–17, 20–22], and 2 articles reported molar intrusion into the MS in the vertical direction [18, 19].

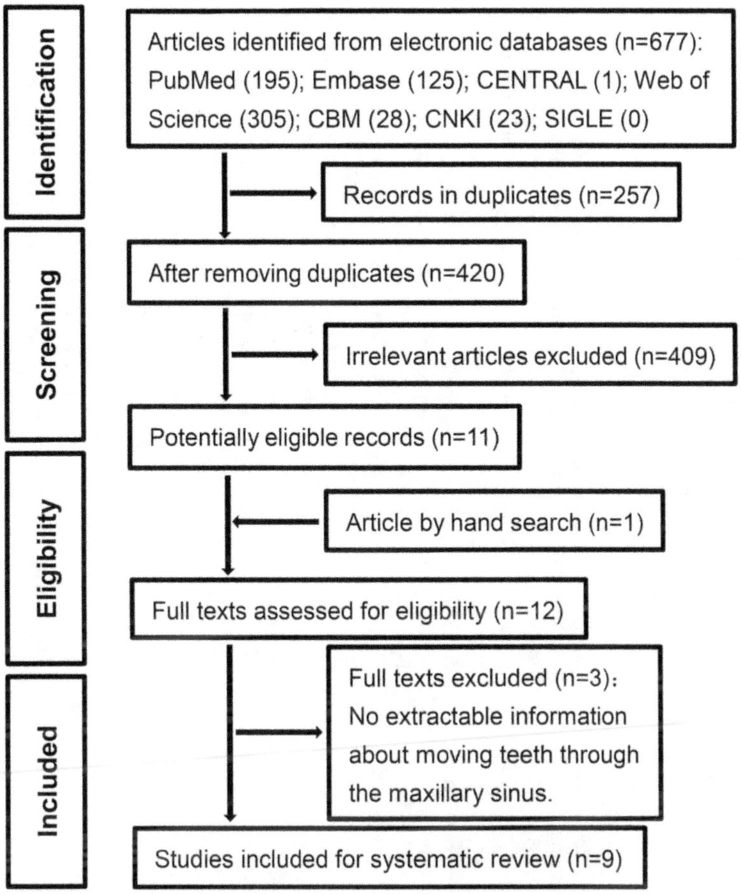

Fig. 1 PRISMA flow diagram showing the search and selection process

For tooth movement in the sagittal direction, all authors reported distal or mesial bodily movement of the target teeth [14–22]. However, Cacciafesta et al. [17], Re et al. [22], Oh et al. [16], Park et al. [15] and Kuroda et al. [14] revealed that the overall translation consisted of processes of initial tipping followed by up-righting. Saglam et al. [21] and Carvalho et al. [20] described distal bodily movement of the second premolars, but no details were provided in their reports. For molar intrusion into the MS, Yao et al. reported intrusion of tooth numbers 26 and 27 with slight distal tipping [19], while Kravitz et al. reported intrusion of tooth number 16 with palatal crown tipping [18].

Duration and rate of tooth movement

For tooth movement in the sagittal direction, Re et al. moved tooth number 25 by 6 mm distally in 6 months [22]. Oh et al. reported distal movement of 5 mm for tooth number 25, mesial movement of 10 mm for tooth number 28, and opposing movement of 10 mm between tooth numbers 15 and 17 in 70 months [16]. Opposing movements of 2–3 mm between tooth numbers 14 and 16 and 1–2 mm between tooth numbers 24 and 26 were achieved in 30 months in Park et al.'s article [15]. Carvalho et al. moved tooth number 15 by 7 mm distally in 6 months [20]. In addition, Kuroda et al. achieved group distalization of the maxillary dentition of 4–5 mm in 28 months [14]. For tooth movement in the vertical direction, 3-mm intrusion in 5 months and 4.4-mm intrusion in 6 months for molars were reported by Yao et al. and Kravitz et al., respectively [18, 19]. Overall, for molar intrusion into the MS, the individual cases showed a rate of 0.6–0.7 mm/month, and for distal-mesial movement, rates of 0.16–1.17 and 0.05–0.16 mm/month were reported for premolars and molars, respectively.

Alveolar bone formation and remolding of the sinus floor

Re et al. [22], Saglam et al. [21], and Carvalho et al. [20] moved the second premolars distally through the MS with pneumatization into the alveolar bone. Alveolar bone formation occurred in the moving direction, along with direct remolding of the sinus lamina dura and sinus lift, and implants were subsequently inserted in the previous positions of the second premolars. Likewise, alveolar bone formation was observed in the studies of Cacciafesta et al. [17] and Oh et al. [16], and signs of sinus wall modeling were also observed in Oh et al.'s

Table 2 Characteristics of included case reports

Author(s)	Country	Age	Sex	Teeth	SRR	Mechanics	Active force system used	Radiographic view	Conclusion
Cacciafesta (2001) [17]	Denmark	25	F	2(27,28)	type-3	segment; multibracket	coil spring	panoramic; periapical film	Teeth can be moved into anatomical sites lacking periodontium provided that the orthodontist uses an appliance that generates both constant forces and constant moment to force ratios.
Re (2001) [22]	Italy	24	F	1(25)	type-4	segment	T-loop	panoramic; periapical film	The clinical findings of this study indicate that with a proper orthodontic force system, a tooth can be displaced through the sinus area, and the sinus lift surgical augmentation procedure can be avoided.
Yao (2004) [19]	Taiwan	31	F	2(26,27)	type-3	segment; miniplate, miniscrew	elastic power chain	panoramic; periapical film 3D digitizer	The biological responses of teeth and the surrounding bony structures to intrusion appeared normal and acceptable. Furthermore, the periodontal health and vitality of the teeth were sufficiently maintained even after a 1-year follow-up.
Kravitz (2006) [18]	USA	44	F	1(16)	type-3	miniscrew	elastic power chain; coil spring	panoramic	A supraerupted maxillary molar can be successfully intruded within the maxillary sinus cortical floor using two orthodontic miniscrews. Short-term molar intrusion can be achieved without clinically detectable apical root resorption.
Oh (2014) [16]	USA	41	F	4(15,17,25,28)	type-2:15,25,28 type-4:17	multibracket	elastic power chain; coil spring; tip-back bend; double helical loop	panoramic; periapical film; CBCT	Successful tooth movement through the maxillary sinus can be achieved without noticeable side effects. New bone formation along the course of tooth movement and changes in the size and shape of the maxillary sinus were observed. Maintaining light continuous forces and moving teeth at a slow rate were key in accomplishing bodily movement and direct bone resorption.
Park (2014) [15]	Japan	31	M	4(14,16,24,26)	type-2:14,24 type-3:16,26	multibracket; TAD	T-loop; Intrusion archwires; TAD	panoramic; CBCT	Spaces from tooth extractions can be closed by bodily movement through anatomic barriers such as the maxillary sinus, but in view of the proximity of the maxillary sinus floor and maxillary root tips, orthodontists must be particularly cautious when doing this.
Saglam (2014) [21]	Turkey	54	M	1(25)	type-3	multibracket	coil spring	panoramic; periapical film;	Modification of the sinus floor by orthodontic treatment may be an alternative treatment strategy for patients requiring a sinus lifting procedure due to pneumatization of maxillary sinus.
Carvalho (2014) [20]	Brazil	38	M	1(15)	type-3	multibracket	unknown	periapical film	Orthodontic movement is a safe and predictable procedure and may replace sinus lift and graft procedures for patients who smoke or for individuals with a history of sinusitis. The procedure also allows implant placement in an area of mature bone rather than in grafted bone, which may be a favorable factor for osseointegration.
Kuroda (2016) [14]	Japan	29	F	9(14,15,16,17,23, 24,25,26,27)	type-2:14 type-3:15,16,17, 23,24,25,26,27	multibracket; TAD	coil spring	panoramic	Interradicular miniscrews are useful for distalizing the maxillary dentition to correct class II malocclusion. With this new strategy, group distalization with miniscrews enables a simpler treatment with greater predictability.

SRR sinus-root relationship, *TAD* temporary anchorage device, *CBCT* cone beam computed tomography

Table 3 Outcomes of the 9 included case reports

Author(s)	SRR	Force magnitude	Moving distance through sinus	Duration	Tooth movement type	Bone forming and remodeling of the sinus floor	Side effects	Follow-up and relapse
Cacciafesta (2001) [17]	type-3	50 g	4–5 mm (half the width of a molar)	unknown	bodily mesially; up-righting	Bone formation took place.	minimal root blunting; No marginal bone loss was visible.	unknown
Re (2001) [22]	type-4	50 g/mm	6 mm	6 months	bodily distally (tipping, translation, root movement)	Alveolar bone formation and direct remodeling of the sinus lamina dura occurred.	Pulp vitality, bone support and normal width of the periodontal ligament were maintained.	unknown
Yao (2004) [19]	type-3	150–200 g	3 mm	5 months	intrusion, slight distal tipping	The lamina dura followed molar intrusion and bone remodeling was achieved.	Periodontal health and vitality of the teeth were maintained.	1 year; Periodontal health and vitality of the teeth were well maintained.
Kravitz (2006) [18]	type-3	100–150 g	4.4 mm	6 months	intrusion, palatal crown tipping	Radiograph showed intact lamina dura around the first molar within the floor.	no radiographically evident root resorption.	unknown
Oh (2014) [16]	type-2:15,25,28 type-4:17	light forces	25: 6 mm; 28: 10 mm; 10 mm (15–17)	70 months	25: bodily distally (tipping, up-righting); 28: bodily mesially (tipping, up-righting); 15: bodily distally; 17: bodily mesially	Signs of sinus wall modeling and new alveolar bone deposition were observed in the direction of tooth movement.	No apparent root resorption was observed, and the alveolar bone level was maintained.	18 months; Occlusion and normal overjet and overbite were maintained.
Park (2014) [15]	type-2:14,24 type-3:16,26	light forces	14–16: (bodily 2–3 mm, up-righting 15–20°) 24–26: (bodily 1–2 mm, up-righting 20–25°)	30 months	14, 24: bodily distally, up-righting; 16, 26: bodily mesially, rotated mesially, up-righting	The floor of the sinus did not displace coronally during orthodontic approximation of these teeth.	Some areas showed signs of apical root resorption.	1 year; Stable occlusion and the orthodontic treatment results were maintained.
Saglam (2014) [21]	type-3	unknown	7 mm	unknown	bodily distally	Alveolar bone formation and remodeling of the sinus floor occurred.	Maintained pulp vitality and bone support without loss of the connective tissue attachment.	2 years; Acceptable intraoral tissue health was observed after 2 years.
Carvalho (2014) [20]	type-3	mild and moderate	7 mm	6 months	bodily distally	The cortical bone and sinus mucosa displaced the maxillary sinus floor during bone and periodontal remodeling.	Radiographically evident root resorption was observed.	unknown
Kuroda (2016) [14]	type-2: 14 type-3:15,16,17, 23,24,25,26,27	200 g	4–5 mm	28 months	bodily distally (tipping, up-righting)	unknown	No serious root resorption.	5 years; Occlusion and facial profile were stable.

SRR sinus-root relationship, *Moving distance through sinus* the distance by which the tooth was moved through the maxillary sinus study. In terms of molar intrusion, Yao et al. and Kravitz et al. found that the lamina dura followed the course of molar intrusion, and bone remolding during intrusion was achieved in Yao et al.'s case [18, 19].

Safety and side effects

First, radiographically evident OIRR was reported by Cacciafesta et al. [17], Park et al. [15] and Carvalho et al. [20], whereas no apparent OIRR was reported by Kravitz et al. [18], Oh et al. [16] and Kuroda et al. [14]. Second, no perforation of the sinus floor or loss of pulp vitality was reported in the 9 cases [14–22]. Third, standard periodontal control measures were adapted by Cacciafesta et al., Re et al., Oh et al., and Saglam et al. [16, 17, 21, 22], and they reported that bone support and periodontal health were maintained. Similar result was observed by Yao et al. [19].

Stability and relapse

Oh et al. [16], Park et al. [15] and Kuroda et al. [14] reported stable occlusion after follow-ups of 1.5, 1 and 5 years, respectively. The periodontal health and vitality of the teeth were maintained in Yao et al.'s case [19]. Saglam et al. reported acceptable intraoral tissue health after 2 years [21].

Discussion

This systematic review intended to determine the feasibility, safety and stability of current interventions for MTTMS. Nine case reports representing the available human clinical studies were included. In general, the present study indicated the feasibility of MTTMS. However, the difficulty of the moving process varied substantially, possibly indicating the heterogeneity among clinical measures and internal anatomic structures and the inherent bias of case reports.

In MTTMS, bodily movement is desired. The key biomechanical objective is uniform distribution of orthodontic forces along the PDL and the line of the active force passing through the center of resistance [29, 30]. Carefully designed segments or TADs can produce approximate determinate force systems and may facilitate bodily movement [9, 17, 31, 32]. Considering the anatomic variability of the MSF and the complexity of the SRR [8], techniques for better control in three dimensions should be developed, especially for patients with primarily regional complaints. To achieve tooth movement by frontal resorption, mild and constant forces (35–60 g, 70–120 g and 10–20 g for tipping, bodily and intrusion movement, respectively) are recommended. However, considering the amount of resistance in sliding mechanics [9, 30], the decay rate of forces and the root numbers of the posterior teeth, the magnitude of 50–200 g of force applied in the included cases seems safe.

In the present study, most cases showed initial stages of tipping through the MS, which is consistent with a previous study [33]. Deviation from ideal bodily movement may reflect expression of a well-designed pure Newtonian mathematical force system applied on the in vivo PDL. Orthodontic forces are derived from deformation of some parts of existing appliances; however, each appliance has a particular load deflection rate, and the decay rates of the counterparts (i.e., the moment of force and the moment of couple) in the equilibrium system are not equal, and consequently, the moment to force ratio constantly changes, resulting in constant changes in the center of rotation and difficulty in maintaining translation [34]. Moreover, in the MS, the distribution of bone density along the axis of a tooth must be considered. The coronal part of the root is more likely to move against cancellous bone while the apical part is more likely to move against cortical bone [9]. Therefore, the tooth is easily tipped toward the moving direction. Furthermore, for molar intrusion, the accompanying tipping may reflect different resistances among roots [19].

Moving at low speeds is a prerequisite for compensatory bone regeneration [16, 35]. Therefore, applying light and continuous forces is the best strategy to achieve the ideal speed for moving teeth. Particularly, the cask effect regarding the moving rate in MTTMS is probably due to cortical anchorage [9]. In Oh et al.'s case, the location of the roots against the cortical bone of the sinus wall provided nearly absolute anchorage in the first 3.5 years [16]. In such cases, only light forces are appropriate as heavy forces against the cortical bone will reinforce the anchorage and cause additional OIRR. However, individual heterogeneity may exist in this regard because no other authors reported such an extreme situation, and a wide range of rate was reported across cases.

According to the theory of tooth movement, new physiological bone along the course of the moved tooth can be harvested [9, 36]. In the past few decades, the development of implant sites with the help of orthodontic tooth movement has been shown to be practical [36], and in several cases, this technique was successfully applied in the MS area [20–22]. One major concern, however, is maintaining the intact membrane of the sinus floor. First, in surgical sinus augmentation procedures, the floor is mechanically and instantaneously lifted by applying graft materials or alveolar bone blocks [37, 38]. This shows the endurance and reparability of the sinus floor as it may adapt to slow and mild tooth movement. Second, recent studies have revealed that under stressful stimulation, bone deposition on the sinus side preceded resorption on the PDL side, and the amount of bone in the sinus wall was maintained or increased. This mechanism may partially account for bone remolding of the sinus floor [11, 12].

Currently, the etiology of OIRR is unclear. However, comprehensive orthodontic treatment, particularly the application of heavy forces, undoubtedly cause increases in the incidence and severity of root resorption [39]. Moving a tooth against the cortical bone is more likely to cause heavy root resorption, but serious OIRR was not reported in any of the included cases, perhaps because of the light forces applied. However, lack of detection of serious OIRR in some cases may reflect a limitation of radiographic approaches [18, 19, 22]. On the one hand, there is hysteresis between histological and radiographical changes, and early root resorption could only be detected on radiographs after 6–12 months [39]. On the other hand, panoramics or periapical films were used in most cases [14, 17–22], but their diagnostic accuracy may be insufficient [39, 40]. For retention, wrap-around or bonded retainers were mainly used for the maxillary teeth, and implants and subsequent prosthetic crowns were installed adjacent to or opposing the moved teeth. All these factors contributed to good retention and stability after MTTMS.

Limitations

Currently, the comprehension of MTTMS is limited. First, prospective controlled clinical trials with large samples are not available, so an optimal orthodontic protocol has not been established. Second, the techniques used to evaluate the SRR, OIRR and perforation of the sinus floor have low accuracy [41] and applying panoramics and periapical films can introduce errors in patient selection or outcome measurements. To improve accuracy, CBCT is an alternative strategy [8, 24, 25, 40, 42]. Third, the results of basic research simulating MTTMS are not necessarily authentic. Although the discovery of recent research was novel and was partly consistent with some clinical observations [11–13], the studies involved only a 2-week observation period on mouse models. And the results were not entirely consistent with the long-term findings in a previous biopsy report in human in which osteoclasts and obvious lamina dura resorption were observed on the sinus side [41]. Therefore, more basic studies with consistent models should be conducted to confirm these results. Lastly, during orthodontic tooth movement, some side effects such as severe root resorption, osseous perforation, and sinus perforation may be beyond orthodontists' control. These cannot be macroscopically or radiologically detected but can be verified histologically. Clinicians should determine accurate diagnoses with consideration of anatomical structures before treatment, execute careful protocols, and conduct progress evaluations throughout treatment [39–41].

Conclusion

At the present stage, no evidence-based protocol could be recommended to guide MTTMS. The empirical application of constant and light to moderate forces (by TAD, segment and multibrackets) to slowly move teeth through or into the maxillary sinus in adults appears to be practical and secure. Bodily movement could be accomplished, but teeth seem to be easily tipped initially, potentially resulting in root resorption. However, this conclusion should be interpreted with caution as the currently available evidence is based on only a few case reports or case series, and longitudinal or controlled studies are lacking in this area.

Abbreviations

CBCT: Cone-beam computed tomography; MS: Maxillary sinus; MSF: Maxillary sinus floor; MTTMS: Moving teeth through the maxillary sinus; OIRR: Orthodontically induced root resorption; SRR: Sinus-root relationship

Funding

The National Natural Science Foundation of China (Nos. 81470722 and 81201379) supported the design of the study and collection, analysis, and interpretation of data and writing and publishing the manuscript.

Authors' contributions

WS, KX, JL conducted the data search, extraction, assessment and the statistical analysis and draft the manuscript. XH made the figures and tables. XC, QL organized the structure of the manuscript and edited the language. WS and JL designed the study and revised the manuscript. All authors read and approved the final version of submission.

Competing interests

The authors declare that they have no competing interests.

Author details

[1]State Key Laboratory of Oral Diseases, National Clinical Research Center for Oral Diseases, Department of Orthodontics, West China Hospital of Stomatology, Sichuan University, Chengdu 610041, China. [2]State Key Laboratory of Oral Diseases, National Clinical Research Center for Oral Diseases, Department of Oral and Maxillofacial Surgery, West China Hospital of Stomatology, Sichuan University, Chengdu 610041, China.

References

1. Rossini G, Parrini S, Castroflorio T, Deregibus A, Debernardi CL. Efficacy of clear aligners in controlling orthodontic tooth movement: a systematic review. Angle Orthod. 2015;85:881–9.
2. Rossini G, Parrini S, Castroflorio T, Deregibus A, Debernardi CL. Diagnostic accuracy and measurement sensitivity of digital models for orthodontic purposes: a systematic review. Am J Orthod Dentofac Orthop. 2016;149:161–70.

3. Cassetta M, Giansanti M, Di Mambro A, Calasso S, Barbato E. Minimally invasive corticotomy in orthodontics using a three-dimensional printed CAD/CAM surgical guide. Int J Oral Maxillofac Surg. 2016;45:1059–64.
4. Melsen B. Adult orthodontics. 1st ed. UK: Wiley-Blackwell; 2012. p. 382–3.
5. von Arx T, Lozanoff S. Maxillary sinus clinical oral anatomy: a comprehensive review for dental practitioners and researchers. Cham: Springer International Publishing; 2017. p. 163–97.
6. Matsuda H, Borzabadi-Farahani A, Le BT. Three-dimensional alveolar bone anatomy of the maxillary first molars: a cone-beam computed tomography study with implications for immediate implant placement. Implant Dent. 2016;25:367–72.
7. Ahn NL, Park HS. Differences in distances between maxillary posterior root apices and the sinus floor according to skeletal pattern. Am J Orthod Dentofac Orthop. 2017;152:811–9.
8. Sharan A, Madjar D. Correlation between maxillary sinus floor topography and related root position of posterior teeth using panoramic and cross-sectional computed tomography imaging. Oral Surg Oral Med Oral Pathol Oral Radiol Endod. 2006;102:375–81.
9. Proffit WR, Fields HW Jr, Sarver DM. Contemporary orthodontics. 4th ed. St Louis: C.V. Mosby; 2007. p. 287-300–331–430.
10. Wehrbein H, Diedrich P. The initial morphological state in the basally pneumatized maxillary sinus–a radiological-histological study in man. Fortschr Kieferorthop. 1992;53:254–62.
11. Maeda Y, Kuroda S, Ganzorig K, Wazen R, Nanci A, Tanaka E. Histomorphometric analysis of overloading on palatal tooth movement into the maxillary sinus. Am J Orthod Dentofac Orthop. 2015;148:423–30.
12. Kuroda S, Wazen R, Moffatt P, Tanaka E, Nanci A. Mechanical stress induces bone formation in the maxillary sinus in a short-term mouse model. Clin Oral Investig. 2013;17:131–7.
13. Daimaruya T, Takahashi I, Nagasaka H, Umemori M, Sugawara J, Mitani H. Effects of maxillary molar intrusion on the nasal floor and tooth root using the skeletal anchorage system in dogs. Angle Orthod. 2003;73:158–66.
14. Kuroda S, Hichijo N, Sato M, Mino A, Tamamura N, Iwata M, et al. Long-term stability of maxillary group distalization with interradicular miniscrews in a patient with a class II division 2 malocclusion. Am J Orthod Dentofac Orthop. 2016;149:912–22.
15. Park JH, Tai K, Kanao A, Takagi M. Space closure in the maxillary posterior area through the maxillary sinus. Am J Orthod Dentofac Orthop. 2014;145: 95–102.
16. Oh H, Herchold K, Hannon S, Heetland K, Ashraf G, Nguyen V, et al. Orthodontic tooth movement through the maxillary sinus in an adult with multiple missing teeth. Am J Orthod Dentofac Orthop. 2014;146:493–505.
17. Cacciafesta V, Melsen B. Mesial bodily movement of maxillary and mandibular molars with segmented mechanics. Clin Orthod Res. 2001;4:182–8.
18. Kravitz ND, Kusnoto B, Tsay PT, Hohlt WF. Intrusion of overerupted upper first molar using two orthodontic miniscrews. A case report. Angle Orthod. 2007;77:915–22.
19. Yao CC, Wu CB, Wu HY, Kok SH, Chang HF, Chen YJ. Intrusion of the overerupted upper left first and second molars by mini-implants with partial-fixed orthodontic appliances: a case report. Angle Orthod. 2004;74:550–7.
20. Savi de Carvalho R, Consolaro A, Francischone CE Jr, de Macedo Carvalho AP. Sinus augmentation by orthodontic movement as an alternative to a surgical sinus lift: a clinical report. J Prosthet Dent. 2014;112:723–6.
21. Saglam M, Akman S, Malkoc S, Hakki SS. Modification of maxillary sinus floor with orthodontic treatment and implant therapy: a case letter. J Oral Implantol. 2014;40:619–22.
22. Re S, Cardaropoli D, Corrente G, Abundo R. Bodily tooth movement through the maxillary sinus with implant anchorage for single tooth replacement. Clin Orthod Res. 2001;4:177–81.
23. Moher D, Liberati A, Tetzlaff J, Altman DG. Preferred reporting items for systematic reviews and meta-analyses: the PRISMA statement. Bmj. 2009; 339:b2535.
24. Shanbhag S, Karnik P, Shirke P, Shanbhag V. Cone-beam computed tomographic analysis of sinus membrane thickness, ostium patency, and residual ridge heights in the posterior maxilla: implications for sinus floor elevation. Clin Oral Implants Res. 2014;25:755–60.
25. Janner SF, Caversaccio MD, Dubach P, Sendi P, Buser D, Bornstein MM. Characteristics and dimensions of the Schneiderian membrane: a radiographic analysis using cone beam computed tomography in patients referred for dental implant surgery in the posterior maxilla. Clin Oral Implants Res. 2011;22:1446–53.
26. Hofmann E. Radiology of the nose and paranasal sinuses for the endoscopic sinus surgeon. In: Stucker FJ, de Souza C, Kenyon GS, Lian TS, Draf W, Schick B, editors. Rhinology and facial plastic surgery. Berlin, Heidelberg: Springer Berlin Heidelberg; 2009. p. 507–12.
27. Fatterpekar GM, Delman BN, Som PM. Imaging the paranasal sinuses: where we are and where we are going. Anat Rec (Hoboken). 2008;291:1564–72.
28. Aimetti M, Massei G, Morra M, Cardesi E, Romano F. Correlation between gingival phenotype and Schneiderian membrane thickness. Int J Oral Maxillofac Implants. 2008;23:1128–32.
29. Cattaneo PM, Dalstra M, Melsen B. Moment-to-force ratio, center of rotation, and force level: a finite element study predicting their interdependency for simulated orthodontic loading regimens. Am J Orthod Dentofac Orthop. 2008;133:681–9.
30. Graber LW, Vanarsdall RL Jr, Vig KWL. Orthodontics: current principles and techniques. 5th ed. Philadelphia: Mosby; 2012. p. 345–80.
31. Kravitz ND, Kusnoto B, Tsay TP, Hohlt WF. The use of temporary anchorage devices for molar intrusion. J Am Dent Assoc. 2007;138:56–64.
32. Manhartsberger C, Morton JY, Burstone CJ. Space closure in adult patients using the segmented arch technique. Angle Orthod. 1989;59:205–10.
33. Wehrbein H, Bauer W, Wessing G, Diedrich P. The effect of the maxillary sinus floor on orthodontic tooth movement. Fortschr Kieferorthop. 1990;51: 345–51.
34. Isaacson RJ, Lindauer SJ, Davidovitch M. On tooth movement. Angle Orthod. 1993;63:305–9.
35. Wingard CE, Bowers GM. The effects of facial bone from facial tipping of incisors in monkeys. J Periodontol. 1976;47:450–4.
36. Somar M, Mohadeb JV, Huang C. Predictability of orthodontic forced eruption in developing an implant site: a systematic review. J Clin Orthod. 2016;50:485–92.
37. Mohan N, Wolf J, Dym H. Maxillary sinus augmentation. Dent Clin N Am. 2015;59:375–88.
38. Jensen OT, Brownd C, Baer D. Maxillary molar sinus floor intrusion at the time of dental extraction. J Oral Maxillofac Surg. 2006;64:1415–9.
39. Huang GJ, Richmond S, Vig KWL. Evidence-based orthodontics. 1st ed. UK: Wiley-Blackwell; 2011. p. 63–87.
40. Yi J, Sun Y, Li Y, Li C, Li X, Zhao Z. Cone-beam computed tomography versus periapical radiograph for diagnosing external root resorption: a systematic review and meta-analysis. Angle Orthod. 2017;87:328–37.
41. Wehrbein H, Fuhrmann RA, Diedrich PR. Human histologic tissue response after long-term orthodontic tooth movement. Am J Orthod Dentofac Orthop. 1995;107:360–71.
42. Lopes LJ, Gamba TO, Bertinato JV, Freitas DQ. Comparison of panoramic radiography and CBCT to identify maxillary posterior roots invading the maxillary sinus. Dentomaxillofac Radiol. 2016;45:20160043.

14

Patient awareness/knowledge towards oral cancer: a cross-sectional survey

Neel Shimpi[1], Monica Jethwani[1,2], Aditi Bharatkumar[1,2], Po-Huang Chyou[3], Ingrid Glurich[1] and Amit Acharya[1,2,3*]

Abstract

Background: Oral cancer (OC) is associated with multiple risk factors and high mortality rates and substantially contributes to the global cancer burden despite being highly preventable.
This cross-sectional study sought to assess current knowledge, awareness, and behaviors of patients in rural communities surrounding OC risk.

Methods: An anonymous 21-question survey was distributed to patients in waiting rooms of a large integrated medical-dental health system serving north-central Wisconsin.
Survey results were summarized via descriptive statistics. Odds ratios surrounding health literacy on OC risk factors were obtained using unconditional univariate logistic regression analysis.

Results: Of 504 dental and 306 medical patients completing the survey, 62.2% were female, Caucasian/White (92%) with 41% having a ≤ high school diploma/equivalent. Current smoker/smokeless tobacco use was reported by 34%, while 39% reported former tobacco exposure. Alcohol use was reported by 54% of respondents at the following frequencies: < once/week, (35%); 1–2 times/week, (16%); 3–4 times/week, (6%); 5–6 times/week, (2%); and daily, (23%). Knowledge about tobacco and alcohol use and increased OC risk was reported by 94 and 40%, respectively. About 50% reported knowledgeability regarding cancer-associated symptomology. Tobacco cessation was reported by 20% of responders. Receipt of education on OC from healthcare providers and human papilloma virus links to OC causation was reported by 38 and 21%, respectively.

Conclusion: Patients who smoked > 20+ cigarettes per day were more knowledgeable about tobacco and OC risk compared to non-smokers and those who smoked ≤ 19 cigarettes/day ($p = 0.0647$). Patients who were alcohol consumers exhibited higher knowledgeability surrounding increased OC risk with alcohol and tobacco exposures compared to alcohol abstainers ($p = 0.06$). We concluded that patients recognized links between tobacco and OC risk but demonstrated lower knowledge of other causal factors. Strategic patient education by providers could increase awareness of OC risk.

Keywords: Oral cancer, Awareness, Knowledge, Attitudes, Community surveys

Background

Oral and oro-pharyngeal cancers (OC) using the World Health Organization (WHO) International Statistical Classification of Disease (ICD-10) definitions are collectively defined by site and include cancers of lip, buccal mucosa, alveolar ridge and gingiva, tongue, floor of mouth and/or unspecified parts of the mouth, tonsil, hard and soft palate and oropharynx [1]. Global annual incidence of these cancers are estimated as 529,500 [2]. Annually in the United States, an estimated 51,540 persons are diagnosed with OCs, which are associated with 25 and 57% 1-year and 5-year mortality rates, respectively. OCs, have shown little improvement in survival statistics across three decades [3, 4]. An estimated 9750 deaths in the upcoming year are predicted in the United States alone [3]. Late-stage diagnosis of OC contributes to poor prognosis.

Upon timely detection, OC is relatively curable. Notably, the rates of poor prognosis are markedly associated with patient delay in health care-seeking behaviors [5–7]. It has been shown that 40% of patients do not present until

* Correspondence: acharya.amit@marshfieldresearch.edu
[1]Center for Oral and Systemic Health, Marshfield Clinic Research Institute, 1000 North Oak Avenue, Marshfield 54449, WI, United States of America
[2]Family Health Center of Marshfield Inc., 1307 N St Joseph Ave, Marshfield 54449, WI, United States of America
Full list of author information is available at the end of the article

progression to an advanced stage (stage 3 or 4) has occurred [8]. Late-stage presentation is associated with metastasis to local lymph nodes, requires aggressive treatment, and is often unsuccessful [6, 8]. A gap in patient knowledge and health literacy surrounding OC, specifically related to risk factors and symptomology, is posited to be among the key modifiable factors contributing to high morbidity and mortality [9].

Historically, the level of risk factor knowledgeability surrounding oral/oropharyngeal cancer has been markedly low, with only one-quarter of individuals recognizing tobacco as an OC-risk factor [10]. Although knowledgeability surrounding tobacco exposure as a dominant risk factor for oral and other cancers is now more pervasive, the relationship between alcohol misuse and OC remains under-appreciated [11]. Tobacco use and alcohol are estimated to play a contributory role to 80% of all incident OCs [12]. Additional contributory risk factors, including oral hygiene and dietary habits are also frequently under-recognized by patients [11].

A growing body of evidence suggests human papillomavirus (HPV) 16 is an important factor associated with OC [13, 14]. Because HPV16 has only recently been identified as a potential risk factor, the level of public knowledgeability surrounding its association with OC emergence has been only infrequently reported to date [15]. Notably, the Oral Cancer Foundation projects that HPV 16, which has also been associated with cervical cancer, may be replacing tobacco use as the primary risk factor for oral OC in individuals younger than 50 years of age [3]. In addition, several factors perceived to be risk factors for OC by patients have not been substantiated, including hereditary causes, marijuana use, HIV infection, and alcohol in mouthwashes [3, 15].

Symptomology surrounding OC also tends to be poorly understood by the patient population [5–7]. Established symptoms of OC include a non-healing ulcer, visible red or white patches, mouth swelling, and tongue soreness. A case study performed by Rogers et al. [7] found that only one in three individuals could correctly identify the hallmark non-healing ulcer as a sign of OC. Among a cohort of individuals diagnosed with OC, less than 50% were aware of oropharyngeal cancers prior to their diagnosis. The majority of subjects were also unable to identify alternative symptoms and tended to view them as non-consequential [7].

Our cross-sectional investigation was designed to assess OC knowledge and awareness among patients presenting for care at Marshfield Clinic Health System (MCHS), a large rural multispecialty clinic. MCHS serves a wide service area encompassing central, northern and western Wisconsin through an integrated network of regionally-based clinics. A survey-based environmental scan was undertaken at five regional medical and nine dental clinics to assess patient knowledgeability and awareness regarding OC. The study additionally screened for lifestyle behaviors associated with OC risk.

Methods

The study was reviewed and granted exempt status by the Marshfield Clinic Research Institute's institutional review board. A cross-sectional study design was applied. All the patients between 18 and 80 years of age in the waiting areas of MCHS five medical and nine dental centers for their appointments were eligible for the survey. A paper-based survey tool at 5th grade readability level, consisting of 21 questions (see Additional file 1: survey instrument) was developed by the study team and organized into subsections including: patient socio-demographics, knowledgeability assessment, and educational outreach surrounding OC from their healthcare provider. Socio- demographic survey questions captured patients' age, gender, race, and ethnicity, educational level and current and historic behavioral habits concerning alcohol and tobacco habits. The knowledgeability assessment consisted of three questions regarding the awareness of alcohol and OC, signs of mouth cancer and actions that may prevent mouth cancer. The educational outreach questions included two questions that captured whether their healthcare providers are educating them about OC and association between HPV and OC. Face validity analysis of the survey was conducted by study team members with appropriate expertise. Content validity analysis of the survey was performed by ten experts from the fields of dentistry, medicine, and statistics prior to dissemination. The survey was also piloted by 12 professionals before dissemination. Time for completion was estimated at 8 to 10 min.

Study participation was voluntary and anonymous. Self-administered surveys were completed by participants in Clinic waiting rooms. Patients presenting to the front desk staff for appointments were approached for completing the survey and hence the survey targeted a convenience sample not driven by a defined sample size. An information sheet was developed for the front desk professionals who administered the survey to the patients. This information sheet included the instructions and script for administering the survey. These also included answers to potential participant questions such as: 'Do I have to take the survey?'; 'How long will the survey take?'; 'Are my answers private/confidential?'; 'What is the survey for?' and 'Do I have to fill it now?'. The instruction sheet also included information to direct any participant comments or questions to research team members. Similarly, the front desk staff also helped in filling out the survey if potential participants could not write. Survey distribution was active for 3 weeks (Jan

2015-Feb 2015) and was collected every weekday. No incentive was offered to the participants.

Surveys were collected by the front desk staff and, placed in an envelope and routed/mailed to the research team on weekly basis. Survey responses were manually entered into a REDCap database [16]. A 10% data validation was performed by second data entry personnel to validate the accuracy of the data entered into the REDCap study database [17]. The data were then exported into Excel (Microsoft Corporation, Seattle, WA) and converted into SAS-formatted dataset (SAS Windows version 9.4, English (SAS Institute Inc., Cary, NC). Rates of missing data are reported for each question represented in the denominator (Total number-missing data). The missing data elements were otherwise excluded from study analyses. For the purpose of the study, tobacco use that included smoking cigarettes, cigars, pipes, and e-cigarettes were categorized as 'smoking tobacco', and tobacco use that included chewing tobacco and using snuff were classified under 'smokeless tobacco'.

All data analyses were carried out using SAS. Descriptive statistics (for any categorical measurements: percentage and corresponding 95% confidence interval (CI); for continuous variables: mean, standard deviation, median, and range) were reported for data surrounding measurements (e.g., cigarettes per day) as well as categorical measurements including patients' attributes (e.g., age, gender, educational level). Educational levels were categorized as I = (no schooling+ Grades 1 to 12), II = (High school diploma+ some college+ Associate degree), III = (Bachelor's degree+ Master's degree+ Professional degree).

Fisher's Exact test was performed for comparing the difference in percentages of reported (a) OC knowledge (defined as yes versus no), (b) partitioned by patients' age grouping (≤ 40 years versus ≥41 years), (c) gender, (d) race, (e)educational level, (f) status of tobacco use (including smoking tobacco and smokeless tobacco), and (g) reported frequency of alcohol use. In addition, Chi square test and odds ratio (ORs) with 95% CI were estimated to examine knowledge concerning specific risk factors in association with OC (defined as 'yes' versus 'no') by using unconditional univariate logistic regression analysis. *P*-values were derived and values of < 0.05 were considered statistically significant.

Results

The data was entered and accuracy was confirmed

Participant demographics

A total of 810 surveys were collected during the 3-week period and included in the analysis. Participants' characteristics are summarized in Fig. 1. Of the participants, 62% (504/806) were female, and 92 and 86% of the participant population was Caucasian and non-Hispanic/Latino respectively, reflecting the regional demographics of the largely rural service area of MCHS spanning central and northern Wisconsin.

Practice behavior

a. Tobacco use Of the 810 participants, 34% (276/810) reported current use of both smoking tobacco and smokeless tobacco, and another 39% (316/810) reported smoking tobacco and smokeless tobacco use in the past. Overall, 20% of participants reported attempted cessation of tobacco product use over the past 12 months. Exposure to passive smoke was reported by 175 participants (22%). The self-reported tobacco use and concurrent use of alcohol is shown in Table 1.

b. Alcohol use The percentage of individuals reporting alcohol consumption was 63% (505/803). The participants reported: 35.4% (283/800) 'less than 1 time a week'; 16.3% (130/800) '1 to 2 times a week'; 6.1% (49/800) '3 to 4 times a week'; 2% (16/800) '5 to 6 times a week'; 2.9% (23/800) 'daily' and 37.3% (299/800) indicated 'never'.

OC knowledge and awareness

Approximately 40% (309/782) of all patients indicated that their healthcare providers (including physicians, nurse practitioners, medical assistants, and health educators) educated them about OC. Approximately 22% (169/787) of all participants indicated that their healthcare providers educated them about the relation of HPV and OC. More than 90% of participants with Educational II (High school diploma+ some college+ Associate degree) and III = (Bachelor's degree+ Master's degree+ Professional degree) correctly identified difficulty in chewing/swallowing as a sign of OC as compared to participants with Education level I (no schooling+ Grades 1 to 12) ($p = 0.0591$). Figure 2 summarizes findings surrounding OC symptomology and risk factors. As shown in this figure, high numbers of participants correctly identified that smoking (728/776 (94%)) and second hand smoke exposure smoke ((622/762) 82%)) were risk factors for OC while lower numbers of participants correctly identified alcohol exposure (601/761 (79%)) and ill-fitting dentures (369/733 (50%)) as OC risk factors. In descending order, signs of OC recognized by participants were a) abnormal mass/lump in mouth (589/766 (77%); b) mouth sore that does not heal 585/771 (76%)); c) white/red patch in mouth (476/759 (63%)); d) difficulty in chewing/swallowing 449/764 (59%)) and e) slow change in voice quality (419/757 (55%)).

Approximately 23% (182/785) reported concurrent use of tobacco (smoking + smokeless) and alcohol. Of these 182, 74 participants (39%) were aware of alcohol contributing to OC risk, while 173 participants (95%) were

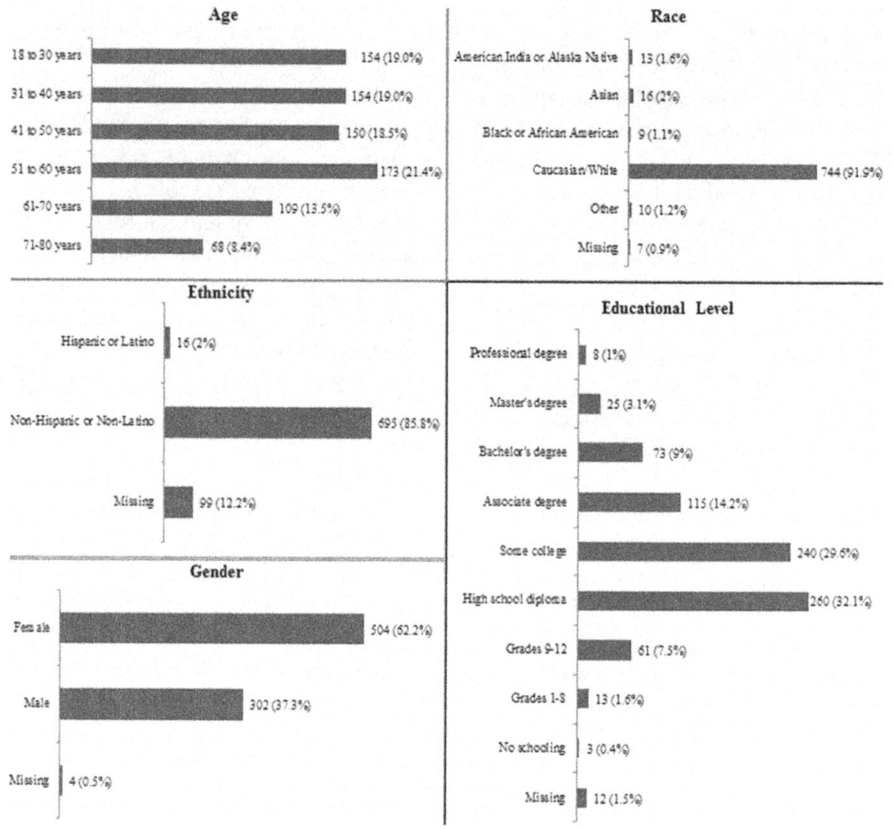

Fig. 1 Characteristics of participants who responded to the survey

aware of tobacco contributing to risk for OC. All alcohol users who were knowledgeable about alcohol-associated risk also indicated knowledgeability of increased risk for OC contributed by smoking.

The present study considered two dependent variables: a. knowledge of tobacco and OC association and b. knowledge of alcohol and OC association. The independent variables that were assessed included age range, gender, educational levels, current smoker, cigarettes/ day, alcohol drinker and number of drinks/week. Table 2 summarizes outcomes of the univariate regression analysis for variables associated with knowledge of tobacco contributing to OC risk.

Study findings also showed that among patients who reported current smoker status, that those that smoked more than 20 cigarettes per day were more knowledgeable about tobacco as a risk factor for oral cancer compared to non-smokers or patients who smoked </= 19 cigarettes/ day ($p = 0.06$). Similarly, participants reporting alcohol consumption were more knowledgeable about tobacco as a risk factor for oral cancer compared to participants who did not drink alcohol ($p = 0.06$). Table 3 summarizes outcomes of the univariate regression analysis for variables associated with knowledge of alcohol and OC association and shows that compared to patients aged 18–30 years, patients aged 31–60 years had significantly lower knowledge of alcohol causing oral cancer. Further, patients with the Educational level III = (Bachelor's degree+ Master's degree+ Professional degree) had significantly lower knowledge of alcohol as an OC risk factor than those with Education level I (no schooling+ Grades 1 to 12) and Education level II = (High school diploma+ some college+ Associate degree) and that education and dental patients had significantly greater knowledge of alcohol as an OC risk than medical patients. Finally no significant associations were observed between gender, current tobacco smoking status, number of cigarettes smoked per day, alcohol drinking status, number of drinks per week and the knowledge of alcohol causing oral cancer.

Discussion

The data collected in the present study indicated that while survey participants were generally aware of the tobacco as a key OC risk factor, knowledge surrounding other associated risk factors, including alcohol, was less extensive. Overall, this study found that the majority of respondents (94%) reported knowing that quitting tobacco can decrease OC risk. However despite knowledge surrounding smoking risk, rate of patients reporting current smoker status or current smokeless tobacco use

Table 1 Overview of self-reported tobacco use and concurrent use of alcohol

		Male			Female		
Type of tobacco and frequency of alcohol use		Current	Former	Nonsmoker	Current	Former	Nonsmoker
Smoking tobacco		33% (97/298)	35% (101/294)	33% (93/289)	35% (155/491)	22% (153/491)	43% (183/491)
	Cigarettes/day	74	[a]N/A	[a]N/A	141	[a]N/A	[a]N/A
	Cigars/day	11	[a]N/A	[a]N/A	4	[a]N/A	[a]N/A
	Pipes/day	3	[a]N/A	[a]N/A	0	[a]N/A	[a]N/A
	E-cigarettes-puffs/day	3	[a]N/A	[a]N/A	4	[a]N/A	[a]N/A
	Cigarettes + cigars/day	2	[a]N/A	[a]N/A	2	[a]N/A	[a]N/A
	Cigarettes + pipes/day	1	[a]N/A	[a]N/A	1	[a]N/A	[a]N/A
	Cigarettes +cigars+ pipes/day	0	[a]N/A	[a]N/A	1	[a]N/A	[a]N/A
	Cigarettes + E-cigarettes-puffs/day	3	[a]N/A	[a]N/A	2	[a]N/A	[a]N/A
Concurrent use of alcohol with smoking tobacco use	Never	27/95	31/101	32/93	60/154	61/153	77/174
	< 1 time a week	26/95	35/101	25/93	54/154	62/153	63/174
	1 to 2 times a week	23/95	16/101	19/93	26/154	18/153	25/174
	3 to 4 times a week	8/95	10/101	9/93	10/154	6/153	5/174
	5 to 6 times a week	1/95	7/101	4/93	2/154	3/153	0/174
	Daily	10/95	2/101	4/93	2/154	3/153	1/174
Smokeless tobacco		10% (31/289)	23% (59/289)	68% (199/289)	1% (5/492)	5% (24/492)	94% (463/492)
	Chew/day	9	[a]N/A	[a]N/A	1	[a]N/A	[a]N/A
	Snuff/day	15	[a]N/A	[a]N/A	2	[a]N/A	[a]N/A
	Snus/day	4	[a]N/A	[a]N/A	0	[a]N/A	[a]N/A
Concurrent use of alcohol with smokeless tobacco use	Never	7/31	21/59	61/196	2/5	13/23	183/455
	< 1 time a week	13/31	23/59	58/196	0/5	7/23	174/455
	1 to 2 times a week	9/31	12/59	33/196	0/5	1/23	69/455
	3 to 4 times a week	1/31	2/59	23/196	1/5	1/23	18/455
	5 to 6 times a week	0/31	0/59	9/196	1/5	0/23	4/455
	Daily	1/31	1/59	12/196	0/5	1/23	7/455

[a]N/A = Please note that the details for smoking and smokeless tobacco represent for current status of tobacco use only Note: For smokeless tobacco data: the total percentage corresponds to all individuals who indicated use of smokeless tobacco but not all indicated the specific type of smokeless tobacco

was 32% (254/792) and 5% (37/794), respectively, exceeding rates most recently reported by the Center for Disease Control (CDC) (15.5 and 3.4%, respectively) [18, 19]. Importantly, patients reported low rates of counseling by healthcare providers surrounding OC risk. Compared to tobacco exposure risk, participants reported lower rates of knowledge surrounding additional risk factors associated with OC including: "brushing and flossing teeth twice daily: 79% (607/764)" and "avoiding contact with second-hand smoke 82% (622/762)", while 79% (601/761) selected "quitting alcohol". Findings from our study support that educational initiatives may be warranted to improve health literacy surrounding risk factors for OC among medical providers as well as patients [20–22].

Participants who lack knowledgeability and are generally unaware of the risk factors contributing to OC put themselves at greater risk for first presenting with disease at an advanced stage when less extensive, highly effective curative treatment is required. Curative treatment of OC generally includes resection for primary tumors whereas those with more extensive involvement may require more extensive surgical procedures and/or intensive, chemotherapeutic intervention, often with concurrent intensive adjunctive treatment [1, 23].

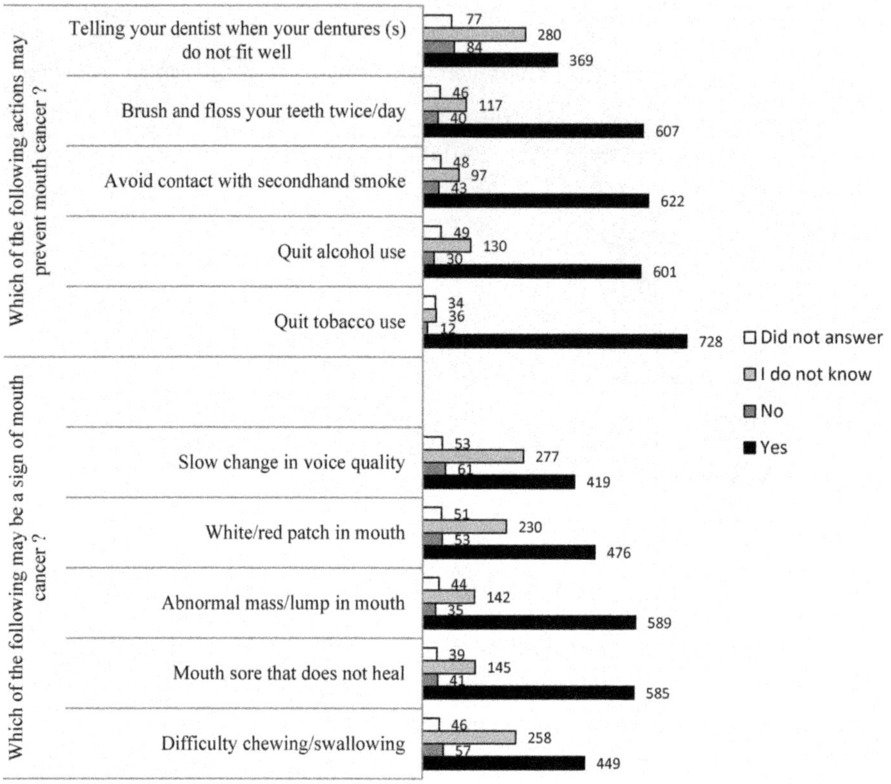

Fig. 2 Summary findings associated with oral cancer knowledge and awareness

Interventional strategies: Tobacco cessation

Notably, only 48% (133/276) of participants who were current tobacco users (smoking and/or smokeless) had received counselling for tobacco cessation from their health care providers following documentation of their tobacco use history. Although this finding suggests potential responsiveness among healthcare providers in establishing a climate promoting and integrating improved tobacco cessation care delivery, the overall survey response indicated that less than half [approximately 40% (309/782)] the participants had received education surrounding their increased risk status for OC by their healthcare provider. Notably, rates surrounding receipt of education regarding smoking cessation to decrease risk for oral cancer reported in the current study (40%) were higher than respective rates reported in the studies conducted in some other countries (e.g.; Lawoyin et al., in Nigeria (20%) [24], Reddy et al., in South India (26%) [25]. By contrast studies that focused on rates of education by dental providers surrounding smoking cessation showed rates as high as 78% in advising patients regarding smoking cessation [26].

One of our previous studies examined the rate of primary care physicians' (PCPs) awareness of OC risk factors and the extent to which they provided patients with OC education. The study found that the self-reported comfort levels of PCPs who had practiced less than 10 years for educating patients about oral cancer was 52%, while 46% of PCPs who practiced more than 10 years indicated being comfortable with this educational process. Further, providers in this prior study attributed the low percentage of comfort levels to the minimal oral health-related training received during their professional medical training [27].

Importance of concurrent use of alcohol and tobacco and OC risk status

The concurrent use of alcohol and tobacco has been recognized to have more detrimental effect as compared to the tobacco use or alcohol use alone [28, 29]. The National Institute on Alcohol Abuse and Alcoholism's 2001–2002 survey reported that approximately 46 million adults used both alcohol and tobacco [28]. The link between concurrent tobacco and alcohol use behavior has been reported previously [29]. People who drink and smoke are at higher risk for certain types of cancer, particularly oral and pharyngeal. Alcohol and tobacco exposure are associated with approximately 80% of cases of OCs in men and about 65% in women [1, 19]. Studies have also shown that the risk of developing OC by using tobacco and alcohol in combination is additive and greater or equal to, alcohol multiplied by risk associated with tobacco [29–33]. In our study about 23% (187/787) were concurrent tobacco and alcohol users and only 39% of

Table 2 Proportions and Predictors of Knowledge of Tobacco Causing Oral Cancer

Characteristics	Knowledge of tobacco causing oral cancer		Odds Ratio	95% CI	*p*-value
	Yes (n/%)	No (n/%)			
Age (years)					
18–30[a]	148 (97.4)	04 (2.6)	1.00		
31–60	449 (95.3)	22 (4.7)	0.54	0.19–1.61	0.2701
61–80	165 (95.4)	08 (4.6)	0.55	0.16–1.86	0.3370
Gender					
Male	285 (96.3)	11 (3.7)	1.20	0.57–2.51	0.6325
Female[a]	476 (95.6)	22 (4.4)	1.00		
Educational level					
I[a]	069 (92.0)	06 (8.0)			
II	585 (96.1)	24 (3.9)	1.85	0.73–4.67	0.1918
III	100 (96.2)	04 (3.9)	1.90	0.52–6.96	0.3333
Current Smoker					
Yes	239 (95.2)	12 (4.8)	0.79	0.38–1.62	0.5080
No[a]	510 (96.2)	20 (3.8)	1.00		
Cigarettes/day					
0[a]	524 (96.5)	19 (3.5)	1.00		
1–19	146 (95.4)	07 (4.6)	0.79	0.33–1.90	0.6014
20+	065 (91.6)	06 (8.4)	0.41	0.16–1.06	0.0647
Alcohol drinker					
Yes	423 (97.0)	13 (3.0)	1.94	0.95–3.95	0.0691
No[a]	336 (94.4)	20 (5.6)	1.00		
Drink/week					
0 to < 1[a]	530 (95.5)	25 (4.5)	1.00		
1 to 4	172 (97.2)	05 (2.8)	1.61	0.61–4.25	0.3379
5 to 7	036 (92.3)	03 (7.7)	0.56	0.16–1.94	0.3617
Dental patient					
Yes	477 (95.8)	21 (4.2)	1.03	0.51–2.09	0.9369
No[a]	287 (95.7)	13 (4.3)	1.00		

[a]'referent' group: I = (no schooling+ Grades 1to 12); II = (High school diploma+ some college+ Associate degree); III = (Bachelor's degree+ Master's degree+ Professional degree)

these concurrently exposed participants reported awareness of the risk for OC contributed by alcohol.

OC screening and symptomology recognition

A preventative approach to oral cancer is posited to be far more cost effective in terms of patient outcomes and associated healthcare costs than a curative model which is associated with high healthcare cost surrounding treatment. Notably, OC screening has prompted considerable debate in the health care realm. In 2014, the United States Preventative Service Task Force issued a report assessing the feasibility of conducting nation-wide screening for asymptomatic OC. Although the report raised concern regarding the OC status and outcomes in the United States, it concluded that the evidence base required to support screening was currently lacking [34]. In the absence of population screening, greater onus is placed on the patient to be informed regarding OC risk and detection, and establishing health literacy around this topic may be especially challenging in underserved populations [35]. Moreover, surveys by the CDC further revealed that the use of e-cigarettes, a type of battery-operated nicotine delivery system, has doubled from 2011 to 2012, thus increasing the risk of developing OC [36, 37]. This observation further emphasizes that despite declines in rates of smoking, alternative forms of tobacco exposure continue to contribute health risk for the general population.

The current study found that around half of respondents possessed adequate oral symptomology knowledge,

Table 3 Proportion and Predictors of Knowledge of Alcohol Causing Oral Cancer

Characteristics	Knowledge of alcohol causing oral cancer		Odds Ratio	95% CI	*p*-value
	Yes (n/%)	No (n/%)			
Age (years)					
18–30[a]	71 (47.0)	80 (53.0)	1.00		
31–60	173 (37.0)	295 (63.0)	0.63	0.45–0.93	0.0187
61–80	75 (43.4)	98 (56.7)	0.84	0.54–1.30	0.4302
Gender					
Male	116 (38.9)	182 (61.1)	0.91	0.68–1.22	0.5170
Female[a]	203 (41.3)	289 (58.7)	1.00		
Education					
I[a]	37 (50.0)	37 (50.0)	1.00		
II	244 (40.3)	361 (59.7)	0.71	0.45–1.12	0.1406
III	36 (34.3)	69 (65.7)	0.55	0.30–0.99	0.0443
Current smoker					
Yes	106 (42.6)	143 (57.4)	1.17	0.86–1.59	0.3203
No[a]	205 (38.8)	323 (61.2)	1.00		
Cigarettes/day					
0[a]	211 (38.9)	311 (61.1)	1.00		
1–19	65 (42.8)	87 (57.2)	1.15	0.80–1.66	0.4436
20+	31 (44.3)	39 (55.7)	1.23	0.74–2.02	0.4252
Alcohol drinker					
Yes	164 (37.5)	273 (62.5)	0.77	0.58–1.02	0.0714
No[a]	154 (43.9)	197 (56.1)	1.00		
Drink/week					
0 to < 1[a]	226 (41.0)	325 (59.0)	1.00		
1 to 4	71 (39.7)	108 (60.3)	0.93	0.66–1.32	0.6942
5 to 7	12 (30.8)	27 (69.2)	0.63	0.31–1.27	0.1976
		Dental patient			
Yes	221 (44.7)	274 (55.3)	1.61	1.19–2.16	0.0019
No[a]	100 (33.4)	199 (66.6)	1.00		

[a]= 'referent' group, I = (no schooling+ Grades 1to 12), II = (High school diploma+ some college+ Associate degree), III = (Bachelor's degree+ Master's degree+ Professional degree)

although less than 50% reported receiving prior education from a primary care provider. A study conducted by Villa et all among dental patients showed that approximately 65 and 80% of participants were aware that white/red patch or mass/ulcer in mouth respectively, were possible signs of oral cancer, while in the present study patient awareness surrounding these lesions was 76 and 62% respectively. Villa et al. [9] also reported that more than 85% of the participants in their study did not receive counseling on oral cancer from dentists, physicians or other healthcare providers.

Human papilloma virus (HPV) and OC risk

Recent research proposes HPV especially HPV 16, as a newly recognized additional risk factor for OC [3]. In the current study which was focused on behavioral risk factors contributing to OC (including tobacco and alcohol exposures), one question was included to explore whether providers were educating patients concerning HPV and risk for OC. About one fourth of participants reported having acquired knowledge about HPV as a risk factor for OPC from their healthcare provider. Our study suggests that further promotion of public awareness concerning OC and HPV as a risk factor.

Study limitations

This study acknowledges some limitations. Since it was focused on quantitative assessment of the knowledge, awareness, and lifestyle behaviors of patients in the context of OC, the survey tool validation was limited to face and content validity. The information provided by the patients was self-reported; hence, our ability to validate findings is limited. Further, data was collected from a single, albeit large, health care system and may not be universally generalizable to other population-based settings beyond the current environment. This raises the potential for selection bias within the targeted population of the current study. The refusal rate for participation was not captured by personnel offering the survey to patients coming through their departments and hence it was not possible to determine a denominator that would permit calculation of response rate. Considering that 97% of the oral cancers are squamous cell carcinomas, this study did not include questions on knowledge surrounding sun exposure as a risk factor for basal cell carcinoma [38]. Further, the study also did not assess patient's oral health literacy and general health literacy. Because the survey was anonymous and voluntary, there was a possibility that a person could have taken the survey more than once. For the question, "during the past 12 months, have you tried to stop using tobacco products?", participants were only given the option to answer as 'yes' or 'no'. Thus the survey did not assess the number of smoking cessation attempts by the participants in the 12 month period.

The study did not access frequency of opportunities for patient education by healthcare providers surrounding HPV and OC since HPV which shows higher association with oropharyngeal cancers. Similarly, the study did not assess the number of times the participants visited the medical providers or the volume of information that was given during the patient education. As reports on chewing areca nut or betel quid use are limited in North America, we did not assess the information on betel quid in our survey [39].Quantification of alcohol was based on number of times a participant reported drinking alcohol in a week and not based on the number of units consumed per day. The study was conducted in a healthcare delivery setting focused on patients rather than community member/population setting. Future studies may target assessment of knowledge and awareness of the community rather than the patient population subset since patients might be more informed on the topic than an average community member who may only infrequently visit a healthcare setting.

Conclusion

Overall, our data supports that patients were generally aware of the OC risk associated with tobacco, but knowledge of other risk factors was more limited. The study looked at health literacy surrounding known risk factors associated with OC. Based on findings in this cross-sectional, population-based study, this research identified that improvement of health literacy surrounding oral cancer may be warranted and has helped to identify that educational initiatives targeting both medical providers and patients are needed to reduce the burden of OC in the current absence of recommendation for population-based screening in order to improve outcomes associated with early detection.

Abbreviations

CDC: Centers for Disease Control and Prevention; CI: Confidence Interval; HPV: Human papillomavirus; SD: Standard Deviation

Acknowledgements

The authors thank Cathy Schneider from the Biomedical Informatics Research Center for her assistance with survey tool formatting and preparation of the data sets for analysis. The authors would also like to thank Dixie Schroeder from Institute for Oral and Systemic Health and Debra Kempf from Division of Education of Marshfield Clinic for their coordination in the project. The authors would also like to thank Jacob Blamer and Marie Fleisner from the Office of Scientific Writing at Marshfield Clinic Research Institute for their assistance with reviewing and editing this manuscript.

Author contributions

All authors contributed equally to this work. NS: Supervised the project and prepared the manuscript draft and conducted data analysis MJ: Conducted the study and participated in reviewing the manuscript. AB: Conducted the study and participated in reviewing the manuscript. PC: Conducted statistical analysis and helped in interpretation of the data. Participated in editing the statistical material of the manuscript. IG: Helped in preparing, editing the manuscript and data analysis. AA: Initiated and oversaw the project conduct. Participated in data analysis and editing the manuscript drafts. All authors read and approved the final manuscript.

Funding

The study was supported, in part, by a grant from Delta Dental of Wisconsin, funds from Marshfield Clinic Research Institute (MCRI), Center for Oral and Systemic Health, Division of Education and Family Health Center of Marshfield. The funding bodies had no role in the design of the study and collection, analysis and interpretation of data and in writing the manuscript.

Competing interests

The authors declare that they have no competing interests.

Author details

[1]Center for Oral and Systemic Health, Marshfield Clinic Research Institute, 1000 North Oak Avenue, Marshfield 54449, WI, United States of America. [2]Family Health Center of Marshfield Inc., 1307 N St Joseph Ave, Marshfield 54449, WI, United States of America. [3]Office of Research Computing and Analytics, Marshfield Clinic Research Institute, 1000 North Oak Avenue, Marshfield 54449, WI, United States of America.

References

1. World Health Organization. International Statistical Classification of Diseases and Related Health Problems-10th Revision (ICD-10)-WHO Version. 2016. http://apps.who.int/classifications/icd10/browse/2016/en#/C00-C14. Accessed 5 Apr, 2018.
2. Shield KD, Ferlay J, Jemal A, et al. The global incidence of lip, oral cavity, and pharyngeal cancers by subsite in 2012. CA Cancer J Clin. 2017;67(1):51–64.
3. Oral Cancer Foundation. Oral Cancer Facts: rates of occurrence in the United States. 2018. https://oralcancerfoundation.org/facts/. Accessed 5 Apr, 2018.
4. American Cancer Society. Oral Cavity and Oropharyngeal Cancer 2016. Atlanta: American Cancer Society. 2018. http://www.cancer.org/acs/groups/cid/documents/webcontent/003128-pdf.pdf. Accessed 5 Apr, 2018.
5. Scott SE, Grunfield EA, McGurk M. Patient's delay in oral cancer: a systematic review. Community Dent Oral Epidemiol. 2006;34(5):337–43.
6. Dobson C, Russell AJ, Rubin GP. Patient delay in cancer diagnosis: what do we really mean and can we be more specific? BMC Health Serv Res. 2014:14–387.
7. Rogers SN, Vedpathak SV, Lowe D. Reasons for delayed presentation in oral and oropharyngeal cancer: the patients perspective. Br J Oral Maxillofac Surg. 2011;49:349–53.
8. Rogers SN, Brown JS, Woolgar JA, et al. Survival following primary surgery for oral cancer. Oral Oncol. 2009;45:201–11.
9. Villa A, Kreimer AR, Pasi M, et al. Oral cancer knowledge: a survey administered to patients in dental departments at large Italian hospitals. J Cancer Educ. 2011;26:505–9.
10. Horowitz AM, Canto MT, Child WL. Maryland adults perspectives on oral cancer prevention and early detection. J Am Dent Assoc. 2002;133:1058–63.
11. Rogers SN, Hunter R, Lowe D. Awareness of oral cancer in the Mersey region. Br J Oral Maxillofac Surg. 2010;49:176–81.
12. National Institute on Alcohol Abuse and Alcoholism. Alcohol and Tobacco. Alcohol Research & Health. 2006; 29(71). https://pubs.niaaa.nih.gov/publications/aa71/aa71.htm. Accessed 5 Apr, 2018.
13. Swanson M, Kokot N, Sinha U. The Role of HPV in Head and Neck Cancer Stem Cell Formation and Tumorigenesis. Cancers (Basel). 2016;8:E24.
14. Chai RC, Lim Y, Frazer IH, et al. A pilot study to compare the detection of HPV-16 biomarkers in salivary oral rinses with tumor p16 (INK4a) expressions in head and neck squamous cell carcinoma patients. BMC Cancer. 2016;16:178.
15. Formosa J, Jenner R, Nguyen-Thi MD, Stephens C, Wilson C, Ariyawardana A. Awareness and knowledge of oral cancer and potentially malignant oral disorders among dental patients in far North Queensland. Australia Asian Pac J Cancer Prev. 2015;16:4429–34.
16. Harris PA, Taylor R, Thielke R, Payne J, Gonzalez N, Conde JG. Research electronic data capture (REDCap)—a metadata-driven methodology and workflow process for providing translational research informatics support. J Biomed Inform. 2009;42:377–81.
17. Kupzy K, Cohen M. Data validation and other strategies for data entry. West J Nurs Res. 2015;37:546–56.
18. Centers for Disease Control and Prevention. Current Cigarette Smoking Among Adults—United States, 2016. MMWR Morb Mortal Wkly Rep. 2018; 67(2):53–59 [accessed 22 Feb 2018].
19. Centers for Disease Control and Prevention. Fast facts and Fact sheet. Smokeless Tobacco Use in the United States. 2014. https://www.cdc.gov/tobacco/data_statistics/fact_sheets/smokeless/use_us/index.htm. Accessed 5 Apr, 2018.
20. Preet R, Khan N, Blomstedt Y, Nilssonn M, Stewart WJ. Assessing dental professionals' understanding of tobacco prevention and control: a qualitative study in Västerbotten County. Sweden BMJ Open. 2016;23(2):16009.
21. Hassona Y, Scully C, Shahin A, Maayta W, Sawair F. Factors influencing early detection of oral cancer by primary health-care profesionals. J Cancer Educ. 2016;31(2):285–91.
22. Nicotera G, DiStasio SM, Angelillo IF. Knowledge and behaviors of primary care physicians on oral cancer in Italy. Oral Oncol. 2004;40(5):490–5.
23. Shah JP, Gil Z. Current concepts in Management of Oral Cancer– Surgery. Oral Oncol. 2009;45:394–401.
24. Lawoyin JO, Aderinokun GA, Kolude B, Adekoya SM, Ogundipe BF. Oral cancer awareness and prevalence of risk behaviours among dental patients in South-Western Nigeria. Afr J Med Med Sci. 2003;32:203–7.
25. Srikanth Reddy B, Doshi D, et al. Oral cancer awareness and knowledge among dental patients in South India. J Craniomaxillofac Surg. 2012;40:521–4.
26. Prakash P, Belek MG, Grimes B, et al. Dentists' attitudes, behaviors, and barriers related to tobacco-use cessation in the dental setting. J Public Health Dent. 2013;73(2):94–102.
27. Shimpi N, Bharatkumar A, Jethwani M, Chyou PH, Glurich I, Blamer J, Acharya A. Knowledgeability, attitude and behavior of primary care providers towards oral Cancer: a pilot study. J Canc Educ. 2018;33(2):359–64.
28. Drobes DJ. Concurrent Alcohol and Tobacco Dependence: National Institute of Health Report; 2002. http://pubs.niaaa.nih.gov/publications/arh26-2/136-142.htm. Accessed 08 Jan 2018
29. Falk DE, Yi HY, Hiller-Sturmhofel S. An epidemiologic analysis of co-occurring alcohol and tobacco use disorders: findings from the National Epidemiologic Survey on alcohol and related conditions. Alcohol Research & Health. 2007;29:162–71.
30. Shingler E, Robles LA, Perry R, et al. Systematic review evaluating randomized controlled trials of smoking and alcohol cessation interventions in people with head and neck cancer and oral dysplasia. Head Neck. 2018; https://doi.org/10.1002/hed.25138.
31. Petti S, Scully C. Determinants of oral cancer at the national level: just a question of smoking and alcohol drinking prevalence? Odontology. 2010;98(2):144–52.
32. Radoi L, Menvielle G, Cyr D, et al. Population attributable risks of oral cavity cancer to behavioral and medical risk factors in France: results of a large population based case-control study, the ICARE study. BMC Cancer. 2015;15:287.
33. Zheng T, Boyle P, Zhang B, et al. In: Boyle P, Gray N, Henningfeld J, Seffrin J, Zatonski W, editors. Tobacco use and risk of oral cancer. IN: Tobacco: Science, Policy and Public Health. Oxford, England: Oxford university press; 2004. p. 399–432.
34. Moyer VA, U.S. Preventative Services Task Force. Screening for oral cancer: U. S. Preventative Services Task Force recommendation statement. Ann Intern Med. 2014;160:55–60.
35. Davis TC, Williams MV, Marin E, Parker RM, Glass J. Health literacy and cancer communication. CA Cancer J Clin. 2002;52(3):134–49.
36. National Institute on Drug Abuse (NIDA). Advancing Addiction Science. National Institutes of Health (NIH); U.S. Department of Health and Human Services. 2016. https://www.drugabuse.gov/. Accessed 30 Aug 2016.
37. Cheng T. Chemical evaluation of electronic cigarettes. Tob Control. 2014; 23(Suppl 2):ii11–7.
38. Feller L, Khammissa RA, Kramer B, Altini M, Lemmer J. Basal cell carcinoma, squamous cell carcinoma and melanoma of the head and face. Head Face Med. 2016;12:11.
39. Centers for Disease Control and Prevention. Betel Quid with Tobacco (Gutka). 2017. Available at https://www.cdc.gov/tobacco/basic_information/smokeless/index.htm. Accessed 8 Jan 2018.

15

Comparison of the occlusal contact area of virtual models and actual models: a comparative in vitro study on Class I and Class II malocclusion models

Hyemin Lee[1], Jooly Cha[1], Youn-Sic Chun[2] and Minji Kim[2*]

Abstract

Backgrounds: The occlusal registration of virtual models taken by intraoral scanners sometimes shows patterns which seem much different from the patients' occlusion. Therefore, this study aims to evaluate the accuracy of virtual occlusion by comparing virtual occlusal contact area with actual occlusal contact area using a plaster model in vitro.

Methods: Plaster dental models, 24 sets of Class I models and 20 sets of Class II models, were divided into a Molar, Premolar, and Anterior group. The occlusal contact areas calculated by the Prescale method and the virtual occlusion by scanning method were compared, and the ratio of the molar and incisor area were compared in order to find any particular tendencies.

Results: There was no significant difference between the Prescale results and the scanner results in both the molar and premolar groups ($p = 0.083$ and 0.053, respectively). On the other hand, there was a significant difference between the Prescale and the scanner results in the anterior group with the scanner results presenting overestimation of the occlusal contact points ($p < 0.05$). In Molars group, the regression analysis shows that the two variables express linear correlation and has a linear equation with a slope of 0.917. R^2 is 0.930. Groups of Premolars and Anteriors had a week linear relationship and greater dispersion.

Conclusions: Difference between the actual and virtual occlusion revealed in the anterior portion, where overestimation was observed in the virtual model obtained from the scanning method. Nevertheless, molar and premolar areas showed relatively accurate occlusal contact area in the virtual model.

Keywords: Digital intraoral scanner, Occlusal contact areas, Virtual occlusion

Background

The development of digital scanners brings about a lot of changes to the dental treatment environment. As a non-invasive method without radiation exposure, the digital scanning method is expected to reduce treatment time and improve the quality of treatment by allowing frequent evaluations according to needs [1]. It is even possible to know the state of occlusal contact by utilizing digital imagery by scanning models using an intraoral scanner. The use of the intraoral scanner offers the advantage of excluding the necessity of the impression process, production of the master cast, errors in the process of mounting on the articulator and errors due to the thickness of the occlusal evaluating paper. The manners of recording the interocclusal relationship include scanning the impression material of the maxillo-mandibular occlusal relationship, and scanning the buccal portion at centric occlusion. There is a risk of movement of the impression material during the scanning process in the former method, so the latter method which offers useful information in the analysis of the state of occlusion in an actual patient without

* Correspondence: minjikim@ewha.ac.kr
[2]Department of Orthodontics, College of Medicine, Ewha Womans University, Seoul, South Korea
Full list of author information is available at the end of the article

the need of any impression materials by directly capturing the occlusion and buccal contact points is preferred.

Digital impressions are divided into a direct method and an indirect method. The direct method is where digital imagery is obtained by scanning the oral environment of the patient, and the indirect method is where images in the form of digital models are obtained by scanning plaster models. Most researches evaluate the reproducibility and accuracy of the scanner by comparing the virtual models obtained from the indirect method with the plaster models. The size of tooth, width of arch etc. are usually compared by comparing the measured values of the plaster model with use of a digital caliper to the values obtained from scanned images [2–4]. But there are many factors which may cause errors in these methods, so as of recently there has been an introduction of analytical methods which employ 3-dimensional superimposition for comparison and analysis [5]. Images obtained from scanners are not only used in the general production of dental prostheses, but also as guides in implant operations and the production of implant prostheses, and more recently, in the diagnosis and planning of orthognathic surgery and orthodontic setups [6–10]. This signifies that operations that analyze the manner of occlusal contacts and the state of the occlusal plane of the complete maxillary and mandibular dentition using digital images has become commonplace.

As a result, new methods that analyze the occlusal points, the occlusal area and the occlusion have surfaced as a research topic. The T-scan and the Prescale are representative [11]. With the T-scan, the patient is instructed to carry out a series of occlusal movements such as lateral movements and anterior movements with a sensor placed in between their upper and lower arches, which is then recorded making it possible to analyze the order of occlusion according to the duration and strength of pressure applied on the tooth. The T-scan is recognized as a reproducible method in the analysis and evaluation of occlusal contacts at maximum intercuspation [12–15]. The Prescale system which was developed in Japan in that early 1990s consists of a pressure sensitive film in which a pressure between 5Mpa and 150Mpa applied to it will result in the destruction of micro capsules within the film, and a red color appears as a colorless dye mixes with a developing solution in the film. The color becomes darker as the pressure applied to it is higher, and the difference in the density of the color is analyzed. Hattori et al. [16] stated that the Prescale was meaningful as scientific data since it is possible to compare data obtained in a large scale research such as cohort studies. Suzuki et al. [17] stated that the speed and duration of the strength of occlusion applied to the Prescale sheet does not influence any changes in its color, and that the Prescale sheet does not get influenced by the moisture in the oral cavity. Also, according to the research conducted by Hidaka et al., [18] it was reported that there was a strong linear relationship between the load applied to the Type-R 50H sheet and the load deciphered from the sheet, making the Prescale it a trustworthy system in measuring the occlusal force.

Orthodontic treatment is the solution of malocclusion and the creation of functional occlusion. For 3-dimensional imagery to be generalized in orthodontic treatment, evaluation of the accuracy of the virtual occlusion obtained from the intraoral scanner is required. Research on the occlusal contact of restorations obtained from single tooth or partial arch scans are ongoing, but research on the occlusal contact of the full arch using virtual occlusion is meager and its accuracy has not been proven [19–21]. Before this study was conducted, clinically when the virtual occlusion was constructed, errors were commonly seen in certain area. Even though there was a lack of contact in the anterior portion of the maxilla and mandible, contact between the two arches was indicated. But because of the limited space when directly scanning the patient's mouth leads to a decrease in accuracy, [22–25] a cast study which can control these conditions and increase reproducibility is in need. Therefore, the aim of this study was to evaluate the accuracy of virtual occlusions obtained by intraoral scanners using plaster dental models in vitro, by comparing virtual occlusal contact area with actual occlusal contact area obtained by prescale method.

Methods

Study materials

Study plaster models

Of the patients that visited the Orthodontics This study Department in Ewha Womans University Mokdong Hospital who were over 19 years of age, before orthodontic treatment, 24 sets of Class I models and 20sets of Class II models were selected. The criteria on model selection were as follows.

(1) Models with an orthodontic base.
(2) Models with Class I or Class II division 1 M occlusal relation.
(3) Models without any fractured cusps or incisal edges.
(4) Models of patients before any orthodontic treatment.
(5) Models containing only permanent teeth, excluding the 3rd molar.
(6) Models without any ankylosed teeth or missing teeth, excluding the 3rd molar.

Models with the following criteria were excluded from this study.

(1) Models with an arch length discrepancy of 5 mm or over due to crowding or spacing.
(2) Patients were excluded when there were additional plaster models and bite materials for Temporomandibular Joint disorder diagnosis and treatment.

Scanning commenced after surface air bubbles and other minor deformations were removed from the selected models.

Method of research

Obtaining the 3D digital scan model

The 3D intraoral scanner used in this study was the 2nd generation Trios®(3 shape dental systems, Copenhagen, Denmark). With the Trios, scanning of the maxilla and mandible, and automatic occlusal setting is possible. By scanning the buccal side when the two arches are in occlusion, the Trios immediately reproduces the occlusive state of the models. Occlusal analysis is carried out in the form of an occlusal map which is presented in different colors depending on the distance from the surface of the tooth to the opposing tooth in the opposing arch (Fig. 1). Using this occlusal map, analysis of the occlusion and interference existing in the maxillo-mandibular complex can be carried out.

Scanning was carried out by one researcher, **HML** after thorough training on the use of the scanner. All the models were scanned in the order suggested by the manufacturer. All the models were scanned to the bucco-lingual boundary of the base, but the floor of the base was not scanned. The direction of the scans were carried out in identical fashion and based on the knowledge that inclusion of the palate influences the accuracy of the scan, the palate was not included in the scans [26, 27]. Scanning was commenced from the right 2nd molar, following the occlusive surface up to the left 2nd molar. Scanning continued onto the palatal surface of the left 2nd molar all the way to the right 2nd molar, including a portion of the occlusal surface. Finally, the buccal surface was scanned from the right 2nd molar to the left 2nd molar. After this primary scan, the final scan was completed by supplementing any insufficient portions. All maxillary and mandibular models were scanned in an identical manner.

Obtaining the occlusal relationship

Obtaining the occlusal contact area using the Prescale The Dental Prescale system (Fuji Film Corp., Tokyo, Japan) consists of a pressure sensitive sheet in the form of the dental arch and a CCD camera which deciphers the sheets. The pressure sensitive sheets are divided into a thin R-type (98 μm thick) and a W-type (800 μm) which is covered in wax. Depending on the range of measurement, they are further divided into a

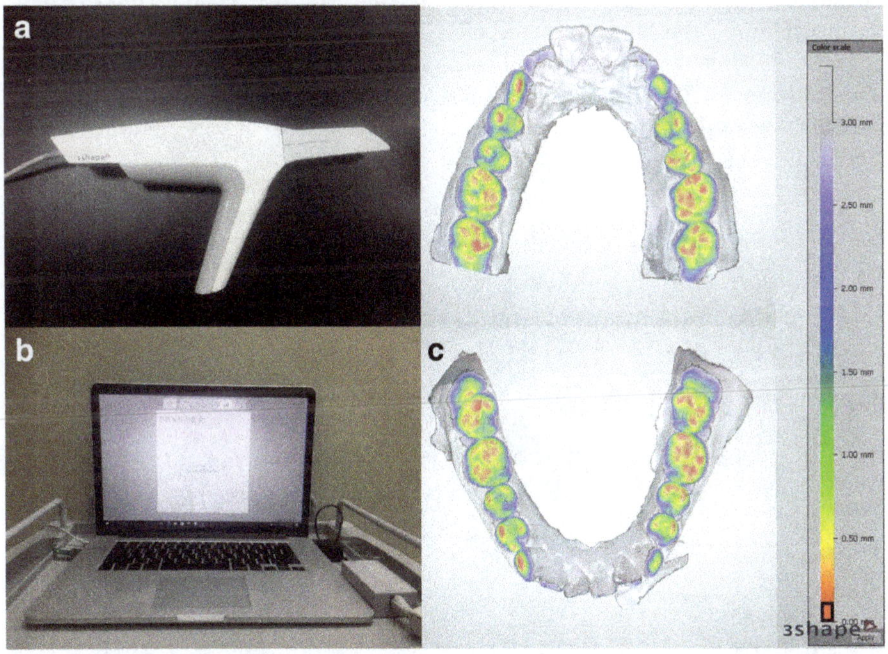

Fig. 1 3D digital intraoral scanner(Trios®). **a** Trios® pod; handheld, lightweight pod of Trios®. **b** Scanner can be connected to personal computer, and therefore easily accessible in clinic. It displays real-time scanning process. **c** Color coded occlusal map and color scale by Orthoanalyzer® program. Color scale indicates a range of distance between maxillary and mandibular teeth. Interocclusal distance increases as the color changes from red to blue scale. The distance values are shown in millimeter

30H type and a 50H type. The 50H, R-type films were used for this study.

The position of different groups of teeth was marked on the empty spaces on the Prescale pressure sensitive sheet. At the position where the maxillary and mandibular 1st molars were occluded, a load of 600 N was applied for 5 s using the Instron. Then the occlusal strength and occlusal area indicated on the pressure sensitive paper was calculated up to a unit of $0.1 mm^2$ using the CCD camera (Occluzer FPD 707, Fuji Film Corp., Tokyo, Japan) (Fig. 2).

The tooth groups were divided and compared as follows.

Molars: 1st and 2nd molars were included. 3rd molars were excluded
Premolars: 1st and 2nd premolars were included
Anteriors: The Central Incisors, Lateral Incisors and Canines were included

Obtaining the occlusal relationship using the scanner
All maxillary and mandibular models were mounted on an articulator (KaVo PROTAR Evo 5®, Kavo Dental GmbH, Riss, Germany). A pilot study was conducted to reproduce the occlusive force exerted onto the plaster models based on the research of Yoon et al. [28] which concluded that the average strength of occlusion in Koreans with malocclusion was 439 ± 229.9 N. Based on this pilot study, a load of 600 N was decided upon for the extent of this research.

With the models in occlusion, the buccal surface of the models were scanned while applying a load of 600 N with the Instron(Instron, Canton, MA, USA). The direction the scans were taken were identical in all the models. Starting from the buccal surface of the right 2nd molars, the scans were continued onto the labial surface of the anterior teeth onto the left 2nd molars. After the scan was completed, a color coded occlusal map of the virtual occlusion was obtained (Fig. 3).

Taking into consideration the 0.098 mm thickness of the Prescale sheet, the area calculated from the scan was 0.098 mm of the interocclusal distance between the maxillary and mandibular teeth. Using Photoshop (Adobe Photoshop CS3 software., Adobe Systems Inc., San Jose, USA) the number of pixels contained in the area corresponding from 0 mm to 0.098 mm on the color coded scale was calculated (Fig. 4).

Comparison of the occlusal contact area
The unit of the occlusal contact area obtained from the Prescale was mm^2 and the unit of the occlusal contact area obtained from the scanner was the pixel. To compare the two methods, the relative ratio of the results obtained from each method was compared. The occlusal contact area obtained from each method was converted to a percentage(%) of the total occlusal contact area in each tooth group.

Statistical analysis The collected data was run through the IBM SPSS Statistics ver. 23.0 (IBM Co., Armonk, NY, USA) for statistical analysis. The paired t-test was carried out in order to compare the occlusal contact area of the virtual occlusion resulting from the 3D intraoral scanner and the occlusal contact area resulting from the Prescale. Simple regression analysis and the Pearson correlation analysis was carried out to determine the correlation between the two groups The confidence interval was set at 95%, and the significance level was set at $p < 0.05$.

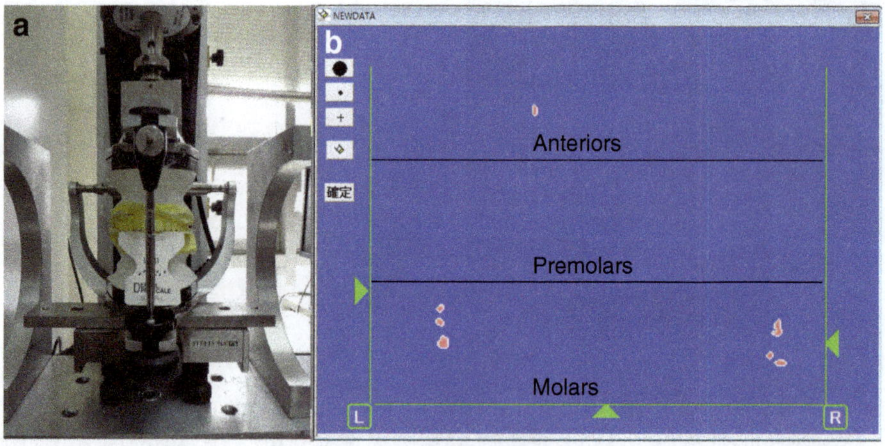

Fig. 2 The occlusal contact area obtained by the prescale. **a** With help of the Instron, models and pressure-sensitive film are applied a compressive force of 600 N for 5 s. **b** Occlusal contact areas were shown by prescale. The area where the anteriors, premolars and molars' position was marked on the space next to the film. The occlusal contact area and the occlusal force are automatically calculated

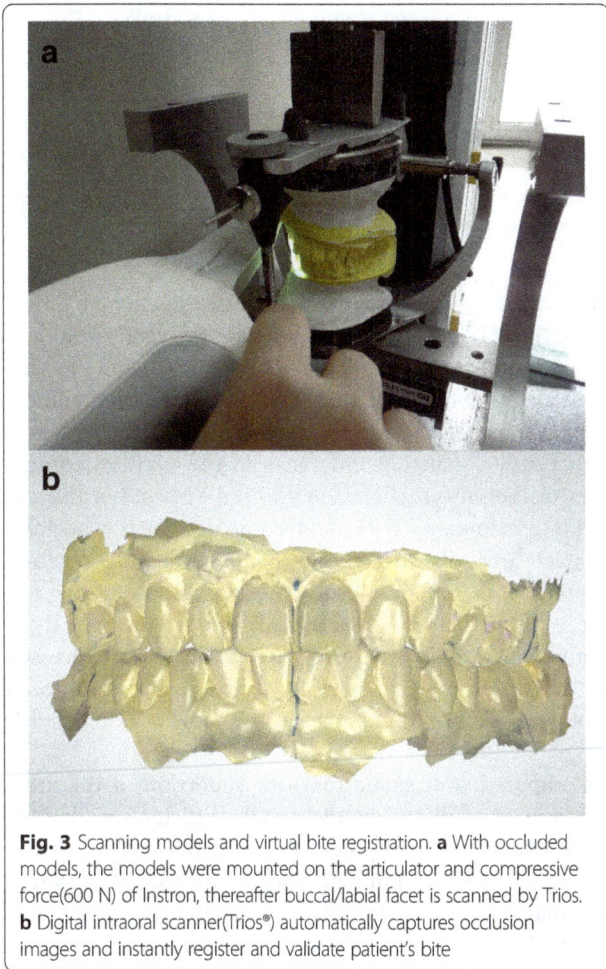

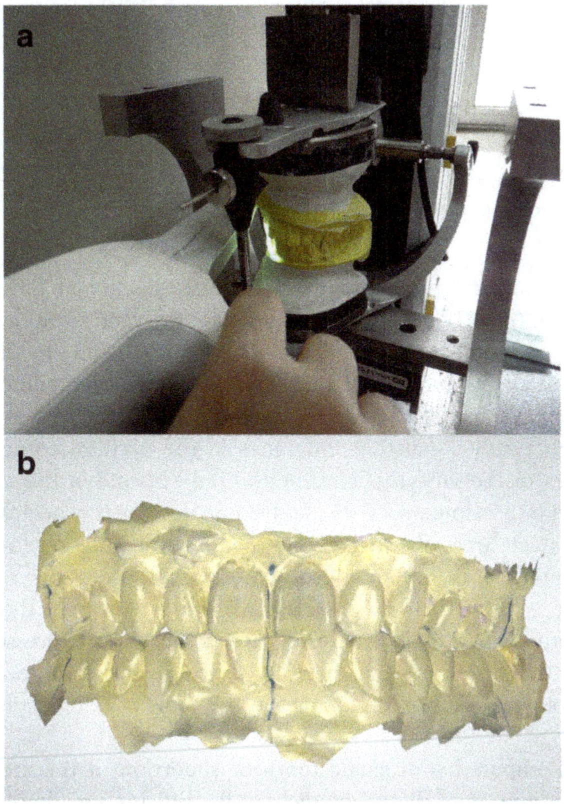

Fig. 3 Scanning models and virtual bite registration. **a** With occluded models, the models were mounted on the articulator and compressive force(600 N) of Instron, thereafter buccal/labial facet is scanned by Trios. **b** Digital intraoral scanner(Trios®) automatically captures occlusion images and instantly register and validate patient's bite

Results

Comparison of the occlusal contact area

The tooth group that showed the least amount of deviation when comparing the occlusal contact area obtained from the Prescale method and the 3D intraoral scanning method was the molar portion. The ratio of the occlusal contact area obtained from the Prescale and the scanner in the molar and premolar groups were similar, and there was no statistically significant difference ($p > 0.05$). The anterior portion showed the highest amount of deviation and a statistically significant difference ($p < 0.05$). Compared to the Prescale, the occlusal contact area resulting from the scanner was overestimated. The occlusal contact area indicated in the scanning method showed overall overestimation in the anterior portion, even in the areas where there was no actual contact (Table 1) (Fig. 5).

Simple regression analysis and correlation analysis

The correlation coefficients (R) of the occlusal contact area resulting from the Prescale and the intraoral scanner in all three groups showed positive correlation and were statistically significant. When comparing the values of each correlation coefficient, the molar group was the largest with a value of 0.964, that of the premolar group was 0.962 and the value of the anterior group was the smallest 0.898. This shows that there is a strong linear relation between the two variables in the molar group. In the molar group which had the highest correlation coefficient, the value of standardized regression coefficient (B) was 0.917. The value of the coefficient of determination (R2) was 0.930 which can be interpreted in a way that it explains 93.0% of this regression model. (Tables 2 and 3).

The level of dispersion of the two types of occlusal contact area and the occlusal contact area from the scanner that was estimated from the occlusal contact area from the Prescale in the molar group showed the most uniform distribution along the regression line. The values appear most scattered around the regression line in the anterior portion, with the premolar portion lying in between the molar portion and the anterior portion. As the values of the occlusal contact area gets smaller in

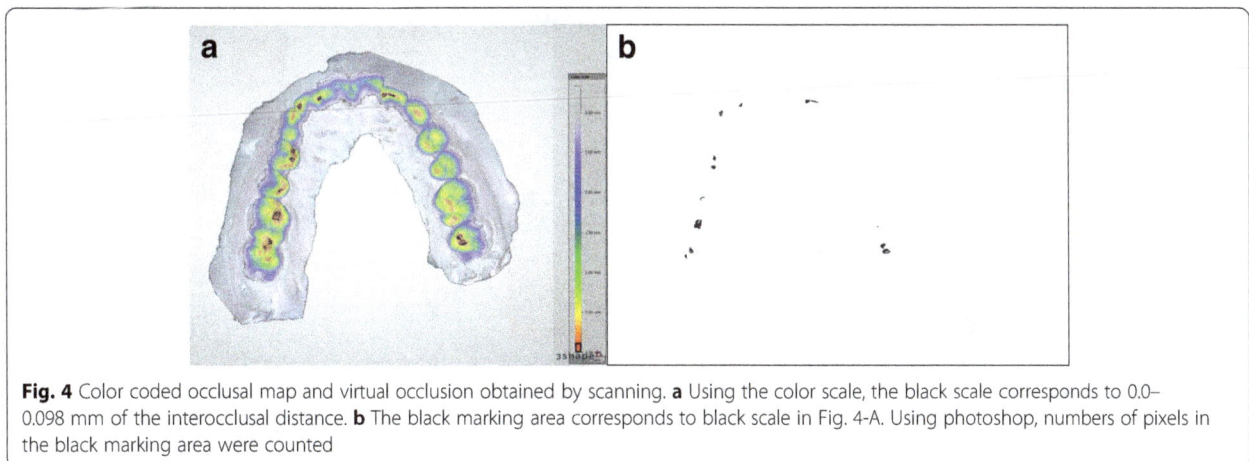

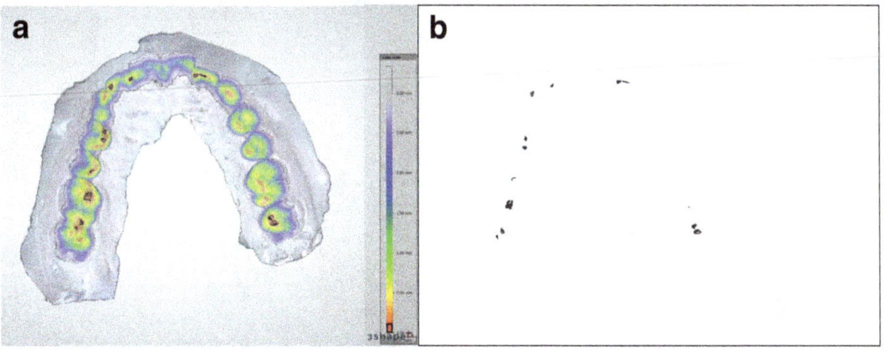

Fig. 4 Color coded occlusal map and virtual occlusion obtained by scanning. **a** Using the color scale, the black scale corresponds to 0.0–0.098 mm of the interocclusal distance. **b** The black marking area corresponds to black scale in Fig. 4-A. Using photoshop, numbers of pixels in the black marking area were counted

Table 1 Comparison of differences between occlusal contact area calculated by intraoral scanner and prescale (prescale-intraoral scanner) (unit:%)

	Difference(SD) (prescale-scanner)	*p*-value
Molars(M)	1.59 (5.67)	0.083
Premolars(P)	1.84 (5.83)	0.053
Anteriors(A)	−3.43 (6.09)	< 0.001*

Difference: occlusal contact area from prescale-occlusal contact area from scanner
SD standard deviation
Significance level: *; $p < 0.05$ by paired t-test

Table 2 Correlation coefficients (R) and *p*-value analysis by tooth groups

Groups	R	*p*-value
Molars	0.964	< 0.001*
Premolars	0.962	< 0.001*
Anteriors	0.898	< 0.001*

Significance level: *; $p < 0.05$ by Pearson correlation analysis

the premolar and anterior group, they are positioned closer to the regression line (Fig. 6).

Discussion

Currently, intraoral scanners are not only used in obtaining images of the single tooth and the dental arch, they are also utilized in the diagnosis and planning of orthognathic surgery and orthodontic setups [7, 9, 10, 29]. Using digital images obtained from scans to analyze the state of occlusal contact as well as the morphology of the occlusal surface of the complete maxillo-mandibular dentition has become more common. For intraoral digital scanners to be used more generally, it must be possible to obtain precise scan images of the full arch and dentition, and the virtual occlusion that results from those images must be able to reproduce the actual occlusion.

This study measured and compared the occlusal contact area of actual models obtained from the Prescale and the virtual occlusion obtained from scanned images. The results show that in the molar portion, there was little difference in the occlusal contact area obtained from the virtual occlusion and that obtained from the Prescale and there was no statistically significant difference. ($p > 0.05$) In the molar portion, the ratio of the occlusal contact area of the virtual occlusion to the Prescale showed a high degree of correlation, almost forming a linear line.($R = 0.964$, $B = 0.917$) There was a statistically significant difference in the occlusal contact area of the virtual occlusion and the Prescale in the anterior portion, ($p < 0.05$) and compared to the occlusal contact area obtained from the Prescale, the occlusal contact area obtained from the virtual occlusion was overestimated. During the course of the research, there were a lot of cases where occlusal contact was expressed in the anterior portion of the virtual occlusion even though there was no contact in the same region according to the Prescale.

Compared to a single tooth or a portion of the arch, scanning the full arch is technically difficult and there is more chance of error when obtaining the images [30]. It has been mentioned in a number of previous studies that the magnitude of these errors are clinically acceptable [5, 30, 31].

The results of superimposition carried out by most of the previous studies in the literature aimed at evaluating the accuracy of the intraoral scanner show a lower degree of accuracy in the distal portion of the molars

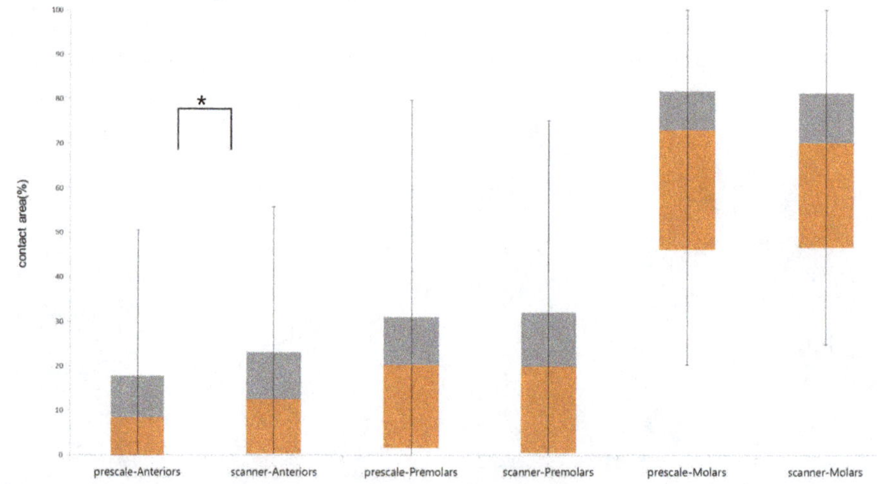

Fig. 5 Comparison of box plots between occlusal contact area by intraoral scanner and prescale. Occlusal contact area (%) by intraoral scanner is similar in prescale for the group of Molars and Premolars. In Anteriors group, occlusal contact area by intraoral scanner is greater than prescale. The plots shows median, 25% quartile, 75% quartile and maximum-minimum range. Significance level: *; $p < 0.05$ by paired t-test

Table 3 Regression of virtual occlusion by intraoral scanner on occlusion by prescale

Group	Regression coefficient		SE	*p*-value	R^2
Molars	*B*	0.917	0.040	< 0.001*	0.930
	constant	3.930	2.807	0.169	

B standardized coefficients, *SE* standard error; R^2, coefficient of determination
Significance level: *; $p < 0.05$ by simple regression analysis

and the incisal surface of the anterior teeth [5, 31, 32]. These errors occur due to the presence of sharp curves in the distal portions of the molars and the incisal portions of the anterior teeth which cause diffraction of light resulting in errors when obtaining images [27, 33]. In other words, precise scan images of complex structures with the presence of undercuts are difficult to obtain. Even in this study, precise scan images could not have been obtained in the anterior portion due to the diverse morphology and tooth crowding present during the individual scanning of the maxillary and mandibular models.

The algorithm involved in the manner of registration of 3-dimensional images of the intraoral scanner could have been the cause of the results in the anterior portion. The scanner used in this study employs the best fit algorithm. There have been many studies on the best fit algorithm [34, 35]. The most representative problem with this method is that the errors that occur in the beginning continue to add up as the scanning process continues. Solaberrieta et al. [36] recommended that in order to reduce the errors in the best fit algorithm, when employing the buccal scan method to produce the virtual occlusion, instead of scanning the full arch, to only obtain three precise scan images (images of the bilateral molar area and the frontal anterior image) of a width of 24 mm and a height of 5 mm. They stated that if these three images can be obtained, a virtual model occlusion that is closest to the actual model occlusion was possible. The important point was that the distance among the sections should be as large as possible, and that precise images of the left and right molars were imperative. In reality, with the models in maximum intercuspation, when the buccal surface is scanned from the molar to the anterior portion, even before the full arch is scanned, the program completes the occlusion. Due to the best fit algorithm, as scanning progressed from the molar portion to the anterior portion, it seems that the errors added up as the scanning process continued to present itself with overestimation in the anterior portion in this study.

Intraoral scanner used in this study employs ultrafast optical sectioning technology based on confocal microscopy, taking more than 3000 2D images per second and then combining them into 3D. In the process of creating the virtual occlusion, the scanner determines the relative position of the maxilla and the mandible through the process of scanning, and depends on the images of the teeth that are already registered, as well as the images of the surface of the maxillary and mandibular teeth in intercuspation. But these images do not include any information on the direction, position or angle in a 3-dimensional space [21, 34]. Due to the lack of 3-dimensional information, it is difficult to position the scanned images of the maxilla or the mandible when there is a partial or complete edentulous area. And detailed registration of superimposed images of two scans is also difficult [34]. As it is shown in the results of this study, when the virtual occlusion is formed from the registration of the two images, the anterior portion is shown to contact more closely than in reality. Also, the maxillo-mandibular labial images that are superimposed as a result of the diverse overbite and overjet in the anterior labial portion may not have supplied adequate

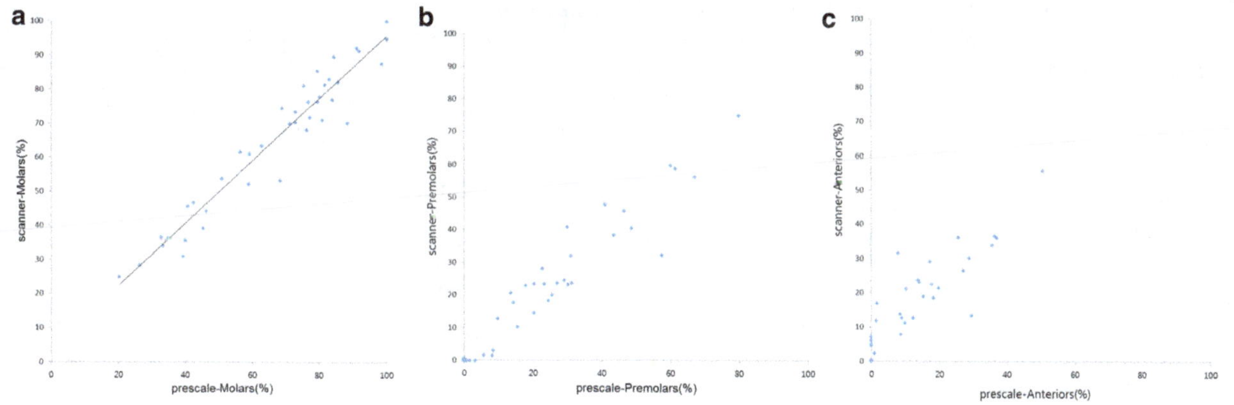

Fig. 6 Scatterplot and regression line comparing the occlusal contact area of intraoral scanner to the occlusal contact area of prescale. **a** In Molars group, the regression analysis shows that the two variables express linear correlation and has a linear equation with a slope of 0.917. R2 is 0.930. **b** Scatterplot of occlusal contact area by intraoral scanner and by prescale in Premolars Group. **c** Scatterplot of occlusal contact area by intraoral scanner and by prescale in Anteriors Group. Groups of Premolars and Anteriors have a week linear relationship and greater dispersion

information in the registration of the maxilla and mandible, which could be the cause of another form of error. In reality, to solve these problems, methods for precise registration are being suggested and effort in developing such software is underway [37, 38]. Research uses the virtual articulator to construct the virtual occlusion from scanned images [37, 39]. Delong et al. [37] demonstrated the possibility of reproducing the functions of the virtual articulator and actually obtaining acceptable results by comparing its accuracy under various conditions, and creating the necessary software to analyze the occlusion from virtual models.

The Prescale which was used as a control group in this study makes it possible to analyze the occlusal contact area of the full arch quantitatively, and is known as a trustworthy system in measuring the occlusive force. It can be with better use as it enables to compare scientific data when large data is collected [15, 17]. The Prescale is a good means to quantitatively evaluate the occlusive force, but it has its limitations in the form of the deformation of its sensors and its thickness. The thickness of the film may interrupt movement onto intercuspation and it has been reported that there is a limitation as a result of the distortion of the pressure sensor [15].

But currently, of the methods of measuring the occlusive force, since there is no golden standard that can represent the occlusal contact points, the Prescale which is a scientific method that can display the occlusive force was used in this study.

Being conducted with plaster models, the results of this study could be different from clinical tests. Errors of the Prescale resulting from the non-uniform pressure upon closing or the position of the head, by applying uniform pressure to the models with the Instron were avoided but it was not possible to express the maximum intercuspation through the opening and closing of the mandible in an actual oral cavity. However it can be a good milestone to develop the software for 3d intraoral scanner. And it can examine the difference between virtual and real occlusal by scanning system as it reduces the errors from intraoral scanned images and imaging skills.

Conclusion

This study evaluated the accuracy of the jaw relation record through the buccal scan method in a state of occlusion by comparison of the occlusal contact area obtained by the Prescale and a 3D intraoral scanner, and whether it could be used clinically. The tooth groups were divided into a molar portion, a premolar portion, and an anterior portion. The occlusal contact area obtained from the Prescale and the 3D intraoral scanner was measured, ultimately comparing the virtual occlusion and the actual occlusion.

In the molar portion and the premolar portion, there was no statistically significant difference between the occlusal contact area obtained from the Presacle method and the scanning method ($p > 0.05$). There was a statistically significant difference between the two methods in the anterior portion where overestimation was observed. ($p < 0.05$).

There was no statistically significant difference between the actual occlusion and the virtual occlusion using 3D scan images in the molar portion, but there was statistically significant difference between the two methods in the anterior portion, which presented with overestimation of the occlusal contact area obtained from the scanning method. The virtual occlusion using scanned images can be used as a reference in the diagnosis and modification of the occlusal contact. But there are limitations to the scanning method, therefore this should be taken into consideration when applying it in the clinical environment. Software and scanning techniques that can more precisely reproduce the patient's jaw relation must be developed.

Abbreviation

3D: 3 Dimensional; Cl: Class; SD: Standard deviation; SE: Standard error

Funding

This work was supported by the National Research Foundation of Korea (NRF) grant funded by the Korea government (MSIP; Ministry of Science, ICT & Future Planning) (No. 2017R1C1B5018349). The funding body had no role in the design of the study or in the collection analysis and interpretation of data, or in writing the manuscript.

Author's contributions

HML designed the study, collected data, performed most of the experiments. JC contributed to data collection, analysis and editing of the manuscript. MJK designed the study and made contributions to conception and design, and interpretation of data. YSC had been involved in revising it critically for important intellectual content. All authors read and approved the final manuscript.

Competing interests

The authors declare that they have no competing interests.

Author details

[1]Graduate School of Clinical Dentistry, Ewha Womans University, Seoul, South Korea. [2]Department of Orthodontics, College of Medicine, Ewha Womans University, Seoul, South Korea.

References

1. Ryeo-Woon K, Geun-Won J, Yu-Ri H, Mee-Kyoung S. Understanding and application of digital impression in dentistry. Kor J Dent Mater. 2014;41(4): 253–61.
2. Leifert MF, Leifert MM, Efstratiadis SS, Cangialosi TJ. Comparison of space analysis evaluations with digital models and plaster dental casts. Am J Orthod Dentofac Orthop. 136(1):16.e11–4. discussion 16
3. Lippold C, Kirschneck C, Schreiber K, Abukiress S, Tahvildari A, Moiseenko T, Danesh G. Methodological accuracy of digital and manual model analysis in orthodontics - a retrospective clinical study. Comput Biol Med. 2015;62:103–9.
4. Sousa MV, Vasconcelos EC, Janson G, Garib D, Pinzan A. Accuracy and reproducibility of 3-dimensional digital model measurements. Am J Orthod Dentofacial Orthop. 2012;142(2):269–73.
5. Patzelt SB, Emmanouilidi A, Stampf S, Strub JR, Att W. Accuracy of full-arch scans using intraoral scanners. Clin Oral Investig. 2014;18(6):1687–94.
6. Kim J, Chun Y-S, Kim M: Accuracy of bracket positions with a CAD/CAM indirect bonding system in posterior teeth with different cusp heights. Am J Orthod Dentofac Orthop, 153(2):298–307.
7. Dauti R, Cvikl B, Franz A, Schwarze UY, Lilaj B, Rybaczek T, Moritz A. Comparison of marginal fit of cemented zirconia copings manufactured after digital impression with lava™ C.O.S and conventional impression technique. BMC Oral Health. 2016;16(1):129.
8. Nedelcu R, Olsson P, Nyström I, Thor A. Finish line distinctness and accuracy in 7 intraoral scanners versus conventional impression: an in vitro descriptive comparison. BMC Oral Health. 2018;18:27.
9. Im J, Kang SH, Lee JY, Kim MK, Kim JH. Surgery-first approach using a three-dimensional virtual setup and surgical simulation for skeletal class III correction. Korean J Orthod. 2014;44(6):330–41.
10. Imburgia M, Logozzo S, Hauschild U, Veronesi G, Mangano C, Mangano FG. Accuracy of four intraoral scanners in oral implantology: a comparative in vitro study. BMC Oral Health. 2017;17(1):92.
11. Ji-Man P, Seong-Joo H, Yoon-Sic C. The methods for occlusal force measurement and their clinical application. J Kor Dent Assoc. 2012;50(1):22–30.
12. Afrashtehfar KI, Qadeer S. Computerized occlusal analysis as an alternative occlusal indicator. Cranio. 2016;34(1):52–7.
13. Jae-Ho Y. A preliminary study on quantitative analysis using the COMPUTERIZED t-scan system. J Kor Dent Assoc. 1989;27(9):861–7.
14. Garrido Garcia VC, Garcia Cartagena A, Gonzalez Sequeros O. Evaluation of occlusal contacts in maximum intercuspation using the T-scan system. J Oral Rehabil. 1997;24(12):899–903.
15. Ando K, Kurosawa M, Fuwa Y, Kondo T, Goto S. A study on measuring occlusal contact area using silicone impression materials: an application of this method to the bite force measurement system using the pressure-sensitive sheet. Dent Mater J. 2007;26(6):898–905.
16. Hattori Y, Okugawa H, Watanabe M. Occlusal force measurement using dental prescale. J Jpn Prosthodont Soc. 1994;38:835–41.
17. Suzuki T, Watanabe T, Yoshitomi N, Ishinabe S, Kumagai H, Uchida T. Evaluation of a new measuring system for occlusal force with pressure sensitive sheet. J Jpn Prosthodont Soc. 1994;38:966–73.
18. Hidaka O, Iwasaki M, Saito M, Morimoto T. Influence of clenching intensity on bite force balance, occlusal contact area, and average bite pressure. J Dent Res. 1999;78(7):1336–44.
19. Nilsson J, Richards RG, Thor A, Kamer L. Virtual bite registration using intraoral digital scanning, CT and CBCT: in vitro evaluation of a new method and its implication for orthognathic surgery. J. Craniomaxillofac. Surg. 2016; 44(9):1194–200.
20. Solaberrieta E, Minguez R, Barrenetxea L, Otegi JR, Szentpetery A. Comparison of the accuracy of a 3-dimensional virtual method and the conventional method for transferring the maxillary cast to a virtual articulator. J Prosthet Dent. 2015;113(3):191–7.
21. Iwaki Y, Wakabayashi N, Igarashi Y. Dimensional accuracy of optical bite registration in single and multiple unit restorations. Oper Dent. 2013;38(3): 309–15.
22. Anh JW, Park JM, Chun YS, Kim M, Kim M. A comparison of the precision of three-dimensional images acquired by 2 digital intraoral scanners: effects of tooth irregularity and scanning direction. Korean J Orthod. 2016;46(1):3–12.
23. Park HR, Park JM, Chun YS, Lee KN, Kim M. Changes in views on digital intraoral scanners among dental hygienists after training in digital impression taking. BMC oral health. 2015;15(1):151.
24. Kim J, Park JM, Kim M, Heo SJ, Shin IH, Kim M. Comparison of experience curves between two 3-dimensional intraoral scanners. J Prosthet Dent. 2016; 116(2):221–30.
25. Jung YR, Park JM, Chun YS, Lee KN, Kim M. Accuracy of four different digital intraoral scanners: effects of the presence of orthodontic brackets and wire. Int J Comput Dent. 2016;19(3):203–15.
26. Gan N, Xiong Y, Jiao T. Accuracy of intraoral digital impressions for whole upper jaws, including full dentitions and palatal soft tissues. PLoS One. 2016; 11(7):e0158800.
27. Gonzalez de Villaumbrosia P, Martinez-Rus F, Garcia-Orejas A, Salido MP, Pradies G. In vitro comparison of the accuracy (trueness and precision) of six extraoral dental scanners with different scanning technologiesJ Prosthet Dent. 2016;116(4):543–550.e541.
28. HR Y, YJ C, KH K, CR C. Comparisons of occlusal force according to occlusal relationship, skeletal pattern, age and gender in Koreans. Korean J Orthod. 2010;40(5):304–13.
29. Adolphs N, Liu W, Keeve E, Hoffmeister B. RapidSplint: virtual splint generation for orthognathic surgery – results of a pilot series. Computer Aided Surgery. 2014;19(1–3):20–8.
30. Ender A, Mehl A. Accuracy of complete-arch dental impressions: a new method of measuring trueness and precision. J Prosthet Dent. 2013;109(2): 121–8.
31. Flugge TV, Schlager S, Nelson K, Nahles S, Metzger MC. Precision of intraoral digital dental impressions with iTero and extraoral digitization with the iTero and a model scanner. Am. J. Orthod. Dentofac. Orthop. 2013;144(3): 471–8.
32. Mangano FG, Veronesi G, Hauschild U, Mijiritsky E, Mangano C. Trueness and precision of four intraoral scanners in oral Implantology: a comparative in vitro study. PLoS One. 2016;11(9):e0163107.
33. Persson AS, Oden A, Andersson M, Sandborgh-Englund G. Digitization of simulated clinical dental impressions: virtual three-dimensional analysis of exactness. Dent Mater. 2009;25(7):929–36.
34. Andriessen FS, Rijkens DR, van der Meer WJ, Wismeijer DW. Applicability and accuracy of an intraoral scanner for scanning multiple implants in edentulous mandibles: a pilot study. J Prosthet Dent. 2014;111(3):186–94.
35. Müller P, Ender A, Joda T, Katsoulis J. Impact of digital intraoral scan strategies on the impression accuracy using the TRIOS pod scanner. Quintessence Int. 2016;47(4)
36. Solaberrieta E, Garmendia A, Brizuela A, Otegi JR, Pradies G, Szentpetery A. Intraoral digital impressions for virtual occlusal records: section quantity and dimensions. Biomed Res Int. 2016;2016:7173824.
37. DeLong R, Ko C-C, Anderson GC, Hodges JS, Douglas W. Comparing maximum intercuspal contacts of virtual dental patients and mounted dental casts. J Prosthet Dent. 2002;88(6):622–30.
38. MS K, SC P. Registration of dental range images from a intraoral scanner. Korean J CDE. 2016;21(3):296–305.
39. DeLong R, Ko CC, Olson I, Hodges JS, Douglas WH. Helical axis errors affect computer-generated occlusal contacts. J Dent Res. 2002;81(5):338–43.

16

Influence of denture surface roughness and host factors on dental calculi formation on dentures

Keisuke Matsumura*, Yuji Sato, Noboru Kitagawa, Toshiharu Shichita, Daisuke Kawata and Mariko Ishikawa

Abstract

Background: Dental calculi formation on dentures can worsen the oral cavity environment by complicating oral hygiene. However, few studies have investigated the effect of how patients use and manage their dentures, denture surface roughness, and host factors such as oral cavity dryness and saliva properties on denture cleanliness and denture dental calculi formation. Accordingly, we conducted the present survey to evaluate these factors to clarify the strength of the influence of each factor.

Methods: We enrolled 53 patients who had used dentures for at least 3 months and used a dental prosthesis that covered at least the six front teeth including the left and right mandibular canines. After staining the dentures, we divided the participants into a group that was positive for dental calculi (DCP group) and a group that was negative for dental calculi (DCN group). After removing all the stains, we evaluated the surface roughness of the dentures. A questionnaire was used to survey how the participants used and managed their dentures. Oral cavity dryness was evaluated, and resting saliva samples were collected to assess saliva properties. Correlations between the presence or absence of dental calculi and denture use and management were evaluated using a chi-square test. Correlations with denture surface roughness, oral cavity dryness, and saliva properties were evaluated using the Mann–Whitney U test. Correlations between the presence or absence of dental calculi and all factors were analyzed using multivariate analysis (quantification II).

Results: Surface roughness was significantly greater in the DCP group ($p < 0.01$), and the DCP group members wore their dentures during sleep significantly more often and used a denture cleaner when storing their dentures significantly less often (both $p < 0.01$). No significant differences were observed for oral cavity dryness or saliva properties. The multivariate analysis showed significant correlations of dental calculi formation with denture surface roughness and items related to denture use and management, but not for oral cavity dryness or saliva properties.

Conclusions: Our findings indicate that dental calculi formation is influenced by how dentures are used and managed and by denture surface roughness, but not by oral cavity dryness and saliva properties.

Keywords: Dental calculi on dentures, Denture surface roughness, Denture management, Denture usage

* Correspondence: k-matsumura@dent.showa-u.ac.jp
Department of Geriatric Dentistry, Showa University, School of Dentistry, 2-1-1 kitasenzoku Ota Ward, Tokyo 145-8515, Japan

Background

The progressive increase in average lifespan, especially in recent years, has resulted in Japan becoming a "super-aged" society, with 26.7%, or more than one in four people, being 65 years of age or older. As the percentage of elderly people increases, the number of people who use dentures is expected to increase as well.

The adhesion of plaque to dentures may worsen a patient's oral environment or general health. Denture plaque adheres more easily to rough denture surfaces, and dental calculi can form when plaque reacts with saliva components. Dental calculi adhere strongly to denture surfaces, making home care difficult and creating new areas for dental plaque formation. This can worsen oral hygiene [1, 2] and adversely affect patients' health by putting them at risk for infections such as pneumonia, which can occur when bacteria enter the lungs along with saliva during silent aspiration [3–5].

Studies investigating the dental calculi formation process have shown that calcium deposits occur from a few hours to 3 days after the appearance of denture plaque [6]. Thus, patients must be instructed how to use and manage their dentures to prevent the long-term adhesion of denture plaque.

The composition of dental calculi resembles that of supragingival calculi that form on natural teeth. Moreover, since saliva components are necessary for dental calculi formation, variations in the oral environment are thought to affect this process [7].

Previous studies have described the relationships between the adhesion of plaque to dentures and factors such as denture surface roughness, methods of denture usage and management, oral cavity dryness, and saliva properties. However, how these factors relate to dental calculi adhesion and how strongly these various factors affect dental calculi formation remain unclear. Therefore, in the present study, we aimed to test the null hypothesis that there is no difference in the degree of influence of these factors on dental calculi formation.

Methods

This cross-sectional study was approved by the Showa University School of Dentistry ethics screening committee (No. 2015-015). Because dental calculi often form on the polished lingual surface of mandibular dentures, we evaluated only the dental calculi formed in this area. To reduce variation in the data, a single practitioner performed all dental calculi identification.

Participants

The participants were denture users who visited the Department of Geriatric Dentistry at the Showa University School of Dentistry, had no limb disabilities, and managed their dentures independently at home. After fully explaining the intent of the study, we obtained consent from 53 people (28 men, 25 women; mean age ± standard deviation 79 ± 7.6 years). The subjects' dentures were full or partial dentures that covered at least the six front teeth including the left and right mandibular canines. People who were in the midst of tissue conditioning or those who had used dentures for less than 3 months prior to the study were excluded, in order to reduce variability within the subject cohort.

Data collection

Five items comprising 16 factors were surveyed or measured once during a regular health check-up (which typically occurs every 3 months): presence or absence of dental calculi on dentures, denture surface roughness, methods of denture use and management, oral cavity dryness, and saliva properties. To determine presence or absence of dental calculi, a plaque disclosing solution (Rondells Blue Disclosing Pellets®, DIRECTA, Upplands Väsby, Sweden) was used to stain the dentures. This solution produces different colored stains depending on the stage of plaque formation (within 3 days of formation: red; longer than 3 days: blue). After cleaning with a sponge brush, we separated the participants into groups based on visual inspection of dental calculi on dentures. Those who exhibited blue stains and white calcifications were classified into the DCP group, while those who did not show any staining or calcifications were classified into the DCN group.

Denture surface roughness was calculated as arithmetic mean roughness (Ra). Dentures that exhibited blue stains and white calcifications were cleaned with a solution for removing dental calculi (Quick Denture®, GC, Tokyo, Japan) followed by a disinfectant solution (Laborac D®, SUNDENTAL, Osaka, Japan) for 5 min each in an ultrasonic cleaning bath. A surface roughness meter (Surftest SJ-210®, Mitutoyo, Tokyo, Japan) was used to measure denture surface roughness on 4-mm areas of dental calculi adhesion in the DCP group, while reference locations, specifically the polished denture surfaces of the midline, and left and right canines, were measured in the DCN group. The surface roughness for each denture was calculated as a mean of three measurements.

Denture use and management was evaluated using a questionnaire based on guidelines for denture cleaning in the clinic and instructions for denture management by dental hygienists from the Japanese Society of Gerodontology [8] (Fig. 1). Interview surveys were conducted after collecting resting saliva.

Oral cavity dryness was evaluated by resting saliva flow rate and oral cavity moisture.

Resting saliva flow rate was measured using the method reported by Fontana et al. [9]. While sitting in a

Answer those that fall under the following items about denture.

1) Denture wearing time
   1: All days
   2: At mealtimes
   3: Only when go out

2) Nighttime wearing
   1: Remove everyday
   2: Remove sometimes
   3: Wearing everyday

3) Method of storage
   1: In water dissolved denture cleanser
   2: In water
   3: In air

4) Denture cleaning methods

Cleaner	Brush
1: Cleaner for denture	1: Cleaner for denture
2: Tooth paste	2: Tooth brush
3: Not use	3: Not use

5) Frequency of denture cleanser usage
   1: Everyday
   2: Sometimes
   3: Not use

6) Denture stabilizer usage
   1: Not usage
   2: Sometimes
   3: Everyday

Fig. 1 Questionnaire for denture usage / management

chair, the participant was instructed to swallow the saliva in the mouth at the start of the measurement, and then to incline the head anteriorly in a resting state. The saliva that accumulated in the mouth was collected in a disposable cup, and the saliva accumulated over 5 min was measured to the 0.1 g using a small electric scale (Pocket Scale® CS-240, COSTOM, Tokyo, Japan). Considering that the specific gravity of saliva is 1.003 [10], the amount of saliva secreted per minute was calculated on the basis of the amount of resting saliva collected over 5 min to obtain the resting saliva flow rate (mL/min).

To measure oral cavity moisture, we used an intraoral moisture meter (Mucus®, Life, Saitama, Japan) that uses a sensor to evaluate the static electric capacity of the moisture in the oral mucosal epithelium. With a specialized cover over it, the sensor was pressed perpendicularly onto the measurement sites: buccal mucosa and lingual mucosa. These sites were chosen because they are areas where people often complain of oral cavity dryness and because they are easily accessible [11]. The buccal mucosa measurement was performed at a site approximately 10 mm medial to the angle of the mouth. A finger was used to hold the site lightly from the outside during the measurements. The lingual mucosa measurement was performed on the dorsum of the tongue, approximately 10 mm from the tip. The participants were asked to stick their tongue out during the measurements. The mean value of three measurements for each participant was used in the analysis.

Saliva properties were evaluated based on spinnbarkeit (saliva spinnability), calcium ion (Ca^{2+}) concentration, and pH and buffer capacity. The spinnbarkeit of saliva, which expresses the level of viscosity, was measured according to the method reported by Yamagaki et al. [12], using a spinnbarkeit meter (NEVA METER®, Co., Ltd. Ishikawa. Kitakyusyu. Japan). After collection, we placed 60.0 μm^3 of saliva in a measurement dish with the device set to wet mode. Seven consecutive measurements were made, and the mean of five measurements was used for further analysis after discarding the maximum and minimum values.

Ca^{2+} was measured in 0.25 mL of saliva using a calcium ion meter (Compact Calcium Ion Meter®, B-751, HORIBA, Kyoto, Japan). The mean of three consecutive measurements was used for subsequent analysis. A pH meter (Compact pH meter®, B-712, HORIBA, Kyoto, Japan) was used to measure the pH in 0.25 mL of saliva. Next, an acid-load solution (pH 3, 0.25 mL) was dropped onto and mixed into the saliva to measure buffer capacity. pH and buffer capacity were measured consecutively for each sample. This process was repeated three times and the mean value was used for further analysis.

Statistical analysis

Presence or absence of dental calculi was compared with the individual measurement and other data items using a chi-square test. Statistical analysis was performed after separating the responses into recommended methods of denture use and management, and other methods. Oral dryness and saliva property items were analyzed using the Mann–Whitney U test. Multivariate analysis (quantification II) was used to examine the correlation between the presence or absence of DC and the factors evaluated.

Results

Of the 53 participants, 19 were in the DCP group and 34 were in the DCN group. The mean duration of denture use in the DCP group (54 months) was not significantly different from that in the DCN group (29 months). The mean use period was about twice as much as DCP than DCN group, but there was no significant difference between groups. Also, the use period was classified based on the median value, and the use and frequency of use of the denture cleanser during storage were equal. It was suggested that adherence in denture care is subtracted regardless of the use period. The subjects were elderly, which means they were likely taking medications or had reduced physical function; however, none reported experiencing oral dryness or a medication-induced decrease in saliva secretion.

As shown in Fig. 2, the denture surface roughness in the DCP group was significantly higher than that in the DCN group (median 2.3 μm vs 1.0 μm and mean 2.6 μm vs. 1.2 μm, respectively; all $p < 0.01$).

With respect to denture usage and management (Fig. 3), the proportion of participants who wore dentures during the day tended to be higher in the DCP group than in the DCN group. Moreover, compared with DCN members, a significantly higher proportion of the DCP members wore their dentures at night ($p < 0.01$) and did not use a denture cleaner at night (p < 0.01).

The proportion of participants who used denture cleaner on their dentures tended to be smaller in the DCP group than in the DCN group, while the proportion who used regular toothpaste tended to be larger in the DCP group. The proportion who used a denture brush tended to be smaller in the DCP group than in the DCN group, while the proportion who used a toothbrush tended to be larger in the DCP group. The proportion of participants who used denture cleaner every day was significantly smaller in the DCP group than in the DCN group ($p < 0.01$).

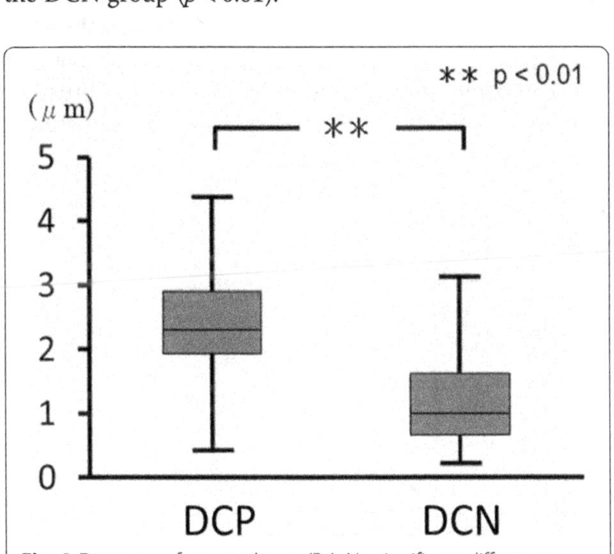

Fig. 2 Denture surface roughness (Ra). No significant differences were observed between the DCP and DCN groups

The proportion of participants who used adhesive regularly was significantly larger in the DCP group than in the DCN group ($p < 0.01$). Some members of the DCP group used adhesive sometimes, but it was used very infrequently in both groups.

With respect to oral cavity dryness, resting saliva flow rate was slightly higher in the DCP group than in the DCN group, but the difference was not significant (Fig. 4). The DCP group had slightly higher moisture values for both buccal and lingual mucosa, but the differences were not significant (Fig. 4). All values, based on the assessment criteria, were either within or close to the normal range.

All values for the measured saliva properties were slightly higher in the DCP group, but none of the differences was significant (Fig. 5).

Figure 6 shows the results of the multivariate analysis (quantification II) in the form of a graph that expresses the degree of influence numerically (= category score). The graph shows correlation coefficients for items with significant correlations. Significant correlations were observed between dental calculi adhesion and denture surface roughness, handling during sleep, denture storage methods, frequency of denture cleaner use, and frequency of dental adhesive use. The strongest correlation was between dental calculi adhesion and surface roughness. Significant correlations were not observed for the oral dryness or saliva property items.

Discussion

The purpose of this study was to clarify the difference of the influence of factors of dental calculi on denture formation. Factors related to dental calculi formation were found to have different degrees of influence, which rejects the null hypothesis. In this cross-sectional study on denture cleaning, participants were selected randomly from among people who used dentures and could manage them independently. The subject dentures were full or partial dentures that covered the mandibular front teeth using a dental plate or artificial teeth. Dental calculi often occur on denture surfaces near the opening of the parotid gland on the maxilla and near the openings of the submandibular and sublingual glands on the mandible. It has been reported that dental calculi are more common on the mandible than on the maxilla [13], so for this study, we chose the lingual side of the mandible to eliminate error due to differences in the dental calculi formation site.

Dental calculi formation is reported to begin with calcification that occurs within 3 days of denture plaque adhesion, with calcification completed by 2 weeks [7]. Because long-term adhesion of denture plaque to the same site can lead to dental calculi formation, it can serve as an indicator of the everyday dental hygiene of denture users. Dental calculi were observed in 36% of

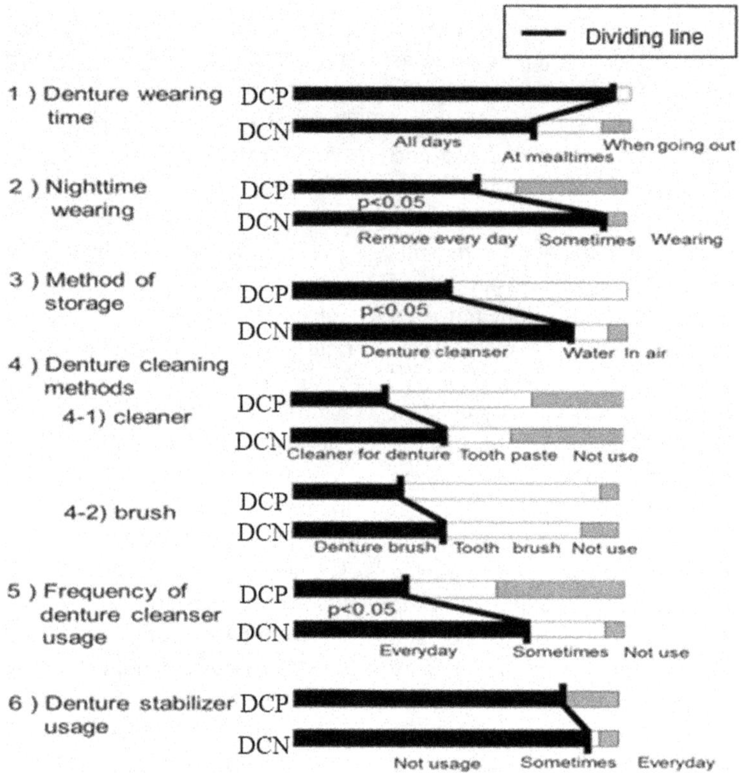

Fig. 3 Denture usage / management. Significant differences were observed between the DCP and DCN groups in denture treatment during sleep, denture storage, and the frequency of denture stabilizer usage

the participants surveyed in this study, which is higher than expected and indicates that improvement in dental hygiene is needed.

A relationship between denture surface roughness and bacterial adhesion to resin has been reported [14]. In this study, abrasive paper was used to modify the surface roughness of dentures and the extent of bacterial adhesion was compared between surfaces with different roughness, revealing significantly more bacterial adhesion on rougher surfaces. Further, cleaning dentures with toothpaste containing an abrasive agent can make the surface even rougher [15], indicating the importance of thorough denture polishing during clinic visits and of recommending against the use of abrasive agents for cleaning dentures.

In previous studies [16–19], recommended methods for using and managing dentures included not wearing them at night, using a denture brush, and using denture cleaner frequently. The usefulness of denture brushes was reported in a study that stained dental plaque and then compared the cleaning effects of a denture brush to that of a toothbrush [19], showing that denture brush

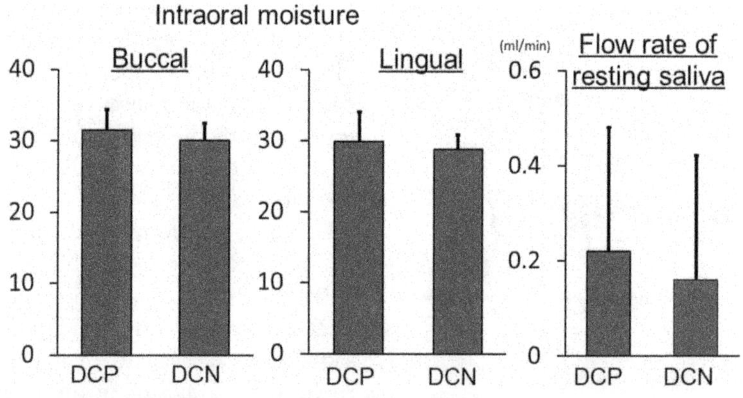

Fig. 4 Oral cavity dryness. No significant differences were observed between the DCP and DCN groups

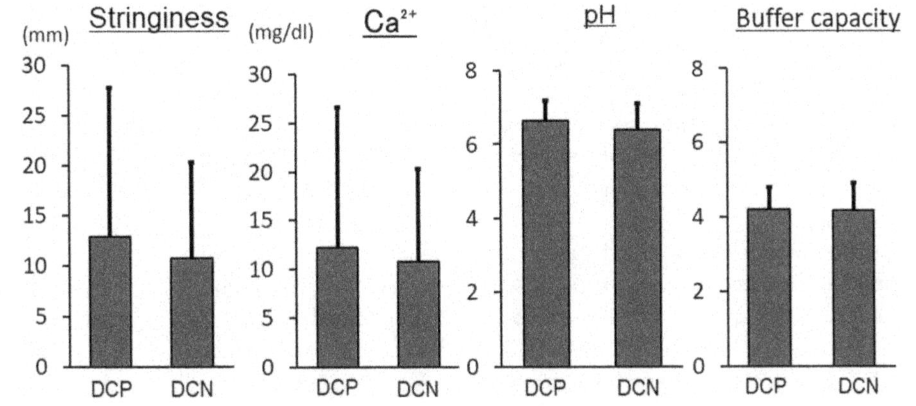

Fig. 5 Saliva properties. No significant differences were observed between the DCP and DCN groups

usage had a greater cleaning effect than toothbrush usage.

In the present study, the use of denture adhesive tended to be more common in the DCP group. Adhesives are used to increase the dentures' retentive force. However, several studies have found that adhesive usage has adverse effects including deviations of the intercuspal position, alveolar ridge absorption, and other issues [20, 21]. Despite these findings, it has been reported recently that adhesives can be used comfortably if they are used properly under the supervision of a dentist [22–24]. However, it should be noted that the denture adhesive itself has no antimicrobial properties [25]. If used improperly, the surface of adhesive can become rough, and if adhesive is not fully removed, it can provide a surface for the rapid growth of oral microbes. Patients need to be sufficiently warned when they are instructed on using adhesives. These reports are consistent with the results of the present study, demonstrating the importance of appropriate instruction and ensuring patient adherence.

Oral dryness is caused by a decrease in saliva in the oral cavity. This can be caused by reduced saliva secretion, dehydration, or other factors. Reduced saliva secretion decreases self-cleaning functions, which can promote plaque buildup and worsen denture cleanliness [26]. In the present study, we examined resting saliva flow rate and moisture of the oral mucosal epithelium as factors that could potentially influence oral dryness.

Various methods for measuring resting saliva secretion have been reported [27–30]. We selected the spitting method because it is the simplest and is commonly used. The normal resting saliva flow rate is approximately 0. 3 mL/min, but is thought to vary widely [31]. Pedersen et al. [32] compared saliva secretion from the submandibular glands in younger people aged 28–39 years with

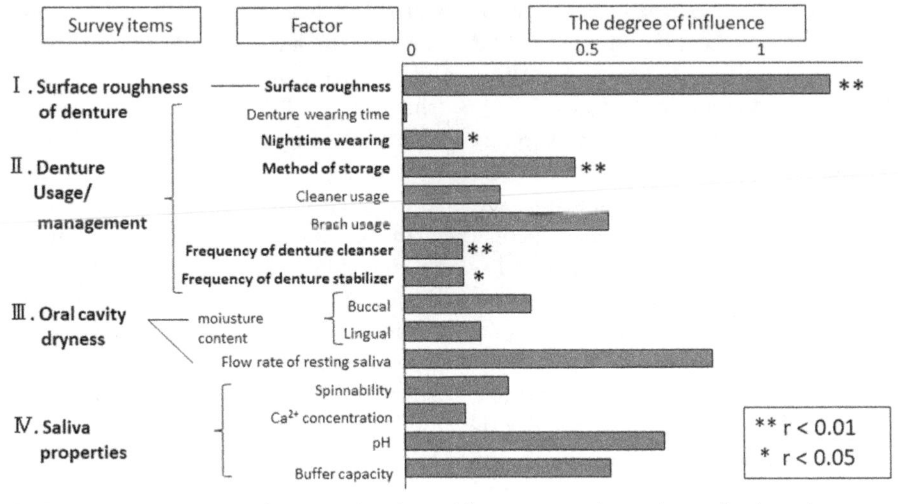

Fig. 6 The degree of influence for denture calculi formation. Significant differences were observed regarding how dentures were treated during sleep, how dentures were stored, frequency of denture cleaner use, and frequency of adhesive use

that in elderly people aged 70–90 years. They found that the resting saliva secretion of elderly people was 80% lower than that of younger people. Bertram et al. [33], Brun et al. [34], Mason et al. [35], and Meyer et al. [36] also reported that total saliva secretion decreases with age. However, even though the average age of the participants in the present study was 79 years, their saliva flow was within the normal range.

The device we used for the measurements is useful for objectively evaluating the dryness and moisture content of mucous membranes, but it cannot directly evaluate the amount of saliva secreted [37]. Fukushima et al. [38] reported the following values for oral moisture: normal: ≥29.6, borderline: 28.0–29.5, moderate oral dryness: 25. 0–27.9, and severe oral dryness: < 24.9.. The mean values obtained in the present study were all ≥28.0, indicating that while some participants had reduced saliva secretion, none had oral dryness. We found no studies in the literature that examined the relationship between the moisture content of the oral mucosal epithelium and oral cavity cleanliness. However, because low saliva secretion can reduce self-cleaning functions, this may be a useful indicator for making chairside risk predictions. The results of this study suggest that the moisture of the oral mucosal epithelium has little effect on dental calculi formation.

Saliva properties that are thought to affect calculi formation in natural teeth include the presence of plaque buildup with supersaturated calcium phosphate, salivary pH, and salivary proteins. The main component of dental calculi is calcium phosphate [7], and the composition and formation process of dental calculi on dentures resemble those of supragingival calculi formed on natural teeth. Thus, we used the factors affecting dental calculi formation in natural teeth as a reference point when selecting saliva properties to measure as potential factors affecting dental calculi formation in dentures.

No significant differences were observed for any of the saliva properties measured in the present study. This suggests that differences in saliva properties have little influence on dental calculi formation in dentures.

We found no studies that describe the factors affecting spinnbarkeit. That said, if the amount of saliva secreted stays relatively stable, changes in the ratio of serous saliva to mucous saliva could affect spinnbarkeit. As people age, the acinus of their salivary glands atrophy and disappear, a tendency that is particularly marked in the parotid glands. Therefore, the flow of serous saliva may start decreasing at an early stage [39].

Salivary mucin, one of the factors that determine spinnbarkeit in natural teeth, is known to react with calcium and promote the formation of dental calculi. In the present study, higher spinnbarkeit levels were observed in the DCP group, which suggests that spinnbarkeit may contribute to dental calculi formation on dentures.

We also investigated the relationship between Ca^{2+} concentration and salivary pH. Above a critical pH (5.5), free calcium in the oral cavity becomes super saturated with respect to calcium phosphate. Moreover, the ratio of free calcium to total calcium is almost the same, which indicates that an increase occurs as the saliva flow rate rises [28]. Salivary pH is generally constant at approximately 7.0 [40], which makes decalcification of dental calculi that have formed unlikely. Our results showed that Ca^{2+} concentration and pH tended to be higher in the DCP group than in the DCN group. Moreover, participants who wore their dentures all day were constantly in a state in which cleaning and decalcification were less likely, which may have promoted dental calculi formation.

The above results indicate the influence of various factors on dental calculi formation in dentures. They suggest a sequence of events in which plaque adheres to rough denture surfaces, and then calcifies when it is left in place for a long time because of inappropriate denture use or management. Moreover, our investigation of oral cavity dryness and saliva suggests that individual differences could make dental calculi formation more likely. These results provide some evidence indicating that dentists should provide their patients with smooth denture surfaces and instruct them in how to use and manage their dentures appropriately.

We designed a cross-sectional study to confirm the relationships among multiple variables simultaneously. It is important to note this limitation when interpreting the results of this study. The properties and components of saliva fluctuate throughout the day. Therefore, performing an accurate saliva survey requires a large number of subjects and collecting saliva samples over several days. However, the number of samples we could collect was limited because our saliva survey was performed during regular health checks, which included a survey of denture use and management. Therefore, while the results of our investigation of saliva and other factors indicate the importance of denture surface roughness and methods of denture use and management, it does not establish proof. A longitudinal study would be necessary to substantiate the relationships suggested by our findings.

In this study, we examined the lingual polished surfaces of mandibular dentures to obtain uniform measurements. In future studies, we plan to examine maxillary dentures. In addition, by expressing the results of questionnaire surveys and host factors numerically, we hope to create assessment sheets that can help improve the oral cleanliness of denture patients.

Conclusions

The results of this study indicate that denture surface roughness and the methods of denture use and management significantly affect dental calculi formation. Furthermore, our findings suggest that oral cavity dryness and saliva properties have little influence on dental calculi formation.

Abbreviations

DCN: Dental calculi negative; DCP: Dental calculi positive

Acknowledgements

We thank the professors of the Department of Geriatric Dentistry at our school of dentistry for their assistance, and the participants for their cooperation with the study. We also express our gratitude to Professor Shoji Hironaka of Showa University's department of oral hygiene for special needs dentistry, Professor Kazuyoshi Baba of the department of dental prosthetics, and Professor Takashi Miyazaki of the department of dental engineering for their helpful advice.

Funding

This study was funded by a grant for developing research on longevity medicine (28-13) from the National Center for Geriatrics and Gerontology.

Authors' contributions

KM was involved in study design and concept, data collection, data analysis and interpretation, and manuscript writing and review. SY participated in study design and concept and reviewed the manuscript. KN reviewed the manuscript and supervised the study. TS collected, analyzed, and interpreted the data. DK collected the data. MI collected, analyzed, and interpreted the data. All the authors approve the submission of the manuscript.

Authors' information

Keisuke Matsumura is a PhD student in the department of Geriatric Dentistry, University of Showa.

Competing interests

The authors declare that they have no competing interests.

References

1. Budtz-Jφrgensen E. The significance of Candida albicans in denture stomatitis. Scand J Dent Res. 1974;82:151–90.
2. Davenport JC, Hamada T. Denture stomatitis–a literature review with case reports. Hiroshima J Med Sci. 1979;28:209–20.
3. Sekizawa K, Ujiie Y, Itabashi S, Sasaki H, Takishima T. Lack of cough reflex in aspiration pneumonia. Lancet. 1990;335:1228–9.
4. Niimi A, Matsumoto H, Ueda T, Takemura M, Suzuki K, Tanaka E, et al. Impaired cough reflex in patients with recurrent pneumonia. Thorax. 2003; 58:152–3.
5. Yoneyama T, Yoshida M, Matsui T, Sasaki H. Oral care and pneumonia. Oral care working group. Lancet. 1999;354:515.
6. Ishikawa C. Electron microscopic study of denture plaque and denture Calculus. J Prosthodont Res. 1997;41:985–97.
7. Hosoi T, Ishikawa C. Formation processes of denture plaque and denture Calculus, and method of the elimination of their deposits. J Prosthodont Res. 1999;43:649–58.
8. http://www.gerodontology.jp/publishing/file/guideline/guideline_2013.pdf. In: http://www.gerodontology.jp/publishing/guideline.shtml. Japan Society of Gerodontology. Accessed 15 Jan 2014.
9. Fontana M, Zunt S, Eckert GJ, Zero D. A screening test for unstimulated salivary flow measurement. Oper Dent. 2005;30:3–8.
10. Shannon IL. Specific gravity and osmolality of human parotid fluid. Caries Res. 1969;3:149–58.
11. Takahashi T, Takahashi M, Toya S, Koji T, Morita O. Clinical usefulness of an oral moisture checking device (Mucas ®). Prosthodont Res Pract. 2006;5:214–8.
12. Yamagaki K, Kitagawa N, Sato Y, Okane M, Mashimo J. The relation between the physical properties of oral moisturizer and denture retention force. Jpn J Gerodontol. 2012;26(4):402–11.
13. Wang YH. Morphological study of calculus deposits on full and partial dentures. I. Structure, distribution and composition. Showa Shigakkai Zasshi. 1985;5:16–23. [Article in Japanese]
14. Yamauchi M, Yamamoto K, Wakabayashi M, Kawano J. In vitro adherence of microorganisms to denture base resin with different surface texture. Dent Mater J. 1990;9:19–24.
15. Harrison Z, Johnson A, Douglas CW. An in vitro study into the effect of a limited range of denture cleaners on surface roughness and removal of Candida albicans from conventional heat-cured a crylicres in denture base material. J Oral Rehabil. 2004;31:460–7.
16. Chan EC, Iugovaz I, Siboo R, Bilyk M, Barolet R, Amesel R, et al. Comparison of two popular methods for removal and killing of bacteria from dentures. J Can Dent Assoc. 1991;57:937–9.
17. Jose A, Coco BJ, Milligan S, Young B, Lappin DF, Bagg J, et al. Reducing the incidence of denture stomatitis: are denture cleansers sufficient? J Prosthodont. 2010;19:252–7.
18. Paranhos HF, Silva-Lovato CH, de Souza RF, Cruz PC, de Freotas-Pontes KM, Watanabe E, et al. Effect of three methods for cleaning dentures on biofilms formed in vitro on acrylic resin. J Prosthodont. 2009;18:427–31.
19. da Silva CH, Paranhos Hde F. Efficacy of biofilm disclosing agent and of three brushes in the control of complete denture cleansing. J Appl Oral Sci. 2006;14:454–9.
20. Zarb G, Bolender C, Hickey J, Carlsson G. Boucher's prosthodontic treatment for edentulous patients. 10th ed. St. Louis: Mosby; 1990. p. 495.
21. Ortman LF. Patient education and complete denture maintenance. In: Winkler S, editor. Essentials of complete denture prosthodontics. Philadelphia: W.B.Saunders; 1979. p. 467–79.
22. Grasso JE, Rendell J, Gay T. Effect of denture adhesive on the retention and stability of maxillary dentures. J Prosthet Dent. 1994;72:399–405.
23. Kelsey CC, Lang BR, Wang RF. Examining patients' responses about the effectiveness of five denture adhesive pastes. J Am Dent Assoc. 1997;128: 1532–8.
24. Berg E. A clinical comparison of four denture adhesives. Int J Prosthodont. 1991;4:449–56.
25. Bartels HA. Bacteriological appraisal of adhesive denture powders. J Dent Res. 1945;24:15–6.
26. Almstahl A, Wikstrom M. Oral microflora in subjects with reduced salivary secretion. J Dent Res. 1999;78:1410–6.
27. Navazesh M, Christensen CM. A comparison of whole mouth resting and stimulated salivary measurement procedures. J Dent Res. 1982;61:1158–62.
28. Ben-Aryeh H, Miron D, Szargel R, Gutman D. Whole-saliva secretion rates in old and young healthy subjects. J Dent Res. 1984;63:1147–8.
29. Flink H, Tegelberg A, Lagerlof F. Influence of the time of measurement of unstimulated human whole saliva on the diagnosis of hyposalivation. Arch Oral Biol. 2005;50:553–9.
30. Woods DL, Kovach CR, Raff H, Joosse L, Basmadjian A, Hegadoren KM. Using saliva to measure endogenous cortisol in nursing home residents with advanced dementia. Res Nurs Health. 2008;31:283–94.
31. Dawes C. Physiological factors affecting salivary flow rate, oral sugar clearance, and the sensation of dry mouth in man. J Dent Res. 1987;66:648–53.
32. Pedersen W, Schubert M, Izutsu KT, Mersai T, Truelove E. Age dependent decreases in human submandibular gland flow rates as measured under resting and poststimulation conditions. J Dent Res. 1985;64:822–5.
33. Bertram U. Xerostomia. Clinical aspects, pathology and pathogenesis. Acta Odontol Scand. 1967;25:1–126.
34. Brun R, Domine E. Study of transpiration. 13. Acta Derm Venereol. 1958;38: 91–103. [Article in French]
35. Mason DK, Chisholm DM. Salivary glands in health and disease. London: WB Saunders Co; 1975. p. 229.

36. Meyer J, Necheles H. Studies in old age: IV. The clinical significance of salivary, gastric and pancreatic secretion in the aged. JAMA. 1940;115:2050–5.
37. Takahashi F, Koji T, Morita O. Oral dryness examinations: use of an oral moisture checking device and a modified cotton method. Prosthodont Res Pract. 2006;5:26–30.
38. Fukushima Y, Yoda T, Araki R, Sakai T, et al. Evalution of oral wetness using an improved moisture-checking device for the diagnosis of dry mouth. Oral Sci Int. 2017;14:33–6.
39. Zwiech AB, Szczepanska J, Zwwiech R. Sodium gradient, xerostomia, thirst and inter-dialytic excessive weight gain: a possible relationship with hyposalivation in patients on maintenance hemodialysis. Int Urol Nephrol. 2014;46(7):1411–7.
40. Jenkins GN. A century of oral physiology. Br Dent J. 1981;151(1):6–10.

17

Osteo-regeneration personalized for children by rapid maxillary expansion: an imaging study based on synchrotron radiation microtomography

Alessandra Giuliani[1*], Serena Mazzoni[1], Carlo Mangano[2], Piero Antonio Zecca[3], Alberto Caprioglio[3], Nicolò Vercellini[3], Mario Raspanti[3], Francesco Mangano[2], Adriano Piattelli[4], Giovanna Iezzi[4] and Rosamaria Fastuca[5]

Abstract

Background: Personalized maxillary expansion procedure has been proposed to correct maxillary transversal deficiency; different protocols of stem cell activation have been suggested and rapid maxillary expansion (RME) is the most commonly used among clinicians. The present study aimed to quantify in three-dimensions (3D) the osteo-regeneration of the midpalatal suture in children submitted to RME.

Methods: Three patients (mean age 8.3 ± 0.9 years) were enrolled in the study to preform biopsy of midpalatal suture. Two patients (subjects 1 and 2) were subjected to RME before biopsy. The third patient did not need maxillary expansion treatment and was enrolled as control (subject 3). Midpalatal suture samples were harvested 7 days after RME in subject 1, and 30 days after RME in subject 2. The samples were harvested with the clinical aim to remove bone for the supernumerary tooth extraction. When possible, maxillary suture and bone margins were both included in the sample. All the biopsies were evaluated by complementary imaging techniques, namely Synchrotron Radiation-based X-ray microtomography (microCT) and comparative light and electron microscopy.

Results: In agreement with microscopy, it was detected by microCT a relevant amount of newly formed bone both 7 days and 30 days after RME, with bone growth and a progressive mineralization, even if still immature respect to the control, also 30 days after RME. Interestingly, the microCT showed that the new bone was strongly connected and cross-linked, without a preferential orientation perpendicular to the suture's long axis (previously hypothesized by histology), but with well-organized and rather isotropic 3D trabeculae.

Conclusions: The microCT imaging revealed, for the first time to the authors' knowledge, the 3D bone regeneration in children submitted to RME.

Keywords: Rapid maxillary expansion, Medical imaging, Bone regeneration, Synchrotron radiation, Microtomography, Midpalatal suture

* Correspondence: a.giuliani@univpm.it
[1]Sezione di Biochimica, Biologia e Fisica Applicata, Department of Clinical Sciences, Università Politecnica delle Marche, Via Brecce Bianche 1, 60131 Ancona, Italy
Full list of author information is available at the end of the article

Background

Personalized maxillary expansion procedure was proposed to correct maxillary transversal deficiency [1, 2] by splitting the midpalatal suture stimulating cell growth towards osteo-regeneration [3]. Different protocol of stem cell activation were suggested and rapid maxillary expansion (RME) is the most spread among clinicians. RME was recently indicated as treatment not only to solve transversal maxillary deficiency but for a variety of clinical conditions [4] since sagittal problems and underdevelopment of the midface might be the consequences of untreated transversal deficiency [5–11]. Moreover, occlusal disharmony and functional problems involving breathing pattern changes might derive from maxillary arch deficiency [12–14]. RME was then underlined to have positive effects not only in increasing maxillary arch perimeter but also on general health of growing patients, then increasing the potential of its indications [4, 15, 16].

When RME is performed, dental and skeletal changes occur producing an increase in the upper arch dimension. The appliance produces midpalatal suture splitting and the defect created is usually filled with new bone [17]. Since the very beginning of its use, the skeletal effects of RME on mid palatal suture were investigated with the means of radiographic techniques in 2-dimensions [18] and 3-dimensions with cone beam computed tomography (CBCT) [19, 20] in order to better understand the processes behind the healing of the suture and then preventing relapse with adequate treatment and retention time. Significant density reduction right after the active phase of expansion with an increase in the sutural density after 6-months retention was showed by Lione [21]. Indeed, the limit of radiographic investigations was the lacking of comprehension of real cellular activity but only the presence/absence of mineralized tissue might be documented. For this reasons morphologic and histologic studies were performed mainly on animals. Several of them [22–25] showed how the healing process is the combination of multiple steps with new bone and connective tissue formation and remodeling. In particular remodeling process were reported to be continuous and 3 to 4 weeks were not enough to restore the initial inter-digitated form of the mid palatal suture [22]. The first investigations on human being performed by Melsen [26, 27] collected samples of growing subjects during RME at different stages of treatment and compared them to autoptic material subjected to no treatment.

Recently, some of the authors of the present study reported a case analysis at 7 and 30 days from RME [28]. The preliminary histological results showed bone growth in the gap already after 7 days, with the healing process still ongoing after 30 days from RME.

Even though some evidence was assessed on the topic no strong conclusions might be drawn according to the results of a recent systematic review [29].

This fact could easily be expected because standard imaging techniques, like radiography and histology, which are routinely implemented for bone analysis, cannot fully match statistical requests, although they provide useful complementary information.

In particular, while histology provides qualitative analysis of the newly formed bone after RME, 3D structural data and the relative quantitative analysis on regenerated bone are difficult to obtain by this technique. Indeed, although in principle the 3D morphology of the new bone could be extracted by the analysis of serial sections of the biopsy, this approach is not the optimum because of the histological decalcification that the sample undergoes before the analysis.

Furthermore, X-ray medical radiology presents several limitations, also in this case due to its 2D nature: radiographs just provide 2D images of a 3D object, not completely reconstructing the anatomy that is being assessed. Anatomical structures give superimposing signals, often with anatomical or background noises inducing difficulties in interpreting data. Usually, 2D radiographs show fewer details than those actually present, precluding also the analysis of the soft-tissue to hard-tissue relationships [30].

In this survey, the impact of the computed tomography (CT) technique has been revolutionary, enabling to study the bone with a contrast discrimination up to three orders of magnitude better than conventional radiography [31].

Absorption-based tomography, at high resolutions, i.e. microtomography (microCT), was demonstrated to give fundamental information on bone tissues microstructure, with images of the 3D spatial organization of the bone in different environmental [32–35] and genetic [36–38] conditions. Moreover, interesting microCT studies have been performed on different biomaterials, indicated as bone-substitute candidates, in dental [39, 40] and orthopedic [41, 42] districts, within an acellular strategy [43, 44] or combining the biomaterial with cells in vitro [45–48].

The availability of synchrotron radiation (SR) x-ray sources has further stimulated research based on the use of microCT. SR shows numerous advantages with respect to laboratory x-ray sources, including higher beam intensity, higher spatial coherence, and monochromaticity. In fact, the polychromatic source and cone-shaped beam geometry, like in CBCT, complicate assessment of bone mineral density. Depending the X-rays absorption on the amount of mineral in bone, a suitable calibration at SR facilities is able to correlate the reconstructed gray levels – in microCT images, obtained using a monochromatic X-ray beam, to the local bone mineral density [49].

The present study aimed to investigate, for the first time to the authors' knowledge by SR-based microCT, the 3D changes in-vivo in midpalatal suture in humans, 7 and 30 days after RME.

This work exploits the monochromaticity property of SR, reducing the beam hardening effects, and simplifying the segmentation process of the images analysis.

We demonstrated that SR-based microCT, combined with a monochromatic X-ray beam, allows to study the early stages of bone regeneration in midpalatal suture, even on a very small cohort thanks to the 3D nature of the microCT analysis.

Methods

Subjects

Subjects presenting at the Division of Orthodontics (University of Insubria, Varese, Italy) and looking for orthodontic care were enrolled in the present study. The research protocol was reviewed and approved by the Ethical Committee of the AO Ospedale di Circolo e Fondazione Macchi (Varese, Italy), with Deliberative Act nr.826 of the 3rd of October, 2013. Moreover, the followed procedures adhered to the World Medical Organization Declaration of Helsinki. The parents of all the patients signed an informed consent for the enrollment of the children in the study and for the release of diagnostic documents for scientific purposes, before entering the treatment. All the patients had to comply with the following inclusion criteria to be enrolled in the study: 1) good general health as assessed with medical history and clinical judgement [50]; 2) patients who presented a supernumerary tooth located at the maxillary midline which had caused anomalies in the position of the upper incisors and for this reason need to be surgically removed. Indeed, the present sample was enrolled for the presence of a median maxillary supernumerary unerupted tooth (mesiodens) in mixed dentition, which had to be removed since causing eruption problems to the upper incisors in each single case.

The surgical procedure of mesiodens extraction was made easier by the maxillary expansion, when needed, since the bone around the mesiodens was softer after the treatment. The bone or woven bone around the mesiodens was collected instead of the traditional demolition due to the bur in order to expose the mesiodens and perform the extraction and used as sample of the present study. Three patients (1 female and 2 males, mean age 8.3 ± 0.9 years) were enrolled in the study. Two patients (1 female, subject 1 and 1 male, subject 2) presented maxillary transverse deficiency that needed to be corrected with RME treatment before the supernumerary tooth extraction thus facilitating surgical procedure by reducing the amount of bone around the extraction site. The third patient did not need RME treatment but was enrolled as control (subject 3) since the supernumerary tooth on the maxillary midline was present. Each patient underwent CBCT recording (CS 9300, Carestream Dental, Atlanta, GA, USA) performed in seated position (120 kV, 3.8 mA, 30 s) [51] prior to the surgical treatment to accurately plan the surgery (Fig. 1).

Hyrax type expander (10-mm screw, A167–1439, Forestadent, Pforzheim, Germany) banded to the upper second deciduous molars as alternative to anchorage on permanent molars or miniscrews [52–54] was employed. The screw of the palatal expander was turned two times the day of its placement (0.45 mm initial transversal activation). Afterwards, parents of the patients were instructed to turn the screw once per each following day (0.225 mm activation per day). The maxillary expansion was performed until dental overcorrection. The expander was then kept on the teeth as a passive retainer and the patients underwent no further orthodontic treatment during retention.

Biopsy procedure of the midpalatal suture

Midpalatal suture biopsies were collected during surgical removal of the supernumerary tooth in each patient. Contamination was avoided as much as possible by removing pathological tissue only after the biopsy of the midpalatal suture. After gathering of the mucous membrane of the hard palate, the biopsy was harvested by means of a cylindrical trephine bur with 7-mm on the midline along the midpalatal suture. Samples included both tissue sutures and one-side bone margin.

The treatment was performed only on subjects 1 and 2, while subject 3, not having received any treatment, was included as control. Each patient underwent a single biopsy collection, 7 days (subject 1) and 30 days (subject 2) after RME. The subject 3 (control) underwent surgery

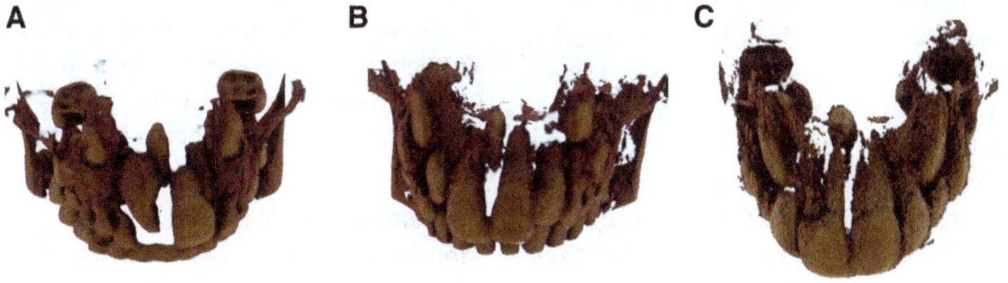

Fig. 1 Volume rendering of the pretreatment cbct: (**a** and **b**) treated patients; (**c**) control patient

for mesiodens extraction and midpalatal suture biopsy, without any other treatment.

Then, the three biopsies were dehydrated in a glycolmethacrylate resin (Technovit 7200 VLC, Kulzer, Wertheim, Germany) to be investigated by microCT.

Synchrotron radiation – based microtomography

The X-ray microCT scans were performed at the SYRMEP beamline of the ELETTRA synchrotron radiation facility (Trieste, Italy). The samples were investigated using isometric voxel with edge size of 4.2 μm; exposure time of 1600 ms/projection; and X-ray beam energy of 21 keV. The sample-detector distance of 50 mm enabled to work in absorption mode, where the resulting images were based solely on attenuation contrast.

The SYRMEP Tomo Project (STP) in-house software suite was used to reconstruct the tomographic slices, applying directly the standard filtered back-projection algorithm [55]. The STP is composed by a newly developed code and by external libraries [56].

The different grey values shown in the histogram of the reconstructed volumes are proportional to the linear attenuation coefficient μ of the different phases included in the sample, in turn proportional to their respective densities. The commercial software VG Studio MAX 1.2 (Volume Graphics, Heidelberg, Germany) was used to generate images for the visualization of the density distribution in 3D. Scatter HQ algorithm and an oversampling factor of 5.0 were considered the best settings to improve the x-ray contrast differences within samples. The volume of the bone was computationally obtained by multiplying the volume of a voxel (~ 74 μm^3) by the number of voxels underlying the peak associated with it, after thresholding of the histograms by the Mixture Modeling Algorithm (MMA-NIH ImageJ Plugin). Indeed, thresholding was performed to automatically separate the newly formed bone phase from background and organic phase.

Structural analysis of the newly formed trabecular bone was performed in order to verify how the 3D morphology modifies from 7 to 30 days after RME. The following morphometric parameters were evaluated: Total Specific Volume (BV/TV – expressed as a percentage); Total Specific Surface (BS/BV – per millimeter); Mean Struts Thickness (BTh - expressed in micrometers); Mean Struts Number (BNr – per millimeter); Mean Struts Separation (BSp - expressed in micrometers); Anisotropy Degree (DA); Connectivity Density, i.e. number of trabeculae per unit volume (Conn.D. – expressed in $pixel^{-3}$).

The Degree of Anisotropy (DA) is a measure of how highly oriented the structures are within a certain volume. Indeed, trabecular bone structures could vary their orientation depending on time from RME. The DA index can vary between 0 (all observation confined to a single plane or axis) and 1 (perfect isotropy). DA of the retrieved samples, that is, the presence of preferential orientations, was analysed using the BoneJ Plugin [57] of ImageJ software (http://imagej.nih.gov/ij) [58], version 3.

For a faster visualization, 3D meshes were also obtained in standard Wavefront OBJ format with the commercial software *Mimics 17* (http://biomedical.materialise.com) and visualized with *Meshlab v1.3.3* (http:(//meshlab.sourceforge.net).

Histological processing

After the microCT imaging, the sample blocks were prepared for the histological analysis. They were sectioned along the longitudinal axis, with a high precision diamond disk at about 150 μm and reduced to about 30 μm of thickness with the grinding machine Precise 1 Automated System (Assing, Rome, Italy). Three slices were prepared for each biopsy, that were stained with acid fuchsin and toluidine blue and imaged with a light microscope (Laborlux S, Leitz, Wetzlar, Germany) equipped with a high-resolution video camera (3CCD, JVC KY-F55B, JVC®, Yokohama, Japan) connected to a dedicated PC (Intel Pentium III 1200 MMX, Intel®, Santa Clara, CA, USA). The system was associated with a digitizing pad (Matrix Vision GmbH, Oppenweiler, Germany) and a software (Image-Pro Plus 4.5, Media Cybernetics Inc., Rockville, MD, USA) dedicated to histomorphometric analysis.

Scanning electron microscopy

The Scanning Electron Microscopy (SEM) analysis of the specimens was carried out at the Laboratory of Human Morphology of the Insubria University. The blocks remaining after the preparation of the ground sections were mounted on appropriate stubs with conductive glue, carbon coated with an Emitech K550 sputter-coater (Quorum Emitech, Ashford, UK) fitted with an Emitech K250 flash evaporator (Quorum Emitech, Ashford, UK) and observed with a FEI XL-30 FEG high resolution Scanning Electron Microscope (FEI, Eindhoven, The Netherland) operating in Backscattered Electrons (BSE) imaging at an acceleration voltage of 20 kV. With this technique, the contrast formation depends on the local composition: in particular, the higher the atomic number the higher the resulting brightness. With an appropriate setting the mineralized regions stand out brightly against the soft matrix and the embedding resin. Pictures were directly obtained in digital format as 1424 × 968, 8bpp TIFF grayscale files.

Data and statistical analysis

Morphometric data were statistically analysed with the support of the SigmaStat 3.5 software (Systat Software, San Jose, California). Statistical significance was assessed by two-tailed t test. *P*-values were considered significant when < 0.05.

Results

Synchrotron radiation - based microtomography

Osteo-regeneration of midpalatal suture sites, 7 and 30 days after RME, was studied by 3D microCT analysis.

Figure 2 (panel a) reports the histogram referred to the bone mineralization degree (BMD- mg/cm^3) study, respectively 7 and 30 days after the RME, comparing these profiles with the control midpalatal site. In these profiles, representing the "Intensity Counts vs. Grey Level", the grey levels - here referred to an unsigned 8-bit scale - are proportional to the linear absorption coefficient μ, that in turn is nearly proportional to the BMD (i.e. the mass density) of the newly formed bone. Two different peaks were segmented, the first corresponding to air and soft tissues, and the other corresponding to the newly formed bone. The histogram area with the grey levels < 100, i.e. the area referred to air and soft tissues, was excluded by the present investigation. Independently from time of observation after RME, it was detected a relevant amount of bone in both the treated biopsies, as shown by the blue and red peaks, corresponding to the linear attenuation coefficient of the newly formed bone in biopsies retrieved 7 and 30 days after RME, respectively. While these peaks lie in a grey level range between 110 and 220, the control biopsy is in the range between 150 and 250, demonstrating that, 30 days after RME, the BMD in the treated sites is still sensibly lower than in the control site. Furthermore, the peaks referred to regenerated sites are broadened respect to the profile referred to the control, indicating a larger distribution of μ values strictly reasoned by the fact that the mineralization level is inhomogeneous during the midpalatal regeneration.

Representative 2D sections of these samples are shown in Fig. 2 (panels b, c, and d). Despite the similarity of the thickness of the suture channel already 7 days after RME compared to that of the control suture (400–700 μm, yellow arrows), the surrounding bone structure presented a storiform shape in the treated palates, against a bulky appearance in the control.

Moreover, as revealed by the 3D reconstructions (Fig. 3) and the Additional file 1: Video 1, the trabecular structures correspond to a sectioned grid of newly formed bone perforated by a regular lattice of spaces, structures that are supposed to maximize the contact of the vascular net with the growing calcified tissue.

In order to estimate the evolution of these structures, a morphometric analysis of the overall 3D mineralized tissues was performed. The results are shown in Table 1.

This characterization showed that, even if not significant differences ($p > 0.05$) between specific volumes (BV/TV), specific surface (BS/BV) and mean trabecular thicknesses (BTh) were detected at the two time-points, the mean struts number (BNr) significantly increased from 7 days to 30 days after RME ($p = 0.013$). Coherently, the spacing (BSp) significantly decreased ($p = 0.028$).

The anisotropy analysis showed that, with respect to this parameter, despite the significant increasing of the struts number, the structure preserved its orientation from 7 days to 30 days from the treatment starting, suggesting a natural evolution of a regeneration process already started after the first week from RME. Furthermore, an average DA value of 0.7–0.8 indicated that the structure was highly isotropic in 3D.

As expected by the increased number of struts, also the Conn.D parameter significantly increased from 7 to

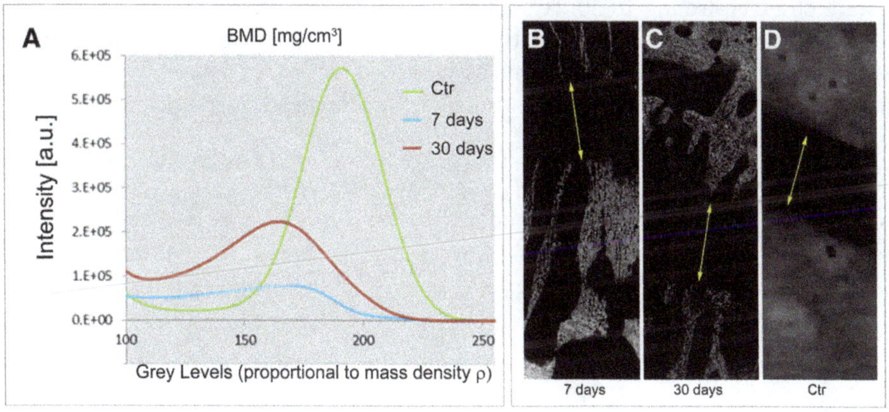

Fig. 2 a Portion of the "intensity vs. gray levels" profile. The grey levels are proportional to the linear attenuation coefficient μ that, in turns, is nearly proportional to ρ, the bone mineral density (BMD). The integrated areas of the represented peaks correspond to the newly formed mineralized bone volume in RME-treated midpalatal sites and in the control. **b-d** Representative 2D sections of the treated palatal sites 7 days (**b**) and 30 days (**c**) after RME, and of the palatal control (**d**). The thickness of the suture channel was similar to that of the control suture (400–700 μm, yellow arrows), showing that the storiform way of remineralization was already started 7 days after RME

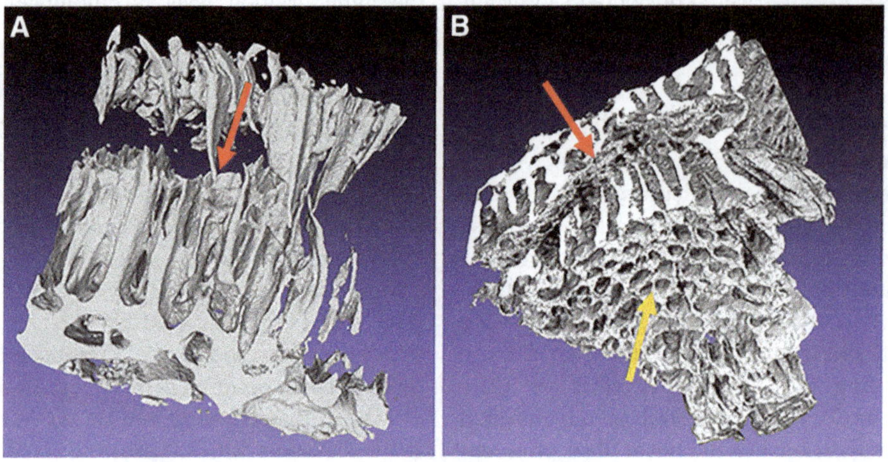

Fig. 3 3D microCT rendering of the biopsies retrieved 7 days (**a**) and 30 days (**b**) after the RME. Both the specimens clearly showed the meshwork of the bone perforated by non-mineralized spaces. The direction indicated by the red arrows corresponded to the section plane of histological and SEM micrographs. The right image offers a better view of the canals (yellow arrows) that cross the whole thickness of the bone to reach the sutural channel

30 days after RME ($p = 0.014$), demonstrating that the structure became more and more bulky, with an expected trend in time towards the control morphology.

To better visualize and compare the newly formed bone at 7 and 30 days after RME, the 3D color maps of the bone thickness distribution were also reconstructed, as shown in Fig. 4 (panels a-f).

The whole biopsies of the samples retrieved respectively 7 and 30 days after the RME treatment were shown in Fig. 3a and d. The same samples were visualized with different orientations respectively in Figs. 4b and 3e, better showing the 3D distribution of trabecular size, in agreement with the color bar in the bottom-center position of Fig. 4. The same information was better displayed in selected 2D slices, 7 (Fig. 4c) and 30 (Fig. 4f) days after the RME. An overall significant increase of the number of trabeculae and a slight increase of the trabecular thickness were observed from 7 to 30 days after RME. Indeed, the color maps demonstrated that there was a slight increase in thickness of the struts (as well as for the BNr) from 7 to 30 days after RME. To confirm this evidence, the "bone thickness distribution vs. the bone volume normalized to the total sample volume" was also assessed. The graph of the bone thickness distribution in both the investigated samples was reported in Fig. 4 panel g. It was shown here that, even if the average bone thickness was calculated to be similar, 7 days after RME there was a 10% of struts in the range between 20 and 96 μm more than 30 days after RME and, in the range between 96 and 172 μm, it was the opposite.

Comparative microscopy results

Light microscopy

Trabeculae apparently having storiform features and connective tissue were observed, 7 days after RME, inside the suture (Fig. 5a). They were composed by newly formed bone, with wide osteocyte lacunae. Small bone fibers were observed close to the blood vessels.

Thirty days after RME, more trabeculae were observed: they are closer than after 7 days from RME and, while in several fields they appeared aligned parallel to each other with a perpendicular orientation to the long axis of the

Table 1 3D morphometric analysis of the constructs retrieved 7 and 30 days after rapid maxillary expansion (RME). The characterization of the 3D mineralized microarchitecture of the newly formed bone showed that the struts number (BNr) significantly increase from 7 to 30 days after RME. Coherently, the spacing (BSp) significantly decrease and the Conn. D significantly increase from 7 to 30 days after RME

Morphometric Parameters	7 days	30 days	Significance Level (*P* value)
Total Specific Volume - BV/TV [%]	22.7 ± 7.3	29.5 ± 2.6	No, $P > 0.05$
Total Specific Surface - BS/BV [mm^{-1}]	47 ± 14	49 ± 7	No, $P > 0.05$
Mean Struts Thickness – BTh [μm]	45 ± 11	42 ± 6	No, $P > 0.05$
Mean Struts Number – BNr [mm^{-1}]	5.3 ± 0.6	7.3 ± 0.6	Yes, $P = 0.013$
Mean Struts Spacing – BSp [μm]	157 ± 30	99 ± 5	Yes, $P = 0.028$
Anisotropy Degree - DA	0.782 ± 0.097	0.758 ± 0.047	No, $P > 0.05$
Connectivity Density - Conn.D. ($\times 10^{-5}$) [μm^{-3}]	3.610 ± 1.651	7.618 ± 0.156	Yes, $P = 0.014$

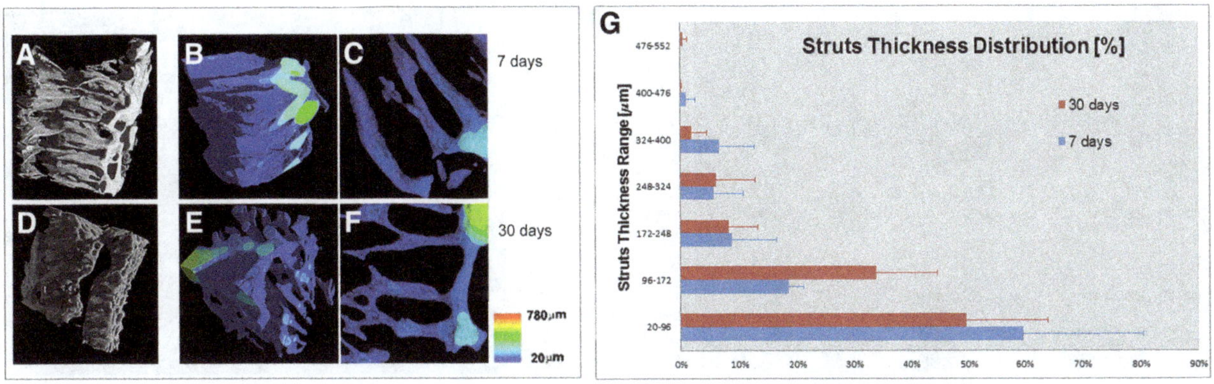

Fig. 4 a-c Biopsy retrieved 7 days after RME: (**a**) 3D microCT reconstruction; (**b**) Study in 3D of the thickness distribution basing on a color map; (**c**) 2D sampling color mapped slice. **d-f** Biopsy retrieved 30 days after RME: (**d**) 3D microCT reconstruction; (**e**) Study in 3D of the thickness distribution basing on a color map; (**f**) 2D sampling color mapped slice. Thickness scale for the color map at the bottom-center position. **g** Histogram of the distribution of the newly formed bone thickness in both the RME-treated midpalatal biopsies. These data demonstrate that there was a slight (not significant; $p > 0.05$) increase in thickness of the struts from 7 days to 30 days after RME

suture, in other few fields they merged into one another (Fig. 5b). However, the rich osteoblastic activity and the detection of osteoid matrix undergoing mineralization in many areas suggested that the osteo-regeneration process was still not ended after 30 days from RME.

Scanning electron microscopy

SEM analysis allowed to achieve high-resolution 2D imaging of the planed face of the specimens, with a mechanism of contrast formation reminiscent of the microCT slices. By analogy with the microCT, with SEM operating in backscattered electron mode, the mineralized portion emerged clearly against the dark backdrop of soft tissue and resin.

The SEM analysis of the biopsy 7 days after RME confirmed the results obtained by microCT and histology. Indeed, the bone matrix was observed to be traversed by dark longitudinal streaks, corresponding to zones of incomplete mineralization; the very high magnifications revealed simultaneous multiple loci of mineralization (Fig. 6a), consistent with a fast neoformation of bone towards the suture channel.

Low magnification images, like Fig. 6 - panel b showing the biopsy at 30 days from RME, were consistent with conventional histology and confirm the presence of elongated bone structures, dendrites, apparently perpendicular to suture axis, pointing towards the sutural space. Indeed, the SEM image in Fig. 6 (panel b), perfectly match the microCT morphologic information shown in Fig. 1c.

At higher magnification (top-left inset of Fig. 6b), in agreement with histologic findings, the calcified tissue exhibited large, irregular osteocyte lacunae, gathered in uneven clusters and suggestive of a fast, storiform growth.

Discussion

Rapid midpalatal expansion effects on suture changes were of great clinical interest in the last years, with

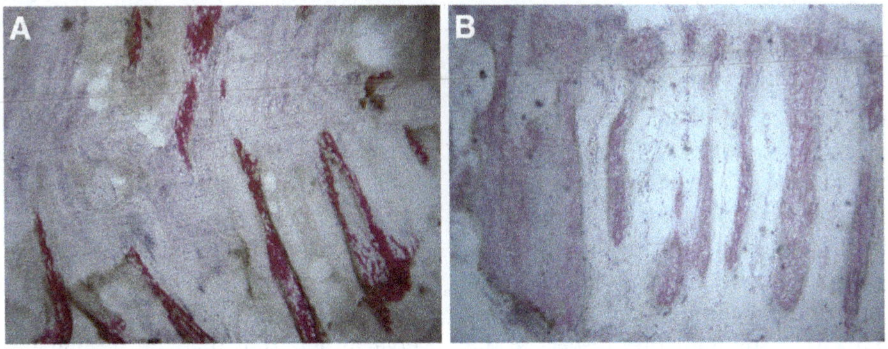

Fig. 5 Light microscopy. **a** 7 days after rapid maxillary expansion: trabecular new bone with storiform appearance was observed. **b** 30 days after rapid maxillary expansion: the newly-formed bone trabeculae were oriented perpendicularly to the long axis of the suture. Toluidine blue and acid fuchsin were used. Original magnification 40×

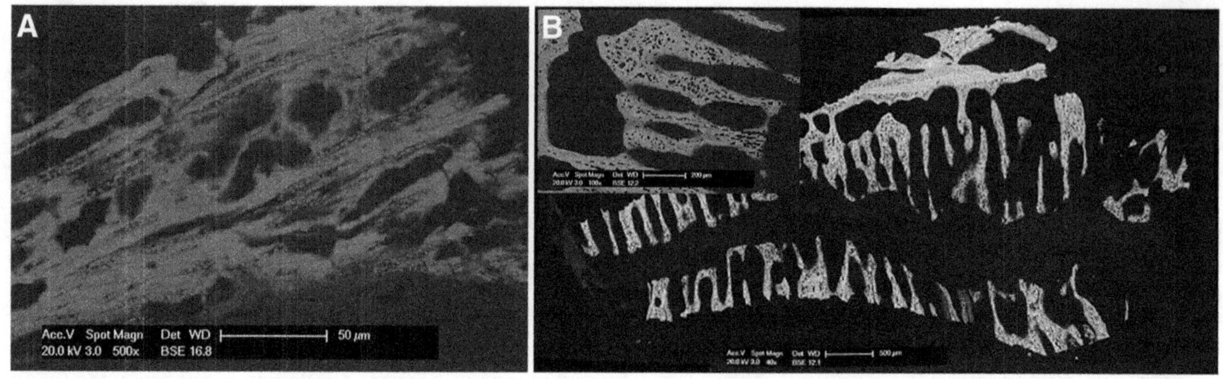

Fig. 6 a Biopsy at 7 days from RME: detail of the tissue at very high magnification. Irregular osteocyte lacunae were interspersed with dark streaks; the tiny dust-like specks were distinct simultaneous loci of mineralization. Bar = 50 μm. **b** Biopsy at 30 days from RME: mosaic of five distinct SEM micrographs of an histological section. The suture, running left to right, was flanked on both sides by elongated streaks, perpendicular to the same suture, separated by empty spaces. Bar = 500 μm. Top-left inset: detail of the mineralized tissue at higher magnification, with irregular osteocyte lacunae. Bar = 200 μm

studies mainly focused on identifying and qualifying the immediate and long-term effects of this treatment in growing teenage or young adults by conventional imaging methods [29]. The specific aim of this case report was to study, for the first time to the authors' knowledge, the short-term 3D quantitative changes after RME by Synchrotron radiation-based microCT.

A similar investigation, enrolling the same subjects, was reported in a previous case report [28]. However, the limit of this study was linked to the high morphometric variability of histological data.

As documented in literature [59], it is often suggested to couple 2D conventional microscopy with advanced 3D quantitative analysis. Indeed, with the use of microCT, it is reasonable to get significant morphometric results on a statistical sample sometimes narrower than the number of patients involved in the histologic study [60, 61], in these cases making no longer necessary the calculation of the statistical power.

In our study, microCT allowed to achieve significant quantitative results in spite of including a single subject for comparisons at 7 days, 30 days after RME, and a control. Indeed, the previous case report [28] on the same subjects was only descriptive and exclusively based on 2D data.

In agreement with histological findings, this microCT study detected a relevant amount of newly formed bone both 7 and 30 days after RME. Furthermore, as previously reported [28], it was observed a progressive mineralization with the peculiar in-plane fishbone appearance of the trabecular bone. As reported in literature [22, 28], the suture mineralization and morphology were confirmed in 3D to be still immature respect to the control, also 30 days after RME.

However, the microCT analysis did not confirm in 3D another finding observed in 2D by light and electron microscopy, i.e. that the newly formed bone trabeculae were oriented perpendicularly to the long axis of the suture and run parallel to each other [28]. Several microCT data contributed to denying in 3D this observation: the calculated value of DA, both 7 and 30 days after the RME, suggests a rather isotropic and poorly oriented structure; the combined significant increase in the number of trabeculae and their connectivity is not compatible with a structure consisting of parallel trabeculae. Moreover, the animation referred to the biopsy got 30 days after RME (delivered as Additional file 1: Video 1), clearly shows a strongly connected and cross-linked structure, similar to the morphology of a bone scaffold, that is expected to become more and more bulky, mimicking the control morphology.

Conclusions

The microCT imaging revealed, for the first time to the authors' knowledge, the following bone regeneration in children submitted to RME: few bone dendrites poorly connected after 7 days from the treatment, more dendrites and more connected after 30 days. Histologic and SEM 2D images showed portions of these dendrites, mainly oriented towards the suture channel, but the 3D microCT observations revealed also the interdendritic connections that, in turn, increased the overall isotropy of the structure, with possible beneficial implications in terms of biomechanical stability.

A drawback of the present study is to have stopped the experimental observations at 30 days from RME, when the microCT and the comparative techniques converge in asserting that the healing process has not yet ended at that time-point.

In synthesis, the morphometric data, as extracted by microCT analysis and 2D microscopy, converge to confirm the progressive healing process, activated by the endogenous stem cells, and the mineralization of trabecular bone structure. These microCT-imaging findings indicated that the new trabeculae might not be oriented perpendicularly to the long axis of the suture, as deduced by 2D microscopy in previous studies.

Abbreviations
(2D): Two-dimensions; (3D): Three-dimensions; (CBCT): Cone beam computed tomograph; (microCT): Microtomography; (RME): Rapid maxillary expansion; (SR): Synchrotron

Acknowledgements
The authors acknowledge the ELETTRA User Office for kindly providing beam-time.

Funding
The present research was not funded, nor supported by any grant; therefore, the authors have no conflict of interest related to the present work.

Authors' contributions
AG, CM and RF made substantial contributions to conception and design, PAZ, AC, NV and RF to acquisition of samples and data on patients, AG and SM to the acquisition of microCT data, GI to the acquisition of histologic data, MR to the acquisition of electron microscopy data; AG and SM to the analysis and interpretation of microCT data; GI and AP to the analysis and interpretation of histologic data; MR and FM to the analysis and interpretation of electron microscopy data; AG, SM, CM, MR,GI have been involved in drafting the manuscript, while RF, FM, PAZ, AC, NV and AP in revising it critically for important intellectual content; All gave the final approval of the version to be published.

Competing interests
The authors declare that they have no competing interests. Francesco Mangano is a Section Editor for BMC Oral Health.

Author details
[1]Sezione di Biochimica, Biologia e Fisica Applicata, Department of Clinical Sciences, Università Politecnica delle Marche, Via Brecce Bianche 1, 60131 Ancona, Italy. [2]Private Practice, Gravedona, CO, Italy. [3]Department of Medicine and Surgery, University of Insubria, Via Guicciardini 9, Varese, Italy. [4]Department of Medical, Oral and Biotechnological Sciences, University of Chieti-Pescara, Via dei Vestini 31, 66100 Chieti Scalo, CH, Italy. [5]Department of Biomedical Sciences, Dentistry and Morphological and Functional Imaging, University of Messina, Messina, Italy.

References
1. Angell EC. Treatment of irregularities of the permanent or adult teeth. Dent Cosmos. 1860;1:540–4.
2. Haas AJ. The treatment of maxillary deficiency by opening the midpalatal suture. Angle Orthod. 1965;35:200–17.
3. Pullen HA. Expansion of the dental arch and opening the maxillary suture in relation to the development of the internal and external face. Dent Cosmos. 1912;54:509–28.
4. McNamara JA Jr, Lione R, Franchi L, Angelieri F, Cevidanes LH, Darendeliler MA, et al. The role of rapid maxillary expansion in the promotion of oral and general health. Prog Orthod. 2015;16:33.
5. Eichenberger M, Baumgartner S. The impact of rapid palatal expansion on children's general health: a literature review. Eur J Paediatr Dent. 2014;15:67–71.
6. Di Blasio A, Mandelli G, Generali I, Gandolfini M. Facial aesthetics and childhood. Eur J Paediatr Dent. 2009;10(3):131–4.
7. Di Blasio C, Di Blasio A, Pedrazzi G, Anghinoni M, Sesenna E. How does the mandible grow after early high condylectomy? J Craniofac Surg. 2015;26(3):764–71.
8. Di Blasio A, Cassi D, Di Blasio C, Gandolfini M. Temporomandibular joint dysfunction in Moebius syndrome. Eur J Paediatr Dent. 2013;14(4):295–8.
9. Zecca PA, Fastuca R, Beretta M, Caprioglio A, Macchi A. Correlation assessment between three-dimensional facial soft tissue scan and lateral cephalometric radiography in orthodontic diagnosis. Int J Dent. 2016: 1473918. https://doi.org/10.1155/2016/1473918
10. Bianchi B, Ferri A, Brevi B, Di Blasio A, Copelli C, Di Blasio C, et al. Orthognathic surgery for the complete rehabilitation of Moebius patients: principles, timing and our experience. J Craniomaxillofac Surg. 2013;41(1):e1–4.
11. Anghinoni ML, Magri AS, Di Blasio A, Toma L, Sesenna E. Midline mandibular osteotomy in an asymmetric patient. Angle Orthod. 2009;79(5):1008–14.
12. Fastuca R, Perinetti G, Zecca PA, Nucera R, Caprioglio A. Airway compartments volume and oxygen saturation changes after rapid maxillary expansion: a longitudinal correlation study. Angle Orthod. 2015a;85(6):955–61.
13. Fastuca R, Meneghel M, Zecca PA, Mangano F, Antonello M, Nucera R, et al. Multimodal airway evaluation in growing patients after rapid maxillary expansion. Eur J Paediatr Dent. 2015b;16(2):129–34.
14. Caprioglio A, Meneghel M, Fastuca R, Zecca PA, Nucera R, Nosetti L. Rapid maxillary expansion in growing patients: correspondence between 3-dimensional airway changes and polysomnography. Int J Pediatr Otorhinolaryngol. 2014;78(1):23–7.
15. Fastuca R, Zecca PA, Caprioglio A. Role of mandibular displacement and airway size in improving breathing after rapid maxillary expansion. Prog Orthod. 2014;15(1):40.
16. Caprioglio A, Bergamini C, Franchi L, Vercellini N, Zecca PA, Nucera R, et al. Prediction of class II improvement after rapid maxillary expansion in early mixed dentition. Prog Orthod. 2017a;18(1):9.
17. Dewey M. Bone development as a result of mechanical force: report on further treatment in attempting the opening of the Intermaxillary suture in animals. Items Interest. 1914;36:420–38.
18. da Silva Filho OG, Montes LA, Torelly LF. Rapid maxillary expansion in the deciduous and mixed dentition evaluated through posteroanterior cephalometric analysis. Am J Orthod Dentofac Orthop. 1995;107:268–75.
19. Franchi L, Baccetti T, Lione R, Fanucci E, Cozza P. Modifications of midpalatal sutural density induced by rapid maxillary expansion: a low-dose computed-tomography evaluation. Am J Orthod Dentofac Orthop. 2010; 137(4):486–8.
20. Acar YB, Motro M, Everdi N. Hounsfield units: a new indicator showing maxillary resistance in rapid maxillary expansion cases? Angle Orthod. 2015; 85:109–16.
21. Lione R, Franchi L, Fanucci E, Laganà G, Cozza P. Three-dimensional densitometric analysis of maxillary sutural changes induced by rapid maxillary expansion. Dentomaxillofac Radiol. 2013;42(2):71798010.
22. Storey E. Bone changes associated with tooth movement: a histological study of the effect of force in the rabbit, Guinea pig and rat. Aust Dent J. 1955;59:147.
23. Cleall JF, Bayne DI, Posen JM, Subtenly JD. Expansion of the Midpalatal suture in the monkey. Angle Orthod. 1965;35:23–35.
24. Murray JM, Cleall JF. Early tissue response to rapid maxillary expansion in the midpalatal suture of the rhesus moneky. J Dent Res. 1971;50:1654.
25. Ohshima O. Effect of lateral expansion force on the maxillary structure in Cynomolgus monkey. J Osaka Dent Univ. 1972;6:11–50.
26. Melsen B. A histological study of the influence of sutural morphology and skeletal maturation on rapid palatal expansion in children. Trans Eur Orthod Sot. 1972;499–507.
27. Melsen B. Palatal growth studied on human autopsy material. Am J Orthod. 1975;68:42–54.
28. Caprioglio A, Fastuca R, Zecca PA, Beretta M, Mangano C, Piattelli A, et al. Cellular Midpalatal Suture Changes after Rapid Maxillary Expansion in Growing Subjects: A Case Report. Int J Mol Sci. 2017b;18(3):E615. https://doi.org/10.3390/ijms18030615.
29. Liu S, Xu T, Zou W. Effects of rapid maxillary expansion on the midpalatal suture: a systematic review. Eur J Orthod. 2015;37(6):651–5.
30. Shah N, Bansal N, Logani A. Recent advances in imaging technologies in dentistry. World J Radiol. 2014;6(10):794–807.
31. Claesson T. A medical imaging demonstrator of computed tomography and bone mineral densitometry. Stockholm: Universitetsservice US AB; 2001.
32. Tavella S, Ruggiu A, Giuliani A, Brun F, Canciani B, Manescu A, et al. Bone turnover in wild type and pleiotrophin-transgenic mice housed for three months in the international Space Station (ISS). PLoS One. 2012;7(3):e33179.

33. Canciani B, Ruggiu A, Giuliani A, Panetta D, Marozzi K, Tripodi M, et al. Effects of long time exposure to simulated micro- and hypergravity on skeletal architecture. J Mech Behav Biomed Mater. 2015;51:1–12.
34. Shiba D, Mizuno H, Yumoto A, Shimomura M, Kobayashi H, Morita H, et al. Development of new experimental platform 'MARS'-multiple artificial-gravity research system-to elucidate the impacts of micro/partial gravity on mice. Sci Rep. 2017;7(1):10837. https://doi.org/10.1038/s41598-017-10998-4.
35. Gerbaix M, Gnyubkin V, Farlay D, Olivier C, Ammann P, Courbon G, et al. One-month spaceflight compromises the bone microstructure, tissue-level mechanical properties, osteocyte survival and lacunae volume in mature mice skeletons. Sci Rep. 2017;7:2659. https://doi.org/10.1038/s41598-017-03014-2.
36. Costa D, Lazzarini E, Canciani B, Giuliani A, Spanò R, Marozzi K, et al. Altered bone development and turnover in transgenic mice over-expressing lipocalin-2 in bone. J Cell Physiol. 2014;228(11):2210–21.
37. Hoshino M, Uesugi K, Yagi N. Phase-contrast X-ray microtomography of mouse fetus. Biology Open. 2012;1(3):269–74. https://doi.org/10.1242/bio.2012430
38. Jiang Y, Zhao J, Liao EY, Dai RC, Wu XP, Genant HK. Application of micro-CT assessment of 3-D bone microstructure in preclinical and clinical studies. J Bone Miner Metab. 2005;23(Suppl):122–31.
39. Iezzi G, Piattelli A, Giuliani A, Mangano C, Barone A, Manzon L, et al. Molecular, cellular and pharmaceutical aspects of bone grafting materials and membranes during maxillary sinus-lift procedures. Part 2: detailed characteristics of the materials. Curr Pharm Biotechnol. 2017;18(1):33–44.
40. Rominu M, Manescu A, Sinescu C, Negrutiu ML, Topala F, Rominu RO, et al. Zirconia enriched dental adhesive: A solution for OCT contrast enhancement. Demonstrative study by synchrotron radiation microtomography. Dent Mater. 2014;30(4):417–23.
41. Cancedda R, Cedola A, Giuliani A, Komlev V, Lagomarsino S, Mastrogiacomo M, et al. Bulk and interface investigations of scaffolds and tissue-engineered bones by X-ray microtomography and X-ray microdiffraction. Biomaterials. 2007;28(15):2505–24.
42. Atwood RC, Jones JR, Lee PD, Hench LL. Analysis of pore interconnectivity in bioactive glass foams using X-ray microtomography. Scripta Mater. 2004; 51:1029–33.
43. Giuliani A, Manescu A, Larsson E, Tromba G, Luongo G, Piattelli A, et al. In vivo regenerative properties of coralline-derived (biocoral) scaffold grafts in human maxillary defects: demonstrative and comparative study with Beta-Tricalcium phosphate and biphasic calcium phosphate by synchrotron radiation X-ray microtomography. Clin Implant Dent Relat Res. 2014;16(5):736–50.
44. Giuliani A, Manescu A, Mohammadi S, Mazzoni S, Piattelli A, Mangano F, et al. Quantitative kinetics evaluation of blocks versus granules of biphasic calcium phosphate scaffolds (HA/β-TCP 30/70) by synchrotron radiation X-ray microtomography: a human study. Implant Dent. 2016a;25(1):6–15.
45. Komlev VS, Peyrin F, Mastrogiacomo M, Cedola A, Papadimitropoulos A, Rustichelli F, et al. Kinetics of in vivo bone deposition by bone marrow stromal cells into porous calcium phosphate scaffolds: an X-ray computed microtomography study. Tissue Eng. 2006;12(12):3449–58. https://doi.org/10.1089/ten.2006.12.3449
46. Manescu A, Giuliani A, Mazzoni S, Mohammadi S, Tromba G, Diomede F, et al. Osteogenic potential of dual-blocks cultured with periodontal ligament stem cells: in-vitro and synchrotron microtomography study. J Periodontal Res. 2016;51(1):112–24.
47. Mazzoni S, Mohammadi S, Tromba G, Diomede F, Piattelli A, Trubiani O, et al. Role of cortico-cancellous heterologous bone in human periodontal ligament stem cell xeno-free culture studied by synchrotron radiation phase-contrast microtomography. Int J Mol Sci. 2017;18(2):364.
48. Komlev VS, Mastrogiacomo M, Pereira RC, Peyrin F, Rustichelli F, Cancedda R. Biodegradation of porous calcium phosphate scaffolds in an ectopic bone formation model studied by X-ray computed microtomograph. Eur Cell Mater. 2010;19:136–46.
49. Kazakia GJ, Burghardt AJ, Cheung S, Majumdar S. Assessment of bone tissue mineralization by conventional x-ray microcomputed tomography: comparison with synchrotron radiation microcomputed tomography and ash measurements. Med Phys. 2008;35(7):3170–9.
50. Biondi K, Lorusso P, Fastuca R, Mangano A, Zecca PA, Bosco M, et al. Evaluation of masseter muscle in different vertical skeletal patterns in growing patients. Eur J Paediatr Dent. 2016;17(1):47–52.
51. Cassi D, De Biase C, Tonni I, Gandolfini M, Di Blasio A, Piancino MG. Natural position of the head: review of two-dimensional and three-dimensional methods of recording. Br J Oral Maxillofac Surg. 2016;54(3):233–40.
52. Fontana M, Cozzani M, Caprioglio A. Non-compliance maxillary molar distalizing appliances: an overview of the last decade. Prog Orthod. 2012; 13(2):173–84.
53. Caprioglio A, Fontana M, Longoni E, Cozzani M. Long-term evaluation of the molar movements following pendulum and fixed appliances. Angle Orthod. 2013;83(3):447–54.
54. Giuliano Maino B, Pagin P, Di Blasio A. Success of miniscrews used as anchorage for orthodontic treatment: analysis of different factors. Prog Orthod. 2012;13(3):202–9.
55. Kak AC, Slaney M. Principles of computerized tomographic imaging. Society of Industrial and Applied Mathematics. 2001. Originally published by IEEE Press at http://www.slaney.org/pct/pct-toc.html.
56. Brun F, Pacilè S, Accardo A. Enhanced and flexible software tools for X-ray computed tomography at the Italian synchrotron radiation facility Elettra. Fundamenta Informaticae. 2015;141:233–43.
57. Doube M, Klosowski MM, Arganda-Carreras I, Cordelières FP, Dougherty RP, Jackson JS, et al. BoneJ: free and extensible bone image analysis in ImageJ. Bone. 2010;47:1076–9.
58. Schneider CA, Rasband WS, Eliceiri KW. NIH image to ImageJ: 25 years of image analysis. Nat Methods. 2012;9:671–5.
59. Giuliani A. Analysis of bone response to dental bone grafts by advanced physical techniques. In: Piattelli A, editor. Bone response to dental implant materials: Elsevier Ltd; 2016. p. 229–46. https://doi.org/10.1016/B978-0-08-100287-2.00012-4.
60. Suresh KP, Chandrashekara S. Sample size estimation and power analysis for clinical research studies. J Hum Reprod Sci. 2012;5(1):7–13.
61. Giuliani A, Iezzi G, Mazzoni S, Piattelli A, Perrotti V, Barone A. Regenerative properties of collagenated porcine bone grafts in human maxilla: demonstrative study of the kinetics by synchrotron radiation microtomography and light microscopy. Clin Oral Investig. 2018;22(1):505–13. https://doi.org/10.1007/s00784-017-2139-6.

18

Prevalence and impact of infant oral mutilation on dental occlusion and oral health-related quality of life among Kenyan adolescents from Maasai Mara

Arthur Kemoli[1], Hans Gjørup[2], Marie-Louise Milvang Nørregaard[3], Mark Lindholm[4], Tonnie Mulli[5], Anders Johansson[6] and Dorte Haubek[3*]

Abstract

Background: Infant Oral Mutilation (IOM) includes germectomy and early extraction of primary and permanent incisors and canines, primarily in the lower jaw.

The aim of the present study was to examine the prevalence and impact of IOM, involving the removal of mandibular permanent incisors and/or canines, on dental occlusion and Oral Health-Related Quality of Life (OHRQoL) among Kenyan adolescents from Maasai Mara.

Methods: In a cross-sectional study, 284 adolescents (14–18 yrs. of age) participated in an oral examination and an interview, using a structured questionnaire on age, gender, medical history, and IOM practice. For the analysis of the dental occlusion, participants with IOM, in terms of absence of two or more permanent teeth in the mandibular incisor and/or canine tooth segments (IOM group), were compared to participants who had all six incisors and canines present in the oral cavity (control group). OHRQoL was assessed using child perception questionnaire (CPQ11–14).

Results: The majority of the participants (61%) had been exposed to IOM, among whom 164 (95%) had absence of two mandibular central incisors. More individuals in the IOM group had maxillary overjet exceeding 5 mm than in the control group (50.9% vs. 20%, $p < 0.001$). Nineteen (11%) subjects in the IOM group had mesial occlusion in contrast to none in the control group ($p < 0.001$). The mean and median total CPQ scores and the mean and median CPQ domain scores were low in both groups with no significant differences between the groups.

Conclusions: Approximately two-thirds of the study population presented with IOM, with the majority of them missing two mandibular permanent central incisors. Although some participants with IOM had substantial maxillary overjet and mesial occlusion, only few of them showed substantial effect on their OHRQoL.

Keywords: Tooth bud, Germectomy, Avulsion, Ebinyo, Malocclusion, Life quality

* Correspondence: dorte.haubek@dent.au.dk
[3]Section for Pediatric Dentistry, Department of Dentistry and Oral Health, Health, Aarhus University, Aarhus C, Denmark
Full list of author information is available at the end of the article

Background

Infant oral mutilation (IOM) is a traditional practice performed in young children, mostly as germectomy of developing primary or permanent mandibular incisors or canines, or early extraction of these tooth types [1–5]. The rationale for IOM can be either therapeutic or ritual [6, 7]. Beyond the removed teeth, dental defects, dental deficiency (aplasia of succedaneous permanent teeth due to IOM on primary teeth), and eruptional disturbances may occur [1, 3, 8]. In addition to these adverse defects and disturbances, unwanted side-effects on dental occlusion may occur due to imbalance of the space in the dental arches as, e.g., development of deep bite by overeruption of the upper incisors without antagonists [9, 10].

IOM is still rampant in several countries in the East African region and has been associated with geographic, cultural, aesthetic, and ritual grounds [1, 5, 8, 11–18]. For example, previous studies in Kenya demonstrate that various types of IOM are still practiced by some tribes in the country [15, 19]. A study by Hassanali and coworkers in a Maasai population from the Kajiado area reported a very high prevalence of removal of primary canine tooth buds in the age group 6 months to 2 years as well as in the age group 3 to 7-years of age (87% and 72%, respectively) [15]. In addition, traditional extraction of mandibular permanent central incisors in Maasai children has been demonstrated [20]. IOM has also been shown to affect the dental arch width [20], the development and eruption of the succedaneous teeth [9], and the dental occlusion [21]. In Kenya, apart from the observations made by Hassanali and coworkers [20], no other studies on the assessment of the long-term effects of IOM on the dental occlusion of the affected children have been found.

Currently, human migration from one part of the world to another is a relatively frequent event [22]. Therefore, subjects with IOM may appear geographically widespread, and hence the phenomenon is of relevance to clinicians all over the world.

The aim of the present study was to examine the prevalence and impact of IOM, involving the removal of mandibular permanent incisors and/or canines, on dental occlusion and Oral Health-Related Quality of Life (OHRQoL) among Kenyan adolescents from Maasai Mara.

Methods

Study population

The study was conducted in January–February 2016 and took place in Mara North Conservancy in Narok County of Kenya. Mara North Conservancy was established in January 2009 through a partnership among eleven member camps and over 800 Maasai landowners with long-term commitments to the environment, wildlife, and local communities.

The study population consisted of adolescents aged 14 to 18 years. They were recruited from the four primary and one mixed secondary schools present in Mara North Conservancy. Out of the total number of teenagers in this age group ($n = 340$), 284 (83.5%) teenagers [mean age: 15.0; SD 1.1; range 14–18 years] were recruited into the study. These were teenagers whose parents/guardians provided a written informed consent for their participation in the study. The teenagers, not included in the study, were those who failed to provide the consent, were absent, or sick on the day of the examination. The age of the participants was determined from the records kept by the schools, except for three of the teenagers, whose age records were missing in the school register. The distribution of the participants according to gender was 153 (55.6%) males and 122 (44.4%) females (information on gender had unintentionally been omitted in the record sheet for nine teenagers). Information on social and economic status of the teenagers and their families was not available to the researchers. The few schools ($n = 5$) in Mara North Conservancy, Narok County, are boarding schools, as the possibilities for transportation within the region is scarce and challenging. Thus, most often parents live far away from the schools. All schools were considered to be at a similar standard and with similar physical and educational possibilities.

The study consisted of two parts, one being a face-to-face interview with the teenagers using structured questionnaires to collect data on age, gender, medical history, IOM practice, and OHRQoL, while the second part included an examination of the participants` teeth present in the oral cavity, including oral photographing of the dentition.

Face-to face interview

Structured questionnaires were used to collect data on age, gender, medical history, IOM practice, and OHRQoL. In order to prevent copying of answers to the questionnaire amongst the participants from the same school class, a clear separation method was applied to prevent intermingling of the participants, until the interviews were finalized.

The OHRQoL part was assessed by the validated Child Perception Questionnaire (CPQ11–14), which is developed to measure the OHRQoL among teenagers [23, 24]. The CPQ includes 37 questions grouped into four domain subscales: oral symptoms, functional limitations, emotional well-being, and social well-being. The response format for all questions is a Likert-like scale. The response options and scores are: "never" (score 0), "once or twice" (score 1), "sometimes" (score 2), "often" (score 3) and "every day or almost every day" (score 4). The range of the additive total CPQ score is 0–148. The ranges of domain subscale scores are 0–24 (oral symptoms), 0–36 (functional limitations and emotional well-being), and 0–52 (social well-being). In addition, the CPQ includes two global questions: Q1) "How would you describe the healthiness of your teeth, mouth, lips or jaws?" (very good, good, okay, or bad) and Q2) "How much does the condition of your teeth, mouth, lips or jaws influence your life?" (not at all, very little, some, a lot, or very much).

The questionnaire for the collection of data on age, gender, medical history, and IOM practice was initially piloted and tested by the two Kenyan authors (AK and TM) concerning the understandability and relevance in a Kenyan context before being used. Further, the Kenyan authors were also the dentists who had the contact with the teenagers when they were interviewed, meaning that the teenagers had the possibility to ask probing questions in English or local languages. The original CPQ questionnaire is written in English [23, 24], and the spoken language in Kenya is English. The English CPQ questionnaire has been validated in other English-speaking communities [23, 24], but it has not been validated specifically in the Kenyan population. As a supplement, the CPQ questionnaire was also translated to the local tribe language of the Maasai population, in case a need arose of having the English version of some or all the questions in the local language for clarification. In addition, the participants did not fill out the questionnaire themselves, but the procedure was carried out by the interviewer and any assistance, if needed, was available from the Kenyan co-authors of the present paper. In practice, there was, however, no need for the translated questionnaire as only probing questions were asked by some participants and subsequently explained by the interviewers. The two interviewers were Kenyan dental researchers from University of Nairobi, Kenya, and they were trained in using the questionnaires, and in addition, they calibrated the interview procedure under field conditions after the finalization of the initial two interviews.

Oral examination

The oral examination was done under field conditions at the respective schools of the teenagers. This means that oral examinations were not performed in a dental office, but in a standard class room with natural lighting. No sophisticated dental equipment was available. The child was made to lie on the top of a table, facing a natural light source. As supplementary light source, a headlamp was used to augment the natural light during the examination of the oral cavity. With clean disposable mouth mirrors and tweezers, an oral examination was carried out to establish the status of the dentition and the dental occlusion. A record on the number of teeth present in the mandibular incisor and canine segments and signs of dental disruption was made on individual forms. Teeth were recorded as present when either partly or fully erupted. A tooth was recorded as having a dental disruption, if the tooth had an abnormal and irregular morphology with unusual hypoplastic defects consistent with previous germectomy in the affected area of the dental arch. Thus, dental disruption was defined as an extrinsic hypoplastic defect or interference with the normal developmental process of the tooth. Dental fluorosis was seen in the study population, but was not an aim to study in the present study. An IOM case was defined as an individual who was missing two or more permanent teeth in the mandibular incisor and/or canine tooth segments, as a result of IOM (also confirmed during interview). Intraoral photographs were taken as a part of the record, with the teeth in occlusion from right, left, and frontal perspective.

The dental occlusion was assessed according to definitions by Bjoerk, Krebs and Solow [25] and included measurement of the horizontal overjet (HO) and the vertical overbite (VO) with a caliper, classification of HO into mandibular overjet ($HO \leq 0$ mm), neutral overjet ($0 \text{ mm} < HO \leq 5$ mm), maxillary overjet ($5 \text{ mm} < HO < 9$ mm), or extreme maxillary overjet ($HO \geq 9$ mm), and classification of VO into neutral overbite ($0 \text{ mm} \leq VO \leq 4$ mm), deep bite (overbite ≥5 mm), or frontal open bite ($VO < 0$ mm). Furthermore, the molar occlusion on each side of the participants was assessed and classified as neutral (the mesiobuccal cusp of the maxillary permanent first molar occludes into the mesiofacial sulcus of the mandibular permanent first molar), distal (mandibular first molar deviates distally to neutral occlusion ½ cusp or more), or mesial (mandibular first molar deviates mesially to neutral occlusion ½ cusp or more). For each side, deviations from normal transverse occlusion was classified as cross bite (the buccal cusp of at least one maxillary canine, premolar, or molar occludes lingual to the buccal cusp of the mandibular teeth) or scissor bite (the lingual cusp of at least one maxillary canine, premolar or molar occludes buccal to the buccal cusps of the mandibular teeth).

Prior to the initiation of the study, training of the researchers, to standardize the methods to be applied, was carried out by studying pictures available in the published literature as well as clinical photos taken of the participants on the first day of the study period. Due to the limited working time at the research site, recall of patients for traditional intra-reliability evaluation was not an option. Only two dentists examined the children (HG, MLMN), while two other dentists (ML, DH) did the recording of the results and the oral photographing. Concerning the inter-rater reliability, the two clinical examiners did an examination twice of

12 participants randomly chosen among the 284 participants. The examinations done twice were executed with four students at the initiation of the study and with two participants another four times during the remaining part of the study. A maximum of (12 × 32 teeth) 384 teeth were included in the double examinations among which a total of 327 (85.1%) were actually found to be present in the oral cavity. Concerning the recording of the teeth present in the oral cavity and the teeth with dental disruption, the percentage agreement between the two examiners were 100%. The missing teeth recorded during the 12 examinations were 35 third molars, 4 s permanent molars, 15 mandibular permanent central incisors, two mandibular permanent canines, and one maxillary permanent canine.

All the children at the participating schools received free education on oral hygiene with a toothbrush and toothpaste provided to them for continued use in school/at home. The participants, who required emergency dental treatment, were referred to the nearest dental clinic or the Dental Hospital of the University of Nairobi.

Data analysis

The data collected were cleaned, coded, and entered into the computer, and analyzed with the use of SPSS 24 (Statistical Package for the Social Sciences, SPSS Inc., Chicago, IL) and STATA 14.0 (StataCorp LLC, Texas, USA). The number of maxillary teeth was compared to the number of mandibular teeth. The total number of missing maxillary incisors and canines was compared to the total number of missing mandibular incisors and canines. For studying the potential consequences of missing teeth due to IOM in the anterior segment of the mandible in relation to the dental occlusion, the IOM group was defined as participants with two or more missing mandibular incisors and/or canines. The group of participants, in whom all mandibular canines and incisors were present, was defined as the control group. Sixteen participants with the absence of only one mandibular permanent incisor or canine were excluded from the comparison between groups due to one missing tooth being below the defined cut-off level.

Overall CPQ11–14 score and domain scores for each participant were calculated by summing the response codes for the questions. If one or more of the questions in a domain were unanswered, the respective domain score as well as the overall CPQ11–14 score was recorded as missing for that participant. The mean additive score of each domain as well as the mean overall CPQ11–14 score were calculated and indicate the severity of impact on OHRQoL in the respective domains [26]. For the CPQ11–14 scale as a whole and for each of the four domains, the number of answers, being reported as "often" or "every-day/almost every day", were counted. The mean of these figures indicate the extent of severe impact on OHRQoL in the respective domains. The percentage of individuals answering "often" or "every-day/almost every day" was calculated and indicate the prevalence of severe impact on OHRQoL in the respective domains [26]. In addition, the median additive scores in the respective domains as well as the median overall CPQ11–14 score were calculated due to the scores not being normally distributed.

Deviations on the dental occlusion and in the answers on IOM and CPQ were assessed according to the defined grouping of participants with or without IOM.

Statistical tests in terms of t-test, Wilcoxon rank sum test (Mann-Whitney), Fischer's exact test, and Chi-square were carried out as appropriate.

Results

Number of teeth present in the oral cavity

Among 283 out of 284 teenagers entered into the study, the overall mean number of permanent teeth present in the oral cavity was 27.9 [SD: 2.0; range: 22–32; 95% CI: 27.7–28.1]. The calculation was based on 283 adolescents only, as one individual, who had only 11 permanent teeth and multiple primary teeth present (most likely due to delayed eruption), was excluded from the calculation of the mean number of the permanent teeth present, but not from other calculations in the study. The number of maxillary teeth [mean 14.5; SD 1.1; 95% CI: 14.4–14.6] exceeds the number of mandibular teeth [mean 13.4; SD 1.3; 95% CI: 13.2–13.5] ($p < 0.001$). The total number of missing mandibular incisors and canines [mean 1.4; SD 1.1; 95% CI: 1.2–1.5] exceeds the total number of missing maxillary incisors and canines [mean 0.1; SD 0.4; 95% CI: 0.1–0.2] ($p < 0.001$).

The distribution of clinically visible teeth as well as the absence of teeth in the mandible according to tooth type is provided in Table 1. A total of 173 out of 284 (61%) teenagers belonged to the IOM group, with bilateral absence of the mandibular central incisors being the dominant finding in relation to the IOM practice (164 out of 173 subjects in the IOM group (94.8%) and 164 out of 284 in the total group (57.7%)) (Fig. 1c and d). Concerning permanent molars, 107, 277 and 276 individuals, respectively, had third molars, second molar and first molars bilaterally present. Third, second, and first permanent molars were absent bilaterally in, 154, three, and two individuals, respectively. Twenty-one, four, and six individuals, respectively, had this status unilaterally.

Disruption of teeth

The distribution of mandibular premolars, canines and incisors with disruption of the tooth crown is also shown in Table 1. Eight individuals (8/284 (2.8%)) had a total of

Table 1 Presence of permanent and primary mandibular teeth and occurrence of dental disruption according to tooth type ($n = 284$)

	DP[a] present	DP absent		dd[b] present	DP with disruption	
Mandibular tooth type	bilateral (n)	bilateral (n)	unilateral (n)	(n)	bilateral (n)	unilateral (n)
Second premolar	280	0	1	3	0	0
First premolar	282	0	1	1	1	0
Canine	267	5	10	2	0	6
Lateral incisor	263	5	14	2	0	3
Central incisor	108	164	12	0	0	0

[a]DP means permanent teeth
[b]dd means primary teeth

11 mandibular premolars, canines, and/or incisors with disruption of the tooth crown. Specifically, one individual had dental disruption of three (tooth no. 34, 44, and 33), one individual had disruption of two (tooth no. 43 and 42), and six individuals had disruption of one tooth crown (three individuals: tooth no. 43; two individuals: tooth no. 32; one individual: tooth no. 33). Thus, in summary a total of 8 individuals had disruption of one or more teeth in the incisor, canine and premolar tooth segments of the mandible.

Dental occlusion

The characteristics of the dental occlusion according to IOM or control group are shown in Table 2. More individuals in the IOM group had maxillary overjet exceeding 5 mm than in the control group (86 (50.9%) vs. 19 (20%), $p < 0.001$). Nineteen (11%) subjects in the IOM group had mesial occlusion in contrast to none in the control group ($p < 0.001$), whereas no significant difference was seen according to findings of distal occlusion, cross bite, and scissor bite. There was no significant difference found in relation to the categories of VO (neutral overbite, deep bite, and frontal open bite) when comparing the IOM group and the control group.

The mean HO was significantly higher in the IOM group compared to the control group ($p < 0.001$), whereas no significant difference in mean VO was found ($p = 0.298$).

Answers to questions on IOM practice

The answers on the subjective aspects of IOM by the 173 (61.1%) teenagers, who had entered the IOM group, are summarized in Table 3. The information on the age at the time of tooth extraction was missing in most cases ($n = 137$). Thus, the possibility that IOM had been carried out at a very early age, exists. The mean age reported as the time point of the extraction for the group ($n = 36$), who remembered the age/occasion, was 7.7 yrs. [SD: 7.7 yrs.; range 3–12 yrs].

The two questions, dealing with the type of person who carried out the tooth removal and how the tooth removal was performed, were in about one third part of the participants answered by "don't know" (31.8% and 35.8%, respectively). Pain control was not used in 60% of the cases. In 87% of the cases, tooth removal was practiced also in siblings. The majority of the adolescents considered tooth removal to be executed for ritual reasons (84%), but in most cases (98%) the participants did not consider tooth removal as a tradition in neither the

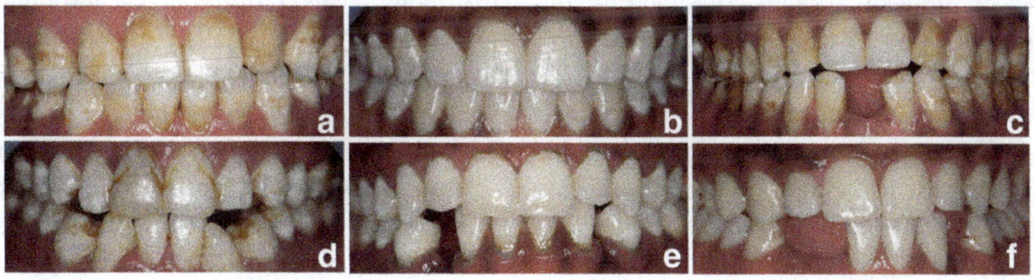

Fig. 1 Kenyan teenagers without IOM (**a** and **b**) and with IOM (**c**, **d**, **e** and **f**). Examples given in **c** and **d** illustrate the traditional type of IOM (two mandibular incisors missing) among adolescents living in Maasai Mara, and the vast majority of the study population (61%) presented with this type of IOM. Space between teeth is seen between mandibular lateral incisors in case C, whereas in case D the space has been closed after removal of mandibular incisors. Cases E and F show uni- and/or bilateral missing permanent canines and/or incisors. Dental fluorosis (variation in severity) is seen on the pictures

Table 2 Characteristics of dental occlusion in the infant oral mutilation (IOM) group compared to the control group

	IOM group (n = 173)[a]	Control group (n = 95)	p
	Number (%)	Number (%)	
Mandibular overjet (HO ≤ 0 mm)	1 (0.6)	0	< 0.001
Neutral overjet (0 < HO ≤ 5 mm)	83 (49.1)	76 (80.0)	
Maxillary overjet (5 < HO < 9 mm)	52 (30.8)	17(17.9)	
Extreme maxillary overjet (HO ≥ 9 mm)	34 (20.1)	2 (2.1)	
Neutral overbite (0 ≤ VO ≤ 4)	139 (83.7)	85 (89.5)	0.226
Deep bite (VO ≥ 5 mm)	17 (10.2)	4 (4.2)	
Frontal open bite (VO < 0)	10 (6.0)	6 (6.3)	
Molar occlusion			
Mesial (one or both sides)	19 (11.0)	0	< 0.001
Distal (one or both sides)	4 (2.3)	4 (4.2)	0.382
Cross bite (one or both sides)	14 (8.1)	12 (12.6)	0.230
Scissor bite (one or both sides)	5 (2.9)	3 (3.2)	0.902
	Mean (SD) [95% CI]	Mean (SD) [95% CI]	p
Horizontal overjet (mm)	5.9 (2.8) [5.5–6.4]	4.1 (SD 1.9) [3.7–4.5]	< 0.001
Vertical overbite (mm)	2.3 (2.4) [1.1–2.6]	2.0 (SD 1.8) [1.6–2.3]	0.298

Comparison by Chi^2-test (HO categories, VO categories, and molar occlusion categories) or t-test (mean HO and mean VO)
Figures in parentheses are percentages of patients with the deviation in the group
Figures in brackets [] are 95% confidence interval (CI)
[a]Missing data on HO of four patients and on VO of seven patients
IOM group: Teenagers missing two to four mandibular incisors and/or canines
Control group: Teenagers with all mandibular incisors and canines present

tribe nor the family. Overall, the majority of the participants (80%) felt happy about the status of their teeth (Table 3).

Answers to CPQ

The numbers of participants completing the specific measures (domains) are given in Table 4. Some answers were missing due to some teenagers refusing to answer the question. In the IOM group, the number of individuals with missing domain scores were respectively two (oral symptoms), five (functional limitations), three (emotional well-being), and one (social well-being). In the control group, the number of individuals with missing domain scores were respectively one (oral symptoms) and two (functional limitations).

The healthiness of teeth and mouth (Q1) was characterized as "very good" or "good" in contrast to "okay" or "bad" by 148 (86%) individuals in the IOM group and by 83 (87%) individuals in the control group ($p = 0.853$). How much the condition of teeth and mouth influenced their lifes (Q2) was answered by "not at all" or "very little" in contrast to "some", "a lot", or "very much" by 156 (91%) individuals in the IOM group and by 85 (89%) in the control group ($p = 0.665$). The mean and median total CPQ scores and the mean and median domain scores were low in both groups, and no significant differences between groups were found ($p \geq 0.191$) (Table 4).

Discussion

The present research project took place in Maasai Mara North Conservancy, a rural Kenyan area that forms part of the Maasai Mara, where the Maasai Mara National Park is situated. The area was chosen as the research site, because it was part of a larger interdisciplinary research project under the auspices of The Maasai Mara Science and Development Initiative (http://maasaimarascience.org/). The indigenous Maasai population living in the area still maintains their traditional life, although human wildlife interaction can be challenging in addition to the interaction with the tourists visiting the national park. It is plausible to expect some changes in the traditions of the Maasai population due to such interactions.

Absence of two mandibular central incisors as a sign of IOM was found in the majority of the teenagers living in Maasai Mara, which was an indication of IOM, in terms of removal of tooth buds or early extraction of mandibular incisors, still being a very common practice in the Maasai Mara area. Other causes than IOM to explain the absence of mandibular incisors could not be fully excluded. The absence of some of the mandibular

Table 3 The answers on aspects related to tooth removal given by 173 adolescents with infant oral mutilation (IOM)

Questions asked	Answers given to questions asked (number (%))				
"Who removed teeth?"	dentist	healer	other person	do not know	not recorded
	4 (2.3)	21 (12.3)	90 (52.0)	57 (33.0)	1 (0.6)
"Which tool was used to remove teeth?"	nail/needle	knife	other	do not know	not recorded
	0 (0)	93 (53.8)	23 (13.3)	55 (31.8)	2 (1.2)
"Who brought you for tooth removal?"	parents	friends	other	do not know	not recorded
	104 (60.1)	0 (0)	6 (3.5)	60 (34.7)	3 (1.7)
"How do you like[a] your teeth?"	happy	do not like (miss)[b]	do not like (other)[c]	do not know	not recorded
	139 (80.4)	27 (15.6)	7 (4.1)	0 (0)	0 (0)
"Why was tooth removal carried out?"	ritual	esthetic	sick	do not know	not recorded
	151 (87.3)	1 (0.6)	1 (0.6)	19 (11.0)	1 (0.6)
"Is pain control used during tooth removal?"	no	yes		do not know	not recorded
	103 (59.5)	5 (2.9)		62 (35.8)	3 (1.7)
"Is tooth removal a tribe tradition?"	no	yes		do not know	not recorded
	170 (98.3)	0 (0)		2 (1.2)	1 (0.6)
"Is tooth removal a family practice?"	no	yes		do not know	not recorded
	146 (84.4)	24 (14.0)		3 (1.7)	0 (0)
"Is tooth removal seen also in siblings?"	no	yes		do not know	not recorded
	21 (12.3)	151 (87.3)		1 (0.6)	0 (0)

Figures given are numbers of adolescents with the specified answer, and the figures in parentheses are percentages of the total group ($n = 173$)
IOM: Absence of a minimum of two mandibular incisors and/or canines according to the cut-off level
[a]The word "like" means "wish to have"/"to take pleasure with"
[b]"I do not like that I have missing teeth in the front"
[c]"I do not like the esthetics of my teeth for other reasons than having missing teeth"

incisors may theoretically be because of dental anomaly, e.g., agenesis of lower incisor(s), deviation of the dental eruption, e.g., retention or impaction of incisors, or avulsion because of traumatic injury. In other populations, agenesis of mandibular incisors is, however, a very rare finding (95% CI: 0.25–0.35%) in comparison to agenesis of mandibular second premolars (95% CI: 2.91–3.22%), maxillary second premolars (95% CI: 1.39–1.61%), and lateral maxillary incisors (95% CI: 1.55–1.78) [27]. Also avulsion of mandibular incisors is rare [28, 29]. Thus, the absence of mandibular permanent incisors found in the present study is most likely explained by IOM. We had, however, only minimal or no information on the dental history of the participants, and radiographic equipment was not available at the research site in Maasai Mara.

Other types of IOM than absence of two mandibular central incisors were also found, for example, a combination of missing lateral incisors and canines (Fig. 1). These types were, however, much less common. According to the present study, the IOM practice impacts on OHRQoL and the dental occlusion to a minor extent only, and according to the questions and aspects assessed in the study, the teenagers were in general satisfied with their dental status.

In the present study, the prevalence of IOM was found to be high (61%). This finding was much higher than the findings in a Sudanese study, reporting 22.4% of children (aged 4 to 8 years) having IOM [30], and in an Ethiopian study, reporting 15% of 2 to 18-year old children having IOM in terms of primary canines extraction and 7% of their permanent canines being affected by the traditional IOM practice [14]. In terms of the missing teeth due to IOM, the present study found the mandibular central incisors to be the most frequently affected tooth type. This result is different from the two above mentioned studies [14, 30], which involved mostly the canines. In contrast, the findings of the present study support previous reports from Maasai Mara, which also describes the absence of mandibular incisors as a dominant and characteristic IOM trait in the Maasai population [7, 20].

In the present Kenyan study, signs of dental disruption during the development of the tooth crowns was seen in few teeth (incisors, canines and/or premolars), and only a minor proportion of the study population (2.8%) showed this deviation of the tooth formation in the mandible. In the previously mentioned Sudanese study on IOM (termed "haifat"), the mandibular permanent canines were found to be the most affected tooth type, primarily with enamel defects on the labial surfaces [30]. In the Sudanese

Table 4 The overall CPQ11–14 score and the four domain scores in 173 adolescents infant oral mutilation (IOM group) compared to 95 adolescents with all mandibular incisors and canines present in the oral cavity (control group)

		CPQ total				Oral symptoms				Functional limitations				Emotional well-being				Social well-being			
	n[a]	Median[b] (P^{10}-p^{90})	Mean[c] (SD)	Prevalence (%)[d]	Extent[e]	Median[b] (P^{10}-p^{90})	Mean[c] (SD)	Prevalence (%)[d]	Extent[e]	Median[b] (P^{10}-p^{90})	Mean[c] (SD)	Prevalence (%)[d]	Extent[e]	Median[b] (P^{10}-p^{90})	Mean[c] (SD)	Prevalence (%)[d]	Extent[e]	Median[b] (P^{10}-p^{90})	Mean[c] (SD)	Prevalence (%)[d]	Extent[e]
IOM group	173	4 (0–18)	6.0 (8.0)	5.5	0.12	2 (0–5)	2.4 (2.3)	3.5	0.04	1 (0–6)	2.1 (3.4)	5.4	0.07	0 (0–3.5)	0.9 (2.9)	1.2	0.02	0 (0–2)	0.7 (2.4)	0.6	0.01
Boys	96	4 (0–20)	7.0 8.9	7.6	0.18	2 (0–6)	2.8 (2.4)	4.3	0.05	1 (0–8)	2.3 (3.5)	6.5	0.09	0 (0–4)	1.0 (3.1)	2.1	0.03	0 (0–2)	0.8 (2.5)	1.0	0.01
Girls	72	4.5 (0–16)	7.6 (8.9)	2.9	0.03	2 (0–6)	2.8 (2.4)	2.8	0.03	1 (0–9)	2.8 (3.7)	4.3	0.06	0 (0–5)	1.2 (2.9)	0	0	0 (0–6)	1.2 (2.8)	0	0
Control group	95	4 (0–14)	5.9 (7.2)	4.4	0.05	2 (0–6)	2.5 (2.2)	3.2	0.04	0 (0–7)	2.1 (3.0)	1.1	0.01	0 (0–2)	0.9 (2.2)	0	0	0 (0–2)	0.7 (2.0)	0	0
Boys	48	4 (0.11)	4.6 (5.0)	2.1	0.02	2 (0–6)	2.4 (2.0)	2.1	0.02	0 (0–6)	1.5 (2.3)	0	0	0 (0–2)	0.6 (1.5)	0	0	0 (0–0)	0.2 (0.7)	0	0
Girls	44	2 (0–13	4.6 (6.1)	7.1	0.10	2 (0–4)	1.9 (2.0)	4.7	0.07	0 (0–5)	1.9 (3.3)	2.3	0.02	0 (0–2)	0.7 (2.5)	0	0	0 (0–0)	0.5 (2.0)	0	0

[a]The number of individuals in the respective groups. Missing data on gender of five IOM individuals and three controls
[b]Median additive score, 10- and 90-percentiles in parenthesis
[c]Mean additive score, standard deviation (SD) in parenthesis (severity of impact)
[d]Prevalence is the percentage of individuals with one or more items scored "often" or "every day/almost every day" in the specified domains
[e]Extent is the mean number of items scored "often" or "every day/almost every day" in the specified domain
IOM: Absence of a minimum of two mandibular incisors and/or canines according to the cut-off level

study, 28.4% of the children with IOM had enamel defects compared to only 8.4% among the controls. In a Tanzanian study, the prevalence of missing and/or disrupted permanent teeth was 8% [12]. All these studies affirm the fact that there is a high risk of damage to tooth germs of permanent teeth while removing other tooth buds or doing early extractions. Dental disruption can be the result of the use of improper instruments to undertake the IOM procedure [3]. Besides the reasons given above, the lack of aseptic procedures could result in local or general infection during the critical period of tooth development and mineralization [19]. This could also result in enamel defects of the tooth crowns. Moreover, a likely explanation to the dental disruption seen on premolars is that 'neighboring' tooth bud(s) to the tooth bud/tooth that was intended to having IOM done, were "hidden" and thereby also damaged, most likely unintentionally.

Dental fluorosis was seen prominently on all teeth of the vast majority of the children participating in the study. Dental fluorosis is endemic in Kenya [31, 32], including the area of Mara North Conservancy. In cases with dental fluorosis, an atypical discoloration of the enamel (from white to brown), is seen. Severe dental fluorosis can, in addition, lead to disintegration of the tooth enamel [33]. However, dental disruption is a quantitative enamel defect, whereas dental fluorosis is a qualitative defect of enamel, eventually complicated by post-eruptive enamel breakdown due to less robust quality of enamel [32]. This circumstance also may need to be taken into consideration while diagnosing tooth anomalies in the population living in Maasai Mara, Kenya. The finding of IOM and enamel defects are, however, not so surprising in the Maasai Mara area, as it is relatively remote and lacks access to the requisite health facilities and oral health education [19].

IOM undertaken as germectomy or early extraction has been found not only to lead to dental disruption of succedaneous or adjacent teeth, but also to affect dental arch width. This has been reported in a study where the oral mutilation involved the extraction of mandibular central incisors [20]. In the present study, the dominant occlusal deviation in the group of participants, who had undergone mandibular incisor removal, was the increased maxillary overjet when compared to the controls without any tooth removal. The difference was statistically highly significant (Table 2), but the overall consequences on the dental occlusion appeared to be at a low to moderate level. However, the presence of mesial molar occlusion is relatively prevalent in the IOM group in contrast to the low prevalence of distal molar occlusion in both IOM group and control group. In Caucasian populations, distal molar occlusion is much more prevalent than mesial occlusion, e.g., in a previous Scandinavian study, which describes mesial molar occlusion in 3–4% and distal molar occlusion in 23–26% of an adolescent population [33, 34]. The prevalent mesial molar occlusion in the IOM group is most likely explained by mesial migration of mandibular teeth after the removal of teeth in the anterior segment of the lower dental arch. Normally, mesial molar occlusion is associated with mandibular overjet, which was present in only one individual of our study population. In general, an increased overjet is associated with distal molar occlusion [34], which was a rare finding in our study group. Thereby, the increased overjet does not seem to be associated with a total retrusion of the mandible or the lower dental arch, but may be explained by a constriction of the anterior segment of the lower dental arch due to removal of incisors in combination with a proclination of the maxillary incisors, eventually because of a forward positioning of the tongue. However, it might be speculated that IOM in terms of incisor removal impacts less on dental occlusion than the absence of canines. In case of missing canines, the occlusal consequences are most likely more extensive. This topic needs to be explored further in a population, where removal of canines is the dominant type of IOM.

In the present study, the exact time when IOM was carried out, was not known, and only a minor proportion of the participants could remember who had performed the IOM (14.3%). However, more than half of the subjects did remember the knife as the tool likely to having been used (Table 3). These findings could be due to the fact that in the majority of the children, the extraction was done early in life. Therefore, they may not be able to recall the incident. Furthermore, the present study showed that the majority (59.5%) of the participants remembered that no form of anesthetics or pain killer tablets was used to obtain pain control. The lack of pain relief may bring children in a condition where they are not able to participate safely in IOM procedures, which could lead to further trauma of other adjacent oral structures. Furthermore, the reason for the dental mutilation carried out might not have been clear to the growing children due to their immaturity. But the majority of teenagers (87.3%) thought that the incident might have been carried out because of tradition or as a ritual. Thus, it was not surprising that the majority of the participants did indicate that their siblings also had experienced tooth removal.

In terms of the effects of IOM on the teenagers daily functioning, most of the teenagers (80.4%) were happy with their dentition irrespective of signs of IOM. Thus, IOM does not seem to have a considerable effect on the OHRQoL. As mentioned in the method section, in order to prevent copying of answers to the questionnaire amongst the participants from the same school class, a clear separation method was applied to prevent intermingling of the participants, until the interviews were finalized. This organization is likely to be a strength of the data collection procedure increasing the validity of the collected data.

The participants came from Mara North Conservancy and were part of the Maasai population with a semi-nomadic lifestyle. The present study sample represents the population living in Maasai Mara only and cannot be extrapolated to Kenya in general. Experienced dental professionals within their dental field collected the data. The clinical examinations were done under field conditions (in class rooms in schools) where lighting was of various quality. This might have affected the results to some extent. However, clinical photos taken were useful as diagnostic supplement to the clinical data collected during the clinical examinations. The lack of radiographic facilities in the area excluded the possibility of diagnosing dental agenesis, impaction of teeth, un-erupted teeth, and other intraosseous structures or pathologies. Nevertheless, except for one subject, all participants had a fully or nearly fully matured permanent dentition minimizing the diagnostic uncertainty due to lack of radiographic equipment. But theoretically, the absence of teeth in the anterior tooth segment of the mandibular arch might be due to other reasons than removal or extraction of incisors. However, previous studies from Maasai Mara have reported on extraction of mandibular incisors as a common tradition [20]. Thus, the vast majority of the absent incisors is likely to be due to germectomy or early extractions.

Oral health education to the community to increase the understanding of the possible long-term effects of IOM practice is needed. This could be done with help from the community health workers and leaders. In addition, there is a need for further studies on appropriate strategies that could be used to "demystifying" the practice and for the development of relevant oral health education programs to address this issue in the tribes that still practice IOM. Future research may include studies on the dental status in young children and qualitative studies focusing attitude to and experiences of IOM in groups of mothers/parents, and elderly people of the Kenyan population. Furthermore, long-term consequences on dental occlusion in populations, where removal of primary and permanent canines are prevalent, need to be explored further, as that type of IOM may impact differently on the dental occlusion than IOM with removal of mandibular incisors.

Conclusions

IOM is still very common in the Maasai Mara region with the extraction of the mandibular central incisors being the most dominant type of IOM. The consequence of the removal of mandibular central incisors is apparently minimal in relation to the dental occlusion and OHRQoL, although some, of course, are more heavily affected than others. Thus, there is still a need for oral health education to the Kenyan communities to increase the understanding of the possible long-term effects of the IOM practice.

Abbreviations

CI: Confidence interval; CPQ: Child Perception Questionnaire; Fig.: Figure; HO: Horizontal Overjet; IOM: Infant Oral Mutilation; no. : number; OHRQoL: Oral Health-Related Quality of Life; p: *p*-value used in the statistical testing; SD: Standard Deviation; VO: Vertical Overbite; vs.: versus; yrs.: years

Acknowledgements

The authors would like to thank the secretary, Gitte Bak Ditlefsen and clinical assistants at Department of Dentistry and Oral Health, Section for Paediatric Dentistry, Aarhus University, Denmark for the assistance in practical matters related to the preparation of questionnaires and examination of the Kenyan adolescents.

Funding

This work was supported by Ingeborg and Leo Dannin foundation. The role of the funding agency was solely financial support, and the agency was not involved in the design of the study or collection, analysis, and interpretation of data or in writing of the manuscript.

Authors' contributions

DH made the overall outline of the present study as a Health representative and part of the interdisciplinary research initiative, Maasai Mara Science and Development Initiative (MMSDI). http://maasaimarascience.org/. DH identified researchers and staff involved in the study in collaboration with AJ. DH wrote the research protocol in collaboration with AK and HG. DH and HG designed and established the aims of the present study. AK took care of the correspondence with the Kenyan ethical committee and other relevant Kenyan authorities. AK and TM recruited the patients from schools in Maasai Mara, Kenya. MLMN and HG clinically examined the study population in collaboration with DH and ML, who recorded the clinical data and took clinical photos of participants. AK and TM collected questionnaire data by interviewing participants. DH entered data into statistical programs and prepared files for further data analyses. HG did the statistical analyses of the collected data. AK, DH and HG wrote the first draft of the manuscript. All authors took part in the interpretation of the data and in the finalization and approval of the submitted version of the manuscript.

Competing interests

The authors declare no potential conflicts of interest with respect to the authorship and/or publication of the present article.

Author details

[1]Department of Paediatric Dentistry, University of Nairobi, Nairobi, Kenya. [2]Center for Oral Health in Rare Diseases, Department of Maxillofacial Surgery, Aarhus University Hospital, Aarhus C, Denmark. [3]Section for Pediatric Dentistry, Department of Dentistry and Oral Health, Health, Aarhus University, Aarhus C, Denmark. [4]Division for Oral Microbiology, Odontology, Umeå University, Umeå, Sweden. [5]Department of Periodontology, University of Nairobi, Nairobi, Kenya. [6]Molecular Periodontology, Odontology, Umeå University, Umeå, Sweden.

References

1. Pindborg JJ. Dental mutilation and associated abnormalities in Uganda. Am J Phys Anthropol. 1969;31:383–9.
2. Hassanali J. Deciduous canine tooth bud removal in infants in East Africa. East Afr Med J. 2007;84:500–1.
3. Girgis S, Gollings J, Longhurst R, Cheng L. Infant oral mutilation – a child protection issue? Br Dent J. 2016;220:357–60.
4. Vukovic A, Bajsman A, Zukic S, Secic S. Cosmetic dentistry in ancient time – a short review. Bull. Int. Assoc. Paleodontology. 2009;3:9–13.
5. González EL, Pérez BP, Sánchez JAS, Acinas MM. Dental aesthetics as an expression of culture and ritual. Br Dent J. 2010;208:77–80.
6. Babe SPS. The mythology of the killer deciduous canine tooth in southern Sudan. The Journal of Pedodontics. 1989;14:48.
7. Garve R, Garve M, Link K, Türp JC, Meyer CG. Infant oral mutilation in East Africa . Therapeutic and ritual grounds. Trop Med Int Health. 2016; 21:1099–105.
8. Holan G, Mamber E. Extraction of primary canine tooth buds: prevalence and associated dental abnormalities in a group of Ethiopian Jewish children. Int J Paediatr Dent. 1994;4:25–30.
9. Bataringaya A, Ferguson M, Lallo R. The impact of Ebinyo, a form of dental mutilation, on the malocclusion status in Uganda. Community Dent Health. 2005;22:146–50.
10. Hassanali J, Odhiambo JW. Analysis of dental casts of 6-8 and 12-year-old Kenyan children. Eur J Orthod. 2000;22:135–42.
11. Mosha HJ. Dental mutilation and associated abnormalities in Tanzania. Odontostomatolgie Tropicale. 1983;6:215–9.
12. Matee MIN, Van Palerstein Helderman WH. Extraction of ′nylon′teeth and associated abnormalities in Tanzanian children. African Dental Journal 1991;5:21–25.
13. Jones A. Tooth mutilation in Angola. Br Dent J. 1992;173:177–9.
14. Welbury RR, Nunn J, Gordon PH, Green-Abate C. "Killer" canine removal and its sequelae in Addis Ababa. Quintessence Int. 1993;24:323–7.
15. Hassanali J, Amwayi P, Muriithi A. Removal of deciduous canine tooth buds in Kenya rural, Maasai Mara. East Afr Med J. 1995;72:207–9.
16. Rodd HD, Davidson LE. 'Ilko dacowo:' canine enucleation and dental sequela in Somali children. Int J Paediatr Dent. 2000;10:290–7.
17. Iriso R, et al. ′Killer′canines: the morbidity and mortality of Ebino in northern Uganda. Trop Med Int Health. 2000;5:706–10.
18. Accorsi S, Fabriani M, Ferrarese N, Iriso R, Lukwiya M, Declich S. The burden of traditional practices, Ebino and tea-tea, on child health in northern Uganda. Soc Sci Med. 2003;57:2183–91.
19. Kemoli AM. Raising the awareness of infant oral mutilation - myths and facts. Contemporary Clinical Dentistry. 2015;6:137–8.
20. Hassanali J, Amwayi P. Biometric analysis of the dental casts of Maasai following traditional extraction of mandibular permanent central incisors and of Kikyu children. Eur J Orthod. 1993;15:513–8.
21. Khonsari RH, Corre P, Perrin JP, Piot B. Orthodontic consequences of ritual dental mutilations in northern Tchad. J. Oral Maxillofac. Surg. 2009;67:902–5.
22. Connor P. At least a million Sub-Saharan Africans moved to Europe since 2010. 2018. www.PewResearchCenter.org.
23. Jokovic A, Locker D, Stephens M, Kenny D, Tompson B, Guatt G. Validity and reliability of a questionnaire for measuring child oral-health-related quality of life. J Dent Res. 2002;81:459–63.
24. Foster Page LA, Thomson WM, Jokovic A, Locker D. Validation of the child perceptions questionnaire (CPQ 11-14). J Dent Res. 2005;84:649–52.
25. Bjoerk A. A method for epidemiological registration of malocclusion. Acta Odontologica Scandinavia. 1964;22:27–41.
26. Slade GD, Nuttall N, Sanders AE, Steele JG, Allen PF, Lahti S. Impacts of oral disorders in the United Kingdom and Australia. Br Dent J. 2005;198:489–93.
27. Polder BJ, Van't hof MA, Van der Linden FP, Kuijpers-Jagtman AM. A meta-analysis of the prevalence of dental agenesis of permanent teeth. Community Dent Oral Epidemiol. 2004;32:217–26.
28. Glendor U. Epidemiology of traumatic dental injuries – a 12 year review of the literature. Dent Traumatol. 2008;24:603–11.
29. Batstone EB, Freer TJ, McNamara JR. Epidemiology of dental trauma: a review of the literature. Aust Dent J. 2000;45:2–9.
30. Rasmussen P, Elhassan E, Raadal M. Enamel defects in primary canines related to traditional treatment of teething problems in Sudan. Int J Paediatr Dent. 1992;2:151–5.
31. Walvekar SV, Qureshi BA. Endemic fluorosis and partial defluoridation of water supplies – a public health concern in Kenya. Community Dent Oral Epidemiol. 1982;10:156–60.
32. Thylstrup A. Posteruptive development of isolated and confluent pits in fluorosed enamel in a 6-year-old girl. Scand J Dent Res. 1983;91:243–6.
33. Helms S. Prevalence of malocclusion in relation to development of the dentition. An epidemiological study of Danish school children. Acta Odontologica Scandinavia. 1970;S58:1+.
34. Helms S. Malocclusion in Danish children with adolescent dentition: an epidemiological study. Am J Orthod. 1968;54:352–66.

Improved anchoring nails: design and analysis of resistance ability

Tensile test and finite element analysis (FEA) of improved anchoring nails used in temporomandibular joint (TMJ) disc anchor

Z. H. Zhou[1†], X. Z. Chen[1†], X. W. Chen[1†], Y. X. Wang[1], S. Y. Zhang[1,3*], S. F. Sun[2*] and J. Z. Zhen[1*]

Abstract

Background: Anchorage is one of the most important treatments for severe temporomandibular joint disorder (TMD). Anchoring nails have shown great success in clinical trials; however, they can break under pressure and are difficult to remove. In this study, we aimed to evaluate an improved anchoring nail and its mechanical stability.

Methods: The experiment consisted of two parts: a tensile test and finite element analysis (FEA). First, traditional and improved anchoring nails were implanted into the condylar cortical bone and their tensile strength was measured using a tension meter. Second, a three-dimensional finite element model of the condyles with implants was established and FEA was performed with forces from three different directions.

Results: The FEA results showed that the total force of the traditional and improved anchoring nails is 48.2 N and 200 N, respectively. The mean (±s.d.) maximum tensile strength of the traditional anchoring nail with a 3–0 suture was 27.53 ± 5.47 N. For the improved anchoring nail with a 3–0 suture it was 25.89 ± 2.64 N and with a 2–0 suture it was above 50 N. The tensile strengths of the traditional and improved anchoring nails with a 3–0 suture was significantly different ($P = 0.033\text{–}< 0.05$). Furthermore, the difference between the traditional anchoring nail with a 3–0 suture and the improved anchoring nail with a 2–0 suture was also significantly different ($P = 0.000\text{–}< 0.01$).

Conclusion: The improved anchoring nail, especially when combined with a 2–0 suture, showed better resistance ability compared with the traditional anchoring nail.

Keywords: Temporalmandibular joint disc anchorage, Mandibular condyle, Anchoring nail, Suture, Tensile test, Finite element analysis, FEA

Background

Temporomandibular joint disorder (TMD) is a common condition, with an approximate prevalence ranging from 13 to 87% [1]. Considering the limitations of non-surgical treatments, including medications [2], splints [3], physical therapy [4], and trigger point injections [5], surgical intervention is needed in severe cases of TMD [6, 7].

Previous clinical reports reveal that the results of surgical temporomandibular joint (TMJ) disc repositioning procedures have been variable due to long-term instability [8]. In 2001, an open joint procedure using Mitek anchoring nails (Mitek mini anchor, Mitek Products Inc., Westwood, Mass) showed great success in both clinical trials and radiography [9]. Despite their success, MiTek anchoring nails still have the following problems: (1) once fixed in the cortical bone, compared with other

* Correspondence: zhangshanyong@126.com; sunshoufu@163.com; zhenlich@163.com
†Z. H. Zhou, X. Z. Chen and X. W. Chen contributed equally to this work.
[1]Department of Oral and Maxillofacial Surgery, School of Medicine, Ninth People's Hospital, Shanghai Jiao Tong University, 639 Zhi Zao Ju Road, Shanghai 200011, People's Republic of China
[2]Department of Stomatology, Tongren Hospital Affiliated to Shanghai Jiao Tong University School of Medicine, Shanghai 200336, People's Republic of China
Full list of author information is available at the end of the article

types of Mitek anchor, Mitek mini anchoring nails tend to break easily under pressure; (2) once the wings are twisted, extraction of the anchoring nail becomes difficult. Spallaccia et al. [10] (2013) described an anchorage surgery using bioabsorbable microanchor nails. Postoperative MRI showed a low reposition rate (65.7% in 35 patients). To improve the success rate, reposition stability and implant safety, He et al. [11] (2015) applied Chinese-made anchoring nails in modified disc anchorage surgery. As the shape of the anchoring nail does not fit perfectly with the anatomical structure of a condyle, 7.47% of patients experienced postoperative friction in the parotideomasseteric region [12]. Our group has previously modified the traditional Chinese-made anchoring nail to reduce discomfort and improve stability. The anchoring nail is designed to be fully threaded, totally implanted in the cortical bone, and fixed with a 2–0 suture. However, the properties and safety of the improved anchoring nail have not yet been studied.

Therefore, in this study, we aimed to assess the mechanical performance of the improved anchoring nail compared with the traditional anchoring nail. In previous studies, tensile tests have been used to estimate the resistance ability of Mitek anchors [9]. With advances in computer science, finite element analysis (FEA) has become a useful tool that addresses the limitations associated with the TMJ structure and has tremendous advantages in many aspects [13, 14]. FEA is capable of modeling and analyzing shape, structure, and resistance ability and has become the most popular numerical theoretical method for TMJ biomechanics analysis. In our study, we used tensile tests and FEA to estimate the resistance ability of the improved anchoring nail. The hypothesis of this study was that the improved anchoring nail would show greater tensile strength compared with the traditional anchoring nail.

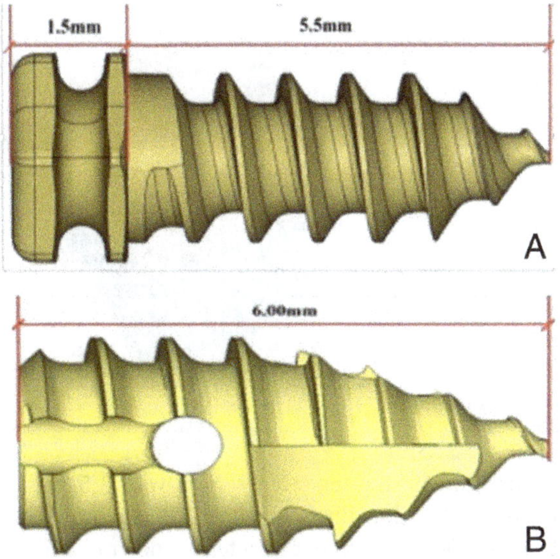

Fig. 1 The two types of anchoring nails. **a** Traditional anchoring nail. **b** Improved anchoring nail

Methods

Tensile test

Subjects

From April 2015 to June 2016, 10 patients (4 males and 6 females, aged 20–72 years old) undergoing TMJ replacement at the Department of Oral Surgery, the Ninth People's Hospital Affiliated to Shanghai Jiaotong University School of Medicine were selected. Condyle specimens were collected, wrapped with wool yarn immersed in normal saline, and preserved at − 20 °C. This study was approved by the Ethics Committee of Shanghai Jiao-Tong University School of Medicine.

Anchoring nails

Both traditional and improved anchoring nails (Cixi City Cibei Dental Instrument Co., Ltd., Cixi, Zhejiang, China) were made of titanium alloy. The total length of the

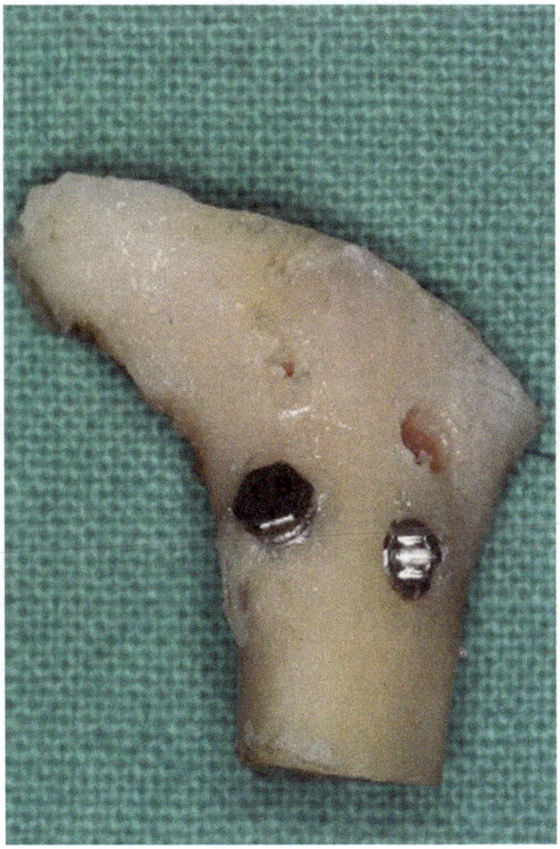

Fig. 2 Condyle specimen. Traditional and modified anchoring nails were implanted in the condyle

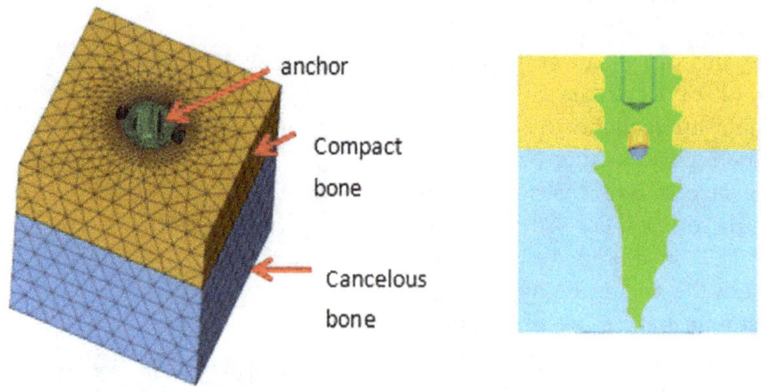

Fig. 3 Finite element computer-aided design model

traditional anchoring nail was 7 mm, with 1.5 mm nut thicknesses, 5.5 mm thread length, 2.8 mm nut diameters, and 2.0 mm thread diameters. The transition between the head and thread was smooth and a groove was designed for the knotting of the suture, which can only be fixed with a 3–0 suture (Fig. 1a). The improved anchoring nail had a length of 6 mm and a diameter of 3.0 mm. There was a small hole in the upper-middle part of the anchoring nail, with two grooves connected to the head. The upper part of the grooves was smooth for the placing and knotting of the suture (Fig. 1b).

Sutures

In this study, 3–0 and 2–0 nylon sutures (Ethibond *Excel, Green Braided Polyester Suture, Ethicon, Inc.) were used. The sutures were 90 cm in length with one suture needle at each end. Each suture was divided into two in the middle.

Implantation procedure

Traditional and improved anchoring nails were implanted 10–15 mm below the inferior margin of the posterior inclined plane of the condylar process. The two anchoring nails were placed symmetrically and the distance between them was more than 3 mm (Fig. 2).

Tensile test

A tension meter ((Cixi City Cibei Dental Instrument Co., Ltd., Cixi, Zhejiang, China) was used for tensile tests. In the lower part, specimens were immobilized with steel wires to a clamping board. In the upper part, the suture was directly immobilized to the clamping board.

Statistical analysis

SPSS 17.0 software (Chicago, IL, USA) was used for statistical analysis. The maximum bearable tension forces of the sutures were analyzed by descriptive statistics and reported as $x \pm s.\ d.$ The difference in tension readings between the two sutures used for the traditional anchoring nail was compared using a *t*-test. (The traditional anchoring nail does not match a 2–0 suture.) The difference in tension readings between the two sutures used for the improved anchoring nail was compared using a Kruskal-Wallis test. $P < 0.05$ was considered significant.

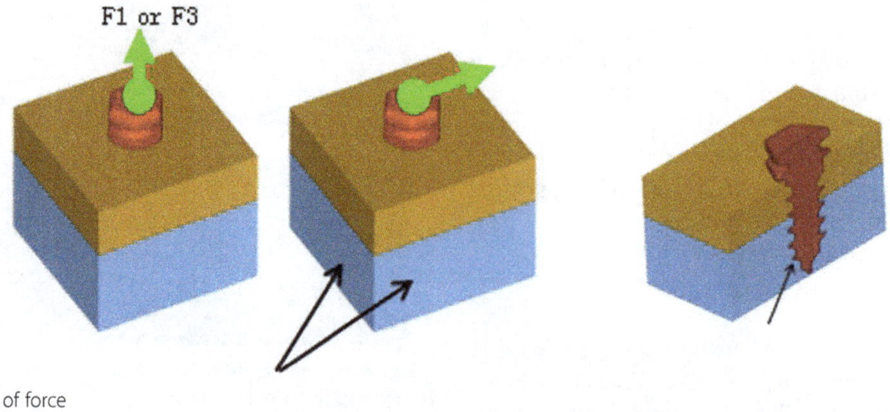

Fig. 4 Three types of force

Table 1 Mean maximum bearable tension forces of sutures under different conditions (*N*, x ± s)

Suture	Number of measurements	Mean maximum bearable tension force (F/N)	Range (F/N)
3–0 suture	20	28.74 ± 3.52	21.15~ 34.17
Conventional anchor nail (with 3–0 suture)	20	27.53 ± 5.47	17.84~ 37.80
Improved anchor nail (with 3–0 suture)	20	25.89 ± 2.64	21.32~ 33.83
Improved anchor nail (with 2–0 suture)	20	50	≥50
2–0 suture	20	50	≥50

Finite element analysis

FEA tool

We used three-dimensional modeling software (Hypermesh, Altair Engineering Inc.) and analysis programs (LS-DYNA, LSTC Inc.) to regulate the network structure and make it more homogeneous, create the solid model, and conduct the stress analysis using the finite element procedure.

Finite element model

A three-dimensional computer-aided design model of the anchoring nails was established and used as the mesh model for the FEA. The finite element model consisted of a first-order tetrahedral mesh, a total of 139,000 units, and 29,000 nodes. (Fig. 3).

Data processing

The FEA results are a stress result accumulated gradually by deformation. Consequently, FEA transforms an engineering stress–strain curve to a true stress–strain curve. The formulae for the transformation are as follows:

True stress = (1 + engineering strain) × engineering stress.

True strain = ln(1 + engineering strain).

Process

The directions of force, including vertical, level, and vertical rotation forces, were selected according to previous studies on TMJ disk movement [15–17]. The main stress point of the anchoring nail was analyzed by FEM.(Fig. 4).

Results

Neither fracture of the cortical bone nor fracture or loosening of the anchoring nails occurred during the implantation, and the anchoring nails were all successfully implanted into the cortical bone of the condylar process. Only sutures were damaged during the tensile tests, and neither the anchoring nails nor the cortical bone were damaged. As the 2–0 suture used for the improved anchoring nail was still not fractured at the maximum tension reading on the tension meter of 50 N, the tensile strength was recorded as above 50 N (Table 1).

According to the FEA of the traditional anchoring nail in condyle, the total vertical force is 481.467 N (Fig. 5), the total level force is 261.587 N (Fig. 6), and the total vertical rotation force is 48.2 N. Therefore, the total force of the traditional nail is 48.2 N. For the improved anchoring nail, the total vertical force is 795.88 N (Fig. 7), the total vertical force is 516 N (Fig. 8) and the total vertical rotation force is 200 N. Therefore, the total force of the improved nail is 200 N, which is twice that of the

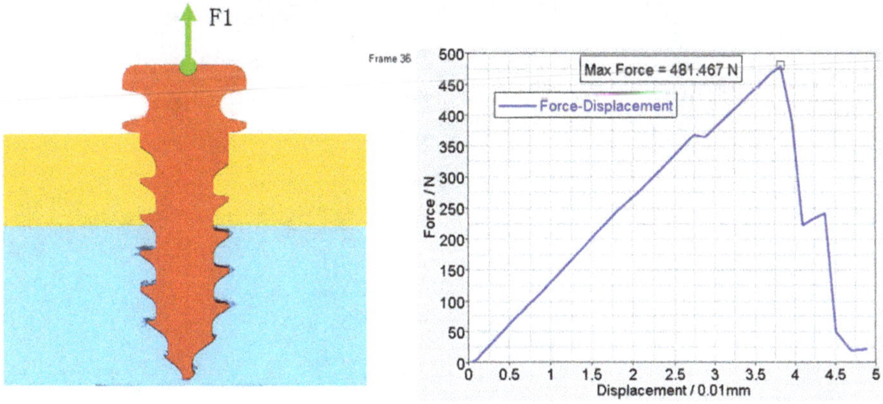

Fig. 5 The total vertical force of the traditional anchoring nail is 481.467 N

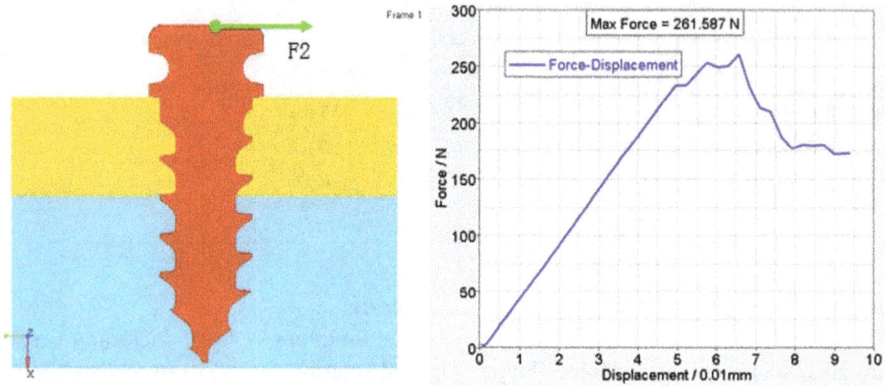

Fig. 6 The total level force of the traditional anchoring nail is 261.6 N

traditional anchoring nail. In the FEA of the different anchoring nail, regardless of the direction the force, the main force points are in the condylar cortical bone rather than the cancellous bone (Fig. 9).

Discussion

Common applications of anchoring nails include repair of the medial canthal ligament, muscle reattachment, TMJ disc repositioning, and other craniofacial surgery [17–19]. Mehra and Wolford [9](2001) reported the first case of using MiTek anchoring nails to reposition the TMJ disc, which achieved good clinical outcomes. However, the specimens they used were from non-living patients. Therefore, the bones had a lower bone density, higher brittleness, and higher risk of fractures, compared with bones taken from living patients, which was the main reason for the frequent bone damage observed. In the tensile test, we performed a control study by implanting the different types of nails in the same fresh specimen to exclude the effect of individual variations and to mimic the real clinical situation. The force applied in the tensile tests was parallel to the long axis of the anchoring nail and the minimum pull-out force was above 50 N. The improved anchoring nail was superior to the traditional anchoring nail.

Both of the anchoring nails used by Mehra and Wolford were implanted into the cortical bone after using a special puncher. If rejection occurs or the anchoring nails are deformed, damaged or misplaced, it is very difficult and traumatic to remove them. Furthermore, a few patients using traditional anchoring nails complained of discomfort in the anterior wall of the external auditory canal, which may be related to the protrusion of the anchoring nail nut. We modified the design of the anchoring nail based on MiTek anchoring nails and the anchoring nails used by He et al. [11](2015). The improved anchoring nail is much easier to implant and extract.

Tensile tests were conducted for the traditional and improved anchoring nails. It was found that the maximum tensile strength of the sutures used in the different anchoring nails varied. For the 3–0 suture, the *t*-test indicated a significant difference in tensile strength between the improved and traditional anchoring nails ($P =$

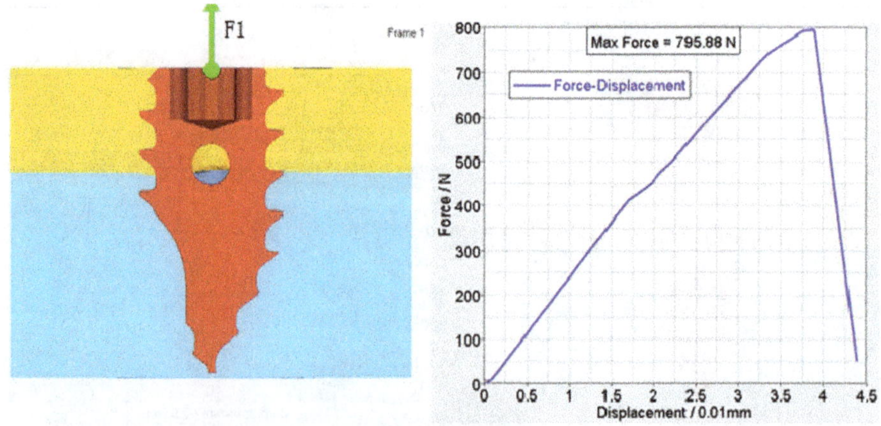

Fig. 7 The total vertical force of the improved anchoring nail is 795.88 N

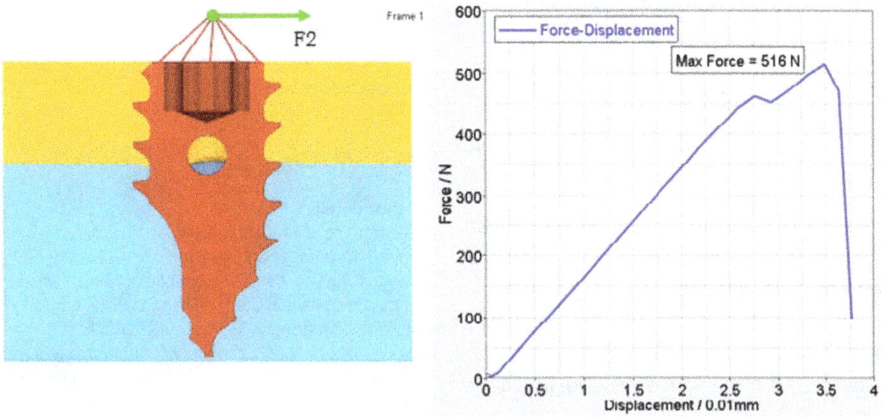

Fig. 8 The total vertical force of the improved anchoring nail is 516 N

0.033–< 0.05). The tensile strength of the conventional anchoring nail with a 3–0 suture was higher than that of the improved anchoring nail with a 3–0 suture. The Kruskal-Wallis test showed that the difference was significant between the 3–0 and 2–0 sutures (P = 0.000–< 0.1). Therefore, the improved anchoring nail with a 2–0 suture was superior to the traditional and improved anchoring nails with a 3–0 suture (Table 2). After implantation, the tensile strength of the 3–0 suture did not vary considerably between the different anchoring nails, and the maximum tensile strength of the sutures in the different anchoring nails was generally smaller than the modulus of elasticity of the sutures. The method of tying sutures to the anchoring nails had little impact on the tensile strength of the sutures.

Compared with larger-suture anchoring nails used in plastic surgery [19] the two anchoring nails in our study had a lower retention force. Other studies have generally been conducted in swine thighbones or in other places in the human body where the bone density is higher. The cortical bone is thicker and the contact area of the anchoring nails was greater. Our measurements indicated that the retention force of the improved anchoring nails was above 50 N, which is higher than the lowest value reported in the above studies. Moreover, the length of the improved anchoring nail embedded in the cortical bone and the thread diameter was larger compared with the traditional anchoring nail.

In the analysis of the finite element model of the two types of anchoring nails, the force and form are given the same analysis. Moreover, we avoided the influence of condylar origin. When the vertical force is applied, the longitudinal pulling out force is often relatively larger compared with the considerable frictional force, due to the limited axial rotation of the anchoring nail. As for the horizontal force, an inversely proportional relationship existed between the lateral force size and force arm L. As the anchoring nail is an asymmetric structure, the lateral pull-out force would be slightly different following the change of lateral forces. When the vertical pull-out force is applied, it is assumed that the coefficient of friction between the anchoring nail and the bone is close to infinity. Furthermore, as both the anchoring nail and the bone have small coefficients of friction, the

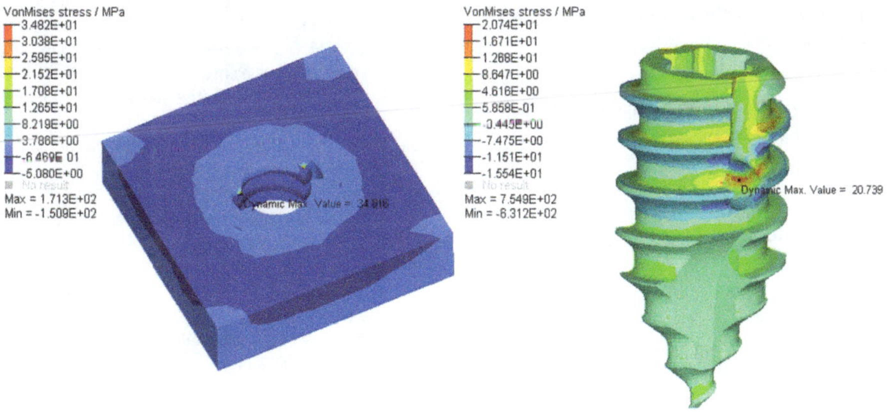

Fig. 9 The stress distribution between the cortical bone and the anchoring nail

Table 2 Comparison of tension forces between traditional and improved anchoring nails

Group	Conventional anchor nail (3–0)/ improved anchor nail (3–0)	Improved anchor nail (2–0)/ conventional anchor nail (3–0)
F (N)	27.53 ± 5.47/25.89 ± 2.64	50/27.53 ± 5.47
P value	0.033	0.000

anchoring nail is mainly planted in the weaker intrinsic bone, which can barely resist anchoring nail rotation. Hence, a small longitudinal tension can make the anchoring nail come out. In the experiment, we used two types of anchoring nail under identical conditions to effectively simulate the actual situation of anchoring nails under stress.

Despite the advantages of this study, there are still some disadvantages. The sample size is small and we aim to enlarge the sample size to obtain more precise results. Moreover, we only performed this study in vitro. In this regard, we aim to verify the effectiveness in vivo and, eventually, in a clinical study.

Conclusion

Both traditional and improved anchoring nails can be successfully implanted into the condyle without fracture of the anchoring nail or destruction of the cortical bone. The improved anchoring nail can resist a stronger pulling-out force compared with the traditional anchoring nail. It can be fixed with 2–0 suture, which substantially improves its resistance ability. It is also more convenient compared with a Mitek anchoring nail in terms of the implant and extraction processes [9].By conducting tensile tests and FEA of the two anchoring nails in the mandibular condyle, we conclude that the improved anchoring nail has better resistance ability compared with the traditional anchoring nail. The improved anchoring nail has the potential for clinical application; however, further research in animals and clinical experience is required.

Abbreviations

FEA: Finite element analysis; FEM: Finite element analysis; TMD: Temporomandibular joint disorder; TMJ: Temporomandibular joint

Acknowledgments

We would like to thank the native English speaking scientists of Elixigen Company (Huntington Beach, California) for editing our manuscript.

Funding

This work was supported by a grant form the Clinical Research Program of 9th People's Hospital, Shanghai Jiao Tong University School of Medicine.

Authors' contributions

SYZ was responsible for the analysis and interpretation of the data; XZC and XWC recorded the data; SFS and YXW built the 3-D model; JZZ collected samples; ZHZ was responsible for the conception, design of the study and critical revision of the manuscript. All authors read the final version of the manuscript and approved the publication of this article.

Competing interest

The authors declare that they have no competing interests.

Author details

[1]Department of Oral and Maxillofacial Surgery, School of Medicine, Ninth People's Hospital, Shanghai Jiao Tong University, 639 Zhi Zao Ju Road, Shanghai 200011, People's Republic of China. [2]Department of Stomatology, Tongren Hospital Affiliated to Shanghai Jiao Tong University School of Medicine, Shanghai 200336, People's Republic of China. [3]Department of Oral Surgery, Shanghai Key Laboratory of Stomatology & Shanghai Research Institute of Stomatology, College of Stomatology, Ninth People's Hospital, Shanghai Jiao Tong University School of Medicine, No. 639, Zhi-Zao-Ju Road, 200011 Shanghai, People's Republic of China.

References

1. Schiffman EL, Friction JR, Haley DP, Shapiro BL. The prevalence and treatment needs of subjects with temporomandibular disorders. Am Dent Assoc. 1990;120:295–303.
2. Dionne RA. Pharmacologic treatments for temporomandibular disorders. Oral Surg Oral Med Oral Pathol Oral Radiol Endod. 1997;83:134–42.
3. Okeson JP, Moody PM, Kemper JT, et al. Evaluation of occlusal splint therapy. J cranio-mandibular Pract. 1983;1:47.
4. Dominique Royle M. TMJ disorders – management of the craniomandibular complex. Physiotherapy 1988, 74:590–590.
5. Mercuri LG, Giobbie-Hurder A. Long-term outcomes after total alloplastic temporomandibular joint reconstruction following exposure to failed materials. J Oral Maxillofac Surg. 2004;62:1088–96.
6. Wilkes CH. Internal derangements of the temporomandibular joint. Pathological variations. Arch Otolaryngol Head Neck Surg. 1989;115(115): 469–77.
7. Zhang S, Liu X, Yang X, et al. Temporomandibular joint disc repositioning using bone anchors: an immediate post surgical evaluation by magnetic resonance imaging. BMC Musculoskelet Disord. 2010;11:262.
8. Kerstens HC, Tuinzing DB, Wa VDK. Eminectomy and discoplasty for correction of the displaced temporomandibular joint disc. J Oral Maxillofac Surg. 1989;47:150–2.
9. Mehra P, Wolford LM. Use of the MITEK anchor in temporomandibular joint disc-repositioning surgery. Proceedings. 2001;14:22.
10. Spallaccia F, Rivaroli A, Basile E, et al. Disk repositioning surgery of the temporomandibular joint with bioabsorbable anchor. J Craniofac Surg. 2013; 24:1792–5.
11. He D, Yang C, Zhang S, et al. Modified Temporomandibular Joint Disc Repositioning With Miniscrew Anchor: Part I—Surgical Technique. J Oral Maxillofac Surg. 2015;73(1):47.e1–9.
12. Li H, Sun S, Fan B, Shen P, Zheng J, Zhang S. Prevention of adhesions in the temporomandibular joint by the use of chitosan membrane in goats ☆. Br J Oral Maxillofac Surg. 2017;55(1):26–30.
13. Roarth CM, Grosland NM. Adaptive meshing technique applied to an orthopaedic finite element contact problem. Iowa Orthop J. 2004;24:21–9.
14. Thresher KW, Saito GE. The stress analysis of humal teeth. J Biomech. 1973;6:443.
15. Tanaka E, Van ET. Biomechanical behavior of the temporomandibular joint disc. Crit Rev Oral Biol Med. 2003;14:138–50.
16. Koolstra JH, van Eijden TM. Combined finite-element and rigid-body analysis of human jaw joint dynamics. J Biomech. 2005;38:2431–9.
17. Liu Z, Fan Y, Qian Y. Comparative evaluation on three-dimensional finite element models of the temporomandibular joint. Clin Biomech. 2008;23:S53.
18. Barnes SJ, Coleman SG, Gilpin D. Repair of avulsed insertion of biceps. A new technique in four cases. J Bone Joint Surg Br. 1993;75:938.
19. Farrall LA. Arthroscopic rotator cuff repairs using suture anchors. AORN J. 1995;62:737–50.

20

Effects of dynamic aging on the wear and fracture strength of monolithic zirconia restorations

Işıl Sarıkaya* and Yeliz Hayran

Abstract

Background: The purpose of this study is to evaluate the wear and fracture strength of crowns and three-unit partial fixed dental prosthesis (FDP) fabricated using by Bruxzir and Incoris TZI as recently introduced monolithic zirconia materials.

Methods: A total of sixteen crowns and sixteen three-unit FDPs were fabricated using Bruxzir and Incoris TZI ($n = 8$). All specimens were subjected to a 2-body wear test in a dual axis chewing simulator for 1,200,000 loading cycles against steatite antagonist balls. The fracture strength and volumetric loss were recorded. The obtained data were statistically analyzed by 2-way ANOVA testing ($\alpha = 0.05$).

Results: The mean volumetric loss of the crowns was higher than that of the three-unit FDPs ($p < 0.05$). Of the two monolithic systems, Incoris TZI exhibited more wear than Bruxzir. The fracture strengths of Bruxzir crowns and FDPs were found to be higher than those of the crowns and FDPs fabricated with Incoris TZI ($p < 0.05$).

Conclusion: In in vitro test conditions, Bruxzir and Incoris TZI monolithic zirconia systems are fracture-resistant for the crown and FDP application against physiologic chewing forces owing to dynamic aging. Among newly developed monolithic zirconia materials, Bruxzir is found to be more resistant to fracture compared to the Incoris TZI.

Keywords: Dynamic aging, Fracture strength, Monolithic zirconia, Wear

Background

Esthetic expectations are the main reason for preferring ceramic restorations, for which the usual processing method is veneering. Major problems associated with multilayered restorations are their low fracture strength and surface chipping. Therefore, new processing techniques have been developed to resolve the chipping problem encountered with ceramic veneering layers [1]. For example, to eliminate the porosity generated within the veneering layer, injection of porcelain over the zirconia framework can be carried out [1]. In addition, CAD-on and rapid layer techniques have become popular in recent years in prosthetic dentistry. Developments in CAD-CAM (computer-aided design, and computer-aided manufacturing) technology have also increased the diversity of materials that can be used for restorations. In this context, new materials, such as PICN (polymer infiltrated ceramic network) materials and monolithic ceramics, are available today for use.

Monolithic restorations aim at improving the final quality of restorations. Further, the problems of surface flaws and chipping problems encountered with veneering can be resolved using monolithic zirconia restorations [2]. Zirconia restorations exhibit good mechanical properties, such as high flexural strength along with good esthetic characteristics and biocompatibility. In order to achieve good results with restorations, the wear properties of restorations should be similar to those of human enamel [3]. Furthermore, restorations should be conservative for antagonist dentition. Although short-term data is available on high-strength zirconia systems, research is still needed on periodontally weakened teeth and bruxism [2].

Physiologic chewing forces are in the range of 10–120 N, while parafunctional forces are greater in the range of 200–800 N [4–8] which both affect biomaterial

* Correspondence: sarikayaisil@gmail.com
Department of Prosthodontics, Tokat Gaziosmanpasa University Faculty of Dentistry, 60100 Tokat, Turkey

survival. Apart from the chewing characteristics and force configuration, clinical parameters, such as moisture, temperature, and pH, also influence the mechanical properties and behavior of materials in the oral cavity [9]. Since the 1940s, chewing-mimicking devices are being used for determining the occlusal wear of restorative materials [10]. Various in-vitro wear tests have been developed to simulate clinical conditions since then. The dual-axis chewing simulator developed by Willytech is often considered as a precise instrument for the fatigue testing of dental materials [10]; several research groups have investigated the wear performance and fracture strength of ceramics with chewing simulators [11–20]. Even today, research is ongoing for new simulators for the preclinical testing of dental materials in vitro chewing simulation conditions [10, 16, 21].

Monolithic zirconia restorations are not preferred when the esthetic function is the priority. However, these systems are beneficial in the case of fixed dental prostheses supported by pathological attrition or severely damaged teeth (FDPs). Adhesive bonding of monolithic restorations is beneficial in various clinical situations, such as excessive unloading forces, compromised mechanical retention, and limited space for adequate tooth preparation [22]. Furthermore, the resin bonding of zirconia restorations is advocated for improving the fracture strength of restorations [22, 23].

The high fracture strength of yttria-stabilized zirconia (YSZ) is attributed to the physical properties of partially stabilized zirconia. In previous studies, the fracture strength of YSZ was reported to vary from 900 N [24] to 2000 N under static loading [25, 26].

Preclinical evaluations help to determine the physical and mechanical behavior of materials. Although the fatigue testing standards (DIN EN ISO 22674) of fixed dental prosthesis materials are established under certain test conditions, it is controversial how much of the intraoral conditions are accurately represented by these standards [27, 28]. Restoration fatigue behavior is required to provide reliable data on the strength characteristics of materials. Usually, universal testing machine data on the fatigue behavior of tested materials are used but oral thermal conditions are not included in this testing.

The aim of this in vitro study is to evaluate the wear and fracture strength of crowns and three-unit partial FDPs fabricated using recently introduced monolithic zirconia materials and subjecting them to 1,200,000 chewing cycle versus steatite balls. The null hypothesis tested was that no difference would be detected in the wear and fracture strength properties of different tested materials.

Methods

Preparation of specimens

In the present study, a mandibular left first molar tooth of the dentulous mandibular cast (Frasaco AG-3 GmbH, Tettnang, Germany) was selected for producing monolithic crown restorations. A mandibular left second premolar tooth (Frasaco AG-3 GmbH, Tettnang, Germany) and a mandibular left second molar tooth (Frasaco AG-3 GmbH, Tettnang, Germany) were selected for fabricating the FDPs. The selected teeth were prepared according to the accepted tooth preparation principles using a chamfer diamond rotary instrument (229-014XC Torpedo, Romidan, Kiryat-Ono, Israel) by adjusting for a 1 mm circumferential chamfer margin, 1.5 mm occlusal reduction, 1 mm axial preparation, and 6° convergence angle. After preparation, the master casts were evaluated using a surveyor to detect undercuts. The prepared teeth were then duplicated as master dies made of Ni-Cr by laser sintering. In total, thirty-two master model dies were obtained, including sixteen master casts that were made as crowns and sixteen master casts that were made as three-unit FDPs; the model dies were fabricated with Bruxzir (Glidewell Laboratories, CA, USA) and Incoris TZI (Sirona Dental Systems GmbH, Bensheim, Germany) ($n = 8$). Bruxzir crowns and three-unit FDPs were fabricated using monolithic zirconium blanks (Bruxzir Solid Zirconia Milling Blanks, 98,5 × 20 mm, Glidewell Laboratories, CA, USA) designed using a Cerec inLab MC X5 system (Sirona Dental Systems GmbH, Bensheim, Germany). Incoris TZI crowns and three-unit FDPs were fabricated from monolithic blocks (40/19 = 40x19x15.5 mm) and designed using a Cerec inLab MC X5 system (Sirona Dental Systems GmbH, Bensheim, Germany). The chemical composition, according to the manufacturer's declaration of investigated Y-TZP ceramics is shown in Table 1. A connector size of 9 mm^2 was selected for FDPs as recommended by the manufacturers. Bruxzir restorations were sintered at a temperature of 1580 °C for 2 h and then glazed with Bruxzir spray glaze powder (Glidewell Laboratories, CA, USA) at a temperature of 830 °C according to the manufacturer's instructions. Incoris TZI restorations were sintered at a temperature of 1510 °C for 2 h and then glazed with Cerec speed glaze spray (Sirona Dental Systems GmbH, Bensheim, Germany) at a temperature of 750 °C according to the manufacturer's instructions. All the restorations and preparations were carried out by the same dentist. Eight crowns and FDPs were created with the two different zirconia materials randomly.

Table 1 Chemical composition of the Y-TZP dental ceramics expressed as weight percent (wt.%)

Ceramic	wt.%						
	Y_2O_3	HfO_2	Al_2O_3	SiO_2	Fe_2O_3	Na_2O	ZrO_2
Bruxzir	4.1	4.0	0.34	< 0.01	< 0.01	< 0.01	Balance
Incoris TZI	4.5–6.0	< 5.0	< 0.05	< 0.05	< 0.05	< 0.05	Balance

Luting of the crowns

All the restorations were adhesively luted on Ni-Cr master cast dies using a dual cure composite material (Panavia F 2.0, Kuraray Medical Co., Tokyo, Japan) according to the manufacturer's instructions. The master cast dies were sun-blasted with 50 μm Al_2O_3 powder at an air pressure of 2.5 bar for 10 s. Equal amounts of Panavia Paste A and B (Panavia F 2.0, Kuraray Medical Co., Tokyo, Japan) were mixed and applied to the intaglio surfaces of the restorations according to the manufacturer's instructions. The restorations were seated onto the dies and held in place by the application of finger pressure. Subsequently, the restorations were cured using a curing light for 20 s. Excess cement was removed with sponge pellets before curing and an air-blocking gel (Oxiguard II, Kuraray Medical Co., Tokyo, Japan) was applied during the setting of the resin cement over 3 min. The obtained specimens were stored for 24 h at 37 °C before being subjected to dynamic aging.

Dynamic aging

All the root surfaces of the metal dies were coated with a 1 mm-thick polyether layer (Impregum Soft, 3 M Espe, St Paul, MN, USA) from the marginal finish line of the restorations to 2-mm apical direction for the purpose of simulating the physiologic mobility of teeth. The metal dies were immersed in a wax bath, which was replaced by polyether in a second fabrication process, as previously described (17,18). Later, restorations on master cast dies were fixed in a resin mold, which acts as the sample holder for the chewing simulator, using a self-curing acrylic resin material (Meliodent, Heraeus Kulzer, Wehrheim, Germany). The specimens underwent thermocycling for 10,000 cycles between 5 and 55 °C over a dwell time of 60 s and a transfer time of 10 s (SD Mechatronik Thermocycler, SD Mechatronik GmbH, Feldkirchen-Westerham, Germany). After thermocycling, the specimens were subjected to a 2-body wear test in a dual axis chewing simulator (CS 4.2, SD Mechatronic GmbH, Feldkirchen-Westerham, Germany). Steatite ceramic balls (Höchst Ceram Tec., Wunsiedel, Germany) of 6 mm diameter were used as the antagonistic abraders. The balls were fixed to the upper sample holders of the chewing simulator using a light-curing composite resin (GC Pattern Resin, GC Corp., Tokyo, Japan). The chewing simulation parameters used are summarized in Table 2. The load was transferred to the center of the central fossa of the mandibular first crowns by opposing steatite balls. To simulate 5 years of clinical service, a total of 1,200,000 cycles were performed (9,10,12). After a 3-dimensional surface analysis using a laser scanner (LAS 20, SD Mechatronic GmbH, Feldkirchen-Westerham, Germany), the volumetric loss (mm^3) in all the specimens was calculated (Fig. 1).

Table 2 The configuration of parameters set for dynamic aging

Parameter	Data
Number of cycles	1.200.000
Force	49 N
Height	3 mm
Lateral movement	1 mm
Descendent speed	60 mm/s
Lifting speed	60 mm/s
Feed speed	40 mm/s
Return speed	40 mm/s
Frequency	1.6 Hz

Fracture strength test

Following the aging procedure, the specimens were tested on a universal testing machine (AGS-X, Shimadzu, Kyoto, Japan) until fracture. They were subjected to a compressive force at a crosshead speed of 1 mm/min with a round shaped modified bur of 4 mm diameter. A metal bar was positioned parallel to the long axes of the crown specimens and the buccal and lingual cusps of the crowns were used to apply the force. Force was transferred to the occlusal connector area of the FDP specimens. The maximum load necessary to fracture each specimen was recorded in Newtons (N).

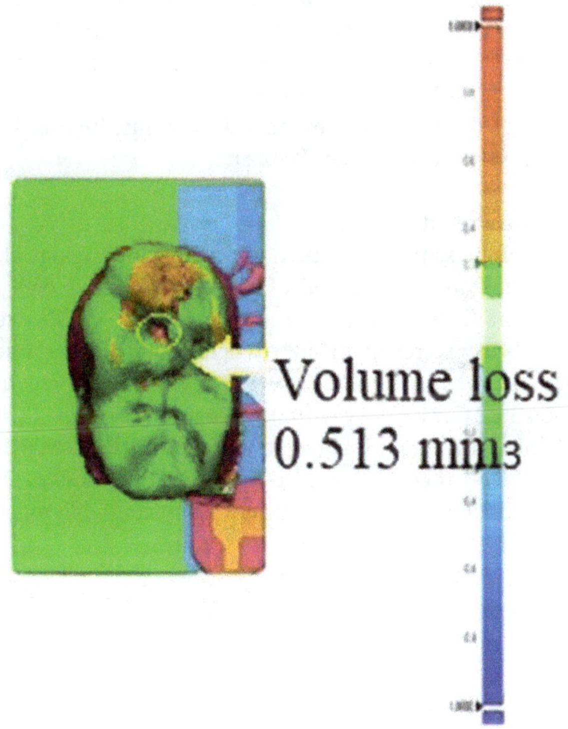

Fig. 1 Laser scanner image of the specimen's with 3-dimensional surface analysis, and the volumetric loss (mm^3)

SEM

To characterize the surface wear patterns, selected specimens were evaluated by a scanning electron microscopy (SEM, Zeiss LEO 440, Oberkochen, Germany), for which the sample surfaces were initially coated with a thin layer of gold. The surfaces were then examined at a magnification of 100X at 25 keV.

Statistical analysis

Statistical analysis was performed using SPSS 20.0 (IBM SPSS Statistics 20, IBM Co., Chicago, IL, USA) for Windows. Having assessed that all the obtained results were normally distributed, the wear and fracture load data were analyzed by two-way ANOVA. Bonferroni adjustment was used for multiple comparisons. Two methods and two monolithic zirconias were used for 4 groups with 80% power, 5% margin of error and effect size of 0.65 with 8 samples in each group, totaling 32 samples. The sampling volume was obtained with the help of the program G * power 3.1.2. The results are expressed as a mean ± standard deviation and the level of significance is set at 5% ($p < 0.05$).

Results

Wear

The mean volumetric loss (mm^3) of the monolithic zirconia specimens is shown in Table 3. Two-way ANOVA showed no statistically significant differences when the wear values of Bruxzir and Incoris TZI crowns after 1,200,000 chewing cycles were analyzed ($F = 10.874$ and $p = 0.003$). The mean volumetric loss of the crowns was observed to be higher than that of three-unit FDPs ($p < 0.05$). Of the two tested monolithic systems, Incoris TZI exhibited more wear than Bruxzir.

Fracture strength

None of the samples fractured during dynamic aging. The mean fracture strength (N) of the monolithic zirconia is shown in Table 4. According to the two-way ANOVA results, Bruxzir crowns exhibited significantly higher fracture strengths (4495 ± 221.33 N) than Incoris TZI crowns (3566.5 ± 217.24 N) ($p < 0.05$). Moreover, Bruxzir FDPs exhibited significantly higher fracture strengths (4506.25 ± 166.44 N) than Incoris TZI FDPs (3327.13 ± 185.81 N) ($p < 0.05$). Besides, no statistically significant differences could be observed between the Bruxzir crowns and FDPs ($p > 0.05$). Representative SEM images of the Bruxzir and Incoris TZI crowns are shown in Fig. 2a and b.

Table 3 Mean values and standard deviations (SD) for volumetric loss (mm^3) of the monolithic zirconias

	Crowns	FDPs	Total
Bruxzir	1,43 ± 0,12(a,x)	1,15 ± 0,17(a,y)	1,29 ± 0,21(a)
Incoris TZI	1,55 ± 0,11(a,x)	1,37 ± 0,16(b,y)	1,46 ± 0,16(b)
Total	1,49 ± 0,13(x)	1,26 ± 0,2(y)	1,38 ± 0,2

Discussion

This in vitro study evaluated the wear and fracture strength of crowns and FDPs fabricated using two recently introduced monolithic zirconia materials. The null hypothesis tested in the present study, which assumed no difference in terms of the wear and fracture strength properties between the two tested materials, was rejected.

Zirconia has been developed with the aim of providing a stronger material for prosthetic dentistry. Ideal restorative materials should exhibit wear properties similar to those of human enamel and should not cause excess antagonist wear. Although short-term data is available on zirconia FDPs, a recent study showed that monolithic polished zirconia crowns caused less wear on antagonist enamel than glazed ceramic metal crowns [29]. In a study on the wear properties of dental ceramics, D'Archangelo et al. [15] reported that the volumetric loss values of IPS e.max Press (0.459 mm^3), IPS e.max CAD (0.355 mm^3), and Vita Mark II (0.472 mm^3) were similar to that of human enamel (0.393 mm^3). However, in the present study, 6 mm-thick disk-shaped specimens and a zirconia antagonist abrader were used. Moreover, the ceramic materials tested in this study exhibited lower hardness than Bruxzir and Incoris TZI monolithic systems.

Parafunctional chewing forces are approximately ten times greater than physiologic chewing forces [4–8]. Day bruxism is reported to affect 20% of the adult population and this number has increased over the past few decades [30]. In patients with bruxism, occlusal wear might be severe and fracture risk of the prosthesis might increase. Therefore, high strength restorative materials resistant to wear and fracture might be required, especially in the posterior region. However, the selected material should not cause temporomandibular joint disorders (TMJ) or increase the degree of dysfunction. Both the monolithic zirconia materials tested in the present study exhibited minimal volumetric loss at their ultimate strength.

The dynamic aging and fracture resistance of monolithic zirconia systems were determined by loading crowns and three-unit FDPs using an SD mechatronic chewing simulator (CS 4.2, SD Mechatronic GmbH). Heintze et al. [16] reported that the SD mechatronic chewing simulator is an adequate and cost-effective tool to test the fatigue strength of layered porcelain fused to metal crowns. The fracture strengths of 3-unit FDPs of different all-ceramic materials were tested using different forces up to 200 N [31–35]. Functional chewing forces were applied to the specimens (49 N) during the fracture

Table 4 Mean values and standard deviations (SD) for fracture load (N) of the monolithic zirconias

	Crowns	FDPs	Total
Bruxzir	4495,00 ± 221,33(a,x)	4507,25 ± 166,44(a,x)	4501,13 ± 189,29(a)
Incoris TZI	3566,5 ± 217,24(b,x)	3327,13 ± 185,81(b,y)	3446,81 ± 231,12(b)
Total	4030,75 ± 524,2(x)	3917,19 ± 632,79(y)	3973,97 ± 574,49

strength test in the present study. The chewing force and characteristics can be changed individually [21]. Under bruxism conditions, teeth are subjected to larger forces over large lateral movement distances [13]. In terms of force configuration, dynamic aging analysis conducted in the present study was carried out in a manner similar to previous studies considering regular occlusal forces and bruxism [10, 15, 16].

It has been reported that almost all materials that have any geometrical shape such as composite, natural teeth, metal, ceramic or steatite can be examined with LAS 20 laser scanner [36]. Advanced users have the possibility to configure many sensor parameters. This includes, for example, median filtering in order to better highlight structures or the setting of the measurement gain in order to maintain the penetration depth of light into the material – and as such the scatter – as low as possible. This allows even the most difficult surfaces such as high gloss ceramics to be analyzed. After laser scanning, the Geomagic Software System allows us to import and export in different CAD data formats and analysis can be carried out beforehand/after comparison scans with matching, 3D-comparison, and 3D-PDFs. 3D analysis of the two scans along with abrasion depth can be seen on a color scale. Preis et al. [14] investigated the two-body wear performance of monolithic dental ceramics subjected to different surface treatments. They determined the vertical substance loss of different CAD/CAM ceramics and used a Laserscan 3D device as an optical profilometer. D'Archangelo et al. [15] used a CAD/CAM Contact Scanner for 3D surface analysis, wear depth, and volumetric loss of ceramics. Laser scanning in prosthetic dentistry is usually used to investigate marginal and internal fit of crown restorations [37]. In the present study, 3D laser images were supported by SEM images.

D'Archangelo et al. [15] reported that when human enamel cusps are used in vitro as antagonistic abraders, standardization of the study might be weak. In this context, steatite balls have been successfully used in the past [14, 17–19]. However, steatite balls cannot accurately mimic the complex enamel structure [14]. In order to overcome this disadvantage of the material, the steatite balls with the closest hardness property to enamel were used in the present study.

On the basis of the obtained findings, almost all the tested monolithic zirconia materials exhibited high load strengths. In a previous study, the fracture strength of YSZ was reported to be in the range of 900–1200 N [24]. In another study, the fracture strength of YSZ-FDPs was reported to be over 2000 N under static loading [25]. Eroğlu et al. [26] studied the fatigue behavior of zirconia-ceramic and reported a fracture strength of 2333 N for three-unit FPDs. Each specimen was subjected to 100,000 chewing cycles at a 50 N load and a 0.5 Hz frequency on the pontic with a 16 mm^2 connector size. No specimen fractured during dynamic loading, similar to the present study. The dimensions of the connector area are crucial for determining the strength of FDPs. In the current study, a connector size of 9 mm^2 was selected according to the manufacturer's suggestion.

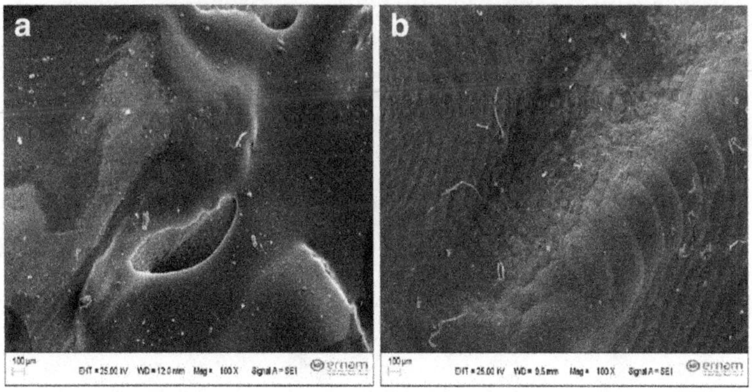

Fig. 2 **a** Exemplary SEM picture (Magnification: 100×) of worn surface of a Bruxzir crown after dynamic aging. **b** Exemplary SEM picture (Magnification: 100×) of worn surface of an Incoris TZI crown after dynamic aging

Apart from the connector design [38], the fracture strength of three-unit FDPs is affected by several factors, such as the FDP location [12], tested chewing parameters, die materials [38], and used antagonist abraders [16]. In the present study, all the monolithic crowns and FDPs were adhesively luted on standardized laser sintering milled-Ni-Cr metal dies instead of polymethyl methacrylate (PMMA) dies. Further, dynamic aging defined in the present study was carried out in a manner similar to previous studies [10, 15, 16, 31, 34].

The major limitation of this study is the difficulty of determining the ideal chewing cycle. In this regard, Özcan and Jonasch [20], in a systematic review on the mechanical durability of all-ceramic single crowns and FDPs, reported that cyclic loading of restorations reduced the material-specific inclination and static fracture strength. However, there is no information on the fracture strength of the currently studied monolithic zirconia crowns and three-unit FDPs in the literature.

A second limitation of the present study is the lack of a secondary higher force against Bruxzir. Considering that Bruxzir material was originally produced against bruxism, bruxzir would have exhibited more strength than 49 N. However, the applied force in the present study was 49 N which is accepted as a normal chewing force in the posterior region, was used for Bruxzir and Incoris TZI restorations. Further studies may be carried out considering chewing forces specific for bruxers.

Conclusions

Based on the findings of this in vitro study, both the monolithic zirconia crowns showed a small but significantly increased volumetric loss compared to three-unit FDPs. Of the two tested monolithic systems, Incoris TZI exhibited greater wear than Bruxzir. The fracture strengths of Bruxzir crowns and FDPs were found to be greater than those of their counterparts fabricated with Incoris TZI. Bruxzir and Incoris TZI monolithic zirconia systems were found to be fracture-resistant for crowns and FDPs against physiologic chewing forces owing to dynamic aging in vitro test conditions.

Abbreviations

%: Percent; 3D: 3-Dimensional; FDP: Fixed dental prosthesis; g: Gram; h: Hour; min: Minute; ml: Milliliter; mm: Millimeter; mm^3: Cubic millimeter; N: Newton; rpm: Revolutions per minute; wt: Weight

Funding

This study was supported by 2014/82 number project by the Gaziosmanpasa University Scientific Research Projects Unit with the used materials.

Role of funder

This study has been supported by only the materials used in the study by Gaziosmanpasa University Scientific Research Projects Unit. Any financial support has not been provided for publication of the study results.

Authors' contributions

IS; Study conception and design, Acquisition of data, Analysis and interpretation of data, Drafting of the manuscript. YH; Study conception and design, Acquisition of data, Analysis and interpretation of data, Critical revision. Both authors read and approved the final manuscript.

Competing interests

The authors declare that they have no competing interests.

References

1. Silva LHD, Lima E, Miranda RBP, Favero SS, Lohbauer U, Cesar PF. Dental ceramics: a review of new materials and processing methods. Braz Oral Res. 2017;28(31):e58. https://doi.org/10.1590/1807-3107BOR-2017.vol31.0058.
2. Raut A, Rao PL, Ravindranath T. Zirconium for esthetic rehabilitation: an overview. Indian J Dent Res. 2011;22:140–3.
3. Seghi RR, Rosenstial SF, Bauer P. Abrasion of human enamel by different dental ceramics in vitro. J Dent Res. 1991;70:221–5.
4. De Boever JA, McCall WDJ, Holden S, Ash MMJ. Functional occlusal forces: an investigation by telemetry. J Prosthet Dent. 1978;40:326–33.
5. Schindler HJ, Stengel E, Spiess WE. Feedback control during mastication of solid food textures- a clinical experimental study. J Prosthet Dent. 1998;80: 330–6.
6. Nishigawa K, Bando E, Nakano M. Quantitative study of bite force during sleep associated bruxism. J Oral Rehabil. 2001;28:485–91.
7. Kohyama K, Hatakeyama E, Sasaki T, Dan H, Azuma T, Karita K. Effects of sample hardness on human chewing force: a model study using silicone rubber. Arch Oral Biol. 2004;49:805–16.
8. Cosme DC, Baldisserotto SM, Canabarro SA, Shinkai RS. Bruxism and voluntary maximal bite force in young dentate adults. Int J Prosthodont. 2005;18:328–32.
9. DeLong R, Douglas WH. An artificial oral environment for testing dental materials. IEEE Trans Biomed Eng. 1991;38:339–45.
10. Kern M, Strub JR, Lü XY. Wear of composite resin veneering materials in a dual-axis chewing simulator. J Oral Rehabil. 1999;26:372–8.
11. Delong R, Douglas WH. Development of an artificial oral environment for testing of dental restoratives: biaxial force and movement control. J Dent Res. 1983;62:32–6.
12. Kheradmandan S, Koutayas SO, Bernhard M, Strub JR. Fracture strength of four different types of anterior 3-unit bridges after thermomechanical fatigue in the dual-axis chewing simulator. J Oral Rehabil. 2001;28:361–9.
13. Heintze SD, Albrecht T, Cavalleri A, Steiner M. A new method to test the fracture probability of all-ceramic crowns with a dual-axis chewing simulator. Dent Mater. 2011;27:10–9.
14. Preis V, Weiser F, Handel G, Rosentritt M. Wear performance of monolithic dental ceramics with different surface treatments. Quintessence Int. 2013;44: 393–405.
15. D'Arcangelo C, Vanini L, Rondoni GD, Pirani M, Vadini M, Gattone M, et al. Wear properties of dental ceramics and porcelains compared with human enamel. J Prosthet Dent. 2016;115:350–5.
16. Heintze SD, Eser A, Monreal D, Rousson V. Using a chewing simulator for fatigue testing of metal ceramic crowns. J Mech Behav Biomed Mater. 2017; 65:770–80.
17. Rosentritt M, Behr M, Gebhard R, Handel G. Influence of stress simulation parameters on the fracture strength of all-ceramic fixed-partial dentures. Dent Mater. 2006;22:176–82.
18. Rosentritt M, Behr M, Scharnagl P, Handel G, Kolbeck C. Influence of resilient support of abutment teeth on fracture resistance of all-ceramic fixed partial dentures: an in-vitro study. Int J Prosthodont. 2011;24:465–8.
19. Stappert CF, Att W, Gerds T, Strub JR. Fracture resistance of different partial-coverage ceramic molar restorations: An in vitro investigation. J Am Dent Assoc. 2006;137:514–22.
20. Özcan M, Jonasch M. Effect of cyclic fatigue tests on aging and their translational implications for survival of all-ceramic tooth-borne single crowns and fixed dental prostheses. J Prosthodont. 2016;23 https://doi.org/10.1111/jopr.12566.
21. Singhatanagit W, Junkaev P, Singhatanagit P. Effect of bidirectional loading on contact and force characteristics under a newly developed masticatory simulator with a dual-direction loading system. Dent Mater J. 2016;35:952–61.

22. Rosenstiel SF, Land MF, Crispin BJ. Dental luting agents: a review of current literature. J Prosthet Dent. 1998;80:280–301.
23. Burke FJ, Fleming GJ, Nathanson D, Marquis PM. Are adhesive technologies needed to support ceramics? An assessment of the current evidence. J Adhes Dent. 2002;4:7–22.
24. Raigrodski A. Contemporary materials and technologies for all-ceramic fixed partial dentures: a review of the literature. J Prosthet Dent. 2001;92:557–62.
25. Tinschert J, Zwez D, Marx R, Anusavice KJ. Structural reliability of alumina, feldspar, leucite, mica, and zirconia-based ceramics. J Dent. 2000;28:529–35.
26. Eroğlu Z, Gurbulak AG. Fatigue behavior of zirconia-ceramic, Galvano-ceramic, and porcelain-fused-to-metal fixed partial dentures. J Prosthodont. 2013;22:516–22.
27. DIN EN ISO 22674 Norm. Metallic materials for fixed and removable restoration application. Berlin: DIN, German Institute for Norming; 2006.
28. Kelly JR, Benetti P, Rungruanganunt P, Bona AD. The slippery slope: critical perspectives on in vitro research methodologies. Dent Mater. 2012;28:41–51.
29. Mundhe K, Jain V, Pruthi G, Shah N. Clinical study to evaluate the wear of natural enamel antagonist to zirconia and metal ceramic crowns. J Prosthet Dent. 2015;114:358–63.
30. Bader G, Lavigne G. Sleep bruxism: an overview of an oromandibular sleep movement disorder. Sleep Med Rev. 2000;4:27–43.
31. Chitmongkolsuk S, Heydecke G, Stappert C, Strub JR. Fracture strength of all-ceramic lithium disilicate and porcelain-fused-to-metal bridges for molar replacement after dynamic loading. Eur J Prosthodont Restor Dent. 2002;10: 15–22.
32. Beuer F, Steff B, Naumann M, Sorensen JA. Load-bearing capacity of all-ceramic three-unit fixed partial dentures with different computer-aided design (CAD)/computer-aided manufacturing (CAM) fabricated framework materials. Eur J Oral Sci. 2008;116:381–6.
33. Kohorst P, Dittmer MP, Borchers L, Stiesch-Scholz M. Influence of cyclic fatigue in water on the load-bearing capacity of dental bridges made of zirconia. Acta Biomater. 2008;4:1140–7.
34. Schultheis S, Strub JR, Gerds TA, Guess PC. Monolithic and bi-layered CAD/ CAM lithium –disilicate versus metal-ceramic fixed dental prostheses: comparison of fracture loads and failure modes after fatigue. Clin Oral Invest. 2013;17:1407–13.
35. D'Arcangelo C, Vanini L, Rondoni GD, De Angelis F. Wear properties of a novel resin composite compared to human enamel and other restorative materials. Oper Dent. 2014;39:612–8.
36. PDF Brochure of SD Mechatronik Dental Research Equipment. http://www.cs-4.de/LAS20-en.pdf Accessed 16 Apr 2018.
37. Luthardt RG, Bornemann G, Lemelson S, Walter MH, Hüls A. An innovative method for evaluation of the 3-D internal fit of CAD/CAM crowns fabricated after direct optical versus indirect laser scan digitizing. Int J Prosthodont. 2004;17:680–5.
38. Oh W, Anusavice KJ. Effect of connector design on the fracture resistance of all-ceramic fixed partial dentures. J Prosthet Dent. 2002;87:536–42.

21

History of periodontal treatment and risk for intrauterine growth restriction (IUGR)

Cande V. Ananth[1,2], Howard F. Andrews[3,4], Panos N. Papapanou[5], Angela M. Ward[6], Emilie Bruzelius[2,6], Mary Lee Conicella[7] and David A. Albert[6*]

Abstract

Background: To explore the hypothesis that maternal periodontitis is associated with increased risk for Intrauterine Growth Restriction (IUGR), we examined the risk of IUGR in relation to periodontal treatment before, during and after pregnancy.

Methods: We conducted a retrospective cohort analysis of insurance claims data from 2009 to 2012 for women who delivered a singleton live birth ($n = 32{,}168$). IUGR was examined as a function of type and timing of dental treatment, adjusting for potential confounders in logistic regression. Sensitivity analysis evaluated the potential effects of unmeasured confounding.

Results: Women who received periodontal treatment after delivery, indicating the presence of untreated periodontal disease during pregnancy, had significantly higher odds of IUGR compared to women who received no periodontal treatment (adjusted OR 1.5, 95% CI 1.2, 1.8).

Conclusions: Periodontal treatment provided in the immediate postpartum period, a proxy for periodontitis during gestation, was associated with increased risk of IUGR.

Keywords: Periodontal treatment, Fetal inflammatory response, Intrauterine growth restriction

Background

In industrialized countries, about four-fifths of low birthweight infants are born preterm and a fifth of these preterm births are due to intrauterine growth restriction (IUGR) [1]. In the absence of congenital malformations and/or chromosomal anomalies, IUGR entails two distinct processes: constitutional smallness, or pathological growth restriction [2]. The prevalence of IUGR varies substantially across populations, but prevalence rates range between 3 and 7%. The etiology of IUGR remains undetermined, but several risk factors for the condition have been identified. These include advanced maternal age, increased parity, smoking during pregnancy, low pre-pregnancy body mass index and low gestational weight gain (due to low energy intake), short maternal stature, poor maternal nutrition, maternal race/ethnicity, and low socioeconomic status being some of the important risk factors [3]. Maternal, placental and fetal infections are strongly implicated in the development of IUGR.

Periodontal diseases are associated with transient bacteremia that may facilitate dissemination of oral bacteria to the uterus, with subsequent infiltration of the amniotic fluid and the umbilical cord and invasion of the placenta. It is believed that hematogenous transport of bacteria and/or pro-inflammatory mediators from sites of periodontal infection into the placenta, fetal membranes, and amniotic cavity induces pathological processes that lead to adverse perinatal outcomes, including IUGR [4–7]. Uteroplacental infection and inflammation are thought to play key roles in the etiology of IUGR [8], with fetal inflammatory response syndrome being characterized as the important cause of IUGR [9]. Collectively, these infections account for up to 15% of IUGR cases [10].

Periodontal infections are associated with an increased risk for adverse pregnancy outcomes, including preterm delivery, and preeclampsia, but whether this increased

* Correspondence: daa1@cumc.columbia.edu
[6]Section of Population Oral Health, College of Dental Medicine, Columbia University, New York, NY 10032, USA
Full list of author information is available at the end of the article

risk also applies to IUGR has not been established. Since infections play an important role in IUGR, we hypothesized that: (i) maternal periodontitis is associated with an increased risk for IUGR; and (ii) treatment for periodontitis in the immediate postpartum period signifies presence of untreated periodontitis during pregnancy, and is associated with elevated risk of IUGR. Furthermore, given the increased risk of recurrence of IUGR and the temporal persistence of periodontal infections, we hypothesized that parity will be an effect modifier of the association between periodontal infection and risk of IUGR.

We tested these hypotheses by examining medical and dental insurance records in a large cohort of 32,168 women, comparing rates of IUGR among women undergoing periodontal care, other types of dental treatment, and those receiving no dental treatment, before, during and after pregnancy.

Methods

Study design and data sources

This retrospective cohort study examined insurance records of women concurrently enrolled in medical and dental insurance plans through Aetna Inc., a nationwide, private health insurer. Aetna's data warehouse holds claim information on members for a four-year period. We therefore restricted the analysis to women that delivered a singleton live-birth between January 2010 and December 2011, and then included claims data for those birth events up to one year before gestation and up to one year after the birth event. We chose to restrict the study to singleton gestations, since the etiology and risk factors for IUGR vary between singleton and multiple births. The study cohort was restricted to women who had both medical and dental insurance, who were between 13 and 50 years of age at the time of delivery, and for whom zip code level data and other covariates were available. The analytic sample included 32,168 women.

Using data from 212,427 dental claim records for the period January 2009 through December 2012, procedures performed before, during and after pregnancy were identified and classified using the Code on Dental Procedures and Nomenclature Current Dental Terminology (CDT) 2009–10 edition for procedures occurring before 2011, and the CDT 2011/2012 edition for procedures from 2011 onwards. Maternal oral treatment type included periodontal treatment, prophylaxis, other dental treatment, or no oral treatment of any kind during the study period. Periodontal treatment was provided by general dentists and periodontists. Oral prophylaxis procedures can be provided by dentists or dental hygienists, however in the United States most oral prophylaxis procedures are provided by dental hygienists. Periodontal treatment included surgical and non-surgical codes (Additional file 1: Table S1). Because the insurance database did not include indicators of conception, the date of conception was estimated from the date of birth. For analytic purposes, each dental treatment category was considered in relation to the time period in which it occurred: pre-conception, during gestation, or after birth. The insurance dataset contained diagnosis codes and treatment codes for medical care, however it was limited to treatment codes for dental services. In the United States, dentists are only required to provide treatment codes for reimbursement via a dental claim. Given that periodontal disease is a chronic condition, periodontal treatment occurring after delivery was considered to indicate that periodontitis was present and untreated during pregnancy.

Using data extracted from 2,622,764 medical claims records, for the period January 2009 through December 2012, presence of IUGR was assumed if one or more International Classification of Diseases (ICD) 9th revision codes indicating slow fetal growth and fetal malnutrition (764.x), or poor fetal growth affecting management of mother (656.5x) had been used. Fetal growth restriction was defined as an IUGR diagnosis within 14 days of delivery; thus, in this study, the term IUGR refers to growth restriction defined accordingly. In each record, both primary and secondary claims were searched. Multiple births were identified and eliminated from the analytic file using supplementary delivery codes V27.2 to V27.9.

Maternal income, race and ethnicity were not available in the insurance database. We therefore imputed these characteristics based on the zip code of residence for each woman at the time of insurance enrollment, and the 2010 United States Census zip code level data for these variables. We identified complications of pregnancy using ICD-9 codes (Additional file 1: Table S2). Because not all women had dental coverage for the entire study period, months of enrollment for each woman was included as a covariate. The sample included women from all 50 states, the District of Columbia, and Puerto Rico.

Statistical analysis

The risk of IUGR was associated with types of dental and periodontal treatment, as previously defined. We fit logistic regression models from which we derived odds ratios (OR) and 95% confidence intervals (CI) to assess the magnitude of the effect. In these models, we adjusted for potential confounding factors including pregnancy complications, maternal age at delivery, primiparity, zip code level income, race, and ethnicity; the models were also adjusted for duration of continuous dental coverage during the study period. Annual income was analyzed in quintiles, and categorized in US dollars as ≤28,125; 28,126 to 33,500; 33,501 to 39,283, 39,284 to 48,831;

and ≥ 48,832. To assess non-linear effects of maternal age on the odds of incident IUGR, we included a quadratic term for age in the regression models.

To test for parity-related effect modification, a two-way interaction term between periodontal treatment and primiparity was included in the logistic regression model. Since the Wald-type chi-square test for the interaction term was significant ($P < 0.01$), we present the results of models stratified by parity.

To determine whether risk of IUGR increases with severity of periodontitis, we examined the rate of IUGR in relation to the number and type of periodontal treatment procedures, and compared women who received surgical as opposed to non-surgical periodontal treatment.

Sensitivity analysis

Since the association between periodontal treatment and IUGR is likely affected by unmeasured confounding, we undertook a sensitivity analysis to evaluate the extent to which unmeasured confounding may have impacted the associations [11]. This sensitivity analysis was based on the following assumptions: (i) the prevalence rates of the unmeasured confounder among pregnancies with and without IUGR were 3% and 6%, respectively; and (ii) the odds ratio of IUGR comparing the presence versus absence of unmeasured confounding was allowed to vary between 0.1 (protective) to 1.0 in 0.1 increments, and 2.0 (increased risk) to 10 in 1.0 increments. The evaluation of the impact of unmeasured confounding was based on fairly conservative assumptions.

Results

Of the 32,168 women in the study, 18,593 (57.8%) received some form of dental treatment during the study period; 9.0% ($n = 2895$) received periodontal treatment, 41.2% ($n = 13,246$) received prophylaxis and 7.6% ($n = 2452$) received some other form of dental treatment (Table 1). The mean maternal age at the time of delivery was 30.8 (standard deviation (SD) = 5.6); subjects lived in zip codes with median Black population of 5% (range 0–99), and median Hispanic population of 8% (range 0–100). Complications of pregnancy were documented for 33.9% of the women in the study. On average, women were enrolled in a dental plan for 27.9 months (SD = 13.3) during the study period. There were relatively small differences between dental treatment groups with respect to each of the above covariates.

Table 2 shows the frequency of each type of periodontal treatment in the cohort. The most frequent non-surgical periodontal procedure was scaling and root planing, which was documented for 7.4% ($n = 2388$) of the women. Full mouth debridement ($n = 584$, 1.8%) and localized delivery of chemotherapeutic agents ($n = 229$, 0.7%) were less frequent. Surgical periodontal procedures occurred only rarely. For over two thirds of the 2895 women who received periodontal treatment during the study period, that treatment occurred only in the period after birth ($n = 1956$, 67.6%). A total of 440 (15.2%) received dental treatment only during gestation, and 343 (11.8%) received treatment in the period prior to conception. 753 (2.6%) received treatment in the gestation and post-gestation periods, 550 (1.9%) received treatment in the pre-gestation and post-gestation periods, and 232 (0.8%) received treatment in the pre-gestation and gestation periods.

IUGR was documented in 2027 fetuses (6.3%). The association between dental treatment before, during and after gestation and the risk of IUGR is shown in Table 3. The incidence of IUGR was 9.2% ($n = 192$) among those receiving periodontal treatment after delivery and 6.1% ($n = 1835$) for those receiving no periodontal treatment. The odds of IUGR for those receiving periodontal treatment post-gestation compared to those receiving no periodontal treatment was 1.5 (95% CI 1.2, 1.8) following adjustment for confounders. The odds of IUGR was elevated among multiparous women who received periodontal treatment post-gestation (OR 1.6, 95% CI 1.3, 1.9). Among primiparous women who received periodontal treatment post-gestation, the risk of IUGR was not elevated (OR 1.3, 95% CI 1.0, 1.8).

The rate of IUGR among those with no dental treatment at any time before, during or after pregnancy was 6.0%, which was marginally but significantly lower than the IUGR rate of those who received any treatment (6.5%; $p = 0.048$); there was also a marginally significant difference in IUGR rates in the post-gestational period between those who received no dental treatment in this period (6.1%) and those who received some form of dental treatment in this period (6.6%; $p = .049$). The slightly elevated IUGR rates of those receiving any form of dental treatment is clearly driven by the increased IUGR rates associated with periodontal treatment, as shown in Table 3.

Sensitivity analysis for unmeasured confounding

The odds ratios corrected for unmeasured confounder(s) are shown in Fig. 1. For instance, if the odds ratio of IUGR comparing the presence versus absence of an unmeasured confounder was 2.0, the bias-corrected odds ratio for each of the three scenarios were 0.7 (95% CI 0.5, 1.1) for pre-gestation periodontal treatment, 1.2 (95% CI 0.9, 1.8) for periodontal treatment during pregnancy, and 1.5 (95% CI 1.3, 1.8) for periodontal treatment post-gestation. For odds ratios of the unmeasured confounder over 5, the bias-corrected odds ratio were enhanced for both periodontal treatment during pregnancy and post-gestation. These findings confirm the confounder-adjusted odds ratios reported earlier (Table 3), and when unmeasured confounding is taken

Table 1 Distribution of maternal sociodemographic characteristics by dental treatment type ($n = 32,168$)

Maternal characteristics	Total (%)	No dental treatment (%)	Periodontal treatment (%)	Prophylaxis (%)	Other dental treatment (%)	*P*-value
Number of subjects (%)	32,168 (100.0)	13,575 (42.2)	2895 (9.0)	13,246 (41.2)	2452 (7.6)	
Maternal age (years)						< 0.01
< 20	2.6	3.4	1.6	1.9	2.7	
20–24	10.8	12.5	13.9	7.6	15.3	
25–29	26.0	26.9	31.8	23.1	29.9	
30–34	34.3	32.7	28.5	37.7	31.5	
≥ 35	26.3	24.4	24.2	29.6	20.6	
Mean age (SD)	30.8 (5.6)	30.4 (5.8)	30.2 (5.5)	31.6 (5.3)	29.9 (5.7)	< 0.01
Primiparity	32.2	31.4	31.8	33.5	30.0	< 0.01
Household Annual income (US $; quintile)						< 0.01
1st (≤28,125)	6.3	6.7	9.0	5.2	6.6	
2nd (28,126 to 33,500)	7.3	7.8	10.5	5.8	8.4	
3rd (33,501 to 39,283)	10.5	11.0	10.7	9.5	13.4	
4th (39,284 to 48,831)	20.6	20.3	22.7	19.9	23.4	
5th (≥48,832)	55.3	54.2	47.2	59.6	48.1	
Median income (US $; range)	50,991 (5000 to 200,000)	50,555 (5787 to 209,001)	47,153 (7436 to 200,001)	52,800 (5000 to 173,368)	47,683 (7236 to 185,466)	< 0.01
Black race (%)						< 0.01
≤ 10	70.0	66.3	71.7	73.8	67.9	
11–35	20.5	21.8	19.7	19.0	22.8	
36–50	2.8	3.1	2.9	2.4	3.6	
≥ 51	6.6	8.8	5.6	4.7	5.8	
Median (range) %	5 (0, 99)	6 (0, 99)	5 (0, 98)	5 (0, 99)	5 (0, 98)	< 0.01
Hispanic ethnicity (%)						< 0.01
≤ 5	40.4	39.1	31.8	44.4	36.8	
6–10	19.8	18.9	22.8	20.1	19.5	
11–20	18.3	18.6	18.9	17.9	18.5	
21–42	13.0	13.3	16.1	11.6	15.0	
≥ 43	8.4	10.1	10.3	6.0	10.2	
Median (range) %	8 (0, 100)	8 (0, 100)	9 (0, 99)	7 (0, 100)	9 (0, 97)	< 0.01
Complications of pregnancy (%)[a]	33.9	34.0	34.6	33.1	36.5	< 0.01
Dental enrollment months, Median (range)	28 (1, 46)	22 (1, 46)	33 (1, 46)	32 (1, 46)	29 (1, 46)	< 0.01

[a]Details of the pregnancy complications are shown in Additional file 1: Table S2

into account, the associations between periodontal treatment both during pregnancy and post-gestation are associated with increased odds of IUGR.

To determine whether severity of post-gestation periodontal care was associated with the likelihood of IUGR, we developed a four-category measure capturing the number of claims for post-gestational maternal periodontal care: zero, one, two, and three or more. The rate of IUGR increased from 6.1% for those with no periodontal care to 8.1% among those with 1 instance of periodontal treatment, 9.8% for those with 2 instances of periodontal treatment, and peaking at 11.1% for those with 3 or more instances of periodontal treatment after birth ($P < 0.01$).

Discussion

The results indicate an association between maternal periodontal disease and odds of IUGR. We observed significantly elevated odds of IUGR among women who experienced periodontal disease during pregnancy, as

Table 2 Frequency (%) of periodontal surgical and non-surgical procedures among women in sample (n = 32,168)[a]

Procedure category	Number	% of total sample
Surgical procedures		
Gingival flap	11	< 0.1
Osseous surgery	40	0.1
Bone replacement graft	58	0.2
Tissue regeneration procedure	61	0.2
Non-surgical procedures		
Scaling and root planing	2388	7.4
Full mouth debridement	584	1.8
Localized chemotherapeutic agents	229	0.7

[a]Number of women who had at least one instance of each procedure; a woman may have had more than one procedure but is counted once in each procedure category

evidenced by periodontal treatment shortly after giving birth. We also found that delivery of a higher volume of periodontal treatment, a possible indicator of more severe periodontal disease, was associated with increased incidence of IUGR. The effect was strongest among those who received periodontal treatment after giving birth, an indication of untreated periodontal disease during pregnancy. While relatively few women received periodontal treatment during pregnancy, the sensitivity analysis suggested that there may be elevated risk of IUGR during this period as well. However, contrary to our initial hypothesis, the risk of IUGR in relation to the timing of the receipt of dental treatment did not vary by parity.

Limitations of the data

Diagnosis of IUGR was based on ICD coding, and this may have introduced some misclassification. Women carrying IUGR fetuses, particularly those that are diagnosed as not being severely growth restricted, are less likely to undergo clinician-initiated obstetrical intervention (labor induction or a prelabor cesarean) and less likely to have a diagnosis of IUGR recorded [12]. However, for severe IUGR (e.g., estimated fetal weight below the third or the first percentiles), misclassification of IUGR status is very unlikely since growth restriction serves as a sentinel cause for obstetrical intervention, and is therefore billed for insurance reimbursement. For the same reason, we believe the recording of the exposure is accurate in this data system because periodontal treatment is the basis for a reimbursable claim.

Second, despite adjustment for several confounders, we lack data on smoking and maternal pre-pregnancy body-mass index. However, the sensitivity analysis conducted to determine the potential effect of unmeasured confounding indicates that our models are robust. Finally, dental data is based on CDT codes that reflect treatment of periodontal disease rather than diagnosis. However, we believe that the treatment codes are sufficiently specific to infer presence of periodontal disease. While women included in this study are from virtually all states in the US, the insured populations are from middle to higher-income socioeconomic strata. This should be considered while generalizing the results from the study; however, it is unlikely that the association between IUGR and infections in general, and periodontal disease in particular, would be any lower among poorer women than among those we studied.

It may appear anomalous in terms of causal reasoning that the relationship we report is between an outcome (IUGR) that occurs *prior* to an exposure (periodontal treatment in the period immediately after birth). However, periodontal disease is a chronic condition. Therefore, it is plausible to assume that women who were treated in the immediate post-gestation period experienced periodontitis and its systemic impact during gestation.

Table 3 Risk of intrauterine growth restriction (IUGR) in relation to timing of dental treatment (n = 32,168)

Treatment	Period of treatment	Number with claims	IUGR n (%)	Adjusted odds ratio (95% confidence interval)		
				Overall	Primiparous women	Multiparous women
Periodontal	Pre-gestation	428	22 (5.1%)	0.7 (0.4, 1.1)	0.5 (0.2, 1.1)	0.9 (0.5, 1.5)
	Gestation	540	40 (7.4%)	1.2 (0.8, 1.7)	1.4 (0.8, 2.4)	1.1 (0.7, 1.7)
	Post-birth	2088	192 (9.2%)	1.5 (1.2, 1.8)	1.3 (1.0, 1.8)	1.6 (1.3, 1.9)
Prophylaxis	Pre-gestation	3387	220 (6.5%)	1.0 (0.8, 1.3)	1.0 (0.7, 1.6)	1.0 (0.7, 1.4)
	Gestation	7043	409 (5.8%)	1.0 (0.8, 1.2)	1.1 (0.8, 1.6)	0.9 (0.7, 1.2)
	Post-birth	11,743	743 (6.3%)	1.0 (0.8, 1.2)	0.9 (0.7, 1.2)	1.0 (0.9, 1.3)
Any dental	Pre-gestation	4655	306 (6.6%)	1.2 (0.9, 1.5)	1.0 (0.7, 1.5)	1.2 (0.9, 1.7)
	Gestation	8986	535 (6.0%)	0.9 (0.7, 1.1)	0.8 (0.6, 1.2)	0.9 (0.7, 1.2)
	Post-birth	14,969	986 (6.6%)	1.1 (0.9, 1.3)	1.2 (0.9, 1.6)	1.1 (0.9, 1.3)

Odds ratios were adjusted for the confounding effects of maternal age, maternal age-square, household income, proportions of African-American and Hispanic ethnicities, and complications of pregnancy. An individual subject may have had a claim in more than one time period, and/or may have received more than one type of treatment in a given time period; the regression models adjust for these instances of multiple treatment exposures

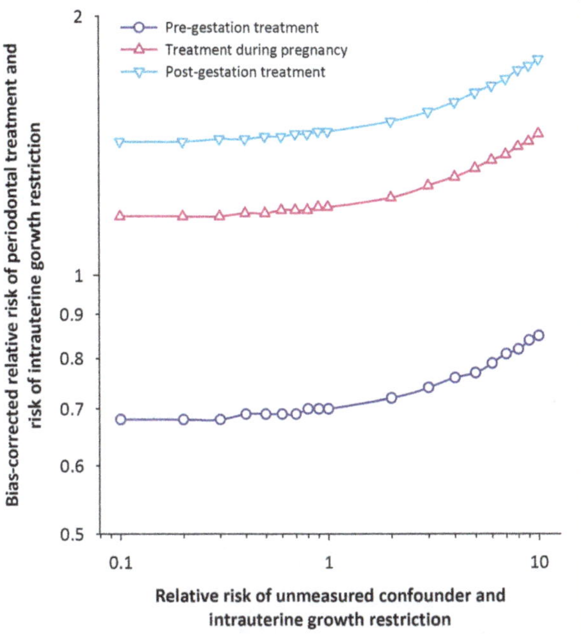

Fig. 1 Sensitivity Analysis for Unmeasured Confounding Between Periodontal Treatment Before, During and Post-Gestation and IUGR. Sensitivity analysis to evaluate the impact of unmeasured confounding of the association between periodontal treatment before (top panel), during (middle panel), and post-gestation (bottom panel) and IUGR. The observed confounder-adjusted odds ratio and 95% confidence interval are also shown for each panel. The unmeasured confounding bias-corrected odds ratio of IUGR for each of the three periodontal treatment periods are shown for prevalence estimates varying from 0.5 to 6.0% of the unmeasured confounder among both the IUGR and non-IUGR groups. The odds ratio of IUGR in relation to the unmeasured confounder is assumed to be 1.25. The red circle for each panel shows the bias-corrected odds ratio for one scenario of the prevalence of the unmeasured confounder of 2% and 4% among IUGR and non-IUGR groups, respectively, and the odds ratio of IUGR in relation to the unmeasured confounder of 1.25. The bias-corrected odds ratio for each of the three scenarios are 0.9 (95% CI 0.6, 1.5) for pre-gestation periodontal treatment, 1.6 (95% CI 1.1, 2.3) for periodontal treatment during pregnancy, and 2.0 (95% CI 1.6, 2.3) for periodontal treatment post-gestation

Finally, while we report that there is an increase in the rate of IUGR as a function of increasing number of treatments for periodontal disease, there are many factors that determine frequency of treatment; therefore, this finding is only suggestive of a relationship between the severity of periodontal disease and increased risk of IUGR.

Strengths of the study

In this study, a large sample of integrated medical and dental claims data provided a unique opportunity to explore the association between IUGR and periodontitis. In addition, the findings appear robust following adjustment for observed confounders, in fact correction for unmeasured confounding makes the associations stronger. Conducting secondary analyses using insurance data to shed light on the possible causes of negative birth outcomes is highly economical, and valuable in suggesting directions for future research.

Biological interpretations

The finding that periodontal treatment post-gestation was associated with an increased risk of IUGR in a large national sample add to the growing body of literature indicating a relationship between periodontal infection and related inflammation with adverse birth outcomes [4–8, 13]. Periodontal treatment in the period immediately following gestation is interpreted as signifying that periodontal disease was present during gestation. The inflammatory process associated with periodontal disease and the presence of periodontal pathogens in the blood can affect the fetus and the placenta [4].

This study utilized periodontal treatment as a proxy for the presence of periodontal disease. Periodontal treatment during gestation was expectedly rare and was also low during the pre-gestational period; our sample size was therefore too small to evaluate effects of treatment during pre-gestation and gestation. We expect that treatment during the pre-gestational and gestational periods to have limited adverse impact on birth outcomes. Tonetti and colleagues observed a short term increase in the systemic inflammatory response immediately following periodontal treatment which was then followed by a decrease in inflammation [14]. The finding that deleterious effects associated with periodontal therapy are short-lived is consistent with our finding of no statistically significant effect of treatment in the period prior to gestation and during gestation. However, periodontal treatment provided immediately following birth, which we found to be significantly related to IUGR appears to be a marker of disease during gestation.

Boggess and colleagues also observed that the incidence of small for gestational age increased with periodontal disease severity [15]. These findings are consistent with observations by several other investigators. In a study of Brazilian women, Siqueria and colleagues found increased odds of IUGR (adjusted OR 2.06, 95% CI 1.07, 4.19) among women diagnosed with periodontitis [16]. Similarly, Kumar and colleagues reported an increased association between periodontitis and IUGR, which was attenuated after adjusting for confounders [17]. The associations that we report are very similar to those of the Brazilian study.

The insured and employed population in our analyses is in the upper quartile of income in the United States and would be expected to have better oral hygiene and prevention practices. In addition, it is expected that utilizing treatment as a proxy for periodontal disease to some extent underestimates the true incidence of periodontal disease. In our analytical sample, maternal periodontal disease, indirectly assessed through the delivery of periodontal treatment in the immediate postpartum period, affected 9% of the women. By comparison, earlier studies have reported prevalence rates of 56–61% for maternal periodontitis [18, 19]. It should be noted that while we and Siquiera and colleagues [16] observed an increased odds for growth restriction with periodontal disease, other studies did not find such a relationship [20].

Conclusions

Periodontal disease manifests itself as destruction of the supporting structures of the teeth and is associated with systemic dissemination of bacteria and bacterial products as well as the release of inflammatory mediators that can adversely impact the placenta resulting in fetal growth restriction. In our analysis, IUGR was present in 6.3% of the sample. In 2012, 46% of the United States adult population was estimated to have experienced periodontal disease [21]. The high prevalence of periodontal disease in adults, and the cost associated with the morbidity and mortality of adverse birth outcomes, justifies further investigation of the systemic impact of periodontal infection/inflammation on the feto-placental unit.

As demonstrated in this study, research that involves the integration of medical and dental records can be informative in elucidating the role of potential exposures on adverse outcomes, and may ultimately lead to improved patient outcomes and more cost-effective care [22]. In particular, the use of combined medical and dental national insurance claims data provides an opportunity to explore the association of birth outcomes with dental health and dental treatment in women of childbearing age. 56% of American adults aged 19–64 had private dental insurance in 2009, and 10% of all procedure types in the dental office were related to periodontics [23, 24]. Data were obtained from a national insurance carrier that provides medical insurance to 23.5 million persons, and dental coverage to about 14.6 million persons across the United States [25].

In this retrospective study we show an association between periodontal treatment as a proxy for the presence of periodontal disease and IUGR, however randomized controlled trials are needed to establish the efficacy of periodontal therapy on pregnancy outcomes such as fetal growth restriction. Periodontal care should be emphasized for women of childbearing age to improve general oral health. Policies encouraging evaluation and early intervention to control/eliminate periodontal pathology prior to pregnancy may be able to reduce the risk of IUGR and related complications in the newborn.

Abbreviations

CDT: Code on Dental Procedures and Nomenclature Current Dental Terminology; CI: Confidence Intervals; ICD: International Classification of Diseases; IUGR: Intrauterine Growth Restriction; OR: Odds Ratio; SD: Standard Deviation

Funding

This study was funded by a grant from Aetna Inc.

Authors' contributions

CA, HA, PP, and DA assisted with the design of the study with intellectual contributions from AW, MC, and EB. HA carried out the statistical analyses. All authors read and approved the final manuscript.

Competing interests

CA, DA, PP, HA, EB and AW declare that they do not competing interests on this data analysis and manuscript. MC is an employee of Aetna Inc.

Author details

[1]Department of Obstetrics and Gynecology, College of Physicians and Surgeons, Columbia University, New York, NY 10032, USA. [2]Department of Epidemiology, Joseph L. Mailman School of Public Health, Columbia University, New York, NY 10032, USA. [3]Department of Biostatistics, Joseph L. Mailman School of Public Health, Columbia University, New York, NY 10032, USA. [4]New York State Psychiatric Institute, New York, NY 10032, USA. [5]Division of Periodontics, Section of Oral, Diagnostic and Rehabilitation Sciences, College of Dental Medicine, Columbia University, New York, NY 10032, USA. [6]Section of Population Oral Health, College of Dental Medicine, Columbia University, New York, NY 10032, USA. [7]Aetna Inc., Pittsburgh, PA 15220, USA.

References

1. Villar J, Belizan JM. The timing factor in the pathophysiology of the intrauterine growth retardation syndrome. Obstet Gynecol Surv. 1982;37: 499–506 PMID: 7050797.
2. Ananth CV, Vintzileos AM. Distinguishing pathological from constitutional small for gestational age births in population-based studies. Early Hum Dev. 2009;85:653–8. https://doi.org/10.1016/j.earlhumdev.2009.09.004 PMID: 19786331.
3. Kramer MS. The epidemiology of adverse pregnancy outcomes: an overview. J Nutr. 2003;133(5 Suppl 2):1592S–6S. https://doi.org/10.1093/jn/133.5.1592S PMID: 12730473.
4. Papapanou PN. Systemic effects of periodontitis: lessons learned from research on atherosclerotic vascular disease and adverse pregnancy outcomes. Int Dent J. 2015;65:283–91. https://doi.org/10.1111/idj.12185.
5. Cetin I, Pileri P, Villa A, Calabrese S, Ottolenghi L, Abati S. Pathogenic mechanisms linking periodontal diseases with adverse pregnancy outcomes. Reprod Sci. 2012;19:633–41. https://doi.org/10.1177/1933719111432871.
6. Ide M, Papapanou PN. Epidemiology of association between maternal periodontal disease and adverse pregnancy outcomes--systematic review. J Periodontol. 2013;84(4 Suppl):S181–94. https://doi.org/10.1902/jop.2013.134009 PMID: 23631578.
7. Vettore MV, Md L, da Silva AM, Lamarca GA, Sheiham A. The relationship between periodontitis and preterm low birthweight. J Dent Res. 2008;87: 73–8. https://doi.org/10.1177/154405910808700113.
8. Madianos PN, Bobetsis YA, Offenbacher S. Adverse pregnancy outcomes (APOs) and periodontal disease: pathogenic mechanisms. J Periodontol. 2013; 84(4 Suppl):S170–80. https://doi.org/10.1902/jop.2013.1340015 PMID: 23631577.
9. Romero R, Mazor M. Infection and preterm labor. Clin Obstet Gynecol. 1988; 31:553–84 PMID: 3066544.

10. Longo S, Borghesi A, Tzialla C, Stronati M. IUGR and infections. Early Hum Dev. 2014;90(Suppl 1):S42–4. https://doi.org/10.1016/S0378-3782(14)70014-3 PMID: 24709457.
11. Vanderweele TJ, Mumford SL, Schisterman EF. Conditioning on intermediates in perinatal epidemiology. Epidemiology. 2012;23:1–9. https://doi.org/10.1097/EDE.0b013e31823aca5d PMID: 22157298.
12. Ananth CV, Vintzileos AM. Maternal-fetal conditions necessitating a medical intervention resulting in preterm birth. Am J Obstet Gynecol. 2006;195:1557–63. https://doi.org/10.1016/j.ajog.2006.05.021 PMID: 17014813.
13. Li X, Kolltveit KM, Tronstad L, Olsen I. Systemic diseases caused by oral infection. Clin Microbiol Rev. 2000;13:547–58 11023956.
14. Tonetti MS, D'Aiuto F, Nibali L, Donald A, Storry C, Parkar M, et al. Treatment of periodontitis and endothelial function. N Engl J Med. 2007;356:911–20. https://doi.org/10.1056/NEJMoa063186 PMID: 17329698.
15. Boggess KA, Beck JD, Murtha AP, Moss K, Offenbacher S. Maternal periodontal disease in early pregnancy and risk for a small-for-gestational-age infant. Am J Obstet Gynecol. 2006;194:1316–22. https://doi.org/10.1016/j.ajog.2005.11.059 PMID: 16647916.
16. Siqueira FM, Cota LO, Costa JE, Haddad JP, Lana AM, Costa FO, et al. Intrauterine growth restriction, low birth weight, and preterm birth: adverse pregnancy outcomes and their association with maternal periodontitis. J Periodontol. 2007;78:2266–76. https://doi.org/10.1902/jop.2007.070196 PMID: 18052698.
17. Kumar A, Basra M, Begum N, et al. Association of maternal periodontal health with adverse pregnancy outcome. J Obstet Gynaecol Res. 2013;39:40–5. https://doi.org/10.1111/j.1447-0756.2012.01957.x PMID: 22845916.
18. Abati S, Villa A, Cetin I, Dessole S, Luglie PF, Strohmenger L, et al. Lack of association between maternal periodontal status and adverse pregnancy outcomes: a multicentric epidemiologic study. J Matern Fetal Neonatal Med. 2013;26:369–72. https://doi.org/10.3109/14767058.2012.733776 PMID: 23039761.
19. Vogt M, Sallum AW, Cecatti JG, Morais SS. Periodontal disease and some adverse perinatal outcomes in a cohort of low risk pregnant women. Reprod Health. 2010;7:29. https://doi.org/10.1186/1742-4755-7-29 PMID: 21047427.
20. Srinivas SK, Sammel MD, Stamilio DM, Clothier B, Jeffcoat MK, Parry S, et al. Periodontal disease and adverse pregnancy outcomes: is there an association? Am J Obstet Gynecol. 2009;200:497. https://doi.org/10.1016/j.ajog.2009.03.003 PubMed PMID: 19375568. e1–8.
21. Eke PI, Dye BA, Wei L, Slade GD, Thornton-Evans GO, Borgnakke WS, et al. Update on prevalence of periodontitis in adults in the United States: NHANES 2009 to 2012. J Periodontol. 2015;86:611–22. https://doi.org/10.1902/jop.2015.140520 PMID: 25688694.
22. Leake JL, Werneck RI. The use of administrative databases to assess oral health care. J Public Health Dent. 2005;65:21–35 PMID: 1751492.
23. Nasseh K, Vujicic M. Dental benefits coverage increased for working-age adults in 2014. Health Policy Institute Research Brief. American Dental Association. 2016. http://www.ada.org/~/media/ADA/Science%20and%20Research/HPI/Files/HPIBrief_1016_2.pdf.
24. Manski RJ, Macek MD, Brown E, Carper KV, Cohen LA, Vargas C. Dental service mix among working-age adults in the United States, 1999 and 2009. J Public Health Dent. 2014;74:102–9. https://doi.org/10.1111/jphd.12032 PubMed PMID: 24032402.
25. Aetna Inc. https://www.aetna.com/about-us/aetna-facts-and-subsidiaries/aetna-facts.html. Accessed 18 Feb 2017.

The efficacy of platelet-rich fibrin as a scaffold in regenerative endodontic treatment

Hongbing Lv[1†], Yuemin Chen[1†], Zhiyu Cai[2*], Lishan Lei[1], Ming Zhang[1], Ronghui Zhou[1] and Xiaojing Huang[1*]

Abstract

Background: Blood Clot (BC) or platelet concentrates have been used as scaffold in regenerative endodontic treatment (RET). The aim of this retrospective study was to compare the performance of platelet-rich fibrin (PRF) with BC in inducing root development and periapical lesion healing after tooth revascularization.

Methods: Five patients receiving RET using PRF as a scaffold were matched 1:1 to a previous cohort of 5 patients who underwent tooth revascularization by provoking periapical bleeding. Clinical signs and symptoms were examined at follow-ups. Periapical lesion healing and root development were monitored radiographically. The resolution of clinical signs and symptoms as well as periapical radiolucency was observed in all patients (100%).

Results: Root elongation, dentinal wall thickening and apex closure were found in most cases (80% in both groups). There was no significant difference between the groups in terms of clinical sign resolution, root development and periapical healing.

Conclusions: Within the limits of this study, PRF achieved comparable outcomes to BC in terms of clinical sign and symptom resolution, periapical lesion healing and continued root development in RET.

Keywords: Apical periodontitis, Human immature permanent tooth, Blood clot, Platelet-rich fibrin, Regenerative endodontic treatment

Background

Traditionally, immature permanent teeth with necrotic pulp have been treated by apexification. In 2001, Iwaya et al. first reported a case involving the revascularization of an immature tooth with apical periodontitis [1]. Since then, a paradigm shift has occurred regarding the treatment of immature permanent teeth with pulp necrosis or apical periodontitis. In the past decade, several reports have described regenerative endodontic treatment (RET) [2–4]. Most of these studies were case reports or case series and presented successful results including the resolution of periapical lesions, continued root development, and even the recovery of tooth sensibility [5]. This accumulating evidence has contributed to the development of the current recommendations of the American Association of Endodontists for RET [6]. However, various protocols have been proposed, which differ regarding the concentrations of sodium hypochlorite (NaOCl) that are used for irrigation [7], the antibiotic regimens that are used for disinfection [5, 8], and the scaffold types that are used for tissue regeneration [9, 10]. Clearly, more evidence is needed to develop future treatment recommendations.

RET is based on the concept of tissue engineering [11], which requires the eradication of pathogens, the preservation of stem cells, and the presence of scaffolds and signal molecules [12]. To create a favourable microenvironment for stem cells to migrate, proliferate and differentiate, an ideal scaffold should facilitate spatial orientation and signal molecule release by cells. In most

* Correspondence: caizhiyu@fjmu.edu.cn; hxiaoj@163.com
†Hongbing Lv and Yuemin Chen contributed equally to this work.
[2]Department of Stomatology, Fujian Medical University Union Hospital, Fuzhou 350001, China
[1]School and Hospital of Stomatology, Fujian Medical University, Fuzhou 350002, China

cases of tooth revascularization/revitalization, an endodontic explorer or file is introduced into the root canal and passes through the apical foramen to provoke bleeding from the periapical tissue into the canal to form a blood clot (BC) below the cemental enamel junction (CEJ) [13]. In general, this technique is effective at forming a BC scaffold. However, this procedure has several disadvantages. Firstly, the manipulation used to induce periapical bleeding is technique-sensitive. Clinically, it is difficult to control the speed and volume of bleeding to achieve the desired level. Too little bleeding would be insufficient to provide the necessary scaffold, whereas too much bleeding might overfill the pulp cavity and the open access, thus contacting the surrounding tooth crown and leading to recontamination of the disinfected root canal system. There are also clinical situations in which it is difficult to induce periapical bleeding [14]. Secondly, even when a BC is formed, such clots are far from ideal according to scaffold criteria. Lastly but most importantly, this procedure carries the risk of injury to the inferior alveolar nerve (IAN) or mental nerve when treating mandibular premolars. Studies have confirmed the proximity of premolar apices to the IAN and mental foramina [15–17]. It has been documented that iatrogenic mental nerve paresthesia can be caused by an overfill of Gutta-Percha or by mechanical instrumentation beyond the root apex [18, 19]. In addition, the presence of apical periodontitis or a radicular lesion might further erode the bone that protects the IAN. Therefore, it is imperative to find scaffold alternatives to a BC in RET.

Previous studies have shown the potential of using platelet concentrates as scaffolding in tissue regeneration. Platelet concentrates are autologous, reasonably easy to prepare in a dental setting, and comprise high concentrations of growth factors including transforming growth factor-beta (TGF-beta), vascular endothelial growth factor (VEGF), and platelet-derived growth factor (PDGF) [20]. In vitro studies have documented the effects of these signalling molecules on cell migration, proliferation, differentiation and matrix synthesis [21]. In recent years, platelet concentrates have been successfully applied as scaffolding in tooth revascularization/revitalization. Platelet-rich plasma (PRP) is a first-generation platelet concentrate [22]. Case reports [3, 23] as well as randomized controlled clinical studies [14, 24] have demonstrated the reliability of PRP in improving periapical healing, apical closure and dentinal wall thickening. Platelet-rich fibrin (PRF), a second-generation platelet concentrate, has many advantages over PRP. Firstly, the preparation of PRF does not require the addition of exogenous agents, such as thrombin. Secondly, PRF forms an organized fibrin network in which platelets and leukocytes are trapped. These entrapped cells serve as a reservoir of various growth factors for long-term release. Important circulating immune cells and various cytokines in PRF clots also act against infection. In addition, the mechanical properties of PRF might facilitate the condensation of overlying MTA. Thus, it is rational to expect PRF to be an optimal bioscaffold for tooth revascularization/revitalization.

However, apart from a few case reports describing the use of PRF as a scaffold [25–30], only one clinical trial [31] compared the efficacy of root development and periapical radiolucency resolution after tooth revascularization/revitalization with PRF and with other scaffolds. More clinical studies are required to evaluate the performance of PRF in RET. In order to test if PRF could enhance root development and periapical lesion healing more than a BC, we conducted a controlled cohort study.

Methods

Study population and design

A retrospective, serial case-control study design was used in this study. Patients having nonvital, immature incisors or premolars with radiographic evidence of periapical lesions were included. From January 2014 to December 2014, five cases of tooth revascularization with PRF application were performed by an experienced endodontist at the School and Hospital of Stomatology, Fujian Medical University. These patients represent an initial series of tooth revascularization cases using PRF as a scaffold that was conducted in our hospital in continuum without selection bias.

From January 2012 and December 2013, 11 conventional tooth revascularizations were performed by the same endodontist at the School and Hospital of Stomatology, Fujian Medical University. From this cohort, we selected 5 patients to serve as a control group (the remaining 6 cases were excluded for the following reasons: three cases involved pulp necrosis without periapical radiolucency; one patient underwent tooth extraction 10 months after RET for orthodontic reasons; in one case, tooth development was at stage 9; and contact was lost with the remaining patient after RET). These 5 patients were specifically matched in a 1:1 ratio to index cases of tooth revascularization using PRF with respect to patient age, gender, aetiology, pulp/periapical conditions, foramina development (All teeth were at stage 8 according to Nolla's scoring system [32]) and tooth position. No consideration or analysis of operative parameters and outcomes was made until after selection of the control population. In all cases, written informed consent was obtained from the guardians of the patients after explaining the detailed treatment protocol as per the patient information sheet. The study design and clinical procedures were performed in accordance with the Helsinki Declaration (revised in 2008) and were approved by the Ethics Committee of the School and Hospital of Stomatology, Fujian Medical University.

PRF preparation

PRF was prepared as described by Choukroun et al. [33]. Immediately before surgery, 5 ml of whole blood was drawn into 10-ml test tubes without anticoagulant reagent and was centrifuged at 400 g for 10 min. After centrifugation, whole blood was divided into three layers: (1) the bottom red blood cell layer; (2) the middle PRF layer; and (3) the top serum layer. The PRF layer was separated using sterile scissors, and PRF clots were pressed into a membranous film with sterile dry gauze (Fig. 1a–c). The PRF membrane was then cut into approximately $3 \times 3\text{-mm}^2$ pieces.

Treatment procedure

The treatment procedure for tooth revascularization has been described in our previous study [5]. An access cavity was prepared under rubber dam isolation using a round diamond and an Endo-Z bur (Dentsply Maillefer, Tulsa, OK). The pulp chamber and root canal were gently irrigated with 20 mL of 1% NaOCl without mechanical instrumentation. The canal was then dried using sterile paper points. Subsequently, an inter-appointment medication of triple antibiotic paste comprising ciprofloxacin, metronidazole, and cefaclor (1:1:1) was placed into the apical portion of the canal and filled to just below the CEJ using a syringe under a microscope. The access cavity was temporarily restored with 3 mm of Cavit (ESPE, Seefeld, Germany) and 2 mm of glass ionomer (Fuji IX, GC, Tokyo, Japan).

Revascularization was performed 4 weeks later. The procedure that was used for conventional tooth revascularization was as follows: 2% lidocaine without adrenaline was infiltrated around the apex of the tooth. After reopening of the access, the antibiotic paste was gently flushed out of the canal with sterile normal saline. The irrigation was finalized with 10 mL of 17% EDTA solution, and the tooth was dried using sterile paper points. Under a surgical microscope (Carl Zeiss Meditac Inc., Dublin, CA), a sterile #35 K-file was introduced into the canal beyond the apical foramen using a push and pull motion to provoke bleeding from the periapical tissue. A sterile moist cotton pellet was placed 3 mm below the CEJ with gentle pressure for 15 min to form a BC in the root canal. The BC was directly covered by a layer of CollaPlug (Zimmer Dental, Carlsbad, CA). Then, 3 mm of ProRoot mineral trioxide aggregate (MTA) (Dentsply Tulsa Dental Specialties, Tulsa, OK) was placed over the CollaPlug. After a moist cotton pellet was placed over the MTA, the access cavity was sealed with Cavit.

Revascularization using PRF as scaffolding was performed as follows: local anaesthesia, access reopening, antibiotic paste removal and root canal irrigation were performed following the same procedure as that described previously. After final irrigation of the root canal with EDTA and drying using paper points, the PRF fragments were placed into the canal space using a Buchanan Hand Plugger Size #2 (Sybron Endo, Orange, CA) up to the CEJ. A 3-mm-thick layer of MTA was placed directly over the PRF, followed by a moist cotton pellet and Cavit. One week later, the Cavit was removed

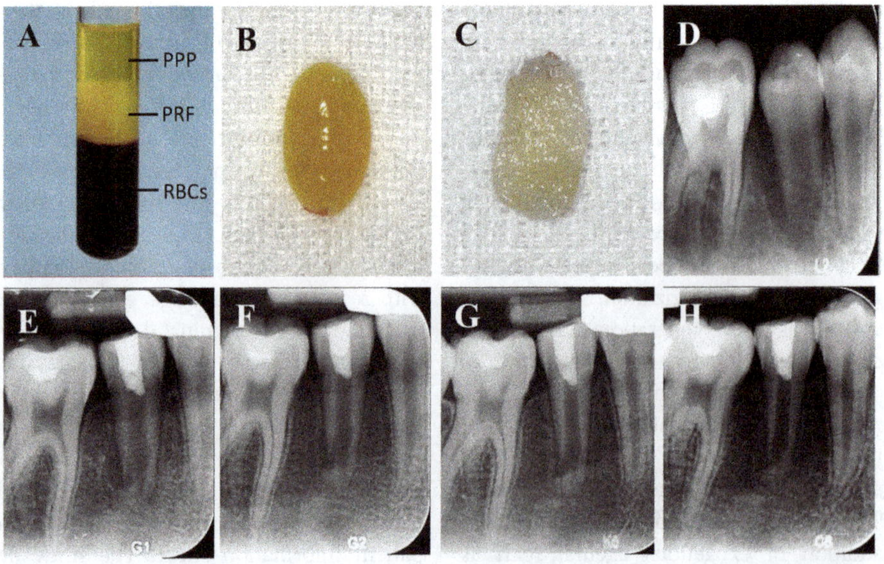

Fig. 1 **a** Peripheral blood after centrifugation: red blood cells at the bottom, PRF in the middle, and platelet-poor plasma at the top. **b** PRF clot. **c** PRF membrane. **d** An periapical radiograph of #45 with apical periodontitis in a 12-year-old girl. The case was treated by RET+PRF in #45. **e** Three-month follow-up periapical radiograph of tooth #45. **f** Six-month follow-up radiograph. **g** Nine-month follow-up radiograph. **h** Twelve-month follow-up radiograph showing complete periapical radiolucency resolution, root apex closure, root elongation and root canal wall thickening

and replaced with a bonded resin restoration (Filtek Z350 XT: 3 M ESPE Dental Products, St Paul, MN).

Postoperative examination and data collection

Recall visits were scheduled at 3, 6, 9, and 12 months. At each appointment, clinical examination as well as a tooth sensibility test including an electronic pulp test (EPT) and a cold test were performed. Root development was monitored by periapical radiography taken with a paralleling technique using the same device (Fig. 1d–h, Figs. 2, 3 and 4).

Statistical analyses

Statistical analyses was performed using SPSS (Statistics software v 19.0; IBV Corp, Armonk, NY). The results were compared between groups using the Chi-Square test. $P < 0.05$ was considered statistically significant.

Results

The results obtained are summarized in Tables 1 and 2. A total of 5 males and 5 females were included in this study. Mean patient ages for the BC and PRF groups were 11.6 (10–12) and 11.4 (9–14) yr., respectively. Compared to the BC group, more males were included in the PRF cohort, but the difference was not significant (60% vs 40%, $P > 0.05$). In each group, one incisor and 4 premolars were treated (Table 1). Postoperatively, resolution of periapical radiolucency was observed in all treated cases (100%). Root elongation, lateral dentinal wall thickening and apex closure were detected in most cases (80% in both groups). Clinical sign and symptom resolution was observed in all patients (100%). There was no significant difference between the groups in terms of root development, periapical healing and clinical sign resolution ($P > 0.05$) (Table 2).

Discussion

The data obtained in the present study showed that tooth revascularization/revitalization using PRF as a scaffold achieved comparable results to the technique of provoking periapical bleeding in terms of periapical lesion healing, continued root formation and clinical sign and symptom resolution. To the best of our knowledge, this is the first retrospective controlled cohort study to compare the efficacy of PRF and BC as a scaffold in RET.

The present study showed no significant difference between PRF and BC groups in terms of periapical lesion healing, root development and clinical sign and symptom resolution. Because we did not provoke periapical bleeding before PRF placement in this study, periapical radiolucency resolution and root development were caused by the presence of the PRF scaffold. Our result is consistent with most previous studies [14, 34, 35] in which PRP served as the only bioscaffold in the treatment protocols. Although another study [24] revealed a remarkable enhancement of periapical healing, apical closure, and dentinal wall thickening in their PRP group, PRP was applied after provoking periapical bleeding in the treatment protocol. The superior performance of the PRP group in that study might be due to the synergistic effects of a BC and PRP in root development. On one hand, the concentrations of CD73 and CD105 mesenchymal stem cells in blood samples taken from immature teeth was up to 600-fold greater than that in circulating blood [36]. The stem cell population in periapically-induced BC should be significantly higher than that in PRF, which is prepared from peripheral blood. On the other hand, compared to a BC, PRF contains a much higher concentration of platelets [37], which might continuously release various growth factors, thereby contributing to tissue regeneration. In a pilot

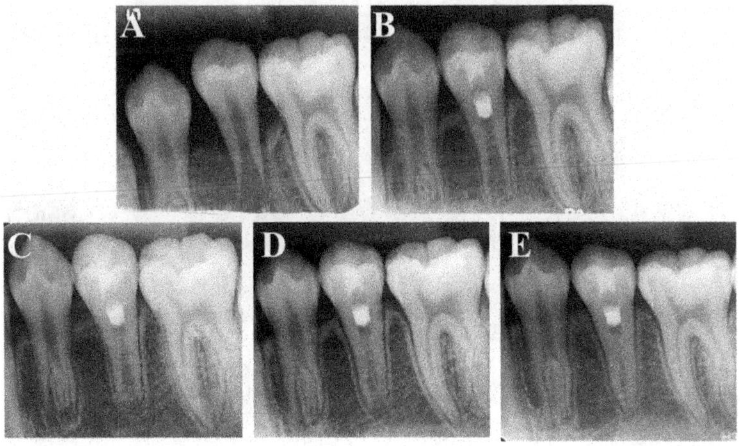

Fig. 2 a An intraoral periapical radiograph of #35 with apical periodontitis in a 12-year-old girl. **b** Three-month follow-up periapical radiograph of tooth #35 after undergoing PRF-aided revascularization. **c** Six-month follow-up radiograph. **d** Nine-month follow-up radiograph. **e** Twelve-month follow-up radiograph showing complete resolution of the periapical radiolucency, thickening of the lateral dentinal walls, and closure of the apex

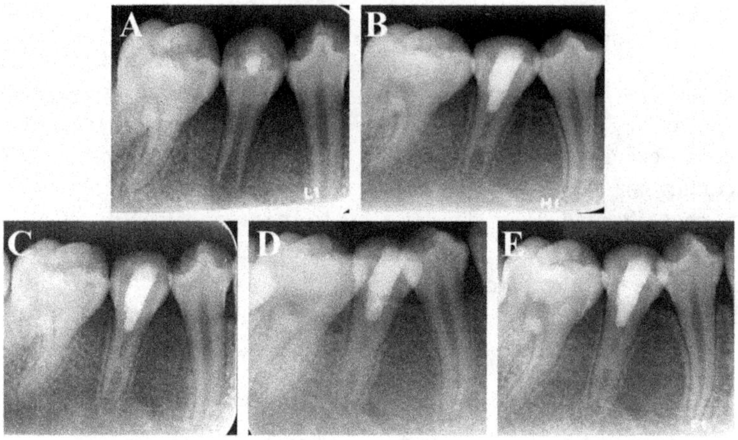

Fig. 3 **a** A periapical radiograph of #45 with apical periodontitis in a 12-year-old girl. In #45, conventional RET was performed. **b** Three-month follow-up periapical radiograph. **c** Six-month follow-up radiograph. **d** Nine-month follow-up radiograph. **e** Twelve-month follow-up radiograph showing healing of the periapical lesion and root development

study, Narang et al. also compared the efficacy of PRF scaffold with that of a BC in RET. It was found that PRF achieved comparable effects in apical closure, dentinal wall thickening and even better results in periapical healing and root lengthening than a BC did [31]. As the patients' ages in their study differed from those in ours, the stem cell concentration in the BC might not be at the same levels. This could possibly affect the results of the treatment. Anyway, our results along with previous studies showed that the effect of PRF as a scaffold in RET was at least comparable, if not superior to that of a BC from the periapical region.

Apart from periapical radiolucency resolution and root development, tooth sensibility recovery has also been reported in many previous studies [1, 3, 13, 38–40]. In these studies, positive responses of teeth to cold and EPT were detected from 5 1/2 months to 2 years postoperatively. In our study, positive responses to the tooth sensibility test were observed between 6 and 9 months after RET. However, because the follow-up period of the present study was only 12 months, tooth sensibility recovery after 1 year was not recorded. Therefore, at this point, we are cautious in drawing conclusions regarding whether PRF scaffold achieves better functional outcomes in terms of pulp sensitivity than a BC. Long-term observations are needed in future studies.

Due to the lack of specimens of human teeth showing revascularization/revitalization, the underlying histological basis for the presence or absence of responses in the tooth sensitivity test remains unclear. Hargreaves et

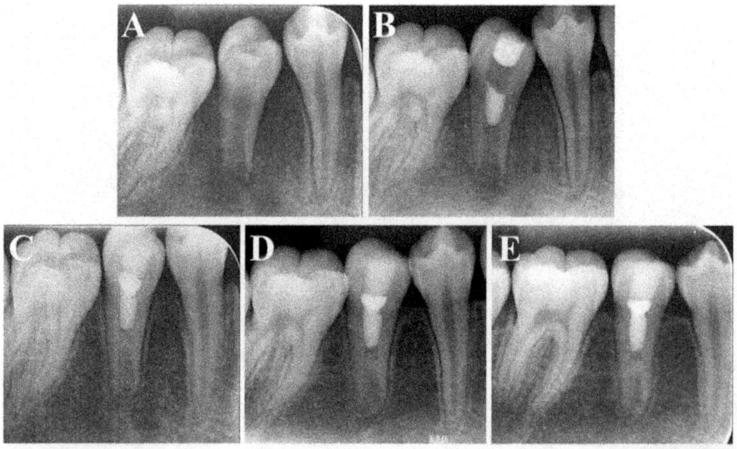

Fig. 4 **a** An intraoral periapical radiograph of a 12-year-old girl showing a wide-open apex of #45 with thin lateral dentinal walls and apical radiolucency. **b** Three-month follow-up periapical radiograph of tooth #45 after undergoing conventional RET. **c** Six-month follow-up radiograph. **d** Nine-month follow-up radiograph. **e** Twelve-month follow-up radiograph showing apical radiolucency resolution, apex closure, root elongation and lateral dentinal wall thickening

Table 1 Clinical and radiographic findings of teeth receiving RET with BC or PRF as scaffold at 1-year Follow-up

Procedure performed	Preoperative variables				Postoperative variables at 1-year follow-up					
					Radiographic findings				Sign and symptom	Sensitivity test
	Tooth# (age/sex)	Aetiology	Pulp/periapical conditions	Foramina development (Nolla's stage)	Periapical healing	Apex closure	Root elongation	Dentinal wall thickening	Resolution	EPT/Cold test (time)
RET with a BC (average age = 11.6 y)	45 (10 y/F)	DE	AP	8	Yes	Yes	Yes	Yes	Yes	+(6 m)
	45 (12 y/M)	DE	AP	8	Yes	Yes	Yes	Yes	Yes	–
	45 (12 y/F)	DE	AP	8	Yes	Yes	Yes	Yes	Yes	–
	45 (12 y/F)	DE	AP	8	Yes	Yes	Yes	Yes	Yes	–
	11 (12 y/M)	Tooth fracture	AP	8	Yes	No	No	No	Yes	–
RET with PRF (average age = 11.4 y)	35 (10 y/M)	DE	AP	8	Yes	Yes	Yes	Yes	Yes	–
	45 (12 y/F)	DE	AP	8	Yes	Yes	Yes	Yes	Yes	+ (6 m)
	35 (12 y/M)	DE	AP	8	Yes	Yes	Yes	Yes	Yes	+ (9 m)
	45 (14 y/F)	DE	AP	8	Yes	No	No	No	Yes	–
	21 (9 y/M)	Tooth fracture	AP	8	Yes	Yes	Yes	Yes	Yes	+ (9 m)

RET regenerative endodontic treatment, *BC* blood clot, *PRF* platelet-rich fibrin, *F* female, *M* male, *DE* dens evaginatus, *AP* apical periodontitis; +, positive; –, negative

Table 2 Comparative evaluation of tooth revascularization with BC and PRF in terms of clinical and radiographic findings at 1-year follow-up (* $P < 0.05$)

Procedure performed	Radiographic findings at 1-year follow-up				Clinical sign and symptom resolution
	Periapical healing	Apical closure	Root lengthening	Dentinal wall thickening	
RET with a BC	5 (100%)	4 (80%)	4 (80%)	4 (80%)	5 (100%)
RET with PRF	5 (100%)	4 (80%)	4 (80%)	4 (80%)	5 (100%)

al. proposed that positive responses to pulp sensitivity tests after tooth revascularization/revitalization indicate the occupation of previously vacant space by innervated tissue [41]. Johns and Vidyanath suggested that thick layers of MTA (3–4 mm) and glass ionomer cement (2 mm) might lead to negative responses to vitality testing [42]. Most recently, we reported a histological study regarding the nature of newly formed tissues after tooth revascularization [5]. In that case, an immature mandibular premolar with apical periodontitis was treated by revascularization/revitalization. Successful treatment results were observed including periapical radiolucency resolution, root development and tooth sensitivity recovery. Ten months later, the tooth was extracted for orthodontic reasons and processed for histological observation. In the canal space, neurons and nerve fibres were observed histologically and were confirmed by immunohistochemical examination. This finding demonstrated the possibility of nerve regeneration after RET, which may play a key role in the recovery of tooth sensitivity.

It has been documented that the mental foramen is located close to the mandibular premolars. In a radiographic study conducted by Fishel D et al. [17], the mental foramina were located at the apices of the first or second premolars in 15.4% or 13.9% of patients, respectively. In another study that aimed to determine the position of the mental foramen in relation to the apex of the second premolar [15], Phillips JL observed that the apex of the second premolar was located anywhere between 2.7 mm mesial, 3.8 mm distal, 3.5 mm above or 3.4 mm below the mental foramen. The author summarized that the apex of the second premolar was located at an average distance of 2.18 mm mesially and 2.4 mm superiorly from the mental foramen. The proximity of the apex of the second premolar and the mental foramen was also confirmed in a cadaver study by Denio D et al. [16]; their study demonstrated that each mental foramen was between 0 mm and 4.7 mm from the respective apex of the second premolar. Obviously, manipulation using needles or files to provoke bleeding beyond the apical foramen of premolars carries the risk of nerve injury. Therefore, it is rational and imperative to find a safe and efficient alternative to periapical bleeding in RET under such situations.

Despite the small number of cases observed, our study provides useful information on the clinical outcome of using PRF in scaffold-enhanced periapical lesion rehabilitation and root development in RET. These data demonstrated the feasibility of using PRF as an alternative scaffold when treating mandibular premolars or when provoking apical bleeding proves difficult. The major disadvantages of using PRF include the need to draw blood in young patients and the need for specialised equipment. However, considering the risks of nerve injury, the advantages of PRF application apparently outweigh its disadvantages in certain cases. Nevertheless, more randomized prospective controlled studies are needed to confirm the reliability of PRF for use as a bioscaffold to aid in developing future guideline recommendations for tooth revascularization/revitalization.

Conclusions

In sum, within the limits of this study, PRF achieved comparable outcomes to BC in terms of clinical sign and symptom resolution, periapical lesion healing and root maturation in RET.

Abbreviations

BC: Blood clot; CEJ: Cemental enamel junction; EPT: Electronic pulp test; IAN: Inferior alveolar nerve; MTA: Mineral trioxide aggregate; NaOCl: Sodium hypochlorite; PDGF: Platelet-derived growth factor; PRF: Platelet-rich fibrin; RET: Regenerative endodontic treatment; TGF: Transforming growth factor; VEGF: Vascular endothelial growth factor

Funding

This work was supported by the Joint Funds for the Innovation of Science and Technology, Fujian Province (grant No. 2016Y9024), Fujian Medical University Professor Academic Development Foundation (grant no. JS14031) and Scientific and Technological Innovation Leading Talent Fund of School and Hospital of Stomatology, Fujian Medical University (grant no. 2015-KQYY-LJ-4).

Authors' contributions

LHB and CYM designed the study, collected data, drafted and wrote the manuscript. CZY participated in the design of the study and helped in collecting the data, writing and reviewing the manuscript. LLS performed the data analysis. ZRH contributed to the data analysis and interpretation. ZM participated in the study design and the preparation of specimens. HXJ contributed to the study design, statistical analyses, and reviewed the manuscript. HXJ also participated in the study design and reviewed the manuscript. All authors read and approved the final manuscript.

Competing interests

The authors declare that they have no competing interests.

References

1. Iwaya SI, Ikawa M, Kubota M. Revascularization of an immature permanent tooth with apical periodontitis and sinus tract. Dent Traumatol. 2001;17:185–7.
2. Jung IY, Lee SJ, Hargreaves KM. Biologically based treatment of immature permanent teeth with pulpal necrosis: a case series. J Endod. 2008;34:876–87.
3. Torabinejad M, Turman M. Revitalization of tooth with necrotic pulp and open apex by using platelet-rich plasma: a case report. J Endod. 2011;37:265–8.
4. Chen MY, Chen KL, Chen CA, Tayebaty F, Rosenberg PA, Lin LM. Responses of immature permanent teeth with infected necrotic pulp tissue and apical periodontitis/abscess to revascularization procedures. Int Endod J. 2012;45:294–305.
5. Lei L, Chen Y, Zhou R, Huang X, Cai Z. Histologic and immunohistochemical findings of a human immature permanent tooth with apical periodontitis after regenerative endodontic treatment. J Endod. 2015;41:1172–9.
6. American Association of Endodontists: Clinical Considerations for Regenerative Procedures. Available at: http://www.aae.org/regeneration/. Accessed 8 June 2016.
7. Law AS. Considerations for regeneration procedures. J Endod. 2013;39:S44–56.
8. Scarparo RK, Dondoni L, Bottcher DE, Grecca FS, Rockenbach MI, Batista EL Jr. Response to intracanal medication in immature teeth with pulp necrosis: an experimental model in rat molars. J Endod. 2011;37:1069–73.
9. Ray HL Jr, Marcelino J, Braga R, Horwat R, Lisien M, Khaliq S. Long-term follow up of revascularization using platelet-rich fibrin. Dent Traumatol. 2016;32:80–4.
10. Rodriguez-Benitez S, Stambolsky C, Gutierrez-Perez JL, Torres-Lagares D, Segura-Egea JJ. Pulp revascularization of immature dog teeth with apical periodontitis using triantibiotic paste and platelet-rich plasma: a radiographic study. J Endod. 2015;41:1299–304.
11. Langer R, Vacanti JP. Tissue engineering. Science. 1993;260:920–6.
12. Hargreaves KM, Giesler T, Henry M, Wang Y. Regeneration potential of the young permanent tooth: what does the future hold? J Endod. 2008;34:S51–6.
13. Banchs F, Trope M. Revascularization of immature permanent teeth with apical periodontitis: new treatment protocol? J Endod. 2004;30:196–200.
14. Bezgin T, Yilmaz AD, Celik BN, Kolsuz ME, Sonmez H. Efficacy of platelet-rich plasma as a scaffold in regenerative endodontic treatment. J Endod. 2015;41:36–44.
15. Phillips JL, Weller RN, Kulild JC. The mental foramen: 2. Radiographic position in relation to the mandibular second premolar. J Endod. 1992;18:271–4.
16. Denio D, Torabinejad M, Bakland LK. Anatomical relationship of the mandibular canal to its surrounding structures in mature mandibles. J Endod. 1992;18:161–5.
17. Fishel D, Buchner A, Hershkowith A, Kaffe I. Roentgenologic study of the mental foramen. Oral Surg Oral Med Oral Pathol. 1976;41:682–6.
18. Knowles KI, Jergenson MA, Howard JH. Paresthesia associated with endodontic treatment of mandibular premolars. J Endod. 2003;29:768–70.
19. Scarano A, Di Carlo F, Quaranta A, Piattelli A. Injury of the inferior alveolar nerve after overfilling of the root canal with endodontic cement: a case report. Oral Surg Oral Med Oral Pathol Oral Radiol Endod. 2007;104:e56–9.
20. Mehta S, Watson JT. Platelet rich concentrate: basic science and current clinical applications. J Orthop Trauma. 2008;22:432–8.
21. Huang FM, Yang SF, Zhao JH, Chang YC. Platelet-rich fibrin increases proliferation and differentiation of human dental pulp cells. J Endod. 2010;36:1628–32.
22. Assoian RK, Grotendorst GR, Miller DM, Sporn MB. Cellular transformation by coordinated action of three peptide growth factors from human platelets. Nature. 1984;309:804–6.
23. Sachdeva GS, Sachdeva LT, Goel M, Bala S. Regenerative endodontic treatment of an immature tooth with a necrotic pulp and apical periodontitis using platelet-rich plasma (PRP) and mineral trioxide aggregate (MTA): a case report. Int Endod J. 2015;48:902–10.
24. Jadhav G, Shah N, Logani A. Revascularization with and without platelet-rich plasma in nonvital, immature, anterior teeth: a pilot clinical study. J Endod. 2012;38:1581–7.
25. Shivashankar VY, Johns DA, Vidyanath S, Kumar MR. Platelet rich fibrin in the revitalization of tooth with necrotic pulp and open apex. J Conserv Dent. 2012;15:395–8.
26. Mishra N, Narang I, Mittal N. Platelet-rich fibrin-mediated revitalization of immature necrotic tooth. Contemp Clin Dent. 2013;4:412–5.
27. Keswani D, Pandey RK. Revascularization of an immature tooth with a necrotic pulp using platelet-rich fibrin: a case report. Int Endod J. 2013;46:1096–104.
28. Johns DA, Shivashankar VY, Krishnamma S, Johns M. Use of photoactivated disinfection and platelet-rich fibrin in regenerative endodontics. J Conserv Dent. 2014;17:487–90.
29. Jadhav GR, Shah D, Raghvendra SS. Autologus platelet rich fibrin aided revascularization of an immature, non-vital permanent tooth with apical periodontitis: a case report. J Nat Sci Biol Med. 2015;6:224–5.
30. Yadav P, Pruthi PJ, Naval RR, Talwar S, Verma M. Novel use of platelet-rich fibrin matrix and MTA as an apical barrier in the management of a failed revascularization case. Dent Traumatol. 2015;31:328–31.
31. Narang I, Mittal N, Mishra N. A comparative evaluation of the blood clot, platelet-rich plasma, and platelet-rich fibrin in regeneration of necrotic immature permanent teeth: a clinical study. Contemp Clin Dent. 2015;6:63–8.
32. Nolla CM. The development of permanent teeth. J Dent Child. 1960;27:254–66.
33. Choukroun J, Diss A, Simonpieri A, Girard MO, Schoeffler C, Dohan SL, Dohan AJ, Mouhyi J, Dohan DM. Platelet-rich fibrin (PRF): a second-generation platelet concentrate. Part V: histologic evaluations of PRF effects on bone allograft maturation in sinus lift. Oral Surg Oral Med Oral Pathol Oral Radiol Endod. 2006;101:299–303.
34. Zhu W, Zhu X, Huang GT, Cheung GS, Dissanayaka WL, Zhang C. Regeneration of dental pulp tissue in immature teeth with apical periodontitis using platelet-rich plasma and dental pulp cells. Int Endod J. 2013;46:962–70.
35. Zhang DD, Chen X, Bao ZF, Chen M, Ding ZJ, Zhong M. Histologic comparison between platelet-rich plasma and blood clot in regenerative endodontic treatment: an animal study. J Endod. 2014;40:1388–93.
36. Lovelace TW, Henry MA, Hargreaves KM, Diogenes A. Evaluation of the delivery of mesenchymal stem cells into the root canal space of necrotic immature teeth after clinical regenerative endodontic procedure. J Endod. 2011;37:133–8.
37. Yamada Y, Ueda M, Naiki T, Takahashi M, Hata K, Nagasaka T. Autogenous injectable bone for regeneration with mesenchymal stem cells and platelet-rich plasma: tissue-engineered bone regeneration. Tissue Eng. 2004;10:955–64.
38. Petrino JA, Boda KK, Shambarger S, Bowles WR, McClanahan SB. Challenges in regenerative endodontics: a case series. J Endod. 2010;36:536–41.
39. Ding RY, Cheung GS, Chen J, Yin XZ, Wang QQ, Zhang CF. Pulp revascularization of immature teeth with apical periodontitis: a clinical study. J Endod. 2009;35:745–9.
40. Iwaya S, Ikawa M, Kubota M. Revascularization of an immature permanent tooth with periradicular abscess after luxation. Dent Traumatol. 2011;27:55–8.
41. Hargreaves KM, Diogenes A, Teixeira FB. Treatment options: biological basis of regenerative endodontic procedures. J Endod. 2013;39:S30–43.
42. Johns DA, Vidyanath S. Revitalization of tooth with necrotic pulp and open apex by using platelet-rich plasma: a case report. J Endod. 2011;37:743; author reply 43–4.

Combining virtual model and cone beam computed tomography to assess periodontal changes after anterior tooth movement

Sun-Hyun Kim[1], Jong-Bin Lee[2], Min-Ji Kim[3] and Eun-Kyoung Pang[4*]

Abstract

Background: Orthodontic force may affect not only periodontal ligaments, but also the alveoloar bone and the gingiva according to the type of tooth movements. The authors assessed changes in gingival thickness (GT) and alveolar bone thickness (ABT) after orthodontic treatment using a new method.

Methods: This study included 408 teeth (208 central incisors, 200 lateral incisors) from the upper and lower 4 anterior teeth of 52 patients who had completed orthodontic treatment. GT and ABT were measured using virtual casts fabricated from impressions and cone beam computed tomography (CBCT). Two sectioned images of every tooth axis were acquired by partitioning each tooth with a line connecting the midpoint of the incisal edge to the midpoint of the cementoenamel junction in the virtual models and the root apex in CBCT images. After superimposing the two sectioned images, GT and ABT were measured before and after orthodontic tooth movement. Correlations between GT and ABT before and after treatment, and changes in GT and ABT associated with sex, tooth arch, tooth position, orthognathic surgery, and tooth inclination and rotation were assessed.

Results: Before orthodontic treatment, GT and ABT were significantly correlated. Patients who underwent orthognathic surgery exhibited an increase in GT thickness compared with those who did not. ABT was significantly decreased in proclined teeth and in rotated teeth.

Conclusions: GT and ABT can be affected by the nature of tooth movement and can be accurately assessed by comparing sectioned CBCT images and virtual models.

Keywords: CBCT, Virtual model, Gingival thickness, Alveolar bone thickness

Background

Recent economic growth has prompted an increase in the demand for orthodontic treatment, particularly, interest in pursuing improvement of the aesthetic aspects of physiognomy. In the past, the purpose of orthodontic treatment was simple tooth alignment; however, aesthetic improvement in physiognomy, completion of occlusion, and the aesthetics of periodontal tissue have also become important factors in responding to patient demands. Therefore, it is necessary to diagnose and prevent undesirable changes in surrounding tissues associated with orthodontic treatment [1–3].

Although orthodontic treatment offers many benefits to patients including tooth alignment, establishment of occlusion, and aesthetic improvement of physiognomy, large amounts of tooth movement can cause unexpected adverse side effects such as root resorption, bone dehiscence, bone perforation, and gingival recession [4, 5]. The loss of alveolar bone is also a potential side effect of orthodontic treatment. When a tooth and its surrounding tissue are moved by orthodontic force(s) and the root compresses the periodontium for a certain period of time, the alveolar bone can be resorbed at that point,

* Correspondence: ekpang@ewha.ac.kr
[4]Department of Periodontology, School of Medicine, Ewha Womans University, 1071 Anyangcheon-ro, Yangcheon-gu, Seoul 07985, Republic of Korea
Full list of author information is available at the end of the article

and bone is deposited where tension is created [6]. Alveolar bone loss can differ in various ways, including magnitude, direction, and duration of orthodontic force(s). Orthodontic force(s) affects not only periodontal ligaments and roots, but also alveolar bone. If it is beyond the physiological range of force suitable for a tooth of a tooth and its surrounding tissues, side effects, such as root resorption and alveolar bone resorption, may occur after orthodontic treatment [7].

It has been reported that in patients with a high alveolar crest and thin alveolar bone, there is a high possibility of recession and loss of alveolar bone at the anterior labial and lingual aspects of the cortical bone [8]. When the anterior teeth move, bone reconstruction occurs in the alveolar crest or bone surrounding the root apex. However, bone reconstruction rarely occurs at the apical region near the cortical plate or mandibular symphysis [9, 10]. From the biological perspective of orthodontic treatment, the thickness of alveolar bone anchoring a tooth, as well as the amount of tooth movement, are important factors when devising an orthodontic plan and choosing an orthodontic treatment method [11]. The thickness of alveolar bone can has been associated with skeletal growth patterns and could be altered by grafting procedures [12, 13].

Many previous studies have measured gingival thickness (GT) and alveolar bone thickness (ABT) [14]. Generally, methods can be divided into those that are invasive and involve tissue damage, such as bone sounding, and those that are non-invasive, such as cone beam computed tomography (CBCT), although radiation exposure may be an issue [15]. One invasive method involves locally anesthetizing the patient's mouth, then measuring thickness directly by inserting a periodontal probe, a needle, or an endodontic instrument [16]. This method has disadvantages in that the patient must endure the pain associated with the anesthesia and measurement; moreover, the results of this method are also prone to inter-observer/operator variation [17]. Conversely, the non-invasive method using CBCT is relatively accurate; however, it may be subject to error when soft tissues, such as the gingiva, are measured due to limits of its resolution [18, 19]. Therefore, we introduce a new method, which combined CBCT imaging to measure ABT and the images generated using a digital intraoral scanner to measure GT. Using measurement data thus acquired, we studied correlations between GT and ABT before and after orthodontic treatment, and the changes in GT and ABT associated with various factors including sex, tooth arch, tooth position, orthognathic surgery, and tooth inclination and rotation.

Methods

This retrospective study involved a total of 408 teeth (208 central and 200 lateral incisors). Specifically, a total of 416 teeth were evaluated from 4 upper and lower anterior teeth of 52 patients who had available records of orthodontic treatment for malocclusion at the Ewha Womans University Mokdong Hospital between January 2009 and April 2016. A total of 408 teeth were selected according to the inclusion criterion that GT and ABT could be measured in natural teeth without defects. Teeth in which GT and ABT could not be measured because of defects, such as those treated with previous orthodontic treatment or periodontal surgery, were excluded. A total of 8 teeth were excluded: 5 that were extracted for treatment; 2 that were replaced by implants; and 1 exhibiting a congenital defect.

This study was approved by the Ethics Committee of the School of Medicine, Ewha Womans University Medical Center (Approval number: EUMC 16–05–032-005).

Measurement of GT and ABT

Cast scanning

After scanning each patient's cast with a digital intraoral scanner (Trios Pod, 3shape dental systems, Copenhagen, Denmark), each anterior tooth in the virtual model was sectioned via a line connecting the midpoint of the incisal edge and the midpoint of the cementoenamel junction (CEJ) (Fig. 1). Tooth section images were acquired for 4 upper and lower anterior teeth. This type of cast scanning is different from intraoral scanning in that patient cast impressions were scanned using an intraoral scanner.

CBCT

CBCT was performed using a Dinnova3 device (HDXWILL, Chung-ju, Korea) with the following operating parameters: current, 10 mA; voltage, 85 kVp; minimum voxel size, 0.15 mm.

Each CBCT image was acquired by sectioning via a line connecting the midpoint of the incisal edge and the root apex using software (OnDemand 3D, Cybermed Co., Seoul, Korea) for each of 4 upper and lower anterior teeth (Fig. 2).

Superimposition

Sectioned CBCT images and those from the virtual models were superimposed to match the shape of the clinical crown of each tooth using software (Photoshop CS, Adobe, San Jose, CA, USA) (Fig. 3). To measure GT and ABT, a perpendicular line was drawn to the tooth axis from a point that was 4 mm apical to the CEJ (Fig. 4). This superimposition method was similar to a technique used in a previous study [14] and has been validated. Furthermore, to ensure reliability, all measurements were performed by the same

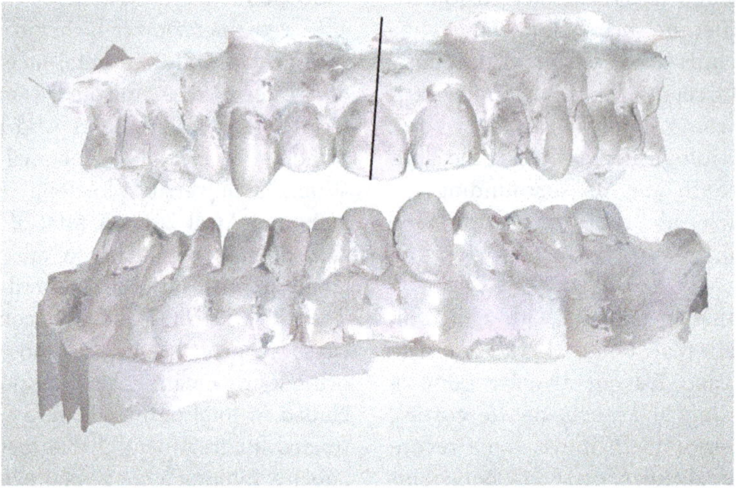

Fig. 1 Tooth sectioning in a cast. After scanning a cast with a digital intraoral scanner, the anterior teeth were sectioned with the line connecting the midpoint of the incisal edge and the midpoint of the cemento enamel junction

trained operator, and repeated 3 times per case for superimposition and measurement of GT and ABT. Sufficiently reliable data were obtained ($p < 0.05$).

Measurement of tooth inclination and rotation

Inclination

To measure tooth inclination, patients were divided into two groups: those who underwent orthognathic surgery and those who did not. In those who underwent orthognathic surgery, the axes of the maxillary teeth were measured in the Frankfort horizontal plane and those of the mandibular teeth were measured in the mandibular plane. In those who never underwent orthognathic surgery, the axes of both the maxillary and the mandibular teeth were measured in the occlusal plane (Fig. 5).

Rotation

To assess the amount of tooth rotation, the angle between the median palatine suture and the extended line of the incisal edge in the maxilla, and the angle between the line connecting both right and left mental foramen and the extended line of the incisal edge in the mandible, was measured. Clockwise tooth rotation

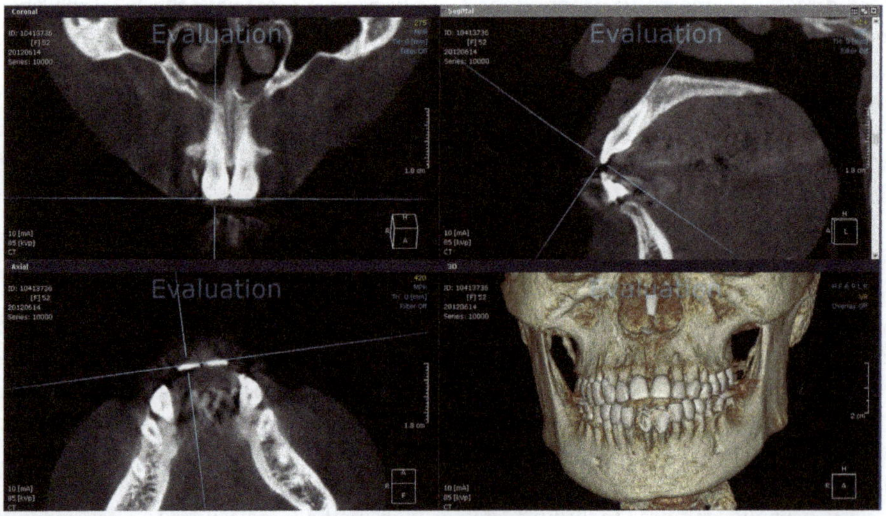

Fig. 2 Tooth sectioning via cone beam computed tomography. The image was obtained by sectioning each tooth along the line connecting the midpoint of the incisal edge and the root apex, using software (OnDemand 3D)

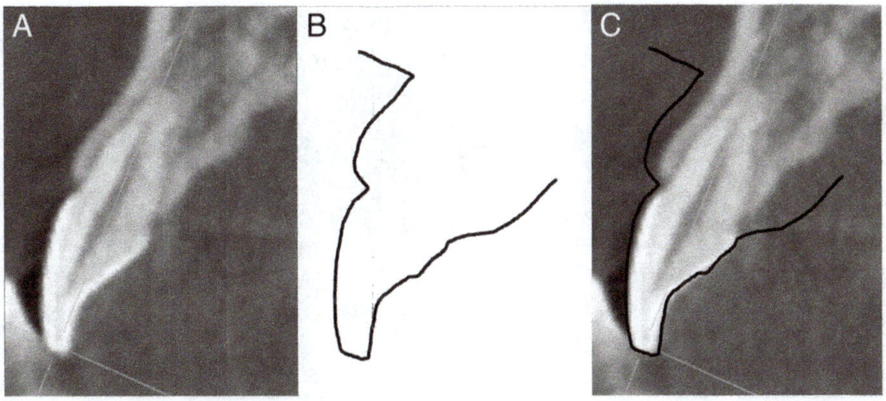

Fig. 3 Superimposition of cast and cone beam computed tomography images. **a** The cone beam computed tomography image. **b** The scanned cast image. **c** Superimposition of (**a**) and (**b**)

was defined as positive (+), while counterclockwise tooth rotation was defined as negative (−). The measured angles before and after orthodontic treatment were analyzed (Fig. 6).

Analysis of GT and ABT

After measuring GT and ABT by superimposing the sectioned image of the virtual model over the CBCT sectioned image, the results were analyzed as described below.

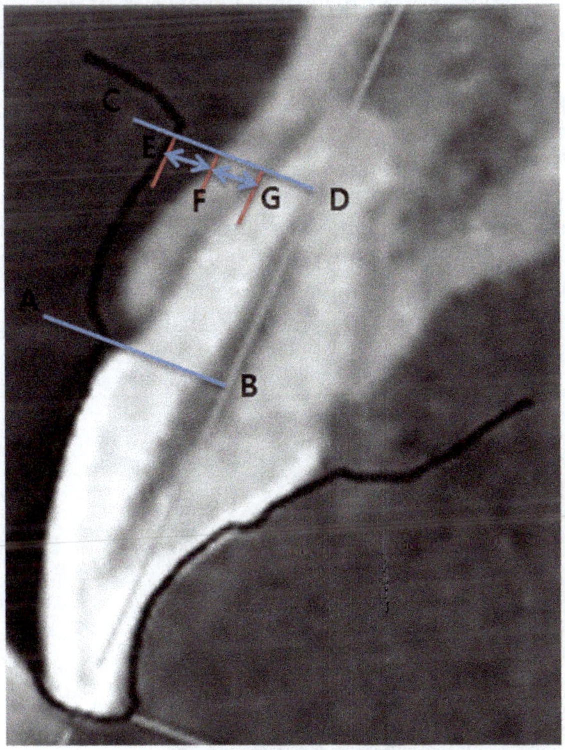

Fig. 4 Measurement of gingival thickness and alveolar bone thickness. **a**, **b**: Perpendicular line from the cemento enamel junction to the tooth axis. **c**, **d** The line incorporating parallel translation of (**a**, **b**) towards its root apex as 4 mm. **e**, **f** Gingival thickness. **f**, **g** Alveolar bone thickness

Correlations between GT and ABT

The correlations between GT and ABT before and after orthodontic treatment were analyzed and compared.

Changes in GT and ABT before and after orthodontic treatment

The changes in GT and ABT associated with sex, tooth arch (maxilla/mandible), tooth position (central/lateral), orthognathic surgery (with/without), and tooth inclination (proclination/retroclination) before and after orthodontic treatment were analyzed and compared.

Changes in GT and ABT associated with tooth movement

After dividing tooth movement according to inclination or rotation, changes in GT and ABT associated with tooth inclination or rotation were analyzed and compared.

Statistical analysis

The data showed normal distribution. Pearson's correlation analysis was performed to analyze correlations between GT and ABT before and after orthodontic treatment. The independent *t*-test was then used to analyze changes in GT and ABT associated with sex, tooth arch, tooth position, orthognathic surgery, and tooth inclination before and after orthodontic treatment. Finally, multi-linear regression analysis was performed to investigate changes in GT and ABT associated with tooth inclination and tooth rotation. All statistical analyses were performed using SPSS version 20 (IBM Corporation, Armonk, NY, USA); $p < 0.05$ was considered to be statistically significant in all tests.

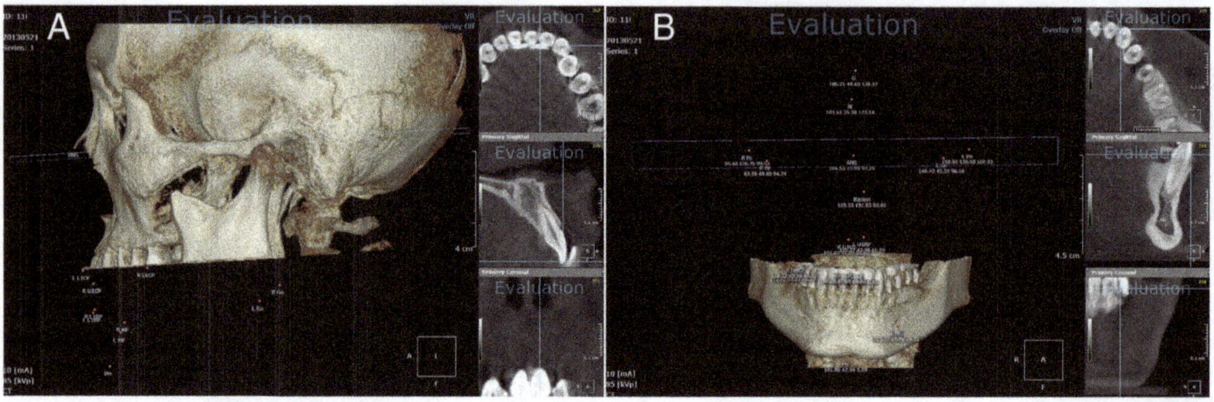

Fig. 5 Measurement of tooth inclination with (**a**) the angle between the Frankfurt horizontal plane and the axis of the tooth in the maxilla, and (**b**) the angle between the mandibular plane and the axis of the tooth in the mandible

Results

A total of 408 teeth, from 4 upper and lower anterior teeth of 52 patients, were analyzed. The mean age of was 22 years, with the following distribution: teenagers (49.5%); twenties (35.0%); thirties (9.8%); and forties and older (5.6%). The mean duration of treatment was 2 years 1 month, and the sex distribution was 80.4% female and 19.6% male (Table 1).

There was a significant correlation between GT and ABT, which was evident only before orthodontic treatment ($p < 0.05$) (Table 2). Changes in GT were not significantly associated with sex, tooth arch (maxilla/mandible), tooth position (central/lateral), or tooth inclination (i.e., proclination/retroclination) before and after orthodontic treatment. However, the change in GT was statistically significant in patients who underwent orthognathic surgery ($p < 0.05$) (Table 3). Changes in ABT were not significantly associated with sex, tooth arch, tooth position, orthognathic surgery, or tooth inclination before and after orthodontic treatment. However, ABT had significantly decreased in teeth that were proclined ($p < 0.05$) (Table 4).

Changes in GT and ABT associated with tooth inclination and rotation were analyzed and compared. In the multilinear regression analysis, GT was not statistically associated with tooth inclination or rotation (Table 5). Similarly, ABT was also not statistically associated with tooth inclination (neither proclination nor retroclination); however, it was significantly associated with tooth rotation ($p < 0.05$). Specifically, greater tooth rotation was associated with a greater reduction in ABT (Table 6).

Discussion

Interest in non-invasive methods to assess and/or measure soft tissue has increased because of patient pain and resistance to orthodontic diagnosis or periodontal treatment [20]. We aimed to measure GT and ABT using non-invasive methods that do not damage

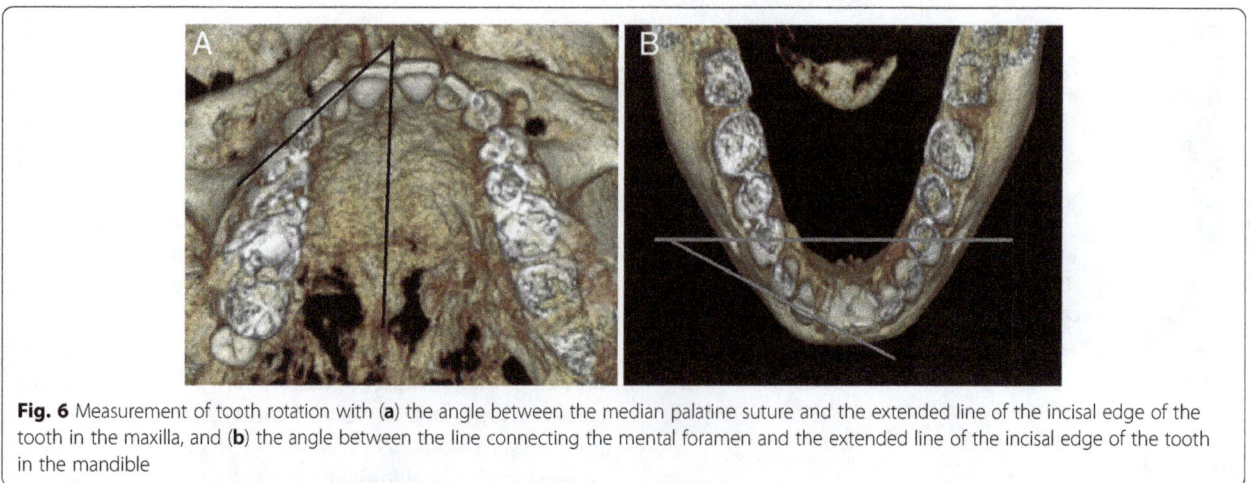

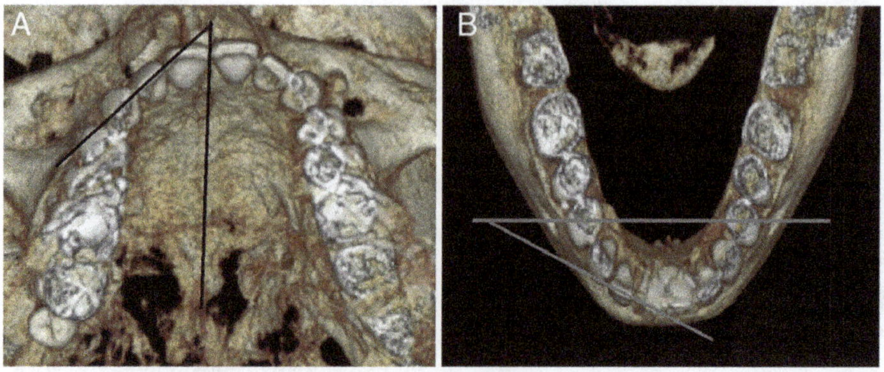

Fig. 6 Measurement of tooth rotation with (**a**) the angle between the median palatine suture and the extended line of the incisal edge of the tooth in the maxilla, and (**b**) the angle between the line connecting the mental foramen and the extended line of the incisal edge of the tooth in the mandible

Table 1 Patient characteristics

Variable	N	%
Age:	mean 21.78 ± 8.77 years	
10–19	202	49.50
20–29	143	35.04
30–39	40	9.80
40 and over	23	5.63
Treatment period	mean 2.19 ± 0.16, years	
Gender		
Male	80	19.60
Female	328	80.39
Tooth arch		
Maxilla	203	49.75
Mandible	205	50.25
Tooth position		
Central incisor	208	50.98
Lateral incisor	200	49.02
Orthognathic surgery of the tooth		
With Surgery	205	50.24
Without surgery	203	49.75

N number of teeth

Table 3 Changes in gingival thickness before and after orthodontic treatment

Variable	Δ	*p* value
Gender		
Male	0.047	0.316
Female	0.103	
Tooth arch		
Maxilla	0.025	0.140
Mandible	0.091	
Tooth position		
Central incisor	0.062	0.867
Lateral incisor	0.054	
Orthognathic surgery of the tooth		
With Surgery	0.143	< 0.001
Without surgery	−0.027	
Translation		
Proclination	0.048	0.597
Retroclination	0.072	

Δ = amount of gingival thickness change after orthodontic treatment

tissue. Although many studies investigating the anatomical shape of the gingiva, the depth of periodontal pockets, and the length of the junctional epithelium have been published [17, 21], relatively few studies examining GT have been reported. It has been suggested that this is partly due to the difficulty of measuring GT [22]. To improve the measurement of GT, we developed a new method using a sectioned image of the patient's virtual dental model. Images acquired using sectioned virtual dental models and volume-rendered CBCT were superimposed, and subtractive analysis was subsequently used to measure GT and ABT. According to previous studies, the alveolar bone crest is usually located 4 mm below the CEJ. Therefore, we drew a perpendicular line to the tooth axis from a point that was 4 mm apical to the CEJ [23], and measured GT and ABT on that line.

Opinions differ as to whether orthodontic treatment causes gingival recession [24–27]. Periodontal disease caused by poor oral conditions during orthodontic treatment may occasionally cause gingival recession; however, loss of alveolar bone due to tooth movement also causes gingival recession. Many previous studies have reported major reasons for gingival recession caused by tooth movement after orthodontic treatment, which included a free gingival margin < 0.5 mm, thin alveolar bone or dehiscence, proclination, and orthognathic surgery [24–27]. Given the

Table 2 Correlations between gingival thickness and alveolar bone thickness before and after orthodontic treatment

	r	*p*-value
Before	0.194	< 0.001
After	0.055	0.268

r Pearson's correlation coefficient

Table 4 Change in alveolar bone thickness before and after orthodontic treatment

Variable	Δ	*p* value
Gender		
Male	−0.013	0.268
Female	0.031	
Tooth arch		
Maxilla	0.002	0.200
Mandible	0.043	
Tooth position		
Central incisor	0.031	0.599
Lateral incisor	0.142	
Orthognathic surgery of the tooth		
With Surgery	0.003	0.223
Without surgery	0.042	
Translation		
Proclination	−0.089	0.021*
Retroclination	0.065	

Δ = amount of alveolar bone thickness changes after orthodontic treatment
*$p < 0.05$

Table 5 Changes in gingival thickness by tooth movement

Variable	Standardized coefficient, β	95% CL		p value
Translation	0.004	0.000	0.008	0.064
Rotation	0.000	−0.003	0.004	0.808

CL confidence limits

results of the present study, we additionally conclude that proclination causes reduced ABT. However, the results relating to changes in GT and ABT before and after orthodontic treatment and their association with sex and orthognathic surgery (with/without) in the current study, differed from those of previous studies. Notably, only 19.2% (80 of 408) of the teeth in the current study were from male subjects, which is one potential reason for the discrepancy in results [15, 28]. With regard to orthognathic surgery, we suggest that the discrepancy may be due to the different measurement method used [29, 30]. In the current study, the angles between the tooth axis and each plane were measured. In patients who underwent orthognathic surgery, the inclination of maxillary teeth was measured in the Frankfort horizontal plane and that of the mandibular teeth was measured in the mandibular plane. In patients who never underwent orthognathic surgery, the inclination of both maxillary and mandibular teeth was measured in the occlusal plane. In contrast, previous studies have used a variety of measurement methods such as ANB (A point, nasion, B point), the angle between the SN line and FH line, among others. We believe that these differences in measurement methods influenced the results [31]. We did not consider the exact type of orthognathic surgery because several previous studies have reported that orthognathic surgery has no effect on the gingiva [32–34].

The current study had some limitations, the first of which was its retrospective design and the use of casts from patients who had already completed orthodontic treatment. If direct intraoral scanning—rather than casting—could have been performed, the results of the study would have been more accurate and reliable. In general, alginate impressions are made at the beginning and at the end of orthodontic treatment. Although possible deformation of casts made from alginate impressions has been reported, it has advantages including convenience and clinically acceptable accuracy [35]. Furthermore, many previous studies have reported high accuracy and reproducibility of digital models obtained by indirectly scanning dental casts [36, 37]. Notably, we suggest that the potential error arising from deformation did not significantly affect the results of the current study. In the future, we believe that further studies can be conducted using scanned images obtained directly from patient mouths via a digital intraoral scanner.

Table 6 Changes in alveolar bone thickness by tooth movement

Variable	Standardized coefficient, β	95% CL		p value
Translation	0.001	−0.004	0.007	0.588
Rotation	−0.004	−0.006	− 0.001	0.005*

CL confidence limits

*$p < 0.05$

Conclusions

In the present study, GT was decreased in patients who underwent previous orthognathic surgery, and ABT was decreased in cases of proclination. GT and ABT can be accurately assessed by comparing sectioned CBCT images and virtual models.

Abbreviations

ABT: Alveolar bone thickness; ANB: A point, nasion, B point; CBCT: Cone beam computed tomography; CEJ: Cemento enamel junction; FH line: Frankfort horizontal line; GT: Gingival thickness; SN line: Sella nasion line

Acknowledgments

This research did not receive any specific grant from funding agencies in the public, commercial, or not-for-profit sectors.

Funding

No external funding was provided in regard with this study.

Authors' contributions

SK contributed to data collection, analysis and development and editing of the manuscript. JL and MK contributed to conception and study design, supervision of data gathering, interpretation of results, and editing of the manuscript. EP was responsible for the study design, development of the research infrastructure, and direct supervision of the data gathering. And she was directly contributed to the data analysis and development and editing of the manuscript. All authors read and approved the final manuscript.

Competing interests

The authors declare that they have no competing interests.

Author details

[1]Department of Clinical Oral Health Science, Graduate School of Clinical Dentistry, Ewha Womans University, Seoul, Korea. [2]Department of Periodontology, Mokdong Hospital, Ewha Womans University, Seoul, Korea. [3]Department of Orthodontics, School of Medicine, Ewha Womans University, Seoul, Korea. [4]Department of Periodontology, School of Medicine, Ewha Womans University, 1071 Anyangcheon-ro, Yangcheon-gu, Seoul 07985, Republic of Korea.

References

1. Reddy MS. Achieving gingival esthetics. J Am Dent Assoc Dent Cosmos. 2003;134:295–306.
2. Addy M, Mostafa P, Newcombe R. Dentine hypersensitivity: the distribution of recession, sensitivity and plaque. J Dent. 1987;15:242–8.
3. Watanabe MG. Root caries prevalence in a group of Brazilian adult dental patients. Brazilian Dent J. 2003;14:153–6.
4. Horiuchi A, Hotokezaka H, Kobayashi K. Correlation between cortical plate proximity and apical root resorption. Am J Orthodont Dentofacial Orthop. 1998;114:311–8.
5. Wainwright WM. Faciolingual tooth movement: its influence on the root and cortical plate. Am J Orthod. 1973;64:278–302.
6. Aass A, Albandar J, Aasenden R, Tollefsen T, Gjermo P. Variation in prevalence of radiographic alveolar bone loss in subgroups of 14-year-old schoolchildren in Oslo. J Clin Periodontol. 1988;15:130–3.
7. Albandar JM, Rise J, Gjermo P, Johansen JR. Radiographic quantification of alveolar bone level changes. J Clin Periodontol. 1986;13:195–200.
8. Wehrbein H, Bauer W, Diedrich P. Mandibular incisors, alveolar bone, and symphysis afterorthodontic treatment. A retrospective study. Am J Orthodont Dentofacial Orthop. 1996;110:239–46.
9. Edwards JG. A study of the anterior portion of the palate as it relates to orthodontic therapy. Am J Orthod. 1976;69:249–73.
10. Mulie R, Hoeve A. The limitations of tooth movement within the symphysis, studied with laminagraphy and standardized occlusal films. J Clin Orthodont. 1976;10:882–93 6-9.
11. Yamada C, Kitai N, Kakimoto N, Murakami S, Furukawa S, Takada K. Spatial relationships between the mandibular central incisor and associated alveolar bone in adults with mandibular prognathism. Angle Orthod. 2007; 77:766–72.
12. Biondi K, Lorusso P, Fastuca R, Mangano A, Zecca PA, Bosco M, Caprioglio A, Levrini L. Evaluation of masseter muscle in different vertical skeletal patterns in growing patients. Eur J Paediatr Dent. 2016;17:47–52.
13. Cutroneo G, Piancino MG, Ramieri G, Bracco P, Vita G, Isola G, et al. Expression of muscle-specific integrins in masseter muscle fibers during malocclusion disease. Int J Mol Med. 2012;30:235–42.
14. Kim YJ, Park JM, Kim S, Koo KT, Seol YJ, Lee YM, et al. New method of assessing the relationship between buccal bone thickness and gingival thickness. J Periodontal Implant Sci. 2016;46:372–81.
15. Müller HP, Schaller N, Eger T, Heinecke A. Thickness of masticatory mucosa. J Clin Periodontol. 2000;27:431–6.
16. Turck D. A histologic comparison of the edentulous denture and non-denture bearing tissues. J Prosthet Dent. 1965;15:419–34.
17. Claffey N, Shanley D. Relationship of gingival thickness and bleeding to loss of probing attachment in shallow sites following nonsurgical periodontal therapy. J Clin Periodontol. 1986;13:654–7.
18. Kydd W, Daly C, Wheeler J 3rd. The thickness measurement of masticatory mucosa in vivo. Int Dent J. 1971;21:430–41.
19. Benavides E, Rios HF, Ganz SD, An C-H, Resnik R, Reardon GT, et al. Use of cone beam computed tomography in implant dentistry: the international congress of Oral Implantologists consensus report. Implant Dent. 2012;21: 78–86.
20. Zecca PA, Fastuca R, Beretta M, Caprioglio A, Macchi A. Correlation assessment between three-dimensional facial soft tissue scan and lateral cephalometric radiography in orthodontic diagnosis. Int J Dent. 2016;2016: 1473918.
21. Goaslind G, Robertson P, Mahan C, Morrison W, Olson J. Thickness of facial gingiva. J Periodontol. 1977;48:768–71.
22. Anderegg CR, Metzler DG, Nicoll BK. Gingiva thickness in guided tissue regeneration and associated recession at facial furcation defects. J Periodontol. 1995;66:397–402.
23. Cook DR, Mealey BL, Verrett RG, Mills MP, Noujeim ME, Lasho DJ, et al. Relationship between clinical periodontal biotype and labial plate thickness: an in vivo study. Int J Periodontics Restorative Dent. 2011;31:345–54.
24. Allais D, Melsen B. Does labial movement of lower incisors influence the level of the gingival margin? A case–control study of adult orthodontic patients. Eur J Orthodont. 2003;25:343–52.
25. Djeu G, Hayes C, Zawaideh S. Correlation between mandibular central incisor proclination and gingival recession during fixed appliance therapy. Angle Orthodont. 2002;72:238–45.
26. Årtun J, Grobéty D. Periodontal status of mandibular incisors after pronounced orthodontic advancement during adolescence: a follow-up evaluation. Am J Orthodont Dentofacial Orthop. 2001;119:2–10.
27. Ruf S, Hansen K, Pancherz H. Does orthodontic proclination of lower incisors in children and adolescents cause gingival recession? Am J Orthodont Dentofacial Orthop. 1998;114:100–6.
28. De Rouck T, Eghbali R, Collys K, De Bruyn H, Cosyn J. The gingival biotype revisited: transparency of the periodontal probe through the gingival margin as a method to discriminate thin from thick gingiva. J Clin Periodontol. 2009;36:428–33.
29. Kim Y, Park JU, Kook Y-A. Alveolar bone loss around incisors in surgical skeletal class III patients: a retrospective 3-D CBCT study. Angle Orthodont. 2009;79:676–82.
30. Kook Y-A, Kim G, Kim Y. Comparison of alveolar bone loss around incisors in normal occlusion samples and surgical skeletal class III patients. Angle Orthodont. 2011;82:645–52.
31. Lee K-M, Kim Y-I, Park S-B, Son W-S. Alveolar bone loss around lower incisors during surgical orthodontic treatment in mandibular prognathism. Angle Orthodont. 2012;82:637–44.
32. Alstad S, Zachrisson BU. Longitudinal study of periodontal condition associated with orthodontic treatment in adolescents. Am J Orthod. 1979; 76:277–86.
33. Zachrisson S, Zachrisson BU. Gingival condition associated with orthodontic treatment. Angle Orthod. 1972;42:26–34.
34. Kloehn JS, Pfeifer JS. The effect of orthodontic treatment on the periodontium. Angle Orthod. 1974;44:127–34.
35. Andlin-Sobocki A, Bodin L. Dimensional alterations of the gingiva related to changes of facial/lingual tooth position in permanent anterior teeth of children. J Clin Periodontol. 1993;20:219–24.
36. Johnson GH, Craig RG. Accuracy of four types of rubber impression materials compared with time of pour and a repeat pour of models. J Prosthet Dent. 1985;53:484–90.
37. Clancy J, Scandrett FR, Ettinger RL. Long-term dimensional stability of three current elastomers. J Oral Rehabil. 1983;10:325–33.

Developmental defects of the enamel and its impact on the oral health quality of life of children resident in Southwest Nigeria

Morenike Oluwatoyin Folayan[1,2*], Nneka Maureen Chukwumah[3], Bamidele Olubukola Popoola[4], Dada Oluwaseyi Temilola[1], Nneka Kate Onyejaka[5], Titus Ayo Oyedele[6,7] and Folake Barakat Lawal[4]

Abstract

Background: Developmental defects of the enamel (DDE) increase the risk for diseases that impact negatively on the quality of life. The objective of this study was to compare the oral health quality of life of children with molar-incisor-hypomineralisation (MIH) and enamel hypoplasia; and assess if caries worsened the impact of these lesions on the quality of life.

Methods: This study recruited 853 6 to 16-years-old school children. They filled the Child-OIDP questionnaire. The MIH, enamel hypoplasia, caries and oral hygiene status was assessed. Poisson regression was used to determine the impact of MIH and enamel hypoplasia on the oral health quality of life, after adjusting for the effect of sex, age, socioeconomic class, oral hygiene and caries status.

Results: The prevalence of MIH and enamel hypoplasia was 2.9% and 7.6% respectively. There was no significant difference in the mean child-OIDP scores of children with or without MIH ($p = 0.57$), children with or without enamel hypoplasia ($p = 0.48$), and children with enamel hypoplasia with and without caries ($p = 0.30$). Children with enamel hypoplasia and caries had worse outcomes for speaking ($p = 0.01$). Children with middle (AOR: 2.74; 95% CI: 1.60–4.67; $P < 0.01$) and low (AOR: 1.75; 95% CI: 1.04–2.95; $p = 0.03$) socioeconomic status, and those with caries (AOR: 2.02; 95% CI: 1.26–3.22; $p = 0.03$) had their oral health quality of life negatively impacted.

Conclusion: MIH and enamel hypoplasia had no significant impact on the overall oral health quality of life of children resident in southwestern Nigeria. However, children with caries and those from middle and low socioeconomic classes had poorer oral health quality of life.

Keywords: Enamel, Hypoplasia, Hypomineralisation, Children, Quality of life, Nigeria

Background

Developmental defects of the teeth are caused by complex interactions between genetic and environmental factors that affect the structure of the enamel during its formation [1]. Developmental defects of the enamel (DDE) can be classified into two distinct categories: those that affect the quality (hypomineralisation) and those that affect the quantity (hypoplasia) of the enamel [2].

One of the most studied forms of hypomineralised enamel is molar hypomineralisation [MIH].

The lesion arises from the disruption of ameloblasts during mineralization and maturation phase of the enamel, thereby giving rise to defective quality of the enamel [3]. The defect affects one to four first permanent molars, and is frequently associated with the affected permanent incisors [4]. A similar lesion has been reported in second primary molars [5, 6]. The defect caused by MIH appears in white, yellow or brown colour, reflecting the hypomineralised nature, while hypoplasia presents as an area of reduced thickness of the enamel in form of pits, grooves, and bands.

* Correspondence: toyinukpong@yahoo.co.uk
[1]Department of Child Dental Health, Obafemi Awolowo University, Ile-Ife, Nigeria
[2]Department of Child Dental Health, Obafemi Awolowo University Teaching Hospitals' Complex, Ile-Ife, Nigeria
Full list of author information is available at the end of the article

The prevalence of MIH ranges between 3.5 and 40.2% [7]. The aetiological factors remain largely unknown, though multiple systemic aetiological factors have been suggested, including the possibility of genetic predisposition [8]. It is an important risk factor for caries in the permanent dentition [9]. The associated post-eruptive breakdown due to soft and porous enamel is associated with tooth sensitivity, disfiguration and rapid plaque retention [3]. Caries [10], dentine sensitivity [11] and poor aesthetics [12] - morbidities associated with MIH – impact negatively on the quality of life of affected individuals. There are however, no studies highlighting the negative impact of MIH on the quality of life, though Arrow [13] reported no impact of enamel defect on the first molars on the quality of life of affected children in Australia.

Unlike MIH whose aetiology remains unclear, enamel hypoplasia is known to be a quantitative defect which results in the formation of clinically visible, localized or generalized pits and grooves on the affected tooth [14]. A high prevalence of the lesion has been observed in children from developing countries [15], children with chronic or acute malnutrition [15], and children with very low birth weight [16]. Enamel hypoplasia has also been associated with increased risk for poor aesthetics [17], caries [18] and poor oral hygiene [19]. We found no study discussing the effect of enamel hypoplasia specifically, on the quality of life of affected individuals. However, Vargas-Ferreira and Ardenghi [17] reported no impact of developmental dental defects on the overall quality of life of affected children, though it caused significant functional limitation.

MIH and enamel hypoplasia both cause discoloration. While discoloration of the posterior teeth may have no significant impact on the psychology of patients, it is expected that discoloration of the anterior teeth – which both MIH and enamel hypoplasia could affect – may negatively impact on the quality of life. Discolorations and aesthetic concerns associated with enamel hypoplasia may however be more severe than that associated with MIH. This increases the possibility of enamel hypoplasia having worse impact on the quality of life when compared with MIH. There is however, no studies to verify this hypothesis.

Past studies conducted in Nigeria showed a high prevalence of MIH [20, 21] and enamel hypoplasia [22, 23]. The prevalence of MIH ranged between 9.7% and 17.7% [20, 21], while that of enamel hypoplasia ranged between 0.13% and 3.6% in the permanent dentition [22–26] and 2.3% to 4.0% in the primary dentition [23, 27]. Co-existence of MIH and enamel hypoplasia had also been described [28]. These lesions were also associated with co-morbidities that affect oral health quality of life [29, 30]. Nigeria therefore provides a good environment to study the impact of MIH and enamel hypoplasia on the oral health quality of life of children. We, therefore, assessed the impact of MIH and enamel hypoplasia on the oral health quality of life of children resident in southwestern Nigeria. We also compared the quality of life of children with DDE with those without DDE and assessed if caries worsened the outcome of DDE on their quality of life.

Methods

Study design

This was a cross-sectional study. Study participants were 6 to 16 years old children and adolescents living in Ile-Ife and Ibadan, Nigeria. Children aged six years were included in the study population because of the possibility of having enamel hypoplasia in the primary dentition [23]. Also, children in the study environment erupt their first permanent molars early: the first permanent mandibular molars are out by 5.68 ± 1.21 years in boys and girls and the first permanent maxillary molars are out by 5.95 ± 0.96 years in girls and 6.15 + 0.93 years in boys [31].

Participants were recruited from public and private secondary schools to ensure representation of all cadres of the socioeconomic strata in the study sample. Socioeconomic status has been associated with the presence of enamel hypoplasia [32]. In Nigeria, children who attend public schools are majorly from the lower socioeconomic strata, while most of those who attend private schools are from the upper socioeconomic strata [33]. Children are taught in English. Public communication is also in English.

Study location

One of the two study locations was Ife Central Local Government Area (LGA), a sub-urban town in south-western Nigeria. The last census showed that the population of the LGA was 138,818, with about 14,000 (10%) being children [34]. The study site also hosts oral health clinics thereby making it possible to refer screened pupils with lesions for oral health care. The second study site was Ibadan, an urban town in southwestern Nigeria. Ibadan the capital city of Oyo State, has a population of about two million, 36% of which are children [35].

Sample size and sampling procedure

The sample size was powered to determine the prevalence of DDE based on the assumption that prevalence of the lesion was 50%. The sample size was calculated using the Cochran formula [36]. This gave a minimum sample size of 384. The sample size was increased by 10% to account for attrition, giving a required sample size of 422 study participants.

A multi-phase sampling method was employed. The first stage involved selection of schools using a simple random sampling technique from a list of 107 registered public and private primary and secondary schools in the Ife-Central LGA and a list of 102 primary and secondary schools in Ibadan North-East LGA. The list was obtained from the Local School Authority. The schools were stratified into public and private schools. Eight (three public and five private) of the 107 schools in Ile-Ife and 12 of the 102 schools in Ibadan were randomly selected by picking blindly from pot containing the names of the schools. A ratio that ensured proportionate representation of both public and private schools in the LGA was used to guide the number of schools to be selected.

The class registration list for each school was then used to determine the specific classes to participate in the study. In each school children aged 6 to 16 years eligible for study participation were enlisted from the study register. Twenty two students were then randomly selected by balloting from the list of eligible students. The recruited students were then met, introduced to the study and given consent forms for their parents to fill. All children eligible to participate in the study who were in school on the day of examination and who had parental consent to participate in the study were enrolled. Children with special care needs were excluded from the study because of an increased likelihood of their having poorer oral health quality of life [37].

Child Oral impact on daily performance (child-OIDP) assessment

The English version of the child version of Oral Impact on Daily Performance (Child-OIDP) questionnaire [38] validated by Chukwumah et al. [30] was used to collect data on oral health quality of life. Trained interviewers administered the questionnaire. It generated information on age, sex, father's occupation, mother's level of education and the oral health quality of life for each child.

Clinical examination

Study procedure

All eligible participants were examined in the classroom in the presence of a teacher. Each child was seated on a chair facing the window to ensure a natural source of light for intra-oral viewing. The dental mirror was used to further provide illumination of the tooth surfaces through reflection of light and sunrays. To ensure privacy, a corner was created in each classroom to conduct the clinical examination.

Diagnosis of caries

Caries was diagnosed using the World Health Organisation Oral Health Survey recommendations [39]. Each tooth was examined for dental caries using the ball tipped WHO dental explorer. Caries status was assessed using the Decayed Missing and Filled Teeth (dmft/DMFT) index. Decayed tooth (d/D) were defined as any tooth whose crown had an unmistakable cavitation on the pits or fissures, or tooth surface, or a filled crown with decay. This implies that caries was diagnosed only when there was dentine involvement. The filled tooth (f/F) was defined as a filled crown with no decay. The missing tooth (m/M) was defined as a tooth extracted due to caries. To arrive at a dmft/DMFT score, the number of teeth with caries, number of extracted teeth due to caries, and the number of teeth with fillings or crowns were summed together [40]. For the purpose of analysis, caries status was further divided into caries present (when dmft/DMFT was 1 or greater) or absent (when dmft/DMFT was 0). Enamel defects were differentiated from carious lesions by their clinical appearance and locations (usually not related to gingival margins or occlusal fissures) [41].

Measuring oral hygiene status

The components of the OHI-S, the Debris Index and Calculus Index, were obtained based on six numerical determinations representing the amount of debris or calculus found on the surfaces of index teeth namely: 11, 16, 26, 31, 36, 46 [42]. Debris and calculus scores were totaled and divided by the number of surfaces scored. Scores were graded as 0.0–1.2 = Good oral hygiene, 1.3–3.0 = Fair oral hygiene and > 3.1 = Poor oral hygiene.

Diagnosis of developmental defects of the enamel

All the teeth were examined wet after debris had been removed with the use of a piece of gauze after the OHI-S assessment. Each surface of the permanent first molar and incisor was screened for demarcated white, yellow or brown opacities, greater or equal to 2 mm in diameter based on European Association of Peadiatric Dentistry's diagnostic criteria for MIH [43]. All the teeth were also examined for enamel hypoplasia. A diagnosis of enamel hypoplasia was made when there was evidence of deficiency in enamel formation seen clinically as localized or generalized pits and grooves on the surfaces of teeth. Both primary and permanent dentitions were examined.

Calibration

The two examiners were trained Paedodontists who had been practicing for a minimum of 10 years. They both undertook a series of calibration exercises to ensure the validity of their diagnosis of dental anomalies; the WHO criteria for the diagnosis of caries [39] and the OHI-S index described by Green and Vermillion [42]. The examiners had several sessions reviewing clinical photographs and repeated practice on examination of lesions, using clinical photographs. The kappa scores for the inter-examiner reliability score for caries, oral hygiene status, MIH and enamel hypoplasia were 0.96, 0.95, 0.50 and 0.72 respectively.

Self report of oral health condition

A checklist of 17 oral conditions was used to assess the child's experience of oral disease in the previous 3 months. Respondents were instructed to answer "yes" if they had experienced any of the disease conditions in the previous 3 months, and "no" if they had not. Oral conditions were described to the children. The 17 checklist conditions were toothache; sensitive tooth; tooth decay or cavity; loss of primary tooth; tooth space (due to non-erupted permanent tooth); fractured permanent tooth; abnormal colour, shape or size of tooth; abnormal position of tooth (e.g. crooked or projecting, gapped); bleeding gums; swollen gums; calculus; oral ulcers; bad breath; deformity of mouth or face (e.g. cleft lip, cleft palate); erupting permanent tooth; and missing permanent tooth.

The impact of oral hygiene, caries and presence of DDE on the child's daily performance using the child-OIDP were also assessed. The child-OIDP assessed the impact of caries on eating, speaking, tooth cleaning, relaxing, emotional status, smiling, studying and social contact. If an impact was reported, the child was asked to grade the severity of the impact on daily life performance in each of the eight items using a four-point Likert-like scale with scores ranging from 0 to 3. A score of 0 meant no impact, 1 meant mild impact, 2 meant moderate impact and 3 meant severe impact.

Children indicated the frequency of an oral health problem by assigning a score from 0 to 3 to each of the items for which they indicated an oral lesion impacted their daily life function. A score of 0 meant no event occurred, 1 meant the event occurred once or twice per month, 2 meant the event occurred once or twice per week and 3 meant the event occurred three or more times per week. The oral impact score for each of the eight daily life performance items was obtained by multiplying the severity scores by the frequency scores. Scores ranged from 0 to 9 per item. The overall impact score was the sum of all eight items (ranging from 0 to 72).

Measure of socioeconomic status

Socioeconomic status was assessed with a multiple item index, combining the mother's level of education with the father's occupation [44]. Each child was allocated into one of five social classes (I–V), with V being the lowest. For ease of analysis, three socioeconomic status groups were established: high (children from the upper and upper middle status), middle (children from the middle status) and low (children from the lower middle and lower status) class.

Data analysis

Data was analysed using the statistical package for social sciences (SPSS) version 17.0. Children were categorized as having or not having MIH, and having or not having enamel hypoplasia. Differences in the item and mean Child-OIDP scores of children with and without MIH; and children with and without enamel hypoplasia were determined respectively. Also, differences in the Child-OIDP scores of children with MIH and enamel hypoplasia who had or did not have caries were also determined respectively. Also, children with MIH were matched with children without any lesion; and children with enamel hypoplasia were matched with children without any lesion. The match was by age, sex and socioeconomic status. Differences in the Child-OIDP scores of matched children were also determined. The McNemar chi square test was used to assess the differences in the mean Child-OIDP scores.

Logistic regression was conducted to determine the impact of the presence of MIH and enamel hypoplasia on the oral health quality of life. Study participants where dichotomized to 'no impact' (when the Child-OIDP was zero) and 'impacted' (when the Child-OIDP ranged from 1 to 72). Adjustment was made for factors that increased the risk for MIH and enamel hypoplasia in the study environment: socio-economic status [45], caries [46] and poor oral hygiene [47]. Also, adjustment was made for oral hygiene status since MIH and enamel hypoplasia both increase the risk for poor oral hygiene, and oral hygiene status can affect the quality of life [9]. Age and gender were also included in the logistic regression model. The goodness of fit for the chi square tests and logistic regression was assessed using the Cox and Snell R square and the Nagelkerke R square. The model was considered to have a good fit if the tests were not statistically significant. A 95% confidence interval was set to confirm if a relationship truly existed within or between variables. The statistical significance level was set at $P \leq 0.05$.

Ethical considerations

Ethical approval for this study was obtained from the Obafemi Awolowo University Teaching Hospitals' Complex Ethics and Research Committee (IRB/IEC/00004553) and the Oyo State Ministry of Health ethical review committee (AD13/479/649). Permission was also obtained from the State Ministry of Education in Ile-Ife and the principals of participating schools. Prior to commencement of the study, informed consent forms were sent to the parents to get their approval prior to recruitment of study participants. Children 12 years and older gave assent for study participation. Students who required treatment were informed and issued a referral letter. No financial compensation was paid for study participation.

Results

Socio-demographic profile of study participants

Table 1 highlights the socio-demographic profile of the study participants. Eight hundred and fifty three participants were recruited for the study. This included 438 (51.3%) males, 428 (50.6%) children aged 6–9 years and 469 (55.0%) children with low socioeconomic status.

Developmental defects of the enamel profile of study participants

Table 1 also highlights the profile of the study participants with DDE. Twenty five (2.9%) children had MIH while 65 (7.6%) children had enamel hypoplasia. One (0.1%) child had both MIH and enamel hypoplasia. Significantly more 6–9 years old children ($p = 0.001$) and children with high socioeconomic status ($p = 0.05$) had MIH. Also, significantly more 10–13 years old children ($p = 0.02$) and children with low socio-economic status ($p = 0.03$) had enamel hypoplasia.

Caries profile of study participants

Table 1 also highlights the caries profile of the study participants. One hundred and two (10.2%) children had caries. Of these, 1 (1.0%) child had MIH while 10 (9.8%) children had enamel hypoplasia. There was no significant difference in the number of children with and those without caries who had MIH ($p = 0.21$) and those who had enamel hypoplasia ($p = 0.38$). The prevalence of caries was higher in children with enamel hypoplasia when compared with children who had MIH ($p = 0.01$).

Table 1 Profile of study respondents ($N = 853$)

Variables	MIH present $N = 25$ n (%)	Enamel hypoplasia present $N = 65$ n (%)	Total $N = 853$n (%)
Age (years)			
6–9	20 (80.0)	22 (33.8)	428 (50.2)
10–13	0 (0.0)	32 (49.2)	302 (35.4)
14–16	5 (20.0)	11 (17.0)	123 (14.4)
P- value	0.001	0.02	
Sex			
Male	10 (40.0)	31 (47.7)	438 (51.3)
Female	15 (60.0)	34 (52.3)	415 (48.7)
P- value	0.25	0.31	
Socio-economic status			
High SES	12 (48.0)	13 (20.0)	241 (28.3)
Middle SES	5 (20.0)	6 (9.2)	143 (16.8)
Low SES	8 (32.0)	46 (70.8)	469 (55.0)
P- value	0.05	0.03	
Caries status			
Caries present	1 (4.0)	10 (15.4)	102 (12.0)
Caries absent	24 (96.0)	55 (84.6)	751 (88.0)
P- value	0.21	0.38	
Oral hygiene Status			
Good	5 (20.0)	19 (29.2)	183 (21.5)
Fair	19 (76.0)	40 (61.5)	600 (70.3)
Poor	1 (4.0)	6 (9.2)	70 (8.2)
P- value	0.71	0.24	

Oral hygiene profile of study participants

Table 1 also highlights the oral hygiene profile of the study participants. One hundred and eighty-three (21.5%) children had good oral hygiene while 70 (8.2%) children had poor oral hygiene. There was no significant difference in the oral hygiene status of children with MIH ($p = 0.71$) and children with enamel hypoplasia ($p = 0.24$).

Effect of developmental dental anomalies on the quality of life of study participants

Table 2 shows the mean child-OIDP scores of children with DDE. There was no significant difference in the mean child-OIDP scores of children with or without MIH ($p = 0.57$) and the mean child-OIDP scores of children with or without enamel hypoplasia ($p = 0.48$). There was also no significant difference in the mean child-OIDP scores of children with and without MIH, and children with and without enamel hypoplasia in the eight items (eating, speaking, contact, schooling, smiling, emotion, relaxing and cleaning) examined.

Difference in the quality of life of study participants with and without MIH

Table 3 compares the mean item and composite child-OIDP scores of children with and without MIH matched for sex, age and socioeconomic status. There was also no significant difference in any of the eight items (eating, contact, schooling, smiling, emotion, relaxing and cleaning) examined between children with and without MIH. There was also no difference in the mean child-OIDP scores of children with and without MIH ($p = 0.86$). The Goodness of fit statistics showed that chi square test = 32.00 ($P < 0.001$), indicating poor model fit.

Difference in the quality of life of study participants with and without enamel hypoplasia

Table 4 compares the mean item and composite child-OIDP scores of children with and without enamel hypoplasia matched for sex, age and socioeconomic status. There was also no significant difference in any of the eight items (eating, contact, schooling, smiling, emotion, relaxing and cleaning) examined between children with and without enamel hypoplasia. There was also no difference in the mean child-OIDP scores of children with and without enamel hypoplasia ($p = 0.96$). The Goodness of fit statistics

Table 2 Mean child-OIDP scores of study participants with developmental enamel defects ($N = 853$)

Characteristics	Eating mean ± SD	Speaking mean ± SD	Contact mean ± SD	School mean ± SD	Smiling mean ± SD	Emotion mean ± SD	Relaxing mean ± SD	Cleaning mean ± SD	C-OIDP mean ± SD
Molar Incisor hypomineralisation (MIH)									
MIH present	0.40 ± 1.29	0.12 ± 0.60	0.00 ± 0.00	0.00 ± 0.00	0.20 ± 0.71	0.00 ± 0.00	0.12 ± 0.60	0.00 ± 0.00	0.68 ± 3.01
MIH absent	0.44 ± 1.40	0.11 ± 0.75	0.01 ± 0.12	0.03 ± 0.36	0.05 ± 0.50	0.02 ± 0.26	0.04 ± 0.49	0.41 ± 1.39	1.09 ± 3.58
P-value	0.88	0.96	0.76	0.72	0.14	0.68	0.44	0.14	0.57
Enamel hypoplasia									
Enamel hypoplasia present	0.45 ± 1.44	0.17 ± 0.84	0.00 ± 0.00	0.00 ± 0.00	0.05 ± 0.37	0.00 ± 0.00	0.05 ± 0.37	0.68 ± 1.85	1.38 ± 3.67
Enamel hypoplasia absent	0.44 ± 1.40	0.11 ± 0.73	0.01 ± 0.12	0.03 ± 0.37	0.05 ± 0.52	0.02 ± 0.27	0.04 ± 0.51	0.37 ± 1.32	1.06 ± 3.55
P-value	0.98	0.52	0.62	0.55	0.91	0.49	0.98	0.09	0.48

showed that chi square test = 22.43 ($P < 0.001$), indicating poor model fit.

Factors that impacted on the quality of life of study participants

Table 5 shows the outcome of the logistic regression analysis to determine factors that impacted on the quality of life of study participants. Children from the middle (AOR: 2.74; 95% CI: 1.60–4.67; $P < 0.01$) and low (AOR: 1.75; 95% CI: 1.04–2.95; $p = 0.03$) socioeconomic classes had increased odds of having their quality of life negatively affected when compared with children with high socio-economic status. MIH ($p = 1.00$) and enamel hypoplasia ($p = 1.00$) had no significant impact on the quality of life of the children. Having one or more DDE had no significant impact on the quality of life of the children ($p = 1.00$). The Goodness of Fit for the logistic regression was 0.051 for the Cox and Snell R square test, and 0.08 for the Nagelkerke R square test indicating a poor fit.

Table 3 Mean child-OIDP scores of study participants with and without molar incisor hypomineralization (MIH) matched for age, sex and socioeconomic status ($n = 50$)

Item	MIH present $n = 25$ Mean ± SEM	MIH absent $n = 25$ Mean ± SEM	*P*-value
Eating	0.12 ± 0.09	0.12 ± 0.09	1.00
Speaking	0.00 ± 0.00	0.00 ± 0.00	–
Cleaning	0.12 ± 0.12	0.08 ± 0.08	0.78
Relaxing	0.00 ± 0.00	0.00 ± 0.00	–
Emotion	0.00 ± 0.00	0.00 ± 0.00	–
Smiling	0.00 ± 0.00	0.00 ± 0.00	–
School	0.00 ± 0.00	0.00 ± 0.00	–
Contact	0.00 ± 0.00	0.00 ± 0.00	–
Child OIDP	0.24 ± 0.14	0.2 ± 0.16	0.86

Discussion

The aim of the study was to assess the impact of DDE on the oral health quality of life of children resident in Ile-Ife and Ibadan, Nigeria. We found that MIH and enamel hypoplasia, with or without caries, had no significant impact on the quality of life of study participants. However, speaking was negatively impacted in children with enamel hypoplasia and caries when compared with children who had enamel hypoplasia but did not have caries. Also, the two significant predictors of oral health quality of life of the study population were socio-economic class and caries: the oral health quality of life of children from the middle and low socio-economic classes, and children with caries was impacted negatively.

The study had some limitations however. The few cases of DDE detected and the low prevalence of caries in the population of children with DDE limited the robustness of the subgroup analysis. Also, prevalence of DDE chosen for the power calculation was high for the study population - higher than the prevalence of DDE identified in prior studies for the population being studied. The use of such a high prevalence implies that the sample size for the study will be less than actually required with implications for under-powering this study. The findings of this study can therefore only be considered an indication of what the probable status of the oral health quality of life of children with DDE could be. An appropriately powered study will give definitive outcomes. In addition, caries was only diagnosed when it affected the dentine. This implies that enamel caries was excluded from the diagnosis of caries in this study thereby leading to an underestimation of the prevalence of caries in the study population. Also, although the results of the chi square tests and logistic regression Goodness of Fit test showed the model was not a good fit, we feel that this may be a type 1 error (incorrect rejection of an acceptable model) due to the low number of observation we had. The hypothesis-testing rationale of this research is more appropriate for testing statistical

Table 4 Mean child-OIDP scores of study participants with and without enamel hypoplasia matched for age, sex and socioeconomic status (*n* = 130)

Item	Hypoplasia present *n* = 65 Mean ± SEM	Hypoplasia absent *n* = 65 Mean ± SEM	*P*-value
Eating	0.58 ± 1.19	0.43 ± 1.12	0.49
Speaking	0.14 ± 0.10	0.29 ± 0.13	0.34
Cleaning	0.74 ± 0.22	0.68 ± 0.23	0.85
Relaxing	0.03 ± 0.02	0.11 ± 0.08	0.33
Emotion	0.03 ± 0.02	0.00 ± 0.00	0.16
Smiling	0.03 ± 0.02	0.05 ± 0.05	0.76
School	0.00 ± 0.00	0.03 ± 0.03	0.32
Contact	0.00 ± 0.00	0.00 ± 0.00	–
Child OIDP	1.55 ± 0.40	1.58 ± 0.42	0.96

significance than evaluating the goodness of fit [48]. Despite these limitations, the study provided some insight into the impact of DDE with and without carious lesions, on the oral health quality of life of children in the study environment.

First, a finding of the study suggests that DDE does not affect the overall quality of life just like Vargas-Ferreira and Ardenghi [17] and Arrow [13] observed. However, unlike Vargas Ferreira and Ardenghi [17] who found that children reported significantly higher impact of DDE on functional limitation, we found no significant impact of DDE on any of the eight functional and social items explored.

DDE are often associated with discoloration. The assumption was that the discoloration associated with MIH and enamel hypoplasia may affect the psychological welfare of study participants enough to affect their quality of life. The study suggests that the discoloration associated with

Table 5 Logistic regression analysis of factors that had impact on the quality of life of children with developmental dental anomalies (N = 853)

Variables	Mean C-OIDP scores	Had impact *N* = 176	Had no impact *N* = 677	Adjusted OR	95% C.I	*P*- value
Age						
6–9	0.68 ± 2.22	68 (38.6)	360 (53.2)	1.00	–	–
10–13	1.57 ± 4.18	81 (46.0)	221 (32.6)	0.91	0.52–1.60	0.75
14–16	1.34 ± 5.23	27 (15.4)	96 (14.2)	0.76	0.46–1.27	0.29
Sex						
Male	1.14 ± 4.23	88 (50.0)	350 (51.7)	1.00	–	–
Female	1.04 ± 2.71	88 (50.0)	327 (48.3)	0.91	0.65–1.27	0.60
Presence of enamel hypoplasia						
Enamel hypoplasia present	1.55 ± 3.21	18 (10.2)	47 (6.9)	1.00	–	–
Enamel hypoplasia absent	1.05 ± 3.60	158 (89.8)	630 (93.1)	0.00	0.00–0.00	1.00
Presence of developmental defect of the enamel						
No DDE	1.08 ± 3.65	155 (20.3)	609 (79.7)	1.00	–	–
1 or 2 DDE	1.20 ± 2.83	21 (23.6)	68 (76.4)	0.00	0.00–0.00	1.00
Presence of MIH						
MIH present	0.24 ± 0.72	3 (1.7)	22 (3.2)	1.00	–	–
MIH absent	1.12 ± 3.62	173 (98.3)	655 (96.8)	0.00	0.00–0.00	1.00
Socio-economic status						
High	0.27 ± 1.08	26 (14.7)	215 (31.8)	1.00	–	–
Middle	0.64 ± 2.01	23 (13.1)	120 (17.7)	2.74	1.60–4.67	< 0.01
Low	1.65 ± 4.55	127 (72.2)	342 (50.5)	1.75	1.04–2.95	0.03
OHI-S						
Good	1.39 ± 3.60	41 (23.3)	142 (21.0)	1.00	–	–
Fair	0.95 ± 3.62	114 (64.8)	486 (71.8)	1.58	0.83–2.99	0.16
Poor	1.51 ± 3.03	21 (11.9)	49 (7.2)	1.55	0.87–2.74	0.13
Caries						
Caries absent	1.02 ± 3.61	68 (66.7)	609 (81.1)	1.00	–	–
Caries present	1.60 ± 3.22	34 (33.3)	142 (18.9)	2.02	1.26–3.22	0.03

OR odds ratio; *C.I* confidence interval

these defects is not significant enough to affect the quality of life of children within this age group [49] in this study population. In Columbia, a significantly high number of children with a form of DDE- fluorosis – actually had psychological impact as a result of the discoloration [50]. This raises the question of possible cultural differences in perception of aesthetics and psychological effect of aesthetics on self-welfare [51].

Second, like Arrow [13] and Chukumah et al. [30], we found that caries had a significant negative impact on the oral health quality of life of the study participants. We also found that caries worsened the impact of enamel hypoplasia on the oral health quality of life of children. The study reinforces previous documentations on the deleterious effect of caries on the oral health of affected persons. Caries is known to negatively impact the quality of life in several ways: untreated caries results in pain and aesthetic issues [49] with pain being the most significant factor that impacts negatively on the quality of life [29].

Third, just like a number of researchers had earlier highlighted [52, 53], we also observed that children with lower socio-economic status experienced more negative impact on their oral health-related quality of life, irrespective of the presence of DDE. In the study environment, a child's socio-economic status does not increase the risk for DDE [30], caries [54] and poor oral hygiene [55]. However, children with low socio-economic status had increased risk for gingivitis [56]. This may be the possible path through which the child's socio-economic status impacts negatively on the oral health. This postulation however, needs to be explored further.

Finally, the study highlighted a few interesting findings about MIH and enamel hypoplasia. Like multiple other studies, the prevalence of enamel hypoplasia was higher than the prevalence of MIH in the study population [22, 23]. Also, the proportion of children with MIH was highest among children of the high socio-economic class, while the proportion of children with enamel hypoplasia was highest among children with low socio-economic status. Oyedele et al. [20] however demonstrated no association between socio-economic status and MIH. Temilola and Folayan [28] also highlighted that socio-economic status cannot be used as a distinguishing feature for MIH and enamel hypoplasia. Multiple studies had highlighted the association between DDEs such as enamel hypoplasia and socio-economic status – with the prevalence of enamel hypoplasia being higher among children with lower socio-economic status [57]. This study finding therefore concurs with findings from prior studies that established an association between enamel hypoplasia and socio-economic status. However, further studies are required to identify if the child's socio-economic status can be used as a distinguishing risk factor for MIH and enamel hypoplasia. We also noticed that the prevalence of caries was higher in children with enamel hypoplasia when compared with children with MIH. These findings highlight the need for further studies on MIH and enamel hypoplasia, especially in communities where the prevalence of these lesions are high.

Conclusion

MIH and enamel hypoplasia do not negatively impact the oral health quality of life of children resident in Southwestern Nigeria. Caries and the socioeconomic status of children were the two factors that had significant impact on the oral health quality of life of children in the study environment. Further studies are however required to explore the similarities and differences in the risk factors and risk indicators for MIH and enamel hypoplasia in the study population.

Abbreviations

Child-OIDP: Child Oral Impact on Daily performance; DDE: Developmental Defects of the Enamel; LGA: Local Government Area; MIH: Molar-Incisor-Hypomineralisation

Acknowledgements

All the study participants who took part in this study are acknowledged for the contributions they have made to the generation of new knowledge in the study environment.

Funding

No grants was received for the study.

Authors' contributions

MOF conceptualise the study. NMC, BOP, DOT, NKO, TAO and FBL were involved with data collection. MOF and NMC conducted the data analysis. MOF developed the framework for the paper. NMC, BOP, DOT, NKO, TAO and FBL contributed to the development of the manuscript, reviewed the final paper and gave consent to its publication. All authors read and approved the final manuscript.

Competing interests

The authors declare they do not have any conflict of interest.

Author details

[1]Department of Child Dental Health, Obafemi Awolowo University, Ile-Ife, Nigeria. [2]Department of Child Dental Health, Obafemi Awolowo University Teaching Hospitals' Complex, Ile-Ife, Nigeria. [3]University of Benin Teaching Hospital, Benin City, Edo State, Nigeria. [4]University of Ibadan, Ibadan, Nigeria. [5]University of Nigeria, Enugu, Nigeria. [6]Department of Surgery, Benjamin Carson, Snr, School of Medicine, Babcock University, Ilisan-Remo, Ogun State, Nigeria. [7]Dental Department, Babcock University Teaching Hospital, Ilisan-Remo, Ogun State, Nigeria.

References

1. Proffit, WR. The development of orthodontic problems. In Contemporary Orthodontics. 2nd edition. Edited by Proffit WR. St Louis: Mosby. 1990:110.
2. Review of the developmental defects of enamel index (DDE Index). Commission on oral health, research & epidemiology. Report of an FDI working group. Int Dent J. 1992;42:411–26.
3. Farah R, Drummond B, Swain M, Williams S. Linking the clinical presentation of molar incisor hypomineralisation to its mineral density. Int J Paediatr Dent. 2010;20:353–60.
4. Weerheijm KL. Molar incisor hypomineralisation (MIH). Eur J Paediatr Dent. 2003;4:114–20.
5. Garot E, Denis A, Delbos Y, Manton D, Silva M, Rouas P. Are hypomineralised lesions on second primary molars (HSPM) a predictive sign of molar incisor hypomineralisation (MIH)? A systematic review and a meta-analysis. J Dent 2018;72:8–13. https://doi.org/10.1016/j.jdent.2018.03.005.
6. Oyedele TA, Folayan MO, Oziegbe EO. Hypomineralised second primary molars: prevalence, pattern and associated co morbidities in 8- to 10-year-old children in Ile-Ife, Nigeria. BMC Oral Health. 2016;16(1):65. https://doi.org/10.1186/s12903-016-0225-9.
7. Jälevik B. Prevalence and diagnosis of Molar-Incisor-Hypomineralization (MIH): A systematic review. Eur Arch Paediatr Dent. 2010;11:59–64.
8. Krishnan R, Ramesh M. Molar incisor hypomineralisation: a review of its current concepts and management. SRM J Res Dent Sci. 2014;5:248–52.
9. Oyedele TA, Folayan MO, Adekoya-Sofowora CA, Oziegbe EO. Co-morbidities associated with molar-incisor hypomineralisation in 8 to 16 year old pupils in Ile-Ife, Nigeria. BMC Oral Health. 2015;15:37.
10. Martins-Junior PA, Oliveira M, Marques LS, Ramos-Jorge ML. Untreated dental caries: impact on the quality of life of children of low socioeconomic status. Paediatr Dent. 2012;34:49–52.
11. Bekes K, Hirsch C. What is known about the influence of dentine hypersensitivity on oral health-related quality of life? Clin Oral Investig. 2012;7:s45–51.
12. Al-Zarea BK. Satisfaction with appearance and the desired treatment to improve aesthetics. Int J Dent 2013: 912368.
13. Arrow P. Child oral health-related quality of life (COHQoL), enamel defects of the first permanent molars and caries experience among children in Western Australia. Community Dent Health. 2013;30(3):183–8.
14. Slayton RL, Warren JJ, Kanellis MJ, Levy SM, Islam M. Prevalence of enamel hypoplasia and isolated opacities in the primary dentition. Pediatr. 2001;23:32–6.
15. Kanchanakamol U, Tuongratanaphan S, Tuongratanaphan S, et al. Prevalence of developmental enamel defects and dental caries in rural pre-school Thai children. Community Dent Health. 1996;13:204–7.
16. Lukacs JR. Localized enamel hypoplasia of human deciduous canine teeth: prevalence and pattern of expression in rural Pakistan. Hum Biol. 1991;63: 513–22.
17. Vargas-Ferreira F, Ardenghi TM. Developmental enamel defects and their impact on child oral health-related quality of life. Braz Oral Res. 2011;25:531–7.
18. Fotedar S, Sogi GM, Sharma KR. Enamel hypoplasia and its correlation with dental caries in 12 and 15 years old students in Shimla, India. J Indian Assoc Public Health Dent. 2014;12:18–22.
19. Masumo R, Bårdsen A, Astrøm AN. Developmental defects of enamel in primary teeth and association with early life course events: a study of 6-36 month old children in Manyara, Tanzania. BMC Oral Health. 2013;13:21.
20. Oyedele TA, Folayan MO, Adekoya-Sofowora CA, Oziegbe EO. Prevalence, pattern and severity of molar incisor hypomineralisation in 8 to 10 year-old children in Ile-Ife, Nigeria. Eur Arch Paediatr Dent. 2015;16(3):277–82.
21. Temilola DO, Folayan MO, Oyedele TA. The prevalence and pattern of deciduous molar hypomineralization and molar-incisor Hypomineralization in children from a suburban population in Nigeria. BMC Oral Health. 2015;15:73.
22. Orenuga OO, Odukoya O. An epidemiological study of developmental defects of enamel in a group of Nigerian school children. Pesq Bras Odontoped Clin Integr João Pessoa. 2010;10:385–91.
23. Temilola DO, Folayan MO, Fatusi O, et al. The prevalence, pattern and clinical presentation of developmental dental hard-tissue anomalies in children with primary and mix dentition from Ile-Ife, Nigeria. BMC Oral Health. 2014;14:125.
24. Salako N, Adenubi J. Chronologic enamel hypoplasia. Tropical Dental Journal. 1984;7(1):29–37.
25. Sawyer DR, Taiwo EO, Mosadomi A. Oral anomalies in Nigerian children. Community Dent Oral Epidemiol. 1984;12(4):269–73.
26. Popoola BO, Onyejaka NK, Folayan MO. Prevalence of developmental dental hard-tissue anomalies and association with caries and oral hygiene status of children in southwestern, Nigeria. BMC Oral Health. 2017;17:8.
27. Adenubi J. Dental status of 4 and 5 year old children in Lagos private schools. Niger Dent J. 1980;1:28–9.
28. Temilola DO, Folayan MO. Distinguishing predisposing factors for enamel hypoplasia and molar-incisor hypomineralization in children in Ile-Ife, Nigeria. Brazilian Journal of Oral Sciences. 2015;14(4). https://doi.org/10.1590/1677-3225v14n4a12.
29. Oziegbe EO, Esan TA, Adesina BA. Impact of oral conditions on the quality of life of secondary schoolchildren in Nigeria. J Dent Child (Chic). 2012;79(3):159–64.
30. Chukwumah NM, Folayan MO, Oziegbe EO, Umweni AA. Impact of dental caries and its treatment on the quality of life of 12- to 15-year old adolescents in Benin, Nigeria. Int J Paed Dent. 2016;26:66–76.
31. Oziegbe EO, Esan TA, Oyedele TA. Brief communication: emergence chronology of permanent teeth in Nigerian children. Am J Phys Anthropol. 2014;153:506–11.
32. Enwonwu CO. Influence of socio-economic conditions on dental development in Nigerian children. Arch Oral Biol. 1976;18(1):95–107.
33. Benson J, Borman G. Family, neighborhood, and school settings across seasons: when do socioeconomic context and racial composition matter for the reading achievement growth of young children? Teach Coll Rec. 2010;112:1338–90.
34. National Bureau of Statistics. 2006 Population Census. 2006. Internet: http://www.nigerianstat.gov.ng/nbsapps/Connections/Pop2006.pdf. Accessed 4 July, 2011.
35. Secretariat. Commission, Statistics section. Ibadan, Nigeria. 2001.
36. Cochran WG. Sampling Techniques. 3rd ed. New York: John Wiley & Sons; 1977.
37. Abanti J, Carvalho TS, Bonecker M, Ortega AO, Ciamponi AL, Raggio RP. Parental reports of the oral health related quality of life of children with cerebral palsy. BMC Oral Health. 2012;12:15.
38. Gherunpong S, Tsakos G, Sheiham A. Developing and evaluating an oral health-related quality of life index for children; the CHILD-OIDP. Community Dent Health. 2004;21:161–9.
39. World Health Organization. Oral health survey-basic method. 4th ed. Geneva: WHO; 1997.
40. Krapp K. Dental Indices. Encyclopedia of Nursing & Allied Health. Ed. Vol. 2. Gale Cengage. eNotes.com. 2002. http:// www. enotes. com/ dental-indices-reference/. Assessed 2 Jan, 2012.
41. Seow WK, Ford D, Kazoullis S, Newman B, Holcombe T. Comparison of enamel defects in the primary and permanent dentitions of children from a low-fluoride district in Australia. Pediatric Dent. 2011;33:207–12.
42. Greene JC, Vermillion JR. The simplified oral hygiene index. J Am Dent Assoc. 1964;68:7–13.
43. Weerheijm KL, Duggal M, Mejare I, et al. Judgement criteria for MIH in epidemiologic studies: summary of the European meeting on MIH held in Athens. Eur J Paediatr Dent. 2003;4:110–3.
44. Folayan M, Idehen E, Ufomata D. The effect of socio-demographic factors on dental anxiety in children seen in a sub-urban Nigerian hospital. Int J Paediatr Dent. 2003;13:20–6.
45. Nakayama, N. The relationship between linear enamel hypoplasia and social status in 18th to 19th century Edo, Japan. 2015. Int J Osteoarchaeol. https://doi.org/10.1002/oa.2515.
46. Petersen PE. Sociobehavioural risk factors in dental caries—international perspectives. Community Dent Oral Epidemiol. 2005;33:274–9.
47. Holst D, Schuller AA, Aleksejuniené J, Eriksen HM. Caries in population—a theoretical, causal approach. Eur J Oral Sci. 2001;109:143–8.
48. Marsh HW, Hau K-T, Wen Z. In search of Golden rules: comment on hypothesis-testing approaches to setting cutoff values for fit indexes and dangers in overgeneralizing Hu and Bentler's (1999) findings. Struct Equ Model Multidiscip J. 2004;11(3):320–41.
49. Peres KG, Latorre Mdo R, Peres MA, Traebert J, Panizzi M. Impact of dental caries and dental fluorosis on 12-year-old schoolchildren's self-perception of appearance and chewing. Article in Portuguese Cad Saude Publica. 2003; 19(1):323–30.
50. Tellez M, Santamaria RM, Gomez J, Martignon S. Dental fluorosis, dental caries, and quality of life factors among schoolchildren in a Colombian fluorotic area. Community Dent Health. 2012;29(1):95–9.
51. Osborne H. Aesthetic experience and cultural value. The Journal of Aesthetics and Art Critic. 1986;44(4):331–7.
52. Leal SC, Bronkhorst EM, Fan M, Frencken JE. Untreated cavitated dentine lesions: impact on children's quality of life. Caries Res. 2012;46:102–6.

53. Paula JS, Meneghim MC, Pereira AC, Mialhe FL. Oral health, socio-economic and home environmental factors associated with general and oral health related quality of life and convergent validity of two instruments. BMC Oral Health. 2015;15:26.
54. Kumar S, Kroon J, Lallo R. A systematic review of the impact of parental socioeconomic status and home environmental characteristics on children's oral health related quality of life. Health Qual Life Outcomes. 2014;12:41.
55. Folayan MO, Kolawole KA, Oziegbe EO, Oyedele T, Oshomoji OV, Chukwumah NM, Onyejaka N. Prevalence, risk factors and predictors of early childhood caries in children resident in sub-urban Nigeria. BMC Oral Health. 2015;15:72.
56. Agbaje HO, Kolawole KA, Folayan MO, Onyejaka N, Oziegbe EO, Oyedele TA, Chukwumah N, Oshomoji OV. Digit sucking, age, gender and socioeconomic status as determinants of oral hygiene status and gingival health of children in suburban Nigeria. J Periodontol. 2016;87(9):1047–56.
57. Vargas-Ferreira F, Salas MM, Nascimento GG, et al. Association between developmental defects of enamel and dental caries: a systematic review and meta-analysis. J Dent. 2015;43(6):619–28.

Satisfaction level in dental-phobic patients with implant-supported rehabilitation performed under general anaesthesia: a prospective study

Louise Sidenö[1,2], Rim Hmaidouch[1*], Jan Brandt[3], Nadine von Krockow[4] and Paul Weigl[1]

Abstract

Background: Phobic patients avoid dental treatment impairing their oral health and making it challenging to offer them prosthetic rehabilitation. This study evaluated patients' experience of implant-supported prosthetic treatment after implantation performed under general anaesthesia due to dental phobia and severe pharyngeal reflexes (SPR). The effect of gender, age and location of implantation on patient satisfaction was tested.

Methods: Two hundred five patients underwent implantation under general anesthesia both in maxilla and mandible, respectively. After a trans-gingival healing period of 6–8 weeks, fixed implant bridges were inserted. Patients completed oral health impact profile questionnaire (OHIP-14). An additional set of six special questions was also developed and considered. Analysis of the OHIP-14 total score was made using logistics regression. Wald chi-square test was used to analyse the effect of age, gender and location of implantation. Effect sizes were estimated as odds-ratios and associated 95% Wald confidence intervals.

Results: Eighty two of 205 patients were included after prosthetic treatment. After start, 38 patients were excluded (4 died and 34 couldn't be reached). OHIP-14-analyses were made by 43 patients (30–90 years). 67% of patients were totally satisfied with the whole implant rehabilitation (scoring 0). Mean of total score was 2.5. Only age affected significantly ($p = 0.014$) patients satisfaction. The obtained data indicate that younger patients (30–64 years) especially women are less satisfied (4.95) than older patients (0.3) for age group (65–90 years).Special questions' data showed that 94.5% were satisfied with their treatment. 77.3% continued regular check-up after treatment and 96.9% would undergo the same treatment again. 95.5% would recommend implants to a friend of colleague.

Conclusion: Gender and location of implantation have no significant influence on patient satisfaction. Younger patients especially women are less satisfied than older patients. Phobic patients are totally satisfied with implant rehabilitation under general anaesthesia which means that this treatment can be considered as a treatment of choice giving these patients the same opportunity like others to improve their oral health and well-being.

Keywords: Patient satisfaction, Dental phobia, Pharyngeal reflex, Dental implants, Prosthetic rehabilitation, general anaesthesia

* Correspondence: hmaidouch@med.uni-frankfurt.de
[1]Department of Postgraduate Education, Master of Oral Implantology, Oral and Dental Medicine at Johann Wolfgang Goethe-University, Theodor-Stern-Kai 7 / building 29, 60596 Frankfurt am Main, Germany
Full list of author information is available at the end of the article

Introduction

Anxious patients due to dental phobia or severe pharyngeal reflexes (SPR) show poorer oral health and more decayed and missing teeth than typical individuals [1]. Prosthetic treatments are needed for recovery of missing teeth in these patients, however, these patients are uncooperative and show poor dental treatment compliance which complicates any treatment; increases risk of failure and makes it difficult to perform implant-supported rehabilitation [2, 3]. A very long procedure is expected if implantation is considered for these patients. Consequently, local anesthesia will be insufficient to perform an adequate operation [4, 5]. In such cases, surgery under general anesthesia could be an option that enables patients undergoing implant treatment to improve their oral health, and well-being.

General anaesthesia makes it convenient for patients to have all surgical procedures carried out in one session and then implants can be installed in the maxilla or mandible or if needed in both jaws in one appointment [6]. As known, rehabilitation with implants prevents continuous alveolar bone resorption, preserves ridge height and width which ensures positive aesthetic outcome [7, 8], comfort and efficacy of prosthetic reconstruction [9–11]. Additional positive factors for patients are increase in self-esteem, and patients' satisfaction [12, 13].

When assessing the outcome of implant treatment, it is important to consider both the clinicians' and the patients' appraisals [14–16]. For the clinicians, implant survival, prosthesis longevity, and the complications are the most important factors. On the other hand, cost effectiveness benefit, social and psychological impact of the treatment are more important for the patients [17, 18]. Patients' satisfaction depends on function, comfort, esthetics and speech disruption [15, 17] and may represent a crucial factor of implant success for the patient [19–22]. Patient satisfaction is seen a vital aspect by evaluating the overall quality of dental rehabilitation and should be made on a regular basis to allow clinical practitioners to assess their services [23–25].

The Oral Health Impact Profile (OHIP) questionnaire is an instrument developed to be used in clinical studies [26–33] to measure Oral Health Quality of Life (OHRQoL). Several short versions of this tool have been developed, such as the version OHIP-14 which consists of seven subgroups with two questions for each one [27, 28, 31].

Most dental satisfaction studies were performed on general dental treatment [34] and patients with dental anxiety have been shown to be significantly associated with greater dissatisfaction [35]. However, no studies have addressed patients' satisfaction suffering from dental phobia and SPR after implantation under general anesthesia; the perception of treatment outcomes by those patients is still missing. The aim of the study is therefore to evaluate satisfaction of partially edentulous patients suffering from dental phobia and SPR with their implant rehabilitation carried out under general anesthesia in one or both jaws. The effect of gender, age and location of implantation will be tested. This study evaluated patients' experience of oral surgical and prosthetic procedures as well as their satisfaction with treatment outcome. The hypotheses of this study are:

- Patients suffering from dental phobia and SPR will experience good patient satisfaction after implant treatment under general anesthesia.
- age, gender and location of implantation will affect patients satisfaction.
- success of rehabilitation with implant fixed bridges by these patients is similar to that by patients treated without general anesthesia.

Methods

The OHIP-14 questionnaire was used to measure patient satisfaction in this investigation. It is a 14-questions survey, grouped as seven domains: functional limitation, physical pain, psychological discomfort, physical disability; psychological disability, social disability, and handicap (Annex). The OHIP-14 has been previously translated into Swedish and the reliability and validity has been tested and recommended for use in studies in the Swedish population [28]. Additionally, a set of six special questions related to patients' dental behaviour and treatment satisfaction (Table 1) was developed in Swedish and used as well. The study proposal was submitted to the ethical committee of Stockholm in Sweden (No 2014/1811–31/1). The board of the ethical committee did not see any ethical research obstacles to this study.

Table 1 Response frequencies for special questions

Question	Response	No. (%)
Are you attending regular check-up at Dentist/Hygienist?	Yes	34 (77.3)
	No	10 (22.7)
Are you satisfied with your implant bridges?	Yes	42 (94.5)
	No	2 (5.5)
Would you recommend implants to friend or colleague?	Yes	42 (95.5)
	No	1 (2.3)
	Don't know	1 (2.3)
Would you recommend narcosis clinic?	Yes	41 (93.2)
	No	2 (4.5)
	Don't know	1 (2.3)
Do you regret the implant treatment?	Yes	2 (6.1)
	No	31 (93.9)
	Missing	11 (–)
Would you do it again?	Yes	31 (96.9)
	Maybe	1 (3.1)
	Missing	12 (–)

Study population

This prospective study involved partially edentulous patients lost their teeth in one or both jaws and treated under general anaesthesia with screw retained fixed implant bridges between 1 January 2006 to 31 December 2012 in a private clinic in Stockholm, Sweden. Informed consent was obtained from all individual participants included in the study. All treated patients had to be in a good general health condition to be eligible for general anaesthesia which was performed and monitored by an anaesthetist. The implant surgery itself did not differ from conventional implant procedure used for non-phobic patients treated without general anaesthesia.

Inclusion criteria

Patients were selected according to the following inclusion criteria:

- Patients with dental phobia and severe pharyngeal reflexes.
- In good general health condition.
- With edentulous maxilla, mandible or both.
- With edentulous jaws minimum 6 months after extraction.
- With no bone augmentation prior or in combination with implant insertion.
- Implantation performed under general anaesthesia:
- With 4–6 Straumann implants (Straumann AG, Basel, Switzerland) in the maxilla.
- With 4–5 Straumann implants in the mandible.
- With screw retained fixed implant bridges.

Exclusion criteria

Patients:

- Treated without general anaesthesia.
- Treated with other implant system than Straumann.
- With other rehabilitation than screw retained fixed implant bridges.
- Treated with bone augmentation were excluded.

Treatment protocol

Patients were treated according to the following protocol:

1) Total extraction due to caries or periodontitis or both was done under general anaesthesia, followed by at least a 6-month healing period.
2) Interim removable dentures were produced in advance and used by the patient during the healing period.
3) Straumann implants were placed under general anaesthesia in the edentulous one jaw or in both (4–6 implants in maxilla, 4–5 implants in mandible).
4) A trans-gingival healing period of minimum 6 to 8 weeks before continuing the treatment (delayed loading).
5) Fixed implant bridge treatment was the final restoration.

Protocol for general anaesthesia

Premedical evaluation of each patient was performed by the anaesthetist. Induction starts preoperatively in a peripheral venous line with 4 mg Betamethason, (Celestone, Merck & Co. Inc., Whitehouse Station, NJ USA), 0.5 mg Atropinesulphate (Myian AB, Stockholm, Sweden) and 2 g Bensylpenicillin (Meda AB, Solna, Sweden). In case of allergy to Bensylpenicillin, clindamycin was used (Clindamycin Orifarm, Stockholm Sweden). Fluid with glucose, Rehydrex 500 ml, was administered during anaesthesia (Fresenius Kabi, Halden Norway). Sedation with Propofol 1,5–2,5 mg/kg (Primex Pharmaceuticals, Helsinki, Finland) followed by Suxameton 25–50 mg (Celocurin Meda AB, Solna Sweden). An analgesic drug Fentanyl was used in doses of 20 microgram (Braun B, Melsungen AB, Germany) and repeated when needed. Intubation was done nasally with a silicon nasal tube, size 6 (Parker Medical, USA Colorado). Before start of surgery the patient is breathing unaided. Throughout the procedure the patient is monitored with ECG (QUIRUMED, Contec, Patient Monitor, Contec Medical Sustem CO LTD;Qinhuangdao, Hebi Province, China), saturation, blood pressure and CO_2 production (Datex Ohmeda 5200 CO2 Capnography Anesterhesia Monitor, DRE Louiville, KY, USA).

Protocol for surgical procedure under general anaesthesia

- Xylocain/adrenalin (Dentsply Pharmaceutical, ONY, United Kingdom) was used as local anaesthesia.
- Surgical flap was designed individually allowing good inspection of the bone and surrounding area.
- Straumann implants 4 to 6 and 4 to 5 were placed in the maxilla and mandible, respectively.
- The implants were inserted with external saline cooling of the drills.
- Healing abutments were applied for external healing.
- Wound closure was done with Vicryl 3–0 (Ethicon, Johnson & Johnson, Diegen, Belgium).
- The patients were allowed to use their soft relined removable dentures directly after implant insertion.
- A minimum of 6 to 8 weeks of healing time before impression taking for prosthetic restoration.

Data collection

Data of the OHIP-14 questionnaire and the set of special questions were collected through follow-up visits at least 3 years after prosthetic treatment. The patients filled the patient consent and the questionnaires at the recall examination under supervision of one of the authors who is not involved in the treatment to avoid bias and any effects of interpersonal reactions. The individuals expressed satisfaction answering questions. The answers have score 0 to 5 where the scoring is distributed as following:

(0) = never, (1) = hardly ever, (2) = occasionally, (3) = fairly often, (4) = very often, (5) = always. According to this scoring procedure low scores represent high patient satisfaction and better quality of life while higher scores gradually show less satisfied patients. As well as this study investigated the success of treatment with fixed full arched implant bridges in the maxilla, mandible or both. Treatment success was defined as functional dental implant bridges from 3 to 9 years after treatment.

Data analysis/statistical methods

The Number of included patients, gender, age, number of installed implants and date of implant surgery were summarised using descriptive statistics, including mean, standard deviation (SD), median, range, frequency, and percentage.

Data of the OHIP-14 questionnaire and the set of special questions were descriptively summarized using descriptive statistics including frequencies, percentage, means and standard deviations as appropriate. Results are presented in tables (2-4) and graphs (1-4) for all patients. The OHIP-14 total score was analysed using logistic regression [36]. A dichotomization of the OHIP-14 total score into 0 vs. > 0 was used as response variable. The predictive ability of age, gender and location of implantation was tested by the use of the Wald chi-square test. Effect sizes were estimated as odds-ratios and associated 95% Wald confidence intervals. The functional success of the restored implant was recorded as either osseointegrated or failure (+/−).

Results

Eighty two patients were treated with implants under general anesthesia between 01.01.2006 to 31.12.2012 and included and treated in this study. After start, 38 patients were excluded (4 died and 34 could not be reached to complete the follow-up after prosthetic treatment). One patient had missing data on several OHIP-14 items. The total patients' number included in the analyses of the OHIP-14 was 43 (30–90 years). Table 2 shows the distribution of gender, age and location of implantation among these patients. The majority of patients were females (63.6%). 47.7% of the implants inserted in the maxilla and 31.8% of the patients had implants installed in both jaws.

Table 2 Background characteristics for included patients ($n = 43$)

Gender	Female, no. (%)	27 (63.6)
	Male, no. (%)	16 (36.4)
Age	Mean (SD)	62.8 (11.2)
	Min., Max	32,90
	Group 30–64 years, no (%)	20 (45.5)
	Group 65–90 years, no. (%)	23 (54.5)
Type of intervention	Maxilla, no. (%)	21 (47.7)
	Mandible, no. (%)	9 (20.4)
	Both, no. (%)	14 (31.8)

The implant treatment of all 43 patients included in this study was successful as far as function and comfort. The follow-up period after the prosthetic reconstruction ranged from 3 to 9 years. Figure 1 shows the OHIP-14 total score distribution for all patients. The OHIP-14 total score was low for the majority of the patients with 67% scoring 0 and with a mean value total score of 2.5. The OHIP-14 total score by subgroups i.e. gender, age and type of intervention group are shown in Figs. 2, 3 and 4 respectively. The graphs seem to suggest some differences. However, the data indicate that younger patients (age group 30–64 years) especially young women are less satisfied (mean = 4.95+/− 9.81) than older patients (age group 65–90 years) with (mean = 0.3+/− 0.76). Logistic regression analysis (Table 3) was used to investigate the relationship between these background variables and the OHIP-14 total score.

Discussion

The literature shows that patients satisfaction has been considered as an important criterion for treatment success since it is associated with compliance and in turn, anticipated treatment quality [9–11, 37]. In this study, the OHIP-14 questionnaire was administered to evaluate the level of satisfaction of patients suffer from dental phobia and SPRs with their implant treatment performed under general anesthesia. The first hypothesis of this study was confirmed because the results clearly demonstrated that the included patients are generally satisfied with their treatment and have good OHRQoL after treatment. The overall of patients have even changed their dental behaviour and continued after the performed oral rehabilitation to visit a dentist or oral hygienist for regular check-ups. The second hypothesis was confirmed in part because the obtained data showed that only age significantly affects patient satisfaction. Younger patients are less satisfied than older patients. But patients' gender and location of implantation do not influence patient satisfaction. Evaluation of the results showed that the implant-supported bridges were successfully maintained in all patients after 3 to 9 years of function which confirm the third hypothesis. The success was measured as the retention of the original screw retained bridges over time. Similar results of success

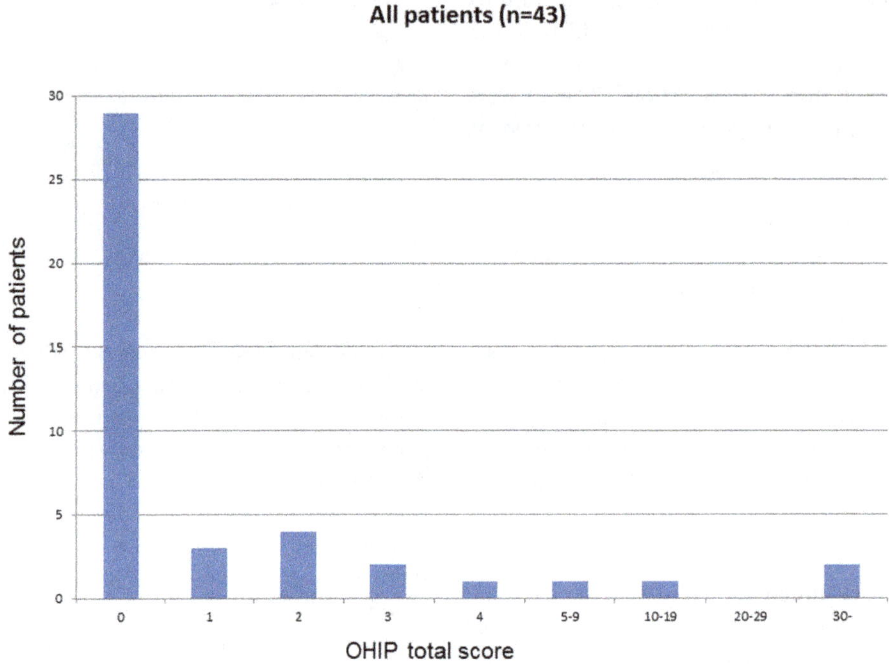

Fig. 1 OHIP-14 total score distribution for all included patients. OHIP-14 total score is presented on the x-axis and number of patients on the y-axis

have been shown in several studies on patients treated without general anesthesia [9, 10, 37–39].

The OHIP-14 used in this investigation was previously validated and recommended for use in clinical studies [27, 28, 31]; it covers a wide range of oral health related problems, i.e. functional limitation, physical discomfort, psychological discomfort, physical disability, psychological disability, social disability and handicap [26, 29–31].

In this study, 43 out of 82 patients returned for regular check-ups which can be considered as a success because it is difficult for this category of patients to change their dental behaviour avoiding visiting a dental clinic. The reason for that could be that through their good satisfaction with their rehabilitation, patients realize the costly investment for the treatment and thus value the return of this investment in the form of sustaining good oral health.

Precise evaluation of the results indicates that only age has a statistically significant effect ($p < 0.05$) on patients' satisfaction, reflecting that the number of patients viewing themselves as "problem free" increased with age. Analyses of data by subgroups indicate that younger patients especially women show more psychological discomfort and are less satisfied than older

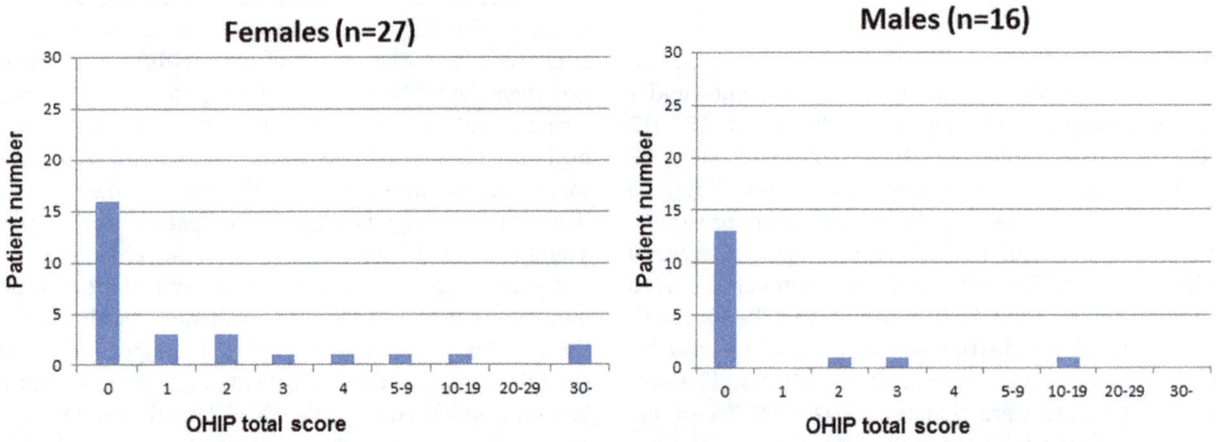

Fig. 2 OHIP-14 total score distribution for female patients and male patients

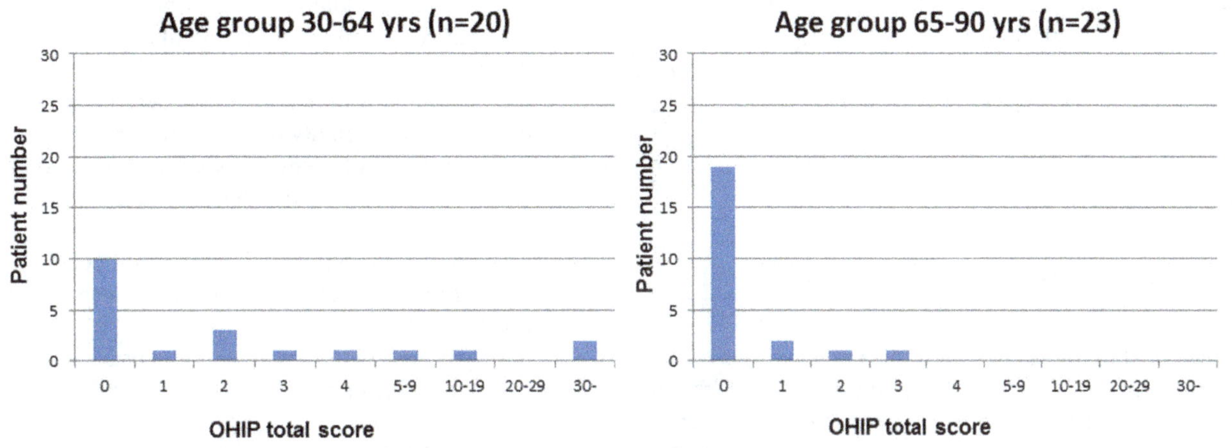

Fig. 3 OHIP-14 total score distribution in age group (30-64) and in age group (65-90)

patients (Figs. 2 and 3). This is an interesting observation and may reflect that aesthetics has become an important issue in modern society [40] and that younger peoples' social life style and attitude differ from older individuals'. These results are in line with a previous study [28] which also shows that oral discomfort has different influences on life depending on gender and age. Gender and location of the intervention showed in this study no significant influence on patients' satisfaction ($P > 0.05$). However, a remarkable aspect is that, in all age groups presented in the graph 2, there are less satisfied women than men.

The results from the special questions showed that almost all patients (94.5%) are satisfied and (95.5%) would recommend the treatment to a friend or colleague.

These data are in accordance with Pjetursson et al. [41] finding; they find that more than 90% of patients treated with crowns or implant-supported fixed partial denture are completely satisfied. The obtained results confirm that 77.3% of the included patients in this study visited a dentist or oral hygienist for regular after treatment check-up. Most patients (93.9%) do not regret this kind of treatment and (96.6%) were willing to have the same treatment performed again if needed.

The findings of this study indicate that the preoperative psychological factors due to dental phobia and SPRs have no effect on post-treatment patients' satisfaction with their implant treatment performed under general anesthesia.

From the results we conclude, with regard to the problem addressed that it is recommended to perform implant treatment on patients with dental phobia and SPR under general anesthesia. Consequently, implant-supported prosthesis would due to the availability of general anesthesia become a treatment option for these patients who otherwise would stay refusing any contact to the dental professionals who in turn have usually excluded implant treatment in cases involving patients with phobia or SPRs.

One question relevant to this topic is the impact of dental phobia from a social economic perspective. The comparably high cost for implant treatment under general anesthesia versus removable dentures could be the major reason for primary limitation for choosing this therapy.

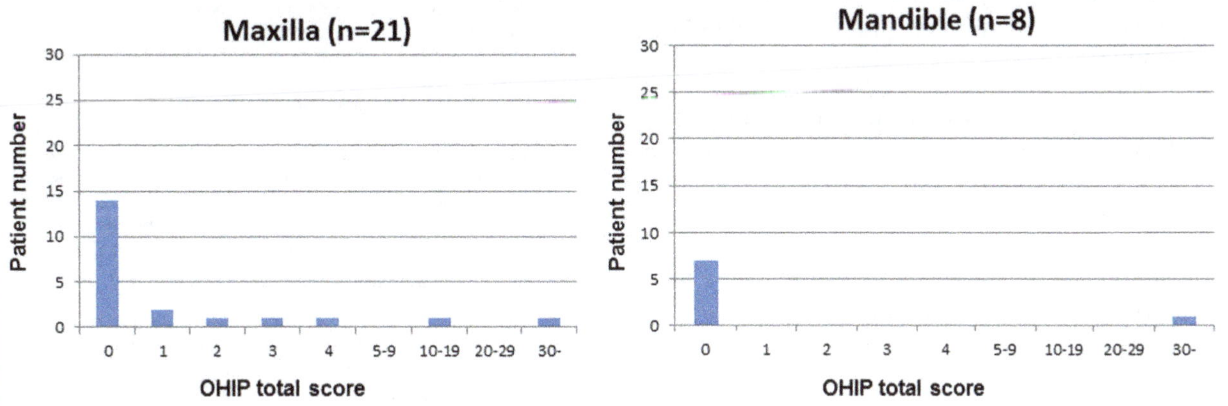

Fig. 4 OHIP-14 total score distribution in maxilla and in mandible

Table 3 Results of logistic regression ($n = 43$). Odds-ratio estimates, associated confidence intervals and p-values

Effect	Estimated odds-ratio	95% confidence, limits	P-value
Gender	3.86	(0.68, 22.1)	0.129
Age	1.10	(1.02, 1.19)	0.014
Type of intervention:			
- both vs. maxilla	0.94	(0.19, 4.57)	0.608
- mandible vs. maxilla	3.49	(0.25, 48.14)	

However, if more patients were able to choose this therapy it could in the long run reduce other costly health care consumption such as depression treatment and medication. This is a discussion worth pursuing in further studies.

Various investigations were made to study satisfaction with implant treatment [41, 42] But to the knowledge of the authors of this study, there is no study investigated satisfaction of patients suffering from dental phobia or SPR after implant treatment under general anesthesia. Therefore, this study fills an important gap in the academic field and should be used to promote a debate.

Conclusion

Based on this study results, it is assumed that treatment using implants is feasible for patients suffering from dental phobia and SPRs. Therefore, these patients can be offered the same implant treatment options as non-phobic patients, with similar success rates.

Annex

OHIP-14 the Oral Health Impact Profile

Dimension Question

Functional

1. Have you had trouble pronouncing any words because of problems limitation with your teeth, mouth or dentures?
2. Have you felt that your sense of taste has worsened because of problems with your teeth, mouth or dentures?

Physical pain

3. Have you had painful aching in your mouth?
4. Have you found it uncomfortable to eat any foods because of problems with your teeth, mouth or dentures?

Psychological discomfort

5. Have you been self-conscious because of your teeth, mouth or discomfort dentures?
6. Have you felt tense because of problems with your teeth, mouth or dentures? Physical disability.
7. Has your diet been unsatisfactory because of problems with your teeth, disability mouth or dentures?
8. Have you had to interrupt meals because of problems with your teeth, mouth or dentures?

Psychological disability

9. Have you found it difficult to relax because of problems with your disability teeth, mouth or dentures?
10. Have you been a bit embarrassed because of problems with your teeth, mouth or dentures?

Social disability

11. Have you been a bit irritable with other people because of problems disability with your teeth, mouth or dentures?
12. Have you had difficulty doing your usual jobs because of problems with your teeth, mouth or dentures? Handicap
13. Have you felt that life in general was less satisfying because of problems with your teeth, mouth or dentures?
14. Have you been totally unable to function because of problems with your teeth, mouth or dentures?

Abbreviations

OHIP: Oral health impact profile; OHRQoL: Oral health quality of life; SD: Standard deviation; SPR: Severe pharyngeal reflexes

Acknowledgements

Co-authors would like to show their gratitude to Dr. Rim Hmaidouch for the preparation of this manuscript.

Funding

All authors declare that this study was not funded by any organization.

Authors' contributions

Contribution of first author LS: 1. Concept/ design of this study, acquisition of data, data analysis, statistics/ interpretation, 2. Drafting article and critical revision of this article, 3. Final approval of the version to be published. 4. Agreement to be accountable for all aspects of the work in ensuring that questions related to the accuracy or integrity of any parts of the work are appropriately investigated and resolved. Contribution of second author RH: 1. Concept/ design of this in vitro study, acquisition of data, data analysis, statistics/ interpretation, 2. Drafting article and Critical revision of this article 3. Final approval of the version to be published 4. Agreement and accountable for all aspects of the work in ensuring that questions related to the accuracy or integrity of any parts of the work are appropriately investigated and resolved. Contribution of third author JB: 1. Concept/ design of this in vitro study, acquisition of data, data analysis, statistics/ interpretation, 2. Critical revision of this article, 3. Final approval of the version to be published, 4. Agreement and accountable for all aspects of the work in ensuring that questions related to the accuracy or integrity of any parts of the work are appropriately investigated and resolved. Contribution of fourth author NK: 1. 1. Concept/ design of this in vitro study, acquisition of data, data analysis, statistics/ interpretation, 2. Drafting article and Critical revision of this article. 3. Final approval of the version to be published. 4. Agreement and accountable for all aspects of the work in ensuring that questions related to the accuracy or integrity of any parts of the work are appropriately investigated and resolved. Contribution of last author PW: 11. Concept/ design of this in vitro study, acquisition of data, data analysis, statistics/ interpretation, 2. Drafting article and Critical revision of this article. 3. Final approval of the version to be published. 4. Agreement and accountable for all aspects of the work in ensuring that questions related to the accuracy or integrity of any parts of the work are appropriately investigated and resolved.

Competing interests

The authors stated explicitly that there are no conflicts of interest in connection with this article and there are no financial or other relationships that might lead to a conflict of interest.

Author details

[1]Department of Postgraduate Education, Master of Oral Implantology, Oral and Dental Medicine at Johann Wolfgang Goethe-University, Theodor-Stern-Kai 7 / building 29, 60596 Frankfurt am Main, Germany. [2]Stockholm, Sweden. [3]Department of Dental Prosthodontics, Faculty of Oral and Dental Medicine at Johann Wolfgang Goethe-University, Theodor-Stern-Kai 7 / building 29, 60596 Frankfurt am Main, Germany. [4]Department of Oral Surgery, Faculty of Oral and Dental Medicine at Johann Wolfgang Goethe-University, Theodor-Stern-Kai 7 / building 29, 60596 Frankfurt am Main, Germany.

References

1. Crofts-Barnes NP, Brough E, Wilson KE, Beddis AJ, Girdler NM. Anxiety and quality of life in phobic dental patients. J Dent Res. 2010;89:302–6. https://doi.org/10.1177/0022034509360189 Epub 2010 Feb 5.
2. Bracha HS, Vega EM, Vega CB. Posttraumatic dental-care anxiety (PTDA): is "dental phobia" a misnomer? Hawaii Dent J. 2006;37:17–9.
3. Smyth JS. Some problems of dental treatment. Part 1. Patient anxiety: some correlates and sex differences. Aust Dent J. 1993;38:354–9.
4. Flick WG, Clayhold S. Who should determine the medical necessity of dental sedation and general anesthesia? A clinical commentary supported by Illinois patient and practitioner surveys. Anesth Prog. 1998;45:57–61.
5. Nick D, Thompson L, Anderson D, Trapp L. The use of general anesthesia to facilitate dental treatment. Gen Dent. 2003;51:464–9.
6. Wolff A, Singer A, Shlomi B. Comprehensive dental treatment under general anesthesia. Dental Cadmos. 2014;82:182–8.
7. Zitzmann NU, Marinello CP. Treatment outcomes of fixed or removable implant-supported prostheses in the edentulous maxilla. Part II: clinical findings. J Prosthet Dent. 2000;83:434–42.
8. Chang M, Odman PA, Wennström JL, Andersson B. Esthetic outcome of implant-supported single-tooth replacements assessed by the patient and by prosthodontists. Int J Prosthodont. 1999;12:335–41.
9. Erkapers M, Ekstrand K, Baer RA, Toljanic JA, Thor A. Patient satisfaction following dental implant treatment with immediate loading in the edentulous atrophic maxilla. Int J Oral Maxillofac Implants. 2011; 26:356–64.
10. Zani SR, Rivaldo EG, Frasca LC, Caye LF. Journal of Oral Oral health impact profile and prosthetic condition in edentulous patients rehabilitated with implant-supported overdentures and fixed prostheses. J Oral Sci. 2009;51:535–43.
11. Martínez-González JM, Martín-Ares M, Cortés-Bretón Brinkmann J, Calvo-Guirado JL, Barona-Dorado C. Impact of prosthetic rehabilitation type on satisfaction of completely edentulous patients. A 5-year prospective study. Acta Odontol Scand. 2013;71:1303–8.
12. Zembic A, Wismeijer D. Patient-reported outcomes of maxillary implant-supported overdentures compared with conventional dentures. Clin Oral Implants Res 2014;25(4):441–450. doi: https://doi.org/10.1111/clr.12169. Epub 2013 Apr 15.
13. Cheng T, Sun G, Huo J, He X, Wang Y, Ren YF. Patient satisfaction and masticatory efficiency of single implant-retained mandibular overdentures using the stud and magnetic attachments. J Dent. 2012; 40(11):1018–23. https://doi.org/10.1016/j.jdent.2012.08.011 Epub 2012 Aug 24.
14. Anderson JD. The need for criteria on reporting treatment outcomes. J Prosthet Dent. 1998;79:49–55.
15. Locker D. Patient-based assessment of the outcomes of implant therapy: a review of the literature. Int J Prosthodont. 1998;11:453–61.
16. Zitzmann NU, Marinello CP. Treatment outcomes of fixed or removable implant-supported prostheses in the edentulous maxilla. Part I: patients' assessments. J Prosthet Dent. 2000;83:424–33.
17. Guckes AD, Scurria MS, Shugars DA. A conceptual framework for understanding outcomes of oral implant therapy. J Prosthet Dent. 1996;75:633–9.
18. Lewis DW. Optimized therapy for the edentulous predicament: cost-effectiveness considerations. J Prosthet Dent. 1998;79:93–9.
19. Allen PF, McMillan AS, Walshaw D. Patient expectations of oral implant-retained prostheses in a UK dental hospital. Br Dent J. 1999;186:80–4.
20. Clancy JM, Buchs AU, Ardjmand H. A retrospective analysis of one implant system in an oral surgery practice. Phase I: patient satisfaction. J Prosthet Dent. 1991;65:265–71.
21. Schropp L, Isidor F, Kostopoulos L, Wenzel A. Patient experience of, and satisfaction with, delayed-immediate vs. delayed single-tooth implant placement. Clin Oral Implants Res. 2004;15:498–503.
22. Assunção WG, Zardo GG, Delben JA, Barão VA. Comparing the efficacy of mandibular implant-retained overdentures and conventional dentures among elderly edentulous patients: satisfaction and quality of life. Gerodontology. 2007;24:235–8.
23. Thanveer K, Krishnan A, Hongal S. Treatment satisfac¬tion among patients attending a private dental school in Vadodara, India. J Int Oral Health. 2010; 2:33–44.
24. Siadat H, Alikhasi M, Mirfazaelian A, Geramipanah F, Zaery F. Patient satisfaction with implant-retained mandibular overdentures: a retrospective study. Clin Implant Dent Relat Res. 2008;10:93–8.
25. Liddelow GJ, Henry PJ. A prospective study of immediately loaded single implant-retained mandibular overdentures: preliminary one-year results. J Prosthet Dent. 2007;97:126–37.
26. Slade GD, Spencer AJ. Development and evaluation of the oral health impact profile. Community Dent Health. 1994;1:3–11.
27. Slade GD. Derivation and validation of a short-form oral health impact profile. Community Dent Oral Epidemiol. 1997;25:284–90.
28. Larsson P, List T, Lundström I, Marcusson A, Ohrbach R. Reliability and validity of a Swedish version of the oral health impact profile(OHIP-S). Acta Odontol Scand. 2004;62:147–52.
29. Pommer B. Use of the oral health impact profile (OHIP) in clinical Oral implant research. J Dent Oral Craniofac Epidemiol. 2013;1:3–10.
30. Slade GD, Spencer AJ, Locker D, Hunt RJ, Strauss RP, Beck JD. Variations in the social impact of oral conditions among older adults in South Australia, Ontario, and North Carolina. J Dent Res. 1996;75:1439–50.
31. Einarson S, Wärnberg Gerdin E, Hugoson A. Oral health impact on quality of life in an adult Swedish population. Acta Odontol Scand. 2009;67:85–93.
32. Locker D, Slade G. Oral health and the quality of life among older adults: the oral health impact profile. J Can Dent Assoc. 1993;59:830–44.
33. Allen F, Locker D. A modified short version of the oral health impact profile for assessing health-related quality of life in edentulous adults. Int J Prosthodont. 2002;15:446–50.
34. Calnan M, Dickinson M, Manley G. The quality of general dental care: public and users' perceptions. Qual Health Care. 1999;8:149–53.
35. Armfield JM, Enkling N, Wolf CA, et al. Dental fear and satisfaction with dental services in Switzerland. J Public Health Dent. 2014;74:57–63.
36. Cox DR, Snell EJ. The analysis of binary data. 2nd ed. London: Chapman and Hall; 1989. p. 26–33.
37. De Liz Pocztaruk R, Da Fontoura Frasca LC, Rivaldo EG, Castro Mattia PR, Vidal AR. Satisfaction level and masticatory capacity in edentulous patients with conventional dentures and implant-retained overdentures Braz. J Oral Sci. 2006;5:1232–8.
38. Fischer K, Stenberg T, Hedin M, Sennerby L. Clin Oral implants res. Five-year results from a randomized, controlled trial on early and delayed loading of implants supporting full-arch prosthesis in the edentulous maxilla. Clin Oral Implants Res. 2008;19:433–41.
39. Zarb AG, Schmitt A. The longitudinal clinical effectiveness of osseointegrated dental implants: the Toronto study. Part II: the prosthetic results. J prosth Dent. 1990;64:53–61.
40. Samorodnitzky-Naveh GR, Geiger SB, Levin L. Patients' satisfaction with dental esthetics. J Am Dent Assoc. 2007;138:805–8.
41. Pjetursson BE, Karoussis I, Bürgin W, Brägger U, Lang NP. Patients' satisfaction following implant therapy. A 10-year prospective cohort study. Clin Oral Implants Res. 2005;16:185–93.
42. Liu Y, Li B, Wang L, et al. Preoperative anxiety decrease the postoperative satisfaction in anterior dental implant surgery. Int J Clin Exp. 2016;9:20044–9.

The association between nutritive, non-nutritive sucking habits and primary dental occlusion

Hiu Tung Bonnie Ling[1†], Fung Hou Kumoi Mineaki Howard Sum[1†], Linkun Zhang[2], Cindy Po Wan Yeung[3], Kar Yan Li[3], Hai Ming Wong[1] and Yanqi Yang[1*]

Abstract

Background: The development of primary dentition can be affected by oral sucking habits. Therefore, this study aims to investigate the association of nutritive and non-nutritive sucking habits with primary dentition development.

Methods: One thousand one hundred and fourteen children aged 2 to 5 years old in Hong Kong were recruited in a cross-sectional study. Information on their nutritive (e.g. breastfeeding and bottle feeding) and non-nutritive sucking habits (e.g. pacifier use and thumb/digit sucking) was collected via questionnaires. The children's primary occlusions were examined in three dimensions.

Results: Children who were breastfed for more than 6 months had a lower proportion of daily pacifier use ($p < 0.05$). Children who used pacifiers daily had a higher proportion of thumb/digit sucking ($p < 0.05$). Children who used pacifiers daily for more than one year had higher chances of developing an anterior open bite ($p < 0.05$) and a reduced overbite ($p < 0.05$). Those exhibiting daily thumb/digit sucking for more than one year had higher chances of developing Class II incisor and Class II canine relationships, an increased overjet and anterior open bite ($p < 0.05$).

Conclusion: Pure breastfeeding for more than 6 months is inversely associated with daily pacifier use and daily pacifier use is positively associated with daily thumb/digit sucking. Children with more than one year of daily pacifier use and thumb/digit sucking have higher chances of developing abnormal dental relationships in the sagittal (i.e. Class II incisor and Class II canine relationships and increased overjet) and vertical (i.e. anterior open bite) dimensions, respectively.

Keywords: Nutritive sucking habit, Non-nutritive sucking habits, Primary dental occlusion

Background

Primary dentition is the foundation for the development of permanent dentition, in terms of determining space and occlusion for future developing teeth. Malocclusion is a developmental disorder of the maxillofacial system that results from genetic and environmental factors and affects the jaw, tongue and facial soft tissues [1]. As sucking habits are variable environmental factors, knowledge of how such behaviour contributes to or prevents malocclusion can help determine better options for children's oral health care. Oral sucking habits, such as breastfeeding and bottle sucking, can be categorised as nutritive habits, which are for feeding children, and non-nutritive habits, such as thumb sucking, finger sucking or pacifier use, which are often used to calm and comfort infants [2]. The calming effects have also been used to provide pain relief during minor procedures such as immunization [3]. Apart from the calming effects and providing a sense of security, pacifier use has been found to be associated with protection of sudden infant death syndrome [3–5].

Breastfeeding is a nutritive sucking habit that has been found to have general, immunological, nutritional and oral benefits for the child [6]. The World Health Organization (WHO) recommends exclusive breastfeeding for the first 6 months of life, with some breastfeeding

* Correspondence: yangyanq@hku.hk
†Hiu Tung Bonnie Ling and Fung Hou Kumoi Mineaki Howard Sum contributed equally to this work.
[1]Department of Paediatric Dentistry and Orthodontics, Faculty of Dentistry, Prince Philip Dental Hospital, The University of Hong Kong, 2/F, 34 Hospital Road, Sai Ying Pun, Hong Kong SAR, China
Full list of author information is available at the end of the article

up to 2 years of age [1, 7]. Our recent study showed that pure breastfeeding is associated with reduced chances of developing abnormal primary dentition, such as lower chances of having a Class II incisal relationship and increased overjet. We also found that children with pure breastfeeding for more than 6 months have wider inter-canine and intermolar widths [8].

Sucking is a natural instinct and is a baby's earliest coordinated muscular activity. The action of breastfeeding uses intensive muscular activity and benefits oral motor development [9, 10]. This repetitive action increases muscle tone and promotes correct development, thus ensuring correct oral function [11]. Other oral habits, such as pacifier use or bottle feeding, produce different functional stimuli [12]. It has been found that those who use pacifiers for more than 6 months and those who bottle feed for over 1 year score lower on masticatory function assessments [12].

When an infant does not breastfeed sufficiently, they may develop other types of sucking habits [13]. Some infants adopt non-nutritive sucking habits to cope with frustration, decreased sense of security or an urge for contact [14]. Certain studies have investigated the association between breastfeeding and non-nutritive sucking habits (i.e. pacifier use and thumb sucking) [2, 15–17]. These studies have reported that breastfeeding is associated with lower chances of pacifier use. However, few have focused on the duration or the frequency of these habits [2, 15, 17]. This is rather important from a dental point of view, because the frequency and magnitude of force are crucial for occlusion development, which may lead to malocclusion in the primary dentition. No study has looked into whether or how non-nutritive sucking habits are interrelated.

Knowing the beneficial oral effects of breastfeeding versus bottle feeding [8], it is also worthwhile to know the effects of non-nutritive oral habits. In contrast to calming and comforting infants, pacifier use is reported to have some unfavourable oral effects. If pacifiers are given to infants when they are learning to suck from their mothers' breasts in the early postpartum period, the use of pacifiers may interfere with proper sucking and cause nipple confusion [18]. Studies have found pacifier use to be associated with an increased prevalence of oral candidiasis, a type of fungal infection [19–22]. Several studies also show that non-nutritive sucking habits are associated with the development of malocclusion in the primary dentition [1, 12, 18]. Nevertheless, the majority of the existing studies do not address the effects of the duration or frequency of non-nutritive sucking habits. However, it is important for dentists and parents to know the frequency and duration of the force required to affect occlusion.

Therefore, the present study aims to (1) determine the associations between nutritive and non-nutritive sucking habits; (2) assess the interrelation between different non-nutritive sucking habits, pacifier use and thumb/digit sucking; and (3) investigate the relationships between various non-nutritive sucking habits and occlusion in the primary dentition. To be representative of having a habit, the frequency and duration of the non-nutritive sucking habits will be emphasised when performing the analyses.

Methods

Samples

A total of 10 kindergartens from different districts of Hong Kong participated in our study. This cross-sectional study was carried out with ethics board approval (HKU/HA HKW IRB: UW12–334) and parental consent forms were collected before the examinations. One thousand one hundred and fourteen children aged 2 to 5 years old participated in the survey. Among the one thousand one hundred and fourteen children, only eight hundred and fifty-one children took part in the oral examination and also completed all the questions in the questionnaires.

Fewer participants were recruited for the oral examinations compared to the surveys, as some did not return consent forms to undergo oral examination, refused examination or were uncooperative upon examination. To maintain the integrity of the study results, participants with severe skeletal discrepancy, with cleft lip or palate, or who were non-Asian were excluded. Only children with primary dentition were included in this study.

In a previous similar study, the probability of the event (Class II canine relationship and increased overjet) is around 20% for those without pacifier/digit-sucking habit and the allocation ratio of having pacifier/digit--sucking habit: no habit is about 1.6:1 [23], it was estimated that a sample of 476 individuals would have 90% chance of detecting an odds ratio of 2 with the two-sided significance level setting at 0.05.

Given this sample size determinations and assuming 20% possible non-responses and loses, the final study population had to be at least 595. As the study recruited 851 subjects who participated in both questionnaires and oral examinations, the sample size was sufficient.

Data collection

The questionnaires were completed by the children's parents or guardians and collected information regarding the frequencies and durations of the children's nutritive and non-nutritive sucking habits. After collecting the questionnaires, those who had left certain sections incomplete were contacted by telephone.

One examiner who had more than 5 years of orthodontic training performed all of the oral examinations throughout the study. The examiner performed calibration with another orthodontist before the study. The examination was carried out in the kindergartens with the children in the lying-down position. The equipment used included oral mirrors, probes and rulers. The children's dental arch relationships were examined in three dimensions (sagittal, vertical and transverse) as listed in Table 1. Duplicated data were collected for 6.23% of the subjects to assess the intra-examiner reliability.

Statistical analysis

The associations between different oral habits and their relationships with occlusion were analysed by multinomial logistic regression, logistic regression and multi-way analysis of variance (ANOVA) using the Statistical Package for the Social Sciences (SPSS) (IBM) version 20.0.

Multinomial logistic regressions were used to investigate the associations between the categorical variables, such as the primary incisal, canine and molar relationships with different sucking habits.

Multivariable logistic regression models were used to investigate the associations between the binary outcome variables, such as the associations between the frequencies of non-nutritive sucking habits and breastfeeding durations, between the different non-nutritive sucking habits and between different non-nutritive sucking habits and overjet, anterior crossbite, open bite, overbite and posterior crossbite.

Multi-way ANOVA using the Bonferroni correction of pairwise comparisons was used to compare the mean intercanine and intermolar widths in children exhibiting different non-nutritive sucking habits.

The significance level was set at $p < 0.05$.

Table 1 Oral examination criteria of the children's three-dimensional dental arch relationships

Sagittal	Vertical	Transverse
Incisal relationship- Classified into three categories: Class I, the lower incisor edges occlude with or lie immediately below cingulum plateau of the upper central incisors; Class II, the lower incisor edges lie posterior to the cingulum plateau of the upper incisors; Class III, the lower incisor edges lie anterior to the cingulum plateau of the upper incisors. The overjet is reduced or reversed [44].	**Overbite**- Coverage of the mandibular incisor by the most protruded fully erupted maxillary incisor and recorded as < 1/2 or ≥ 1/2 [11].	**Intermolar width**- Distance between mesiobuccal cusp tips of the maxillary second primary molars [40].
Canine relationship- Classified into three categories: Class I, the tip of the maxillary primary canine tooth is in the same vertical plane as the distal surface of the mandibular primary canine; Class II, the tip of the maxillary primary canine tooth is mesial to the distal surface of the mandibular primary canine; Class III, the tip of the maxillary primary canine is distal to the distal surface of the mandibular primary canine [11].	**Anterior openbite**- When there are no vertical contacts between upper and lower incisal edges [9].	**Intercanine width**- Distance from cusp tip to cusp tip of the maxillary primary canines [40].
Molar relationship - Classified into three categories: Flush terminal, where the distal surfaces of the upper and lower second primary molars are in the same vertical plane in a centric occlusion; Distal step, where the distal surfaces of the lower primary second molar are in a posterior relationship to the distal surface of the upper second molars in centric occlusion; Mesial step, the distal surfaces of the lower primary second molar are in an anterior relationship to the distal surface of the upper second molars in centric occlusion [11].		**Posterior crossbite**- Recorded when one or more of the maxillary primary canines or molars occluded lingual to the buccal cusps of the opposing mandibular teeth [11].
Anterior crossbite – It was recorded when one or more of the maxillary incisors occluded lingual to the mandibular incisors [45].		
Overjet- Measured from the palatal surface of the mesial corner of the most protruded fully erupted maxillary incisor to the labial surface of the corresponding mandibular incisor [11]. The degree of overjet was recorded in millimeters. In this study, an overjet of greater than 3.5 mm was considered an increased overjet.		

Results

Sample characteristics and measurement error

The survey included 1114 children aged 2 to 5 years old. The boy ($n = 609$, 54.7%) to girl ($n = 500$, 44.9%) ratio was 1.22. Five children's parents did not answer the question on the children's gender.

Regarding the intra-examiner reliability, the Cohen's kappa coefficients ranged from 0.70 to 1.00 and the Interclass Correlation Coefficient (ICC) ranged from 0.89 to 0.98, indicating that the categorical data were in substantial to perfect agreement and the continuous data had excellent reproducibility [24, 25].

Correlations between nutritive and non-nutritive sucking habits

Among the 1114 children who had participated in the survey, 80 participants did not provide complete answers to questions on duration of breastfeeding, frequency of pacifier use or frequency of thumb/digit sucking. Therefore, only 1034 children were included in the analysis (Tables 2 and 3).

Significant association was found between the duration of breastfeeding and the frequency of pacifier use ($p = 0.000$). The children who had experienced pure breastfeeding for more than 6 months had a significantly lower chance of daily pacifier use (multinomial logistic regression: $p = 0.000$; adjusted odds ratio [OR] = 0.412, 95% confidence interval [CI] 0.259–0.655). However, no association between the duration of pure breastfeeding and the development of habitual thumb/digit sucking was found (multinomial logistic regression $p > 0.05$). The associations between the duration of breastfeeding and the frequency of pacifier and thumb/digit sucking are presented in Table 2.

Correlations between non-nutritive sucking habits

Children who used pacifiers daily had significantly higher chances of having daily thumb/digit sucking habits (logistic regression: $p = 0.023$; adjusted OR = 2.136, 95% CI 1.112–4.103) (Table 3).

Associations between non-nutritive sucking habits and primary dental relationships

Among the 1114 children who had participated in the survey, 851 children took part in the oral examination and also completed all the questions in the questionnaires. Hence, the following tables (Tables 4, 5, 6 and 7) are analysis based on the 851 children.

Sagittal dimension

In terms of frequency, the children with daily thumb/digit sucking habits had significantly higher chances of developing Class II incisor relationships (multinomial logistic regression: $p = 0.008$; adjusted OR = 2.237, 95% CI 1.290–3.877), Class II canine relationships (multinomial logistic regression: $p = 0.036$; adjusted OR = 2.595, 95% CI 1.117–6.025) and overjets > 3.5 mm (logistic regression: $p = 0.000$; adjusted OR = 2.879, 95% CI 1.624–5.101) than those without daily thumb/digit sucking habits (Table 4). However, the frequency of pacifier use was not associated with primary incisor, primary canine or primary molar relationships (multinomial logistic regression: $p > 0.05$) (Table 4).

Regarding duration, the children who exhibited daily thumb/digit sucking for more than a year had significantly higher chances of developing Class II incisor relationships (multinomial logistic regression: $p = 0.001$; adjusted OR = 2.930, 95% CI 1.628–5.274), Class II canine relationships (multinomial logistic regression: $p = 0.005$; adjusted OR = 3.483, 95% CI 1.312–9.245) and overjets > 3.5 mm (logistic regression: $p = 0.000$; adjusted OR 3.603, 95% CI 1.987–6.533) than those without daily thumb/digit sucking habits (Table 5). Similar to the analysis of frequency, the duration of daily pacifier use was found to have no association with primary incisor, primary canine or primary molar relationships (multinomial logistic regression: $p > 0.05$) (Table 5).

Vertical dimension

In terms of frequency, the children who used pacifiers daily had significantly higher chances of developing an anterior open bite (logistic regression: $p = 0.000$; adjusted OR = 10.149, 95% CI 3.798–27.122) and significantly

Table 2 Association between the duration of breastfeeding and frequency of non-nutritive sucking habits ($n = 1034$)

			Daily pacifier vs non daily pacifier			Daily thumb/digit sucking vs non daily thumb/digit sucking		
	n	%	OR	95% CI	*p*-value	OR	95% CI	*p*-value
Duration of breastfeeding					**0.000***			0.143
> 6 months	**246**	**23.8**	**0.412**	**0.259–0.655**	**0.000***	0.599	0.318-1.128	0.112
0-6 months	471	45.6	0.840	0.598–1.180	0.134	1.042	0.645–1.683	0.867
Never	317	30.7	1	–	–	1	–	–

OR odds ratio, *CI* confidence interval
[a] Adjusted for background information (age and gender)
* $p < 0.05$
Boldface data are variables with $p < 0.05$ or OR (95%CI) < 1

Table 3 Association between the frequency of pacifier use and frequency of thumb/digit sucking (n = 1034)

Frequency of pacifier use			Daily thumb/digit sucking vs non daily thumb/digit sucking		
	n	%	OR	95% CI	*p* value
Daily pacifier	**212**	**20.5**	**2.136**	**1.112–4.103**	**0.023***
Non daily pacifier	822	79.5	1	–	–

OR odds ratio, *CI* confidence interval
[a] Adjusted for background information (age and gender) and duration of pure breastfeeding
* $p < 0.05$
Boldface data are variables with $p < 0.05$ or OR (95%CI) < 1

lower chances of developing an overbite greater than half of the lower incisor (logistic regression: $p = 0.004$; adjusted OR = 0.555, 95% CI 0.373–0.825) than those who did not use pacifiers daily. In addition, children with daily thumb/digit sucking habits had significantly higher chances of developing an anterior open bite (logistic regression: $p = 0.046$; adjusted OR = 3.440, 95% CI 1.020–11.597) (Table 6). The frequency of thumb/digit sucking was not associated with the extent of the anterior overbite formed (logistic regression: $p > 0.05$) (Table 6).

The results of the duration analyses were very similar to those of frequency analyses. The children who experienced daily pacifier use for more than 1 year had significantly higher chances of developing an anterior open bite (logistic regression: $p = 0.000$; adjusted OR = 15.171, 95% CI 5.298–43.446) and significantly lower chances of developing an overbite greater than half of the lower incisor (logistic regression: $p = 0.045$; adjusted OR = 0.577, 95% CI 0.340–0.890) than those who never had the habit of daily pacifier use (Table 7). In addition, children who displayed daily thumb/digit sucking for more than 1 year had significantly higher chances of developing an anterior open bite (logistic regression: $p = 0.006$; adjusted OR = 6.383, 95% CI 1.689–24.120) than those who had never displayed daily thumb/digit sucking habits (Table 7).

Transverse dimension

The frequency and duration of pacifier use and thumb/digit sucking were neither associated with the development of posterior crossbite (logistic regression: $p > 0.05$) nor the intercanine (ANOVA: $p > 0.05$)/intermolar widths (ANOVA: $p > 0.05$).

Discussion

First, this study assessed the association between nutritive and non-nutritive sucking habits. It was found that children who were breastfed for more than 6 months had significantly less daily pacifier use. No relationship was found between breastfeeding and thumb/digit sucking. The relationship between breastfeeding and pacifier use is consistent with previous studies [17, 26]. Breastfeeding has been found to use more musculature and facilitates the development of the correct orofacial muscles [11, 12, 27]. With unrestricted breastfeeding infants experience improved safety and satisfaction, and thus no other sucking actions are needed, which leads to less pacifier use [11]. One study found increased digit sucking when breastfeeding lasted less than 6 months [15]. However, another study focusing on the frequency of thumb sucking found no relationship to breastfeeding [18], which is similar to our results. The variability between studies may be due to whether the frequency of thumb sucking was taken into account when the data were analysed.

Second, this study assessed the interrelation between different non-nutritive sucking habits. It was found that more daily pacifier use increased the chances for more thumb/digit sucking habits. Not many studies have focused on the relationship between pacifier use and thumb sucking, apart from a study done in 1977 that found an inverse association between the two habits [28]. A possible explanation as to why pacifier use increased thumb/digit sucking in our study is that adaptation to one habit may increase the urge for and addiction to the sucking sensation. In addition, when infants are not sufficiently satisfied by thumb/digit sucking, they may develop other habits to help them to fulfil their needs.

Third, this study investigated the effects of non-nutritive sucking habits on primary dental relationships. In the sagittal dimension, the results of this study agree with previous studies in that thumb sucking is associated with Class II incisor relationships, Class II canine relationships and also increased overjet [29–35]. The higher incidence of increased overjet may be due to proclination of the maxillary incisors and forward displacement of the maxillary base as a result of the pressure of the thumb [36–38]. The overjet may also be worsened by retroclination of the lower incisors due to the lever action of the thumb [39]. The increase in Class II canine relationships may be due to the forward displacement of the anterior maxillary base [35, 39].

Some existing studies have found that pacifier use is associated with increased overjet [11, 40, 41]. Nevertheless, this study did not find any association between pacifier use and the development of primary dentition in the sagittal dimension. The difference may be because the previous studies have not assessed the frequency or duration of pacifier use. Furthermore, most studies have

Table 4 Association between frequency of different non-nutritive sucking habits and primary dental relationships in sagittal dimension ($n = 851$)

	Incisor relationship					Canine relationship					Molar relationship					Overjet		
	p-value	Class II incisor vs Class I incisor		Class III incisor vs Class I incisor		*p*-value	Class II canine vs Class I canine		Class III canine vs Class I canine		*p*-value	Bilateral Flush vs Bilateral Mesial step		Bilateral Mesial step vs Bilateral Distal step		*p*-value	Overjet > 3.5 mm vs non overjet > 3.5 mm	
		OR	95% CI	OR	95% CI		OR	95% CI	OR	95% CI		OR	95% CI	OR	95% CI		OR	95% CI
Frequency of pacifier use	0.490					0.108					0.168					0.495		
Daily		1.292	0.837–1.996	0.981	0.543–1.773		1.656	1.016–2.699	1.204	0.515–2.813		1.508	0.860–2.647	1.688	0.926–3.077		1.191	0.720–1.970
Non-daily		1	–	1	–		1	–	1	–		1	–	1	–		1	–
Frequency of thumb/digit sucking	**0.008***					**0.036***					0.622					**0.000***		
Daily		**2.237**	**1.290–3.877**	0.765	0.287–2.044		**2.595**	**1.117–6.025**	1.806	0.215–5.478		1.182	0.536–2.607	1.494	0.671–3.325		**2.879**	**1.624–5.101**
Non-daily		1	–	1	–		1	–	1	–		1	–	1	–		**1**	**–**

OR odds ratio, *CI* confidence interval
[a] Adjusted for background information (age and gender) and duration of pure breastfeeding
* $p < 0.05$
Boldface data are variables with $p < 0.05$ or OR (95%CI) < 1

Table 5 Association between duration of different non-nutritive sucking habits and primary dental relationships in sagittal dimension ($n = 851$)

	Incisor relationship					Canine relationship					Molar relationship					Overjet		
	p-value	Class II incisor vs Class I incisor		Class III incisor vs Class I incisor		*p*-value	Class II canine vs Class I canine		Class III canine vs Class I canine		*p*-value	Bilateral Flush vs Bilateral Mesial step		Bilateral Mesial step vs Bilateral Distal step		*p*-value	Overjet > 3.5 mm vs non overjet > 3.5 mm	
		OR	95% CI	OR	95% CI		OR	95% CI	OR	95% CI		OR	95% CI	OR	95% CI		OR	95% CI
Duration of daily pacifier use	0.483					0.063					0.183					0.448		
> 1 year		1.416	0.881–2.276	0.988	0.520–1.878		1.995	1.162–3.425	1.003	0.371–2.708		1.111	0.588–2.099	1.711	0.896–3.267		1.417	0.826–2.430
< 1 year		1.960	0.683–5.626	1.121	0.229–5.480		1.426	0.371–5.477	2.77	0.432–17.873		4.459	0.836–23.793	3.158	0.511–19.513		1.058	0.291–3.846
Never		1	–	1	–		1	–	1	–		1	–	1	–		1	–
Duration of daily thumb/digit sucking	**0.001***					**0.005***					0.455					**0.000***		
> 1 year		**2.930**	**1.628–5.274**	0.966	0.354–2.635		**3.483**	**1.312–9.245**	0.658	0.073–5.967		1.005	0.415–2.434	1.663	0.715–3.867		**3.603**	**1.987–6.533**
Never		1	–	1	–		1	–	1	–		1	–	1	–		**1**	**–**

OR odds ratio, *CI* confidence interval
[a] Adjusted for background information (age and gender) and different oral habits
* $p < 0.05$
Boldface data are variables with $p < 0.05$ or OR (95%CI) < 1
The group for < 1 year of daily thumb/digit sucking was excluded since the number of subjects were not sufficient to perform the test

Table 6 Association between frequency of different non-nutritive sucking habits and primary dental relationships in vertical dimension (n = 851)

	Anterior openbite			Anterior overbite		
	p-value	Anterior openbite vs non-anterior openbite		*p*-value	Overbite ≥ ½ vs overbite < ½	
		OR	95% CI		OR	95% CI
Frequency of pacifier use	**0.000***			**0.004***		
Daily		**10.149**	**3.798–27.122**		**0.555**	**0.373–0.825**
Non-daily		1	–		1	–
Frequency of thumb/digit sucking	**0.046***			0.128		
Daily		**3.440**	**1.020–11.597**		0.653	0.377–1.130
Non-daily		1	–		1	–

OR odds ratio, *CI* confidence interval
[a] Adjusted for background information (age and gender) and duration of pure breastfeeding
* $p < 0.05$
Boldface data are variables with $p < 0.05$ or OR (95%CI) < 1

not considered thumb/digit sucking as a confounding factor. In addition, there are different types of pacifiers on the market; different pacifier designs may affect the results.

In the vertical dimension, the results of this study agree with those of existing studies in that thumb/digit sucking and pacifier use are associated with increased open bite [42]. Pressure from the thumb or pacifier hinders the downward growth of the maxillary base and delays the anterior teeth from erupting while the posterior teeth continue to erupt. This results in overeruption of the posterior teeth and the formation of an anterior open bite [11, 33, 35, 36, 43].

Multiple studies have found that non-nutritive sucking habits are associated with smaller maxillary intercanine and intermolar widths and increased posterior crossbite [29, 41]. Nevertheless, this study found no association between non-nutritive sucking habits in the transverse dimension of the primary dentition. These inconsistent findings can be explained by the fact that most of the studies have not accounted for confounding factors, such as age, gender and other non-nutritive sucking habits, in their statistical analyses. Furthermore, many studies have not investigated the frequency or duration of the habits.

The results of this study show that pure breastfeeding for more than 6 months lowered pacifier use, which was associated with less thumb/digit sucking. Together, less pacifier use and less thumb/digit sucking benefited primary dental relationship development in the sagittal and vertical dimensions. These results raise three important points. First, pure breastfeeding for more than 6 months prevents non-nutritive sucking habits. Second, there is a correlation between variable non-nutritive sucking habits. Thus, preventing or breaking a non-nutritive sucking habit may prevent or break others. Third, preventing or breaking non-nutritive sucking habits is important for the development of primary dentition.

This study did have its limitations. The random selection of subjects was difficult, as we needed approval

Table 7 Association between duration of different non-nutritive sucking habits and primary dental relationships in vertical dimension (*n* = 851)

	Anterior openbite			Anterior overbite		
	p-value	Anterior openbite vs non-anterior openbite		*p*-value	Overbite ≥ ½ vs overbite < ½	
		OR	95% CI		OR	95% CI
Duration of daily pacifier use	**0.000***			**0.045***		
> 1 year		**15.171**	**5.298–43.446**		**0.577**	**0.374–0.890**
< 1 year		0.000	0.000–0.000		0.881	0.302–2.570
Never		1	–		1	–
Duration of daily thumb/digit sucking	**0.006***			0.122		
> 1 year		**6.383**	**1.689–24.120**		0.631	0.352–1.131
Never		1	–		1	–

OR odds ratio, *CI* confidence interval
[a] Adjusted for background information (age and gender) and duration of pure breastfeeding
* $p < 0.05$
Boldface data are variables with $p < 0.05$ or OR (95%CI) < 1
The group for < 1 year of daily thumb/digit sucking was excluded since the number of subjects were not sufficient to perform the test

from their schools to take part in the study. Effort was made to spread out the samples across the main territories of Hong Kong. As this is a retrospective study, recall bias is possible. As parents are unable to monitor their children for 24 h each day, there may be an underestimation of thumb/digit sucking habits. Furthermore, the survey questions may have had overlapping response options (e.g. '0–6 months' and '6–12 months'). During the oral examinations, the children were all in the lying-down position to prevent them from moving around; however, it may have been more accurate if they were sitting down instead. Finally, it was difficult to assess whether the child had mild skeletal discrepancy without the use of radiographs.

Conclusion

Breastfeeding for more than 6 months is negatively associated with pacifier use. Pacifier use is positively associated with thumb/digit sucking. Pacifier use and thumb/digit sucking are associated with higher chances of malocclusion in the sagittal (i.e. Class II incisal relationships, Class II canine relationships and increased overjet) and vertical (i.e. anterior open bite) dimensions of the primary dentition.

Abbreviations

ANOVA: Analysis of variance; ICC: Interclass Correlation Coefficient; OR: Odds ratio; SPSS: Statistical Package for the Social Sciences; WHO: World Health Organization

Acknowledgements

We thank the ten nursery schools who participated in the study and extend special thanks to Hong Kong Society for the Protection of Children. Dr. Karen Yuet Wa Hung's support to this project is much appreciated. We also thank the helpers' contribution during the outreach survey.

Funding

The project was supported by the Seed Funding for Basic Research, the University of Hong Kong (201611159297). The funding body played no role in the design of the study and collection, analysis, and interpretation of data and in writing the manuscript.

Authors' contributions

All authors read and approved the final manuscript. HTBL: Questionnaire design, write up of the manuscript. FHKMHS: Examination form design, data analysis, write up of the manuscript. LZ: Examination of participants, manuscript write up especially on section of oral examinations. CPWY: Examination arrangement, data input, manuscript write up especially on section of data collection. KYL: Data analysis, manuscript write up especially on section of statistical analysis. HMW: Questionnaire design, manuscript write up especially on section of analysis of questionnaires. YY: Study design and organization, calibration for the examiner, write-up of the manuscript.

Competing interests

The authors declare that they have no competing interests.

Author details

[1]Department of Paediatric Dentistry and Orthodontics, Faculty of Dentistry, Prince Philip Dental Hospital, The University of Hong Kong, 2/F, 34 Hospital Road, Sai Ying Pun, Hong Kong SAR, China. [2]Department of Orthodontics, Tianjin Stomatological Hospital of Nankai University, 75 Dagu Road, Tianjin, China. [3]Translational Research Laboratory, Faculty of Dentistry, Prince Philip Dental Hospital, The University of Hong Kong, Room 7A26, 7/F, 34 Hospital Road, Sai Ying Pun, Hong Kong SAR, China.

References

1. Peres KG, Barros AJD, Peres MA, Victoria CG. Effects of breastfeeding and sucking habits on malocclusion in a birth cohort study. Rev Saúde Pública. 2007;41(3):343–50.
2. Moimaz SA, Zina LG, Saliba NA, Saliba O. Association between breast-feeding practices and sucking habits: a cross-sectional study of children in their first year of life. J Indian Soc Pedod Prev Dent. 2008;26(3):102–6.
3. Gederi A, Coomaraswamy K, Turner PJ. Pacifiers: a review of risks vs benefits. Dental Update. 2013;40:92–101.
4. Çinar ND. The advantages and disadvantages of pacifier use. Contemp Nurse. 2004;17(1–2):109–12.
5. Adair SM. Pacifier use in children: a review of recent literature. Pediatr Dent. 2003;25(5):449–58.
6. Jackson KM, Nazar AM. Breastfeeding, the immune response, and long-term health. J Am Osteopath Assoc. 2006;106(4):203–7.
7. Exclusive breastfeeding. http://www.who.int/nutrition/topics/exclusive_breastfeeding/en/. Accessed 29 June 2016.
8. Sum FHKMH, Zhang L, Ling HTB, Yeung CPWY, Li KY, Wong HM, Yang Y. Association of breastfeeding and three-dimensional dental arch relationships in primary dentition. BMC Oral Health. 2015;15:30.
9. Narbutytė I, Narbutytė A, Linkevičienė L. Relationship between breastfeeding, bottle-feeding and development of malocclusion. Stomatologija. 2013;15(3):67–72.
10. Rochelle IMF, Da Silva Tagliaferro EP, Pereira AC, De Castro Meneghim M, Nóbilo KA, Ambrosano GMB. Breastfeeding, deleterious oral habits and malocclusion in 5-year-old children in São Pedro, SP, Brazil. Dental Press J Orthod. 2010;15(2):71–81.
11. Xiaoxian C, Bin X, Lihong G. Effects of breast-feeding duration, bottle-feeding duration and non-nutritive sucking habits on the occlusal characteristics of primary dentition. BMC Pediatr. 2015;15:46.
12. Pires SC, Giugliani ER, Caramez Da Silva F. Influence of the duration of breastfeeding on quality of muscle function during mastication in preschoolers: a cohort study. BMC Public Health. 2012;12(1):934.
13. Turgeon-Obrien H, Lachapelle D, Gagnon PF, Maheu-Robert LF. Nutritive and non-nutritive sucking habits: a review. ASDC J Dental Child. 1996;63(5): 321–7.
14. Jyoti S, Pavanalakshmi GP. Nutritive and non-nutritive sucking habits – effect on the developing oro-facial complex: a review. Dentistry. 2014;4:203.
15. Agarwal SS, Nehra K, Sharma M, Jayan B, Poonia A, Bhattal H. Association between breastfeeding duration, non-nutritive sucking habits and dental arch dimensions in deciduous dentition: a cross-sectional study. Prog Orthod. 2014;15:59.
16. Luz CL, Carib DG, Arouca R. Association between breastfeeding duration and mandibular retrusion: a cross-sectional study of children in the mixed dentition. Am J Orthod Dentofac Orthop. 2006;130(4):531–4.
17. Solanki G, Kachhawaha B, Solanki R. Thumb sucking and pacifier use: its relationship with breastfeeding patterns. Int J Current Pharm Research. 2014;4(3):148–9.
18. Aarts C, Hörnell A, Kylberg E, Hofvander Y, Gebre-Medhin M. Breastfeeding patterns in relation to thumb sucking and pacifier use. Pediatrics. 1999; 104:e50.
19. Canadian Paediatric Society. Recommendations for the use of pacifiers. Paediatr Child Health. 2003;8(8):515–9.
20. Sexton S, Natale R. Risks and benefits of pacifiers. Am Fam Physician. 2009; 79(8):681–5.
21. Sio JO, Minwalla FK, George RH, Booth IW. Oral candida: is dummy carriage the culprit? Arch Dis Child. 1987;62(4):406–8.
22. Comina E, Marion K, Renaud FN, Dore J, Bergeron E, Freney J. Pacifiers: a microbial reservoir. Nurs Health Sci. 2006;8(4):216–23.
23. Jabbar NS, Bueno AB, Silva PE, Scavone-Junior H, Inês Ferreira R. Bottle feeding, increased overjet and class 2 primary canine relationship: is there any association? Braz Oral Res. 2011;25(4):331–7.

24. Landis JR, Koch GC. The measurement of observer agreement for categorical data. Biometrics. 1977;33(1):159–74.
25. Rosner B. Fundamentals of biostatistics. 7th ed. Belmont: Duxbury Press; 2011. p. 568–71.
26. Moimaz SA, Saliba O, Lolli LF, Garbin CA, Garbin AJ, Saliba NA. A longitudinal study of the association between breast-feeding and harmful oral habits. Pediatr Dent. 2012;34(2):117–21.
27. Carrascoza KC, Possobon RF, Tomita LM, Moraes AB. Consequences of bottle-feeding to the oral facial development of initially breastfed children. J Pediatr. 2006;82(5):395–7.
28. Zadik D, Stern N, Litner M. Thumb- and pacifier-sucking habits. Am J Orthod. 1977;71(2):197–201.
29. Murray JJ, Nunn JH, Steele JG. The Prevention of Oral Disease. 4th ed. New York: Oxford; 2003. p. 158.
30. Bowden BD. The effect of digital and dummy sucking on arch widths, overbite, and overjet: a longitudinal study. Aus Dent J. 1966;11(6):396–404.
31. Warren JJ, Bishara SE. Duration of nutritive and non-nutritive sucking behaviours and their effects on the dental arches in the primary dentition. Am J Orthod and Dentofacial Orthop. 2002;121(4):347–56.
32. Ozawa N, Hamada S, Takekoshi F, Shinji H. A study on non-nutritive sucking habits in young Japanese – relationships among incidence, duration, malocclusion and nursing behavior. Pediatr Dent J. 2005;15(1):64–71.
33. Al-Dawoody AD. Finger sucking: prevalence, contributing factors and effect on occlusion. Al-Rafidain Dent J. 2004;4(2):135–42.
34. Duncan K, McNamara C, Ireland AJ, Sandy JR. Sucking habits in childhood and effects on the primary dentition: findings of the Avon longitudinal study of pregnancy and childhood. Int J Paediatr Dent. 2008;18(3):178–88.
35. Fukata O, Braham RL, Yokoi K, Kurosu K. Damage to the primary dentition resulting from thumb and finger (digit) sucking. ASDC J Dent Child. 1996; 63(6):403–7.
36. Bisharra SE, Larsson E. Finger habits: their effects and their treatments – part 2. Dent Assist. 2007;76(2):16–22.
37. Proffit WR. The orthodontic problem - the development of orthodontic problems. In: Proffit WR, Fields HW, Sarver DM, editors. Contemporary Orthodontics. Philadelphia: Mosby; 2007. p. 3–23. 130–161.
38. Kato M, Watanabe K, Kato E, Hotta H, Daito M. Three dimensional measurement of the palate using the semiconductor laser: on the influences of the palate of maxillary protrusion with finger sucking. Ped Dent J. 2009;19(1):25–9.
39. Subtelny JD, Subtelny JD. Oral habits – studies in form, function and therapy. Angle Orthod. 1973;43(4):347–83.
40. Warren JJ, Bishara SE, Steinbock KL, Yonezu T, Nowak AJ. Effects of oral habits' duration on dental characteristics in the primary dentition. J Am Dent Assoc. 2001;132(12):1685–93. 1726
41. Aznar T, Galan AF, Marin I, Dominguez A. Dental arch diameters and relationships to oral habits. Angle Orthod. 2006;76(3):441–5.
42. Ngan P, Fields HW. Openbite: a review of etiology and management. Pediatr Dent. 1997;19:91–8.
43. Larsson E. Artificial sucking habits: etiology, prevalence and effect on occlusion. Int J Orofacial Myology. 1994;20:10–21.
44. Mitchell L. The aetiology and classification of malocclusion. An introduction to orthodontics. 3. New York: Oxford University Press; 2007. p. 9–10.
45. Bhat SS, Rao HT, Hegde KS, Kumar BS. Characteristics of primary dentition occlusion in preschool children: an epidemiological study. Int J Clin Pediatr Dent. 2012;5(2):93–7.

27

The effect of bitewing radiography on estimates of dental caries experience among children differs according to their disease experience

L. A. Foster Page[1*], D. Boyd[2], K. Fuge[5], A. Stevenson[3], K. Goad[4], D. Sim[6] and W. M. Thomson[2]

Abstract

Background: Radiography is a regularly used and accepted adjunct to visual examination in the diagnosis of dental caries. It is assumed that not using radiographs can lead to underestimation of dental caries experience with most reports having involved studies of young adults or adolescents, and been focused on the permanent dentition. The aim of this study was to determine the relative contributions of bitewing radiography and clinical examination in the detection of dental caries in primary molars and to determine whether those contributions differ according to caries experience.

Methods: A cross-sectional study was conducted, involving examinations undertaken in dental clinics. Bitewing radiographs taken at the time of the clinical examination were developed and read later, with the data from those used at the analysis stage to adjust the caries diagnosis for the mesial, occlusal and distal surfaces of the primary molar teeth. Children's clinically determined dmfs score was used to allocate them to one of three caries experience groups (0 dmfs, 1–8 dmfs, or 9+ dmfs).

Results: Of the 501 three-to-eight-year-old children examined, nearly three-quarters were younger than six. Caries prevalence and mean dmfs after clinical examination alone and following radiographs were 63.1% and 4.6 (sd, 6.2), and 74.7% and 5.8 (sd, 6.5) respectively. Among children with a dmfs of 1–8, the number of lesions missed during the clinical examination was greater than the number of 106 (25.6%) in children with a dmfs of 9+. In the 185 children with no apparent caries at clinical examination, 124 lesions were detected radiographically, among 58 (46.8%) of those.

Conclusions: Taking bitewing radiographs in young children is not without challenges or risks, and it must be undertaken with these in mind. Diagnostic yields from bitewing radiographs are greater for children with greater caries experience. The findings of this study further support the need to consider using bitewing radiographs in young children to enhance the management of lesions not detected by a simple visual examination alone.

Keywords: Children, Bitewing radiography, Caries status

* Correspondence: lyndie.fosterpage@otago.ac.nz
[1]Department of Oral Sciences, Faculty of Dentistry, University of Otago, PO Box 56, Dunedin 9054, New Zealand
Full list of author information is available at the end of the article

Background

Radiography is a regularly used and accepted adjunct in the diagnosis of dental caries. Early studies found using the traditional clinical examination alone that a much lower sensitivity and specificity occurred than when combined with the use of radiographs [1–3]. Not using radiographs has been shown to lead to underestimation of dental caries experience, especially for that in approximal and occlusal surfaces [4–14]. Even in an ideal clinical environment (with good light, and clean and dry teeth), clinical examinations conducted without adjunctive radiography have been shown to underestimate the actual disease level [15]. However, recent studies have questioned whether using radiographs to increase the sensitivity of visual inspection have concomitantly reduced its specificity and introduced a high number of false positives, leading to an overestimation of caries and then overtreatment [16–19].

Most reports on the underestimation of caries without radiographs have involved studies of young adults or adolescents, and have focused on the permanent dentition. In a study of 12-year-old Lithuanian children, the clinical examination alone detected only 60% of approximal cavitated dentine lesions, while, with radiographic examination alone, 90% of lesions were detected. The diagnostic yield improved significantly when the clinical examination was supplemented with radiographs [6]. In young Chinese adults, the use of clinical examination without the use of bitewing radiographs in the posterior teeth led to an underestimation of the number of carious lesions by approximately 50% [11]. Hopcraft and Morgan (2005) investigated the additional diagnostic yield from bitewings for occlusal and approximal dental caries in adults aged 17–30 years. They found the largest underestimation to be for approximal surfaces, where more than two-thirds of approximal dentine caries lesions went undetected by clinical examination. Other studies have focused on populations with high caries experience [2, 13]. In New Zealand adolescents with high caries experience, approximately 40% of carious lesions were missed when radiographs were not used in the caries diagnosis [13].

There have been fewer such investigations in the primary dentition. Newman et al. (2009) investigated the benefits of bitewing radiography in detecting caries in primary teeth in 6–12-year-olds in a non-fluoridated Australian city. They found that visual examination and radiographs detected 48% more proximal primary molar lesions than visual examination alone. In a study of 267 Swedish 5-year-olds with low caries experience (dmfs = 0.4, 85% caries-free) when bitewing radiography was added to the clinical examination, the dmfs rose to 1.2 and only 67% of children were determined to be caries-free. This included adding both enamel and dentine lesions found on radiographs to the clinical examination [8]. Similar findings were reported for Swedish 9-year-olds, with 29% of the children whose primary molars were classified as caries-free using clinical examination found to have caries involving dentine or enamel on bitewing radiographs [10]. In a Dutch study of 50 six-year-old children with high caries experience (mean dmfs of 7.8), clinical examination alone missed approximately 50% of approximal lesions involving dentine [14]. These studies indicate that radiography is also very important for caries diagnosis in primary teeth, but that its yield may differ according to disease level. Many studies that have investigated caries detection methods have not considered the prevalence of the disease in the interpretation of their findings. The increase in sensitivity provided by using radiographs consequently decreases the specificity at times with the number of errors being higher in populations with low caries experience [16].

The American Dental Association and the European Academy of Paediatric Dentistry have produced best-practice guidelines for bitewing radiography in young children [20, 21]. For the primary dentition, it is recommended that individualised radiographic examination be undertaken if proximal surfaces are unable to be scrutinised. Subsequent sets of radiographs should be taken at intervals determined by the child's caries risk and dentition stage. If the timing of future sets of radiographs is to be determined by the child's caries status, it is imperative to attempt to take a set of radiographs at an age when the clinician can take advantage of the diagnostic yield that radiographs offer. Although there is evidence to support the use of bitewing radiographs in all children regardless of caries experience, there is debate about the value they provide in the primary dentition, particularly in children who present for clinical examination with an apparently sound dentition. There appears to be concern about the risks of radiation exposure in young children.

The aim of this study was to determine the relative contributions of bitewing radiography and clinical examination in detecting dental caries in primary molars in children in a community with high caries experience, in order to determine whether those contributions differ according to caries experience.

Methods

A cross-sectional study design was used. Ethical approval for the study was obtained from the Northern B Health and Disability Ethics Committee (14/NTB/39). All three to eight-year-old children attending 37 schools and preschools in New Zealand's Whanganui region were invited to participate in the study when they attended for their routine clinical examination. Children were excluded if they had recently (within the previous 6 months) had a set of bitewing radiographs taken, had open contacts present between their primary molars, were medically compromised, unable to have radiographs taken, did not have parent consent, or did not assent to participation in the study.

Information on child age, address and ethnicity was obtained from parents. Other socio-demographic information collected included an area-based deprivation score, the NZDep2013. This combines a number of variables measured in the 2013 Census which reflect aspects of social and material deprivation, with each Census meshblock having been allocated a deprivation score [22]. In the current study, the area-based deprivation score was then determined by geocoding each child's street address and matching it (via meshblock number) to the NZDep2013 data-base. The NZDep2013 allocates each address a deprivation score, ranging from 1 (least deprived) to 10 (most deprived).

Each child underwent a clinical examination in Community Oral Health Service Clinics by one of 13 calibrated dental therapists. Visual examination was conducted under a dental light using a flat dental mirror, explorer and triplex air syringe [23]. Caries status was systematically recorded for each surface. Only the clinical status of the primary dentition was recorded. A carious lesion was counted if cavitation was present. Children's clinically determined dmfs score was used to allocate them to one of three caries experience groups (0 dmfs, 1–8 dmfs, or 9+ dmfs).

Bitewing radiographs were taken at the time of the clinical examination. Conventional radiography was used, employing the following technical equipment: Belmont Belray 096-C; Girardelli X-30 for the developer; Carestream Insight IP-21 for the film; and Carestream Readymatic for the developer and fixer. Radiographs were developed and read later by two dental specialists (one in paediatric dentistry, the other in dental public health. There is no training of dental radiography specialists in New Zealand, nor anyone registered as a specialist in dental radiography. No magnification was used in reading radiographs, and surfaces that could not be read were recorded as such. The radiographic examiners were calibrated prior to reading radiographs. Radiograph readings for a randomly selected subset of 23 children were used to determine inter-examiner reliability. To determine intra-examiner reliability, each of the two examiners re-read radiographs on a randomly selected subset of 21 children. The intraclass correlation coefficient for dmfs for inter-examiner reliability score was 0.87, and the intra-examiner scores were 0.92 and 0.89, respectively. Children were excluded from the study if the quality of the film was poor or if there was substantial overlap present on the proximal surfaces, making a diagnosis difficult. The radiography data were entered into a separate data-set which was then merged and used at the analysis stage to adjust for the caries diagnosis of the mesial, occlusal and distal surfaces of the primary molars. Only lesions involving dentine were used in the radiographic adjustment.

Data were entered and analysed using the Statistical Package for the Social Sciences (version 23). Following the computation of univariate descriptive statistics, differences among proportions were tested for statistical significance ($\alpha = 0.05$) using χ^2 tests; differences with continuous variables were tested for statistical significance using the Wilcoxon signed ranks test.

Results

Of the 556 children for whom consent was obtained, 55 (9.9%) were excluded following their clinical examination. The final sample comprised 501 three-to-eight-year-old children, of whom approximately one-third were Māori (Table 1). Females comprised almost half of the sample. Nearly three-quarters of the children were under the age of six, and two-fifths resided in a highly-deprived area.

Summary estimates of the prevalence and severity of dental caries experience—from the clinical examination only, and then from the clinical examination combined with radiography—are presented in Table 2. The use of radiographs resulted in higher estimates for almost all indicators, except for those involving filled or missing surfaces, and missing teeth. The percent difference between the estimates (computed by dividing the difference between them by the clinical examination value and multiplying the result by 100) ranged from – 12.5 to 90.0%. For the whole-mouth estimates, there were statistically significant differences between the clinical-only and radiographically-adjusted estimates for mean dmft, dt, ft., dmfs, and ds, as well as the whole-mouth caries prevalence estimate, which was higher by 18.2% after radiographic adjustment. For the mesial and distal surfaces only, the prevalence and severity estimates were significantly greater, with almost a one-surface difference (on average) in mean ds

Table 1 Sociodemographic characteristics of the sample (parentheses contain row percentages unless otherwise indicated)

	Sex[a]		All[a]
	Female	Male	
Ethnicity			
Māori	78 (32.8)	85 (32.3)	163 (32.5)
NonMāori	160 (67.2)	178 (67.7)	338 (67.5)
Age group (years)			
3–4	35 (14.8)	48 (18.5)	83 (16.7)
5–6	140 (59.3)	146 (56.2)	286 (57.1)
7–8	61 (25.8)	66 (25.4)	127 (25.4)
NZ deprivation score[b]			
1–3 (low)	45 (10.0)	72 (27.4)	117 (23.4)
4–7 (medium)	90 (38.0)	96 (36.5)	186 (37.2)
8–10 (high)	102 (43.0)	95 (36.1)	197 (39.4)
All combined	238 (47.5)	263 (52.5)	501 (100.0)

[a]Column %

[b]This is an area-based SES measure which allocates scores ranging from 1 (lowest deprivation) to 10 (highest deprivation)

Table 2 Comparison of clinical and radiographically adjusted dental caries estimates (brackets contain standard deviation unless otherwise indicated)

	Clinical examination only	Clinical examination and radiographs	Percent difference	*p* value
Whole-mouth estimates				
Prevalence[a]	316 (63.1%)	374 (74.6%)	18.2	< 0.001
Severity				
Mean dmft	2.4 (2.8) 0–16	3.3 (3.0) 0–16	37.5	< 0.001
Mean dt	1.6 (2.2) 0–13	2.6 (2.5) 0–13	62.5	< 0.001
Mean mt	0.0 (0.3) 0–5	0.0 (0.3) 0–5	0.0	> 0.009
Mean ft	0.8 (1.4) 0–7	0.7 (1.2) 0–6	−12.5	< 0.001
Mean dmfs	4.6 (6.2) 0–44	5.8 (6.5) 0–45	26.1	< 0.001
Mean ds	2.1 (3.3) 0–26	3.3 (3.8) 0–30	57.1	< 0.001
Mean ms	0.1 (0.3) 0–5	0.1 (0.3) 0–5	0.0	> 0.009
Mean fs	2.5 (5.0) 0–44	2.5 (5.0) 0–44	0.0	> 0.009
Mesial and distal surfaces of molars only				
Prevalence[b]	266 (53.1%)	343 (68.45)	28.8	< 0.001
Severity				
Mean dfs	2.0 (2.7) 0–17	2.9 (3.1) 0–17	45.0	< 0.001
Mean ds	1.0 (1.6) 0–11	1.9 (2.1) 0–15	90.0	< 0.001
Mean fs	1.0 (2.1) 0–17	1.0 (2.1) 0–17	0.0	> 0.009
Occlusal surfaces of molars only				
Prevalence[b]	250 (49.9%)	283 (56.5%)	13.2	< 0.001
Severity				
Mean dfs	1.6 (2.2) 0–8	1.8 (2.2) 0–8	12.5	< 0.001
Mean ds	0.6 (1.3) 0–8	0.8 (1.4) 0–8	33.3	< 0.001
Mean fs	1.0 (1.7) 0–8	1.0 (1.7) 0–8	0.0	> 0.009

Shown as mean (SD) with range unless otherwise specified
[a]One or more dmft. [b]One or more dfs

being the largest difference observed. With the occlusal surfaces only, there was a significant difference in the prevalence and severity estimates, with a one-third-surface difference in mean ds.

Summary data on the number of lesions detected in the primary molars are presented in Table 3. The total number of lesions detected by clinical examination and radiography was 1245, and the total number of lesions detected by clinical examination alone was 694; 55.7% were detected with both methods. Thus, 44.3% of the lesions present were missed during the clinical examination. Overall, the greatest discrepancy was for approximal surfaces, with clinical examination alone accounting for 49.3% of the number of surfaces detected with clinical examination and radiography (438 out of 889); for occlusal surfaces, clinical examination alone accounted for 74.0% of the number of surfaces detected with clinical examination and radiography (256 out of 346).

In order to determine whether the relative contributions of clinical examination and radiography differed according to caries experience, children were allocated to the following ordinal categories of caries experience: 0 dmfs, with 185 children (43.5%); 1–8 dmfs, with 218 children (36.9%); and 9+ dmfs, with 98 children (19.6%). The mean dmfs score for children who were determined at clinical examination to be caries-free (dmfs = 0.0) was actually 5.9 (sd, 6.0) following radiographic adjustment. Determined at clinical examination to be 3.8 (sd, 2.3), the mean dmfs of the medium group (dmfs between 1 and 8) was 6.1 (sd, 7.1) following radiographic adjustment. That for the high–caries-experience group (dmfs 9+) rose from 15.1 (sd, 5.7) to 16.3 (sd, 5.7) following radiographic adjustment.

Data are presented in Table 4 on the number of lesions detected in primary molars in the children in those three different caries experience groups. For those with no apparent caries experience, radiographs detected 124 lesions, of which nearly two-thirds (62.1%) were detected on the distal surface of the first molars. That raised the prevalence of caries in that group from 0.0 to 31.4%. Among children with 1–8 dmfs, the total number of lesions missed during the clinical examination was 214

Table 3 Number of lesions detected with clinical examinations only (a) and clinical and radiographic examination (b), by tooth and surface[1] in all children

Upper right quadrant							Upper left quadrant					
(b)	7	45	80	123	33	22	16	26	132	72	45	7
(a)	3	28	24	58	24	7	5	18	71	35	32	0
	D	O	M	D	O	M	M	O	D	M	O	D
2nd molar			1st molar				1st molar			2nd molar		
	D	O	M	D	O	M	M	O	D	M	O	D
(a)	2	43	25	84	38	7	4	34	85	24	39	4
(b)	6	56	55	142	41	18	20	41	145	46	58	8
Lower right quadrant							Lower Left quadrant					

D Distal, *O* Occlusal, *M* Mesial

[1]Total number detected with radiography alone = 551; total number of lesions detected with clinical examination alone = 694 (55.7% of those detected with both methods)

Table 4 Number of lesions detected (a) by clinical examination alone and (b) by clinical examination and radiography, by molar tooth and surface, and by caries experience group

Children (*N* = 185) clinically diagnosed with 0 dmfs:

	Upper right quadrant						*Upper left quadrant*					
(b)	0	4	9	20	2	1	0	3	21	7	4	0
(a)	0	0	0	0	0	0	0	0	0	0	0	0
	D	O	M	D	O	M	M	O	D	M	O	D
	Second molar			First molar			First molar			Second molar		
	D	O	M	D	O	M	M	O	D	M	O	D
(a)	0	0	0	0	0	0	0	0	0	0	0	0
(b)	0	1	3	19	2	3	1	1	17	2	3	1
	Lower right quadrant						*Lower left quadrant*					

Total number detected with clinical examination and radiography = 124; number detected with clinical examination alone = 0 (0.0% of the latter)

Children (*N* = 218) clinically diagnosed with 1–8 dmfs:

	Upper right quadrant						*Upper left quadrant*					
(b)	7	45	80	123	33	22	16	26	132	72	46	7
(a)	3	28	24	58	24	7	5	18	71	35	32	0
	D	O	M	D	O	M	M	O	D	M	O	D
	Second molar			First molar			First molar			Second molar		
	D	O	M	D	O	M	M	O	D	M	O	D
(a)	2	43	25	84	38	7	4	34	85	24	39	4
(b)	6	56	55	142	41	18	20	41	145	46	58	8
	Lower right quadrant						*Lower left quadrant*					

Total number detected with clinical examination and radiography = 556; number detected with clinical examination alone = 342 (61.5% of the latter)

Children (*N* = 98) clinically diagnosed with 9+ dmfs:

	Upper right quadrant						*Upper left quadrant*					
(b)	4	17	25	34	18	7	5	13	31	30	14	5
(a)	2	14	12	24	17	4	4	12	24	21	14	0
	D	O	M	D	O	M	M	O	D	M	O	D
	Second molar			First molar			First molar			Second molar		
	D	O	M	D	O	M	M	O	D	M	O	D
(a)	1	18	16	23	22	4	2	17	22	15	17	3
(b)	4	21	31	28	22	4	11	17	31	19	19	4
	Lower right quadrant						*Lower left quadrant*					

Total number detected with clinical examination and radiography = 414; number detected with clinical examination alone = 308 (74.4% of the latter)

(38.5%), with the mesial surface of the maxillary right second molar and distal surfaces of the first primary molars showing the greatest discrepancy. The clinical examination alone accounted for only 55.7% of the number of approximal surfaces detected with clinical examination and radiography (234 out of 420), and clinical examination alone accounted for 79.4% of the number of occlusal surfaces detected with clinical examination and radiography (108 out of 136). Among children with a dmfs of 9+, the total number of lesions missed during the clinical examination was 106 (25.6%). Overall, the discrepancy was greatest for approximal surfaces, with clinical examination alone accounting for only 64.8% of the number of surfaces detected with clinical examination and radiography (177 out of 273). For occlusal surfaces, clinical examination alone accounted for 92.9% of the number of surfaces detected with clinical examination and radiography (131 out of 141).

Discussion

This study set out to determine the relative contributions of bitewing radiography and clinical examination in the detection of dental caries lesions in primary molars in children in a community with high caries experience, and to explore this in groups of children with different caries experience. It found that less caries experience was detected when radiographs are not used in caries diagnosis in these young children. When the total number of lesions was taken into account, the actual difference was 44% less disease experience detected. A number of children who were determined to be caries-free at the time of the clinical examination were found not to be so following the reading of radiographs. The extent of the under-estimation of caries experience differed according to how much overall caries experience the child had, with those in the medium caries group (1–8 dmfs) having the greatest underestimation, and those in the highest group having the least.

It is important to consider the study's strengths and weaknesses. Among the former are the sample's large size (501 young children) and representativeness, and the comprehensiveness of the data collected. Caries data were collected at surface level rather than tooth level, and the clinical examinations were undertaken in appropriate conditions by trained calibrated clinicians. Radiographs were read by two calibrated dental specialists to ensure accuracy, with inter- and intra-examiner reliability being excellent. Another strength of this study is that it takes a pragmatic approach to the research question in reporting data from a number of clinicians working in a community setting rather than data from a small number of trained examiners in an ideal clinical environment, as used in other studies [17]. A weakness was the lack of data on examiner reliability for the dental therapists conducting the clinical examinations. The burden on the young children to have to participate in another examination (for examiner calibration) was felt to be unfair due to their very young age and lower ability to cooperate.

This is the first study to report on the contribution of bitewing radiography to caries diagnosis in children as young as three and on whether those contributions differ according to caries experience on presentation at clinical examination. A hierarchical model of efficacy exists for appraising the literature on the efficacy of imaging. This study reports at Level 2. This addresses diagnostic accuracy, sensitivity, and specificity associated with interpretation of the images, and it includes the person(s) interpreting the image as well as the images per se [24]. Some 369 of the children were six years old or younger and able to have a set of quality radiographs taken. Of the 55 children excluded, only 20 were unable to have radiographs taken or the films could not be read (4% of the overall sample of 521). This differs from a previous study, where it was found impossible to take bitewing radiographs for 18% of 5-to-6-year-olds, with a further 14% of the surfaces being unreadable on those which were taken [14]. By contrast, all clinicians in the current study had training in beam angulation when using adhesive soft foam bitewing tabs; these have been shown to be well-tolerated by young children [17], and may have been responsible for both the high number of bitewing films being taken and their excellent quality.

The findings indicate that using a simple visual clinical examination alone in young children is likely to lead to substantial underestimation of caries experience, and that this effect differs with the extent of the clinically-apparent caries experience. At whole-mouth level, radiographic diagnosis made a moderate difference to the estimates of caries experience, but the surface-specific caries experience data indicate that radiographic diagnosis made a considerable difference, particularly for approximal surfaces. When the total number of lesions involving dentine was taken into account, clinical examination alone resulted in underestimation by 44%. This differential is similar to that observed with a group of 242 Australian 6-year-olds, where a 48% underestimation was found with lesions that involved the inner half of enamel and dentine [2].

Previous studies have suggested that bitewing radiography has the greatest value in children with the highest susceptibility to caries [2]. However, findings with apparently low-caries-risk children have shown that, even if they were diagnosed as caries-free following a clinical examination, nearly one-quarter were found to present with a caries lesion following a bitewing radiograph [8, 10]. Other studies in low-caries-risk populations suggest that taking radiographs does not improve the ability to detect caries lesions when operative treatment is to be undertaken, and that the caries experience of the wider community should be considered in developing locally appropriate guidelines on the use of radiographs [17, 20, 21]. In the current study, almost one-third of those who were apparently "caries-free" were found on radiographic examination to actually have dental caries lesions. This finding is similar to those from a smaller study from the Netherlands where, of the 13 children residing in a high-caries-experience community who were found to be caries-free after a clinical examination, 5 (38%) actually had one or more caries lesions involving dentine [14]. Our study did not include caries lesions limited to the enamel, so the findings may have substantially underestimated the true disease level.

For children with greater caries experience, the differences observed were even more marked, with approximately one-quarter of lesions missed in children presenting with high caries experience. In terms of differences by tooth surface type, the distal surface of the first primary molar consistently yielded the greatest underestimation of dental caries, with 45% of lesions at that site missed. That children who presented with the greatest disease levels had the lowest number of extra lesions found with radiographs is not surprising, given that most will have presented with primary molars that are cavitated or already restored, both of which are more easily identified during the clinical examination. The majority of lesions were found on approximal surfaces, supporting previous studies showing these to be the most commonly missed [8–13, 25]. Identifying such lesions early in young children is important because it allows non-operative preventive measures to be undertaken, and also so that children can be more accurately assigned a caries risk status. This suggests that a simple clinical examination alone does not give a true representation of a young child's caries status, especially for approximal surfaces. A thorough visual and tactile examination using criteria that take the dynamic nature of the disease into consideration and evaluate its activity needs to be considered, because this has been shown to be the method of choice in daily practice for detecting caries in primary teeth [18].

In considering the relevance of these findings in relation to the sensitivity and specificity of diagnostic tests, it has to be remembered that caries diagnosis at the person level is not an "all or nothing" event. That is, it may be so at the individual surface level, but the summary measure (dmfs) is aggregated up at the person level as a continuum (albeit one based on a count variable). Thus, we have a binary event (sound versus decayed) at the surface level, but a continuous variable at the person level. What does this mean? Consider the first group of children in Table 4: those 185 individuals were deemed to be caries-free in the clinical examination, yet 58 (31.4%) actually had one or more carious lesions. Calculating the sensitivity and specificity of the clinical examinations alone (and treating the clinical examination plus radiography as the true situation) at the person level gives 100% specificity and 0% sensitivity, which is not very useful. We cannot do a similar calculation for the other two groups because the person-level prevalence of the condition is 100% in each of those groups anyway. Another key issue is the relative importance of a false positive and a false negative: for a given surface, a false positive may result in a surgical intervention through the placement of the restoration that was not actually needed; a false negative may result in disease progression and sequelae such as pain, infection, the collapse of the tooth structure, the loss of the tooth through extraction, and so on.

Further research that involves clinical trials (not just cross-sectional studies) to explore how radiographic examination impacts on diagnosis (and the treatment decisions) for caries lesions in primary molars of children with different caries experience would be of benefit [26], as would meta-analysis and synthesis of the findings of studies such as the current one.

Finally, it should be borne in mind that the focus of this study was the lesions themselves rather than their prevention or restorative treatment. We are not necessarily advocating restoration of all of the extra lesions discovered through using radiography. Whether that takes place remains a clinical decision to be made by the treating clinician. After all, it is not possible to determine from a radiograph whether a lesion has cavitated (unless it is very advanced), and so it would be incumbent upon the treating clinician to confirm the extent of the lesion before deciding on the most appropriate way to manage it. Nevertheless, it is likely that a considerably higher proportion of such lesions in the primary dentition will have cavitated. The main focus of our paper is on the diagnostic yield, irrespective of the action implications of that yield.

Conclusion

Taking bitewing radiographs in young children is not without challenges or risks, and it must be undertaken with these in mind. Diagnostic yields from bitewing radiographs are greater for children with greater caries experience. The findings of this study further support that using bitewing radiographs in young children detect more lesions than a simple visual examination alone. Children residing in a community with high caries experience, who present with no clinically detected caries lesions following a simple visual examination and who are unable to tolerate bitewing radiographs being taken, may best be considered at risk of caries when determining the timing of recall. They should be managed preventively until a set of radiographs can confirm that they have no caries lesions present.

Abbreviations

dmfs: decayed missing and filled surfaces in the primary dentition; NTB: Northern B Health and Disability Ethics Committee; NZDep2013: New Zealand deprivation scores based on 2013 Census data; χ2 tests: chi squared tests

Acknowledgments

We are grateful to the dental therapists and children of Whanganui District Health Board.

Funding

This study was funded by Cure Kids (New Zealand). This helped with the study collection and analysis of the data.

Author contributions

LFP, DB and WMT sought the funding and designed the study. DB and KF read all the radiographs and DS, KG and AB analysed the data with support from LFP and WMT. All authors were involved in writing and editing the paper. All authors read and approved the final manuscript.

Competing interests

All authors declare they have no competing interests.

Author details

[1]Department of Oral Sciences, Faculty of Dentistry, University of Otago, PO Box 56, Dunedin 9054, New Zealand. [2]Department of Oral Sciences, University of Otago, Dunedin, New Zealand. [3]Hutt Valley District Health Board, Wellington, New Zealand. [4]Waikato District Health Board, Hamilton, New Zealand. [5]Community Oral Health Service, Hutt Valley Hospital, Wellington, New Zealand. [6]Southern District Health Board, Dunedin, New Zealand.

References

1. Kidd E, Pitts N. A reappraisal of the value of bitewing radiograph in the diagnosis of posterior approximal caries. Br Dent J. 1990;169:195–200.
2. Newman B, Seow W, Kazoullis S, Ford D, Holcombe T. Clinical detection of caries in the primary dentition with and without bitewing radiography. Aust Dent J. 2009;54:23–30.

3. Ketley CE, Holt RD. Visual and radiographic diagnosis of occlusal caries in first permanent molars and in second primary molars. Br Dent J. 1993;174: 364–7.
4. Ruiken R, Konig K, Truin JG, Plasschaert F. Longitudinal study of dental caries development in Dutch children aged 8-12 years. Community Dent and Oral Epidemiol. 1986;14:53–6.
5. de Vries HC, Ruiken HM, König KG, van't Hof MA. Radiographic versus clinical diagnosis of approximal carious lesions. Caries Res. 1990;24:364–70.
6. Machiulskiene V, Nyvad B, Baelum V. A comparison of clinical and radiographic caries diagnoses in posterior teeth of 12-year-old Lithuanian children. Caries Res. 1999;33:340–8.
7. Poorterman J, Aartman I, Kieft J, Kalsbeek H. Value of bite-wing radiographs in a clinical epidemiological study and their effect on the DMFS index. Caries Res. 2000;34:159–63.
8. Anderson M, Stecksen-Blicks C, Stenlund H, Ranggard L, Tsilingaridis G, Mejare I. Detection of Approximal caries in 5-year-old Swedish children. Caries Res. 2005;39:92–9.
9. Hopcraft M, Morgan M. Comparison of radiographic and clinical diagnosis of approximal and occlusal dental caries in a young adult population. Community Dent and Oral Epidemiol. 2005;33:212–8.
10. Lillehagen M, Grindefjord M, Mejare I. Detection of Approximal caries by clinical and radiographic examination in 9-year-old Swedish children. Caries Res. 2007;41:177–85.
11. Chu C, Chung B, Lo E. Caries assessment by clinical examination with or without radiographs of young Chinese adults. Int Dent J. 2008;58:265–8.
12. Holt RD, Abdulkarim NT, Rule DC. An evaluation of bitewing radiographs in 5-year-old children. Community Dent Health. 1990;7:389–94.
13. Gowda S, Thomson WM, Foster Page LA, Croucher N. What difference does using bitewing radiographs make to epidemiological estimates of dental caries prevalence and severity in a young adolescent population with high caries experience? Caries Res. 2009;43:436–41.
14. Poorterman JH, Vermaire EH, Hoogstraten J. Value of bitewing radiographs for detecting approximal caries in 6-year-old children in the Netherlands. Int J Paediatr Dent. 2010;20:336–40.
15. Kidd EA, Ricketts DN, Pitts NB. Occlusal caries diagnosis: a changing challenge for clinicians and epidemiologists. J Dent. 1993;2:323–31.
16. Baelum V. What is an appropriate caries diagnosis? Acta Odontol Scand. 2010;68:65–79.
17. Baelum V, Hintze H, Wenzel A, Danielsen B, Nyvad B. Implications of caries diagnostic strategies for clinical management decisions. Community Dent Oral Epidemiol. 2012;40:257–66.
18. Mendes FM, Novaes TF, Matos R, Bittar DG, Piovesan C, Gimenez T, Imparato JC, Raggio DP, Braga MM. Radiographic and laser fluorescence methods have no benefits for detecting caries in primary teeth. Caries Res. 2012;46: 536–43.
19. Bussaneli DG, Restrepo M, Boldieri T, Albertoni TH, Santos-Pinto L, Cordeiro RC. Proximal caries lesion detection in primary teeth: does this justify the association of diagnostic methods? Lasers Med Sci. 2015;30:2239–44.
20. American Academy of Pediatric Dentistry (AAPD). Guideline on prescribing dental radiographs for infants, children, adolescents and persons with special health care needs. Pediatr Dent. 2012;34:319–21.
21. Espelid I. Meja're I, Weerheijm K. EAPD guidelines for use of radiographs in children. Eur J Paediatr Dent. 2003:40–8.
22. Atkinson J, Salmond C, Crampton P. NZDep2013 index of deprivation. 2014. Dunedin. University of Otago.
23. World Health Organization. Oral health surveys : basic methods. 5th ed. Geneva: World Health Organization; 2013.
24. Fryback DG, Thornbury JR The efficacy of diagnostic imaging. Med Decis Mak. 1991;11:88–94.
25. Chawla N, Messer L, Adams G, Manton D. An in vitro comparison of detection methods for Approximal carious lesions in primary molars. Caries Res. 2012;46:161–9.
26. Mendes FM, Pontes LR, Gimenez T, Lara JS, de Camargo LB, Michel-Crosato E, Pannuti CM, Raggio DP, Braga MM, Novaes TF, CARDEC Collaborative Group. Impact of the radiographic examination on diagnosis and treatment decision of caries lesions in primary teeth--the Caries Detection in Children (CARDEC-01) trial: study protocol for a randomized controlled trial. Trials. 2016;17:69.

Influence of povidone-iodine on micro-tensile bonding strength to dentin under simulated pulpal pressure

Najlaa M. Alamoudi[1*], Alaa M. Baik[2], Azza A. El-Housseiny[1,3], Tariq S. Abu Haimed[4] and Ahmed S. Bakry[5,6]

Abstract

Background: Previous studies had reported that bond strength deteriorate over time following the dentin surface pretreatment with chlorhexidine. Therefore, further investigations are needed to evaluate the effect of other materials such as povidone iodine.

The purpose of this study was to investigate the effects of 10% povidone-iodine pretreatment on the resin-dentin micro-tensile bond strength of a single bond adhesive system in permanent teeth over time, and compare it with 2% chlorhexidine.

Methods: Flat dentin surfaces were prepared in 63 extracted permanent teeth. Teeth were randomly assigned to a 10% povidone-iodine pretreatment, a 2% chlorhexidine pretreatment, or a control group. Composite resin blocks were built up over treated surfaces under pulp pressure simulation. The prepared specimens were assigned to three storage time, 24 h, 1 week, and 2 months. Samples were vertically sectioned to obtain specimens of 0.7 to 1.2 mm^2 cross-sectional area.

Results: No significant reduction of bond strength of povidone iodine group was found among the three storage times ($p = 0.477$). A significant reduction of bond strength for both chlorhexidine and control groups was found in the three storage times ($p < 0.001$).

Conclusion: Povidone iodine pretreatment of etched dentin was effective in reducing the loss of bond strength over time, while the chlorhexidine pretreatment and negative control showed significant deterioration in micro-tensile bond strength over time in permanent teeth.

Keywords: Matrix metalloproteinase, Micro-tensile bond strength, Povidone-iodine, Chlorhexidine

Background

A current area of interest in adhesive dentistry is the durability of resin restorations [1]. The generation of resin-dentin bonds entails various challenges, including the preservation of structural integrity and strength. The bonds between resin and dentin using dentin adhesive systems can become damaged over time [2]. Aged composite resin bonded to dentin reportedly exhibited hydrolytic degeneration of collagen [1] without any bacterial enzymes [2].

Matrix metalloproteinases (MMPs) are part of the composition of dentin structure [3]. They are a group of proteases that can destroy the organic matrix of etched dentin [4]. All MMP family members are secreted as inactive proenzymes (Pro-MMPs). Pro-MMPs can be activated by proteases, other members of the MMP family, acids, reactive oxygen, and denaturants [2]. These Pro-MMPs need calcium ion (Ca^{2+}) for their activation. Following bacterial demineralization, Ca^{2+} ions are released and act as a cofactor for the Pro-MMPs activation. These MMPs lead to dentin destruction. Similarly, following acid etching demineralization, MMPs are released and activated [2].

Establishing adhesion to mineralized tissue is based on the reaction of biologic apatite with acids. Etching dentin with 37% phosphoric acid lead to hydroxyapatite crystals dissolution, demineralization of the surface of the dentin matrix, exposure of the underlying collagen

* Correspondence: nalamoudi@kau.edu.sa; nalamoudi2011@gmail.com
[1]Pediatric Dentistry Department, Faculty of Dentistry, King Abdulaziz University, P.O. Box 80209, Jeddah 21589, Saudi Arabia
Full list of author information is available at the end of the article

and creates porosities within that collagen matrix. A demineralized microporous area composed of organic dentin material mainly collagen fibrils is formed. This allows solvated monomers to infiltrate around and into spaces of collagen fibrils to obtain retention for resin-composite materials. However, acid etchings release the Ca^{2+} ions and activate MMPs. These MMPs lead to collagen destruction leading to enzymatic degradation of hybrid layer and subsequently endanger resin-dentin bonding longevity [4]. In order to prevent enzymatic degradation, inhibitors of MMP activity have been applied during adhesive application [5]. One such enzymatic inhibitor is chlorhexidine [2].

Povidone-iodine (PVP-I) was introduced as an antiseptic agent in the 1950s, and is as effective as iodine alone against a broad spectrum of disease-causing microorganisms [6, 7]. It is an organic water-soluble complex that contains molecular iodine and the solubilizing agent polyvinyl pyrrolidone. It is less irritating to the skin than iodine, and unlike iodine it does not require iodides or alcohol to dissolve. Moreover, PVP-I stains are water-soluble.

It has been claimed that PVP-I can induce an endogenous proteinase inhibitor capable of blocking enzymatic activity [8, 9]. Reductions in the collagenolytic activity of MMP-9 by 83% and MMP-2 by 88% were reported after 24 h of PVP-I application on nitrogen and sulfur mustard-induced skin lesions. When skin was analyzed 48 and 72 h after exposure, a similar trend of PVP-I-induced reduction in the two types of collagenase activity was found [8].

The hydrolytic and enzymatic stability of dental adhesives in the oral environment is a concern because the oral environment can severely compromise the durability of resin-dentin bonds. A literature review was performed prior to the current study, to investigate the effects of using chlorhexidine as a MMP inhibitor on dentin substrates, and the influence of chlorhexidine application on the preservation of dentin bond durability. Previous studies have reported that bond strength deteriorated over time following dentin surface pretreatment with chlorhexidine [10, 11]. This suggested that further investigations were needed to evaluate the effects of other materials such as PVP-I on the durability of dentin micro-tensile bond strength (MTBS).

The aim of this study was to evaluate the effects of 10% PVP-I pretreatment on dentin MTBS, and compare it with 2% chlorhexidine pretreatment and no pretreatment in permanent teeth over a period of 2 months.

Methods

Specimen preparation

The protocol of this study was approved by the ethics committee, King Abdulaziz University, Jeddah, Saudi Arabia. This is a randomized experimental in vitro study. Collecting bottles containing 0.5% Chloramine T were distributed to different private and governmental clinics in Jeddah to collect the freshly extracted sound teeth on it. Contact information was given to the dental assistant in charge for each clinic to contact us as soon as the teeth are extracted. Informed consent form was obtained and signed from patients to use their teeth for this research. Sixty-three extracted intact, non-carious, non-restored human permanent third molars were collected. The molars were mounted in 2-cm-diameter cylindrical customized molds using chemically cured acrylic resin (Major Prodotti Dentari Spa, Moncalieri, Italy). The roots were embedded 3 mm below the cementoenamel junction with the long axis of each tooth parallel to the walls of the mold. Each tooth was transversally cut in two steps using a slow speed diamond saw (TECHCUT 4™, Allied High Tech Products, Inc., USA) under copious water irrigation. The first cut was perpendicular to the long axis of each tooth at the coronal part of the crown, to remove the occlusal surfaces of the crowns leaving flat mid-coronal dentin. The subsequent cut was at a level approximately 1 mm below the cementoenamel junction and parallel to the flat dentin surface, to remove the root portion and expose the pulp chamber, from which the pulp tissue was carefully removed using tweezers.

Simulating pulpal pressure

In an attempt to simulate intra-oral conditions, simulated pulp pressure was employed (Fig. 1). All restorative procedures including dentin adhesive bonding were performed under simulated dentinal hydrostatic pressure. Each segment was attached to a petri dish from the pulpal area and penetrated by a 21-gauge stainless steel needle. A flexible tube was connected and sealed to the stainless steel needle and to the back of the petri dish using cyanoacrylate adhesive (Zapit; DVA, Corona, CA, USA). The other end of this tube was sealed to a plastic syringe to maintain an airtight seal. The plastic syringe and the flexible tube were then filled with distilled water. The 1-mm root of the crown segment was bonded and sealed to the inner side of the petri dish using a cyanoacrylate adhesive. The intra pulpal pressure assembly was fixed to a burette stand. To generate an intra-pulpal pressure of 15 cm H_2O, the level of distilled water in the 10-mL plastic syringe was adjusted 15 cm vertically above the flat dentin surface of the tested tooth.

Acid etching and pretreatment

The teeth were randomly assigned to three groups according to the pretreatment solution. Each group had 21 teeth. The teeth were etched with 35% phosphoric acid gel (Scotchbond Universal Etchant, 3 M ESPE, St Paul, MN, USA) for 15 s and rinsed with water for 10 s. They were then placed in 10% PVP-I solution for 60 s in group

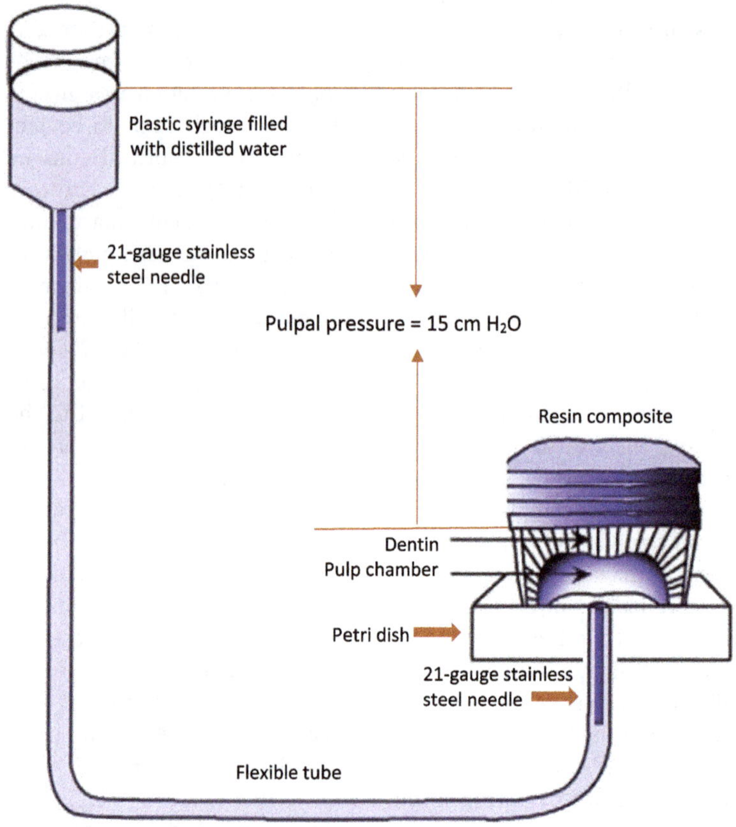

Fig. 1 Illustration depicting the intra-pulpal pressure simulation apparatus used in this study

1, 2% chlorhexidine solution for 60 s in group 2, and in water in the control group (no pretreatment). The dentin surface was dried for 10 s with an oil-and-water-free air source with pressure to remove excess water and pretreatment solutions. Two coats of the single bond (Adper Single Bond 2, 3 M ESPE, St Paul, MN, USA) were applied to the entire flat occlusal surface of the dentin with 5 s of air-drying after each application, before being cured for 10 s with a quartz-tungsten-halogen light-curing unit (Curing Light 2500, 3 M EPSE) delivering 600 mW/cm^2. A composite resin (Filtek Z250, 3 M ESPE, St Paul, MN, USA) crown of 4 mm in height was incrementally applied to the bonded dentin surface in 1-mm increments. A celluloid strip was used to separate the composite and the light curer tip. Each composite increment was light-cured for 30 s.

The prepared specimens were randomly assigned to three storage time subgroups containing 7 teeth each: 24 h, 1 week, and 2 months. Samples were stored in distilled water and placed in an incubator at 37 °C, and the distilled water was changed periodically.

Sample preparation for MTBS

At each designated time-point (24 h, 1 week, 2 months), the teeth in the relevant subgroups were vertically sectioned across the bonded interface (in the occluso-gingival direction) into multiple serial sections using a low speed saw (TECHCUT 4™, Allied High Tech Products, Inc., USA) at a cutting speed of 200 rpm. Each crown segment was sectioned into two or three slabs, then each slab was rotated 90 degrees in the same plane and another two or three sections were made perpendicular to the slabs, resulted in four to six sticks. The cross-sectional areas of the selected specimens were measured using a digital caliper to the nearest 0.01 mm for subsequent bond strength evaluation.

MTBS

To test MTBS, the end of each stick was fixed to the flat stainless steel microgrip of a universal testing machine (Micro-tensile Tester; Bisco, Schaumburg, IL) using cyanoacrylate glue (Zapit; DVA, Corona, CA, USA). The specimens were tension-stressed until failure occurred, using a simplified universal testing machine at a crosshead speed of 1 mm/minute. MTBS was calculated as the maximum load at failure divided by the cross-sectional area of each stick, and was recorded in MPa. The mean MTBS for each group was calculated and the three groups were compared.

Failure mode analysis

The fractured specimens were kept in distilled water for 24 h. All debonded surfaces (dentin and resin) were

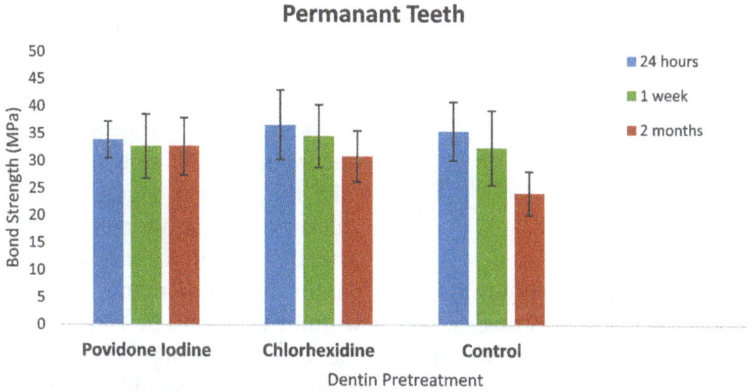

Fig. 2 Means and Standard Deviations of the Micro-tensile bond strengths of the different groups at different storage periods in permanent teeth, Mega pascal (MPa). Within povidone iodine group ($F = 0.746$; $p = 0.477$), within chlorhexidine group and control group ($F = 9.482$, $p < 0.001$ and $F = 46.036$, $p < 0.001$, respectively)

evaluated under a stereomicroscope (Meiji Techno Co. Ltd., Tokyo, Japan) at 50x magnification to assess the mode of failure. The failure modes of the fractured specimens were categorized as adhesive failure when the fracture occurred between adhesive and dentin, cohesive failure in dentin when dentin covered the two fractured parts of the specimen, cohesive failure in resin material when the two parts of the specimens were fully covered with composite resin, or mixed failure when there were two or more of the types of fractures described above.

Statistical analysis

The data were tested for normality using the Shapiro-Wilks test. One-way analysis of variance was conducted to assess the pretreatment effect on resin-dentin bond strength at each storage time-point, and to evaluate the effect of storage time on the resin-dentin bond strength within each pretreatment group (i.e., assuming the samples were independent). The post-hoc Bonferroni test was used for multiple pairwise comparisons to identify any significant differences between groups. All tests employed a 0.05 level of statistical significance.

Results

A total of 376 specimens were subjected to MTBS testing and fracture mode analysis. There were 38 cohesive failures among the 376 sticks. These cohesive failures were either in dentin or in resin material, which does not represent the actual resin-dentin bond strength. Therefore, it was not included in the statistical analysis [12]. The remaining 338 specimens were included in the statistical analysis. The power of the sample size at an alpha value of 0.05 was 1.00. Figure 2 present the mean and standard deviation of each group.

One-way analysis of variance revealed that there was no significant reduction in resin-dentin bond strength in the PVP-I surface pretreatment group at any of the three storage time-points ($F = 0.746$; $p = 0.477$). Conversely, there were significant reduction in resin-dentin bond strength in the chlorhexidine surface pretreatment group and the control group (no pretreatment) at the three storage time-points ($F = 9.482$, $p < 0.001$ and $F = 46.036$, $p < 0.001$, respectively). The post-hoc Bonferroni test indicated that there was no significant loss of resin-dentin bond strength between 24 h and 1 week in the chlorhexidine group. In the control group, the mean bond strength at 1 week was significantly lower than that at 24 h. Additionally, in both the chlorhexidine group and the control group the mean bond strength at 2 months was significantly lower than those at 1 week and at 24 h. Detailed results from the post-hoc Bonferroni test are shown in Tables 1 and 2.

The analyses revealed significant associations between storage time and failure mode within the PVP-I group and the chlorhexidine group. Table 3 shows the associations between storage time and failure mode within each study group.

Discussion

In the present study, only freshly extracted, non-carious, permanent molars were utilized in an attempt to standardize the dentin substrates used. Intact resin-bonded teeth were stored in distilled water under simulated pulpal pressure. The water exposure of intact resin-bonded teeth may resemble a more realistic clinical situation in terms of hydrolytic

Table 1 Post-hoc test for resin-dentin micro-tensile bond strength in the chlorhexidine group

Post-hoc[a]		p value
24 h	1 week	0.386
1 week	2 months	0.021*
2 months	24 h	< 0.001*

[a]Bonferroni test
*Statistically significant at $p < 0.05$

Table 2 Post-hoc test for resin-dentin micro-tensile bond strength in the control group

Post-hoc[a]		p value
24 h	1 week	0.049*
1 week	2 months	< 0.001*
2 months	24 h	< 0.001*

[a]Bonferroni Test
*Statistically significant at $p < 0.05$

degradation than smaller resin-dentin specimens directly exposed to water. Simulated pulpal pressure was used in this in vitro study in an attempt to achieve reliable results that were relevant to real clinical conditions. Simulated pulp pressures ranging from 30 to 37 cm H_2O have been used in many studies investigating the influence of intra-pulpal pressure on the bonding effectiveness of adhesives to dentin [13–15]. In the current study, a lower intra-pulpal pressure was utilized because the intra-pulpal pressure in normal pulp is not as high as previously established [16]. Previous in vivo studies have reported that values of approximately 15 cm H_2O should be used to simulate normal pulp pressure [16, 17].

In the current study, conventional two step etch-and-rinse adhesive was used (Single Bond, 3 M ESPE, St. Paul, MN, USA) which has a pH of 3.6 [18]. Previous studies have suggested that low pH (4.5) acids are capable of activating MMPs [4, 19]. Therefore, it was hypothesized that this adhesive would be capable of activating dentin proteolytic enzymes derived from the underlying partially-demineralized dentin [20].

In the current study, we used 10% PVP-I and 2% chlorhexidine as therapeutic primers of etched dentin. The PVP-I and chlorhexidine were applied to etched dentin before bonding, and the excess was air-dried without rinsing. The technique used in this experiment was a wet bonding technique. PVP-I and chlorhexidine digluconate are soluble in water. The differences in the binding performances of PVP-I and chlorhexidine to collagen and hydroxyl apatite are unknown.

Chlorhexidine has a high affinity to dentin. It can bind electrostatically to the phosphate groups of dentin and to carboxyl groups of collagen fibers. However, chlorhexidine composed of a large water-soluble molecule that might be leaded out of dentin over time [21]. Moreover, the binding mechanism between the PVP-I and the dentinal structure is not clear. However, the application of a miscible (capable of mixing in any ratio without separation of two phases) solution to water-saturated dentin

Table 3 Associations between storage time and failure mode in permanent teeth in each group

Dentin surface pretreatment	Type of failure	Storage time			Total (%)	p value+
		24 h (%)	1 week (%)	2 months (%)		
Povidone-iodine	Adhesive failure	38 (88.4)	32 (82.1)	26 (60.5)	96 (76.8)	0.007*
	Cohesive in dentin	0 (0)	0 (0)	4 (9.3)	4 (3.2)	
	Cohesive in composite	0 (0)	4 (10.3)	5 (11.6)	9 (7.2)	
	Mixed failure	5 (11.6)	3 (7.7)	8 (18.6)	16 (12.8)	
	Total	43 (100)	39 (100)	43 (100)	125 (100)	
Chlorhexidine	Adhesive failure	36 (90.0)	33 (84.6)	24 (61.5)	93 (78.8)	0.013*
	Cohesive in dentin	0 (0)	1 (2.6)	1 (2.6)	2 (1.7)	
	Cohesive in composite	2 (5.0)	0 (0)	5 (12.8)	7 (5.9)	
	Mixed failure	2 (5.0)	5 (12.8)	9 (23.1)	16 (13.6)	
	Total	40 (100)	39 (100)	39 (100)	118 (100)	
Control	Adhesive failure	37 (84.1)	36 (81.8)	30 (66.7)	103 (77.4)	0.053
	Cohesive in dentin	3 (6.8)	1 (2.3)	0 (0)	4 (3.0)	
	Cohesive in composite	1 (2.3)	3 (6.8)	8 (17.8)	12 (9.0)	
	Mixed failure	3 (6.8)	4 (9.1)	7 (15.6)	14 (10.5)	
	Total	44 (100)	44 (100)	45 (100)	133 (100)	
Total	Adhesive failure	111 (87.4)	101 (82.8)	80 (63.0)	292 (77.7)	< 0.001*
	Cohesive in dentin	3 (2.4)	2 (1.6)	5 (3.9)	10 (2.7)	
	Cohesive in composite	3 (2.4)	7 (5.7)	18 (14.2)	28 (7.4)	
	Mixed failure	10 (7.9)	12 (9.8)	24 (18.9)	46 (12.2)	
	Total	127 (100)	122 (100)	127 (100)	376 (100)	

+Fisher's exact test
*Statistically significant at $p < 0.05$

after etching and rinsing should maximize chlorhexidine concentration within the hybrid layer [21]. Without rinsing, excess PVP-I and chlorhexidine may be incorporated into the primer, and released slowly over time [21]. Previous studies have reported that PVP-I has the capacity to be slowly released over time [22–24].

In the present study, the PVP-I group showed no significant reduction in dentin bond strength at the 24 h, 1 week, or 2 months time-points. In contrast, the chlorhexidine and control groups showed significant reductions in dentin bond strength at 1 week and at 2 months. The differences in mean dentin bond strength in the chlorhexidine and control groups between 24 h and 2 months were approximately 6 MPa and 11 MPa, respectively, while the corresponding reduction in the PVP-I group was only ~ 1 MPa. This finding may be explained by the superior water solubility of PVP-I compared to chlorhexidine, and the capacity of PVP-I to slowly release iodine over time [25], which ensures the establishment of a nontoxic, optimal concentration of iodine [26, 27]. This may have resulted in better penetration of PVP-I and inhibition of the MMPs within dentin.

In accordance with the results of previous studies [28–32], in the current study chlorhexidine application after acid etching had no effect on immediate or 1-week resin-dentin bond strength. This is concordant with previous in vitro [33] and in vivo [34] studies using an etch-and-rinse adhesive. Carrilho et al. [33] [34] found that treating etched dentin surfaces of permanent teeth with 2% chlorhexidine did not affect the in vitro or in vivo MTBS of specimens tested at 24 h. Furthermore, a meta-analysis of the effects of 2% chlorhexidine vs. control at baseline (immediate bond strength) revealed no statistically significant difference between groups [35].

In the current study, all the teeth were subjected to pulpal pressure simulation. Campos et al. [36] studied the effects of 0.2% and 2.0% chlorhexidine on dentin bonding durability. Two-step etch-and-rinse (Single-Bond) and all-in-one self-etch adhesive (Clearfil Tri S Bond) were used, and all the teeth were subjected to 30 cm H_2O pulpal pressure and thermo-mechanical stressing. They reported that MTBS was significantly higher in the groups treated with two-step etch-and-rinse adhesive associated with 0.2% and 2.0% chlorhexidine than it was in the control group without chlorhexidine. Additionally, there were no significant differences in MTBS between the group treated with Clearfil Tri S Bond, the control group, and the group treated with 0.2% chlorhexidine after 6 months. Chlorhexidine was reportedly able to reduce the loss of bond strength of single bond adhesive, but not all-in-one self-etch adhesive, after storage for 6 months under simulated pulpal pressure. Those results are concordant with the results of the current study.

The current study had some limitations. The etch-and-rinse system was used in the current study to bond to sound dentin, and thus it may be that the hybrid layer in the current study was infiltrated by the water [37] utilized to exert the pulpal pressure on the dentin surface. However, the presence of an enamel rim sealing the boundaries of the specimens prevented the leaching out of any plasticized adhesive monomer into the storage media [36], and thus diminished the effect of pulpal pressure on the observed bond strength. Additionally, being an in vitro study the results do not directly reflect the clinical conditions of actual teeth, however, simulated pulp pressure was used during bonding and ageing to simulate in vivo conditions. Further clinical studies are needed to confirm the results of the current study.

To the best of our knowledge, this is the first report of data on the effects of PVP-I as a MMP inhibitor on the preservation of dentin bond durability. The results showed that PVP-I, an experimental therapeutic primer, also prevented bond strength deterioration over 2 months of aging. Further studies are needed to explore the reasons behind the preservation of the bond strength. Additionally, long-term studies are needed to evaluate the effects of PVP-I on bond strength. Further studies are also needed to study the inhibitory effects of PVP-I on MMPs directly.

Conclusion

Povidone iodine pretreatment of etched dentin was effective in reducing the loss of bond strength over time, while the chlorhexidine pretreatment and negative control showed significant deterioration in micro-tensile bond strength over time in permanent teeth.

Abbreviations

MMPs: Matrix metalloproteinases; MTBS: Micro-tensile bond strength; PVP-I: Povidone-iodine

Acknowledgments

The authors acknowledge with thanks the Deanship of Scientific Research DSR for their technical and financial support and Dr. Faisal Dardeer for his assistance with sample preparation. We would also like to thank Editage (https://www.editage.com) for English language editing.

Funding

This research received a grant from the Deanship of Scientific Research (DSR) with grand G-41-165-38.

Authors' contributions

NMA made substantial contributions to the conception and design of the study and the development of the survey instrument, analyzed and interpreted the data, and was a major contributor in writing the manuscript, AMB Literature search, study selection, eligibility criteria, data extraction, AAE Analyzing data and manuscript writing, TSA participated in the design, and critically reviewed the manuscript and reviewed data extraction and manuscript writing, ASB participated in the design, and critically reviewed the manuscript and reviewed data extraction and manuscript writing. All authors read and approved the final manuscript.

Competing interests
The authors declare that they have no competing interest.

Author details
[1]Pediatric Dentistry Department, Faculty of Dentistry, King Abdulaziz University, P.O. Box 80209, Jeddah 21589, Saudi Arabia. [2]Pediatric Dentistry Department, King Abdulaziz University Dental Hospital, Jeddah, Saudi Arabia. [3]Pediatric Dentistry Department, Faculty of Dentistry, Alexandria University, Alexandria, Egypt. [4]Biomaterial Department, Faculty of Dentistry, King Abdulaziz University, Jeddah, Saudi Arabia. [5]Operative Dentistry Department, Faculty of Dentistry, King Abdulaziz University, Jeddah, Saudi Arabia. [6]Conservative Dentistry Department, Faculty of Dentistry, Alexandria University, Alexandria, Egypt.

References

1. Hashimoto M, Ohno H, Kaga M, Endo K, Sano H, Oguchi H. In vivo degradation of resin-dentin bonds in humans over 1 to 3 years. J Dent Res. 2000;79:1385–91.
2. Pashley DH, Tay FR, Yiu C, Hashimoto M, Breschi L, Carvalho RM, et al. Collagen degradation by host-derived enzymes during aging. J Dent Res. 2004;83:216–21.
3. Palosaari H, Pennington CJ, Larmas M, Edwards DR, Tjäderhane L, Salo T. Expression profile of matrix metalloproteinases (MMPs) and tissue inhibitors of MMPs in mature human odontoblasts and pulp tissue. Eur J Oral Sci. 2003;111:117–27.
4. Tjäderhane L, Larjava H, Sorsa T, Uitto VJ, Larmas M, Salo T. The activation and function of host matrix metalloproteinases in dentin matrix breakdown in caries lesions. J Dent Res. 1998;77:1622–9.
5. Breschi L, Mazzoni A, Nato F, Carrilho M, Visintini E, Tjäderhane L, et al. Chlorhexidine stabilizes the adhesive interface: a 2-year in vitro study. Dent Mater. 2010;26:320–5.
6. Siggia S. The chemistry of polyvinylpyrrolidone-iodine. J Am Pharm Assoc Am Pharm Assoc. 1957;46:201–4.
7. Shelanski HA, Shelanski MV. PVP-iodine: history, toxicity and therapeutic uses. J Int Coll Surg. 1956;25:727–34.
8. Wormser U, Brodsky B, Reich R. Topical treatment with povidone iodine reduces nitrogen mustard-induced skin collagenolytic activity. Arch Toxicol. 2002;76:119–21.
9. Shi L, Ermis R, Kiedaisch B, Carson D. The effect of various wound dressings on the activity of debriding enzymes. Adv Skin Wound Care. 2010;23:456–62.
10. Sadek FT, Braga RR, Muench A, Liu Y, Pashley DH, Tay FR. Ethanol wet-bonding challenges current anti-degradation strategy. J Dent Res. 2010;89:1499–504.
11. Pashley DH, Tay FR, Imazato S. How to increase the durability of resin-dentin bonds. Compend Contin Educ Dent. 2011;32:60–4.
12. De Munck J, Van Meerbeek B, Yoshida Y, Inoue S, Vargas M, Suzuki K, et al. Four-year water degradation of total-etch adhesives bonded to dentin. J Dent Res. 2003;82:136–40.
13. Gernhardt CR, Schaller HG, Kielbassa AM. The influence of human plasma used for dentin perfusion on tensile bond strength of different light-curing materials. Am J Dent. 2005;18:318–22.
14. Moll K, Haller B. Effect of intrinsic and extrinsic moisture on bond strength to dentine. J Oral Rehabil. 2000;27:150–65.
15. Moll K, Park HJ, Haller B. Effect of simulated pulpal pressure on dentin bond strength of self-etching bonding systems. Am J Dent. 2005;18:335–9.
16. Ciucchi B, Bouillaguet S, Holz J, Pashley D. Dentinal fluid dynamics in human teeth, in vivo. J Endod. 1995;21:191–4.
17. Vongsavan N, Matthews B. Fluid flow through cat dentine in vivo. Arch Oral Biol. 1992;37:175–85.
18. Abu Nawareg M, Elkassas D, Zidan A, Abuelenain D, Abu Haimed T, Hassan AH, et al. Is chlorhexidine-methacrylate as effective as chlorhexidine digluconate in preserving resin dentin interfaces? J Dent. 2016;45:7–13.
19. Vuotila T, Ylikontiola L, Sorsa T, Luoto H, Hanemaaijer R, Salo T, et al. The relationship between MMPs and pH in whole saliva of radiated head and neck cancer patients. J Oral Pathol Med. 2002;31:329–38.
20. Perote LC, Kamozaki MB, Gutierrez NC, Tay FR, Pucci CR. Effect of matrix metalloproteinase-inhibiting solutions and aging methods on dentin bond strength. J Adhes Dent. 2015;17:347–52.
21. Carrilho MR, Carvalho RM, Sousa EN, Nicolau J, Breschi L, Mazzoni A, et al. Substantivity of chlorhexidine to human dentin. Dent Mater. 2010;26:779–85.
22. Durani P, Leaper D. Povidone-iodine: use in hand disinfection, skin preparation and antiseptic irrigation. Int Wound J. 2008;5:376–87.
23. Stadelmann WK, Digenis AG, Tobin GR. Impediments to wound healing. Am J Surg. 1998;176:39S–47S.
24. Quirynen M, Teughels W, De Soete M, van Steenberghe D. Topical antiseptics and antibiotics in the initial therapy of chronic adult periodontitis: microbiological aspects. Periodontol 2000. 2002;28:72–90.
25. Thomas GW, Rael LT, Bar-Or R, Shimonkevitz R, Mains CW, Slone DS, et al. Mechanisms of delayed wound healing by commonly used antiseptics. J Trauma. 2009;66:82–90.
26. Pallasch TJ, Slots J. Antibiotic prophylaxis and the medically compromised patient. Periodontol 2000. 1996;10:107–38.
27. Demir A, Malkoc S, Sengun A, Koyuturk AE, Sener Y. Effects of chlorhexidine and povidone-iodine mouth rinses on the bond strength of an orthodontic composite. Angle Orthod. 2005;75:392–6.
28. Breschi L, Cammelli F, Visintini E, Mazzoni A, Vita F, Carrilho M, et al. Influence of chlorhexidine concentration on the durability of etch-and-rinse dentin bonds: a 12-month in vitro study. J Adhes Dent. 2009;11:191–8.
29. Perdigao J, Denehy GE, Swift EJ Jr. Effects of chlorhexidine on dentin surfaces and shear bond strengths. Am J Dent. 1994;7:81–4.
30. Meiers JC, Shook LW. Effect of disinfectants on the bond strength of composite to dentin. Am J Dent. 1996;9:11–4.
31. de Castro FL, de Andrade MF, Duarte Junior SL, Vaz LG, Ahid FJ. Effect of 2% chlorhexidine on microtensile bond strength of composite to dentin. J Adhes Dent. 2003;5:129–38.
32. Pappas M, Burns DR, Moon PC, Coffey JP. Influence of a 3-step tooth disinfection procedure on dentin bond strength. J Prosthet Dent. 2005;93:545–50.
33. Carrilho MR, Carvalho RM, de Goes MF, di Hipolito V, Geraldeli S, Tay FR, et al. Chlorhexidine preserves dentin bond in vitro. J Dent Res. 2007;86:90–4.
34. Carrilho MR, Geraldeli S, Tay F, de Goes MF, Carvalho RM, Tjäderhane L, et al. In vivo preservation of the hybrid layer by chlorhexidine. J Dent Res. 2007;86:529–33.
35. Montagner AF, Sarkis-Onofre R, Pereira-Cenci T, Cenci MS. MMP inhibitors on dentin stability: a systematic review and meta-analysis. J Dent Res. 2014;93:733–43.
36. Campos EA, Correr GM, Leonardi DP, Barato-Filho F, Gonzaga CC, Zielak JC. Chlorhexidine diminishes the loss of bond strength over time under simulated pulpal pressure and thermo-mechanical stressing. J Dent. 2009;37:108–14.
37. Yuan Y, Shimada Y, Ichinose S, Tagami J. Qualitative analysis of adhesive interface nanoleakage using FE-SEM/EDS. Dent Mater. 2007;23:561–9.

Characterization of oral polymorphonuclear neutrophils in periodontitis patients

Elena A. Nicu[1,2*†], Patrick Rijkschroeff[1†], Eva Wartewig[1], Kamran Nazmi[3] and Bruno G. Loos[1]

Abstract

Background: Maintaining oral health is a continuous and dynamic process that also involves the immune system. Polymorphonuclear neutrophils (PMNs) migrate from blood circulation and become apparent in the oral fluid. Controversies exist regarding the specific role of the oral PMNs (oPMNs) in the presence of chronic oral inflammation, such as periodontitis. In this study we characterized cell counts, activation status, apoptosis, and reactive oxygen species (ROS) generation by oPMNs and circulatory (cPMNs), and the salivary protease activity, in subjects with and without periodontitis.

Methods: Venous blood and oral rinse samples were obtained from 19 patients with untreated periodontitis and 16 control subjects for PMN isolation. Apoptosis and expression of cell activation markers CD11b, CD63, and CD66b were analyzed using flow cytometry. Constitutive ROS generation was detected using dihydrorhodamine123. Additionally, ROS production in response to stimulation was evaluated in samples incubated with 10 μM phorbol myristate acetate (PMA) or *Fusobacterium nucleatum*. Total protease activity was measured using substrate PEK-054.

Results: Periodontitis patients presented with over 4 times higher oPMN counts compared to controls ($p = 0.007$), which was a predictor for the total protease activity ($r^2 = 0.399$, $P = 0.007$). More oPMNs were apoptotic in periodontitis patients compared to the controls ($P = 0.004$). All three activation markers were more expressed on the oPMNs compared to the cPMNs ($p < 0.05$), and a higher expression of CD11b on the oPMNs from periodontitis patients was observed compared to the control subjects ($P = 0.024$). Constitutive ROS production per oPMN was higher compared to the cPMN ($P < 0.001$). Additional analysis showed that the oPMNs retained their ability to respond to stimulation, with no apparent differences between the periodontitis and control subjects.

Conclusions: Higher numbers of oral PMNs, being more apoptotic and having increased levels of degranulation markers were found in periodontitis compared to periodontal health. However, since the oPMNs in periodontitis were responsive to ex vivo stimulation, we conclude that the oPMNs are active in the oral ecosystem. It is currently unknown whether the oPMN counts, which correlated with the detected protease levels, are detrimental in the long term for the oral mucosa integrity.

Keywords: Periodontitis, Polymorphonuclear neutrophilic granulocytes, Reactive oxygen species, Apoptosis, Degranulation

* Correspondence: e.nicu@acta.nl
†Elena A. Nicu and Patrick Rijkschroeff contributed equally to this work.
[1]Department of Periodontology, Academic Centre for Dentistry Amsterdam (ACTA), University of Amsterdam and VU University Amsterdam, Gustav Mahlerlaan 3004, 1081, LA, Amsterdam, The Netherlands
[2]Opris Dent SRL, Sibiu, Romania
Full list of author information is available at the end of the article

Background

Oral health is often confused with the absence of oral disease. However, oral health is a dynamic state, maintained as long as the active equilibrium between oral microbiota, salivary defense mechanisms, and host immune responses exists [1, 2]. Despite the heavy colonization with oral microorganisms, overt infections rarely occur in the oral cavity.

Polymorphonuclear neutrophils (PMNs) are primary determinants in the host response to microbes. They constitute the most abundant population of white blood cells, and are capable of recognizing, binding, internalizing and killing microorganisms [3]. PMNs are recruited to inflammatory sites and are crucial for the clearance of infection. The majority of the existing studies focused on PMNs retrieved from venous blood, which may not necessarily reflect the PMNs' functional contribution on the mucous membranes within the oral cavity. Importantly, the current knowledge is mainly derived from studying PMNs in diseased states, and little is known about their contribution to oral health maintenance [4–10].

Previously, our group characterized PMNs in the oral cavity (oPMNs) from a large group of systemically and orally healthy young individuals [11]. There, we established that on average 1.0×10^6 oPMNs can be purified after 4 rinses, and the PMNs were capable of reactive oxygen species (ROS) production in response to bacterial stimulation ex vivo. We also studied the oPMN in edentulous subjects and found that in the absence of teeth, the number of oPMNs was significantly decreased [12]. Moreover, the oPMNs in edentulous individuals were basically non-functional, being either apoptotic or impaired and not capable of responding to bacterial stimulation ex vivo. The absence of functional oPMNs might compromise the resilience of the edentulous oral cavity.

In a healthy mouth, low numbers of PMNs constantly migrate through the oral epithelia and become apparent in the oral fluid. The sulci around the teeth form an important source for oPMNs; for a long time it has been known that with gingival inflammation the number of oPMNs is increased [4, 7, 13]. Interestingly, Dutzan et al. characterized PMNs in biopsies of both gingiva and buccal mucosa. They concluded that the PMN numbers were correlated with the levels of chemotactic factors in the tissues and found higher PMN numbers in periodontitis patients compared to non-periodontitis at both of these locations [14].

Periodontitis is a chronic inflammatory disease of the supporting tissues of the teeth, initiated in susceptible subjects by an aberrant immune response to dental plaque, and exacerbated by a dysbiotic biofilm. Although the PMN's primary role is protective against microbial invasion, continuous recruitment and migration of PMNs through the periodontal tissues might contribute to the collateral damage and tissue breakdown in periodontitis [15]. Our knowledge about the PMNs that have "travelled" from the gingiva into the periodontal pocket, along the biofilm, into the oral cavity is limited and it is not known whether the oPMN in periodontitis patients can still contribute to oral health maintenance. Older studies only reported on oPMN numbers in periodontitis [13, 16], while more recent studies showed the possibility to study the phenotype and functional capabilities of oPMNs [6, 8, 17, 18]. The oPMNs may represent a distinct subset of peripheral PMNs, which acquire specific traits in periodontitis patients.

To gain more knowledge on the role of oPMNs in periodontitis, this study aimed to characterize the oPMNs numbers and function, in patients with untreated periodontitis and compare those to cells from subjects without periodontitis. Since all oPMNs are migrated cells from the peripheral blood circulation, we also included the analysis of circulatory PMNs (cPMNs) to investigate possible changes of PMN features that may occur when PMNs journey from blood into the oral cavity.

Methods

The study was approved by the Medical Ethical Committee of the *VU* University Medical Center, The Netherlands (2012–210#B2012406, March 29th 2013) and conducted in accordance to the Declaration of Helsinki [19]. All subjects were informed about the purpose of the study, received written information and had given written consent prior to inclusion. This study was retrospectively registered at the ISRCTN registry (trial ID ISRCTN15252886). Registration date August 11, 2017.

Study participants

Participants were recruited from October 2014 until May 2016, at the Academic Centre for Dentistry Amsterdam (ACTA). Patients referred to the Department of Periodontology with untreated periodontitis were selected based on the presence of radiographic bone loss of ≥1/3 of the root length on minimum 2 non-adjacent teeth, on peri-apical long cone radiographs. Control subjects were screened for their periodontal condition using the Dutch Periodontal Screening Index (DPSI) [20]. Healthy controls were defined as subjects having a maximum probing depth of 4–5 mm in the absence of gingival recession (≤ DPSI 3-). Additionally, the absence of alveolar bone loss was confirmed on bitewing radiographs not older than 12 months. Subjects were excluded if they presented with a history of pathologic conditions that are known to systemically affect PMN numbers and function (such as hematological disorders, diabetes mellitus, antibiotics use within the last 6 months, recent history of illness or fever, allergies, alcoholism and pregnancy). Furthermore, individuals with less than 20 teeth, removable partial dentures, night guards, orthodontic banding, (peri) oral piercings or apparent oral lesions were also excluded.

Bacterial culture

Fusobacterium nucleatum (*F.n.*) strain DSM 20482 was grown anaerobically (80% nitrogen, 10% carbon dioxide and 10% hydrogen) in brain-heart infusion (BHI) broth supplemented with 5 μg/ml hemin (Sigma-Aldrich Chemie B.V., Zwijndrecht, Netherlands) and 1 μg/ml menadione (Sigma). Bacteria were isolated from broth cultures by centrifugation, washed twice in sterile phosphate-buffered saline (PBS), prior to dilution with sterile PBS to give a final suspension of 4×10^8 cells/ml which was stored at – 20 °C.

Isolation and purification of PMNs

For each participant, the oPMNs and cPMNs were isolated and subsequently analyzed on the same day without delay. The collection procedure was based on previously described protocol [11]. All participants were instructed neither to gargle nor to clear their throat during the sampling procedure. The oPMNs were obtained by 4 serial rinses of the oral cavity with 20 ml of sterile sodium chloride solution (0.9% NaCl) for 30 s, with a 4½ min intermission. The pooled sample was kept on ice in a 50 ml centrifuge tube (Sigma) until the end of the collection procedure. One ml from the first rinse of each participant was pipetted into a 2 ml microtube and stored at – 80 °C for further analysis (see below *Protease activity*). Venous blood samples were drawn from the antecubital fossa of all subjects into 9 ml sodium heparin blood collection tubes (BD Vacutainer™, Breda, the Netherlands) and maintained at room temperature until the PMN isolation procedure. The isolation procedure of oPMNs and cPMNs was carried out as described before [11]. Cell counts were obtained using a Muse® Cell Analyzer (Merck Millipore, Darmstadt, Germany) and verified with a Bürker-Türk counting chamber and Trypan Blue exclusion for the viability of the PMNs.

Analysis of PMN apoptosis

Cell death was analyzed by means of flow cytometry, using the commercially available apoptosis detection kit *(BD Pharmingen™ FITC Annexin V Apoptosis Detection Kit, BD Biosciences, San Diego, CA, USA).* In brief, PMNs were incubated for 15 min in the dark at room temperature and fixated according to the manufacturer's instructions. Flow cytometric analysis was performed within 1 h *on* a BD Accuri™ C6 flow cytometer (BD Biosciences) and the Accuri CFlow Plus software was used for data acquisition and analysis. The percentages of propidium iodide positive (PI^+) PMNs were calculated, indicating apoptotic or damaged cells.

Analysis of membrane-bound markers of PMN activation

PMN activation was analyzed for the expression of clusters of differentiation (CD) markers CD11b, CD63, and CD66b on the Accuri C6 flow cytometer (BD Biosciences). The low affinity immunoglobulin-Fcγ receptor IIIb (CD16b) was used as a PMN identification marker. PMNs were gated according to CD16 expression and the sideward scatter profile, and analyzed for the mAb of interest as described previously [12]. Briefly, PMNs were incubated on ice for 30 min with phycoerythrin (PE)-conjugated monoclonal antibodies anti-CD11b and anti-CD63 (BD Pharmingen, Breda, Netherlands) or fluorescein isothiocyanate (FITC)-conjugated monoclonal antibody anti-CD66b (BD Pharmingen) according to the manufacturer's instructions. FITC and PE conjugated mouse IgG1 were used as isotype control antibodies with the same concentration as the specific antibodies. After incubation, PMNs were washed with PBS and resuspended in PBS containing 1% paraformaldehyde. CD16 positive PMNs were gated and analyzed for the expressions of the mAb of interest (CD11b, CD63, or CD66b). Data are expressed as mean fluorescence intensity (MFI) after correction for the non-specific binding of the isotype controls.

ROS analysis

Non-stimulated samples were incubated for 30 min with 2 mM dihydrorhodamine123 (DHR) in PBS, in a shaking (50 rpm) waterbath at 37 °C. Stimulation was achieved by adding phorbol myristate acetate (PMA, Sigma) at a final concentration of 0.1 μg/ml or non-opsonized *F.n.* to the cell suspension in a ratio of PMN:*F.n.* of 1:20. Results were expressed as the MFI or the fold increase in MFI (the ratio of MFI of the PMA or *F.n.*-stimulated samples divided by the MFI of samples without stimulation).

Protease activity

To quantify the protease activity in the oral rinses, one ml aliquots from the first rinses of each participant were retrieved from – 80 °C storage and thawed on ice. The protease activity was determined using black 96-wells microplates (F Bottom, Greiner Bio- One GmbH, Frickenhausen, Germany). Each microwell was filled with 70 ml of PBS, and 8 μM protease substrate PEK-054 ([FITC]-NleKKKKVLPIQLNAATDK-[KDbc]), a substrate for total protease activity [21]. As a positive control, trypsin from bovine pancreas was added in duplicate in two-fold serial dilutions, and sterile PBS was used as a negative control. Samples from periodontitis patients and controls were defrosted and 30 μl was added to each microwell. The increase in fluorescence was monitored over 60 min using a fluorescence microplate reader (Fluostar Galaxy, BMG Laboratories, Offenburg, Germany) with an excitation wavelength of 485 nm and an emission wavelength of 530 nm. Relative fluorescence (RF) values were obtained for periodontitis patients and controls. The total protease activity was defined in RF per Unit (RF U).

Statistical analysis

All analyses were performed with the SPSS Statistics 23.0 software (IBM, Chicago, Illinois, USA). Means, standard deviations (SD), range and frequency distributions were calculated. Normal distribution of data was tested with the Kolmogoroff-Smirnov test and when needed, log transformation of data sets was performed before proceeding with parametric statistics. The characteristics of patient and control groups were compared with the Student's T-test or the chi-square test, where appropriate. Within groups, comparisons between non-stimulated and stimulated samples (PMA or *F. nucleatum*) were performed using the Paired T-test. A further, linear regression analysis was performed to explore a possible relationship between the oPMN numbers and the measured PMN parameters. In these analyses, the log-transformed experimental data for oPMN counts were entered as dependent variables, and total protease activity was entered as the independent variable. A *P*-value < 0.05 was considered statistically significant.

Results

Study population

A total of 19 periodontitis patients and 16 control subjects were included in this study. A description of the characteristics of the participants is provided in Table 1. No significant differences were observed between the two groups in relation to age, sex distribution and number of teeth. Periodontitis patients were more often of non-Caucasian descent, smoked and had a higher body mass index (BMI) than the control group. Within the periodontitis group, an average of 9.8 teeth showed a radiographic bone loss of ≥50% of the root length.

Table 1 Characteristics of the study population stratified according to periodontal condition

	Control (*n* = 16)	Periodontitis (*n* = 19)	*p*-value
Age	44.1 ± 11.6	47.9 ± 12.4	0.354
Sex (male)	8 (50%)	11(55%)	0.765
Ethnicity (Caucasian)	12 (75%)	7 (37%)	**0.024**
Smoking (current smoker)	4 (25%)	11 (58%)	0.050
Body mass index	23.5 ± 2.2	27.9 ± 5.0	**0.006**
# of teeth	27.7 ± 3.0	26.6 ± 3.3	0.303
# of teeth with > 50% bone loss	0	9.8 ± 6.0	–
Counts (× 10^6)			
cPMNs[a]	19.3 ± 11.2	17.6 ± 9.0	0.873
oPMNs[b]	1.8 ± 3.2	8.1 ± 11.5	**0.007**

Results for demographic, dental characteristics and counts of oPMNs and cPMNs. Values represent means ± standard deviations, or numbers (%) of subjects. *P*-values calculated by χ^2-test or Student's T-test; (n/a = not applicable). *P*-values < 0.05 were considered statistically significant and are shown in bold

[a]Total cPMNs obtained from a 6 ml tube of blood, after the isolation and purification steps

[b]Total oPMNs collected after 4 × 30 s rinsing with 4½ minutes intermission, after the isolation and purification steps

Isolation of PMNs

The yield of cPMN from venous blood was comparable in healthy controls and periodontitis patients (mean 19.3 versus 17.6 × 10^6, P = 0.873, Table 1). On average, 4.5 times more oPMN were retrieved from periodontitis patients (mean 8.1 × 10^6 cells per sample) than from the control group (mean 1.8 × 10^6 cells per sample, P = 0.007, Table 1).

Apoptosis assay

The apoptotic cPMNs (PI^+) accounted for a mean of 2.8% in the control group. The periodontitis patients showed a higher mean percentage of PI^+ cPMNs compared to the control group (mean 12.3%, P = 0.026, Fig. 1). Similar to the profile of the circulatory cells, the PI^+ oPMNs percentages were higher in periodontitis patients (56.2%) than in controls (39.9%, P = 0.004, Fig. 1). Additionally, more PI^+ cells were found amongst the oPMNs compared to the cPMNs in both patients and controls ($P < 0.001$, Fig. 1).

Degranulation assay

The expression of CD11b, CD63, and CD66b on the cPMNs was low and comparable in healthy controls and in periodontitis patients ($p > 0.05$, Fig. 2a, b, and c, respectively). The oPMNs were more activated than cPMNs, as they expressed 3 to 36-fold higher levels of all three activation markers than the cPMNs, both in healthy controls and in periodontitis patients (all $P < 0.001$, Fig. 2). CD11b was more expressed by oPMNs derived from periodontitis patients than by oPMNs derived from controls (P = 0.024, Fig. 2a). The expression of CD63 and CD66b on the oPMNs was not statistically different between the periodontitis patients and controls (CD63 P = 0.054, Fig. 2b; CD66b P = 0.483, Fig. 2c).

ROS assay

Non-stimulated cPMNs demonstrated comparable levels of ROS production between the control group and the periodontitis group (Fig. 3a). Upon stimulation with either PMA or *F. nucleatum*, ROS production from the cPMNs increased 24–26 fold for the control subjects (both $P < 0.001$, Fig. 3b), whereas the periodontitis patients showed an increase of 33–34 fold compared to the non-stimulated cPMNs (both $P < 0.001$, Fig. 3b). The same pattern was observed for the oPMNs' non-stimulated and stimulated ROS production levels. Comparable ROS levels were produced by oPMNs originating from controls and

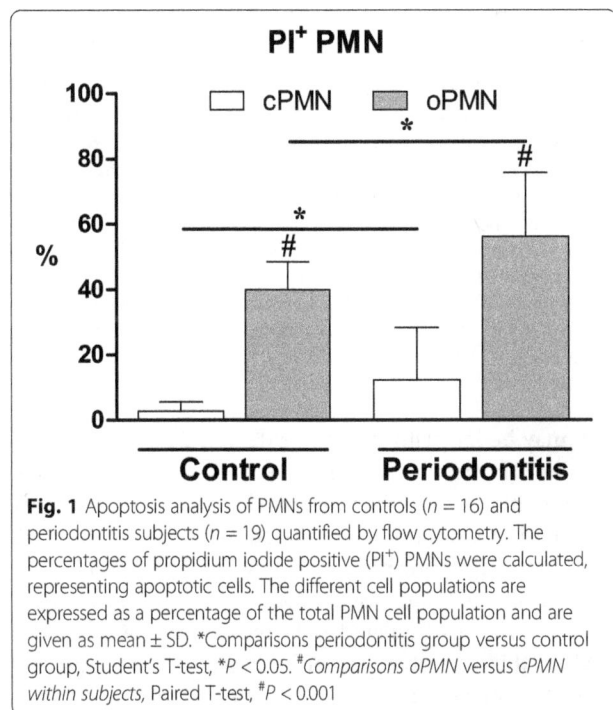

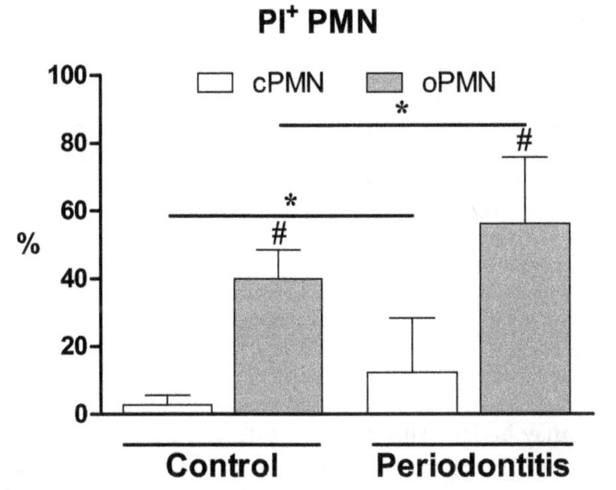

Fig. 1 Apoptosis analysis of PMNs from controls (n = 16) and periodontitis subjects (n = 19) quantified by flow cytometry. The percentages of propidium iodide positive (PI^+) PMNs were calculated, representing apoptotic cells. The different cell populations are expressed as a percentage of the total PMN cell population and are given as mean ± SD. *Comparisons periodontitis group versus control group, Student's T-test, *$P < 0.05$. #*Comparisons oPMN* versus *cPMN within subjects,* Paired T-test, #$P < 0.001$

periodontitis patients (Fig. 3a and c). The oPMNs non-stimulated ROS levels were 3–5 higher compared to the non-stimulated ROS levels produced by cPMNs (both $P < 0.001$, Fig. 3a). Upon stimulation with PMA, only the oPMNs' from the periodontitis group showed a significant increase of ROS production (2 fold increase, $P = 0.012$, Fig. 3c), while ROS levels were not significantly induced by PMA in the control group. Upon bacterial stimulation with *F. nucleatum*, oPMNs from both the control group and the periodontitis group produced higher levels of ROS (control 2.4 fold increase, $P < 0.001$; periodontitis 2.2 fold increase, $P = 0.038$, Fig. 3c).

Protease activity

The total protease activity was analyzed from the first rinse samples and showed a 3.1 times higher activity in the periodontitis group compared to the control group ($P < 0.001$, Fig. 4a). Additionally, the number of oPMNs was a significant predictor for the total protease activity ($r^2 = 0.386$, $P < 0.001$). Further subanalysis revealed that this relation was only found amongst the periodontitis patients ($r^2 = 0.399$, $P = 0.007$, Fig. 4b), and not in the control subjects ($r^2 = 0.063$, $P = 0.349$, Fig. 4b).

Discussion

The purpose of the current investigation was to study the numbers and function of the oPMNs in subjects with periodontitis. Normally, oPMNs contribute to oral health maintenance and form a part of the innate oral defense mechanisms. However in periodontitis these

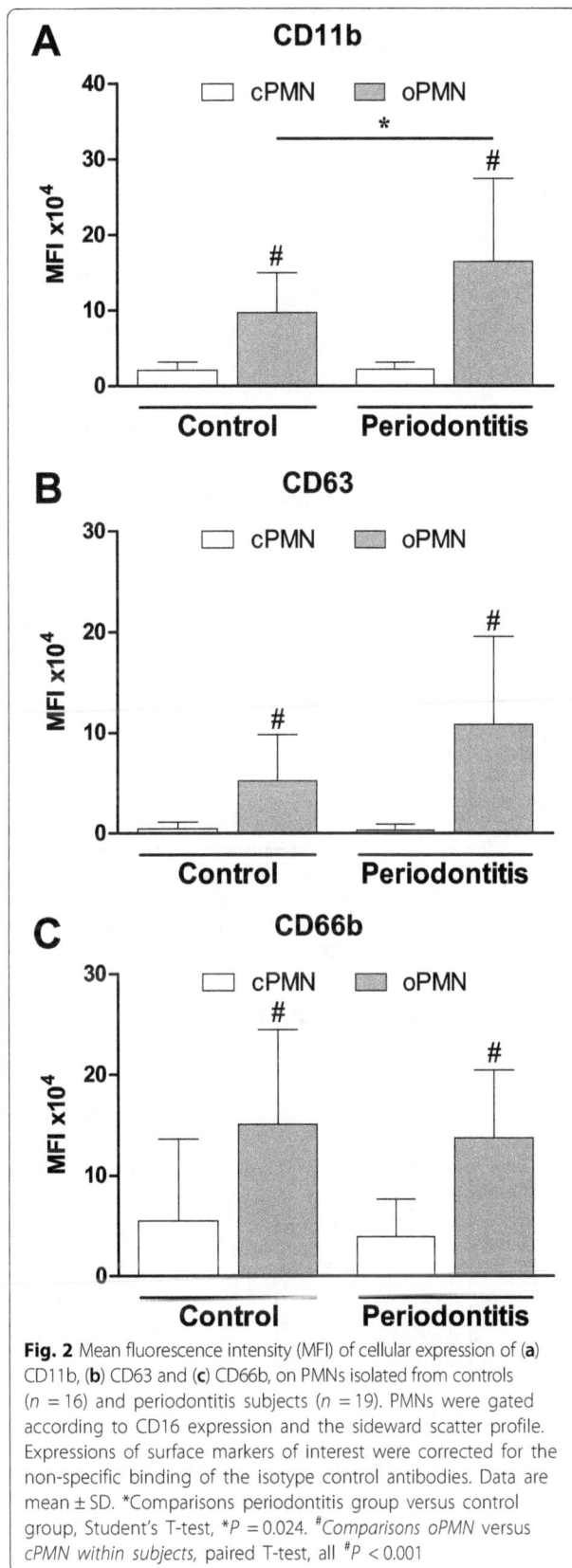

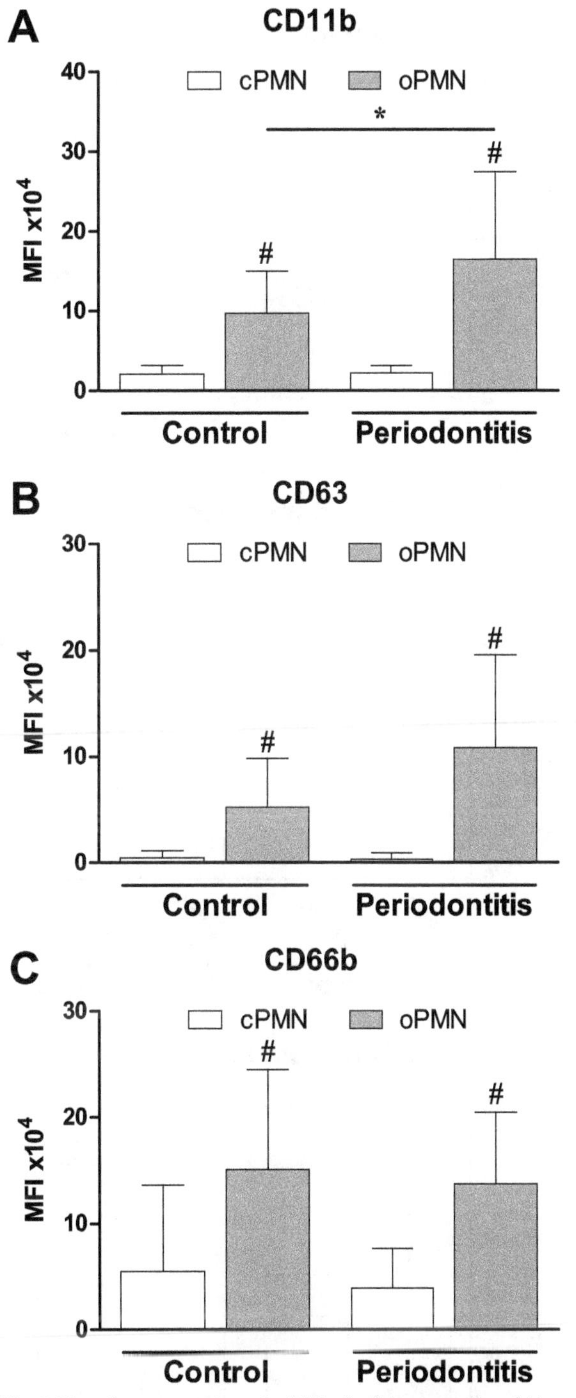

Fig. 2 Mean fluorescence intensity (MFI) of cellular expression of (**a**) CD11b, (**b**) CD63 and (**c**) CD66b, on PMNs isolated from controls (n = 16) and periodontitis subjects (n = 19). PMNs were gated according to CD16 expression and the sideward scatter profile. Expressions of surface markers of interest were corrected for the non-specific binding of the isotype control antibodies. Data are mean ± SD. *Comparisons periodontitis group versus control group, Student's T-test, *$P = 0.024$. #*Comparisons oPMN* versus *cPMN within subjects,* paired T-test, all #$P < 0.001$

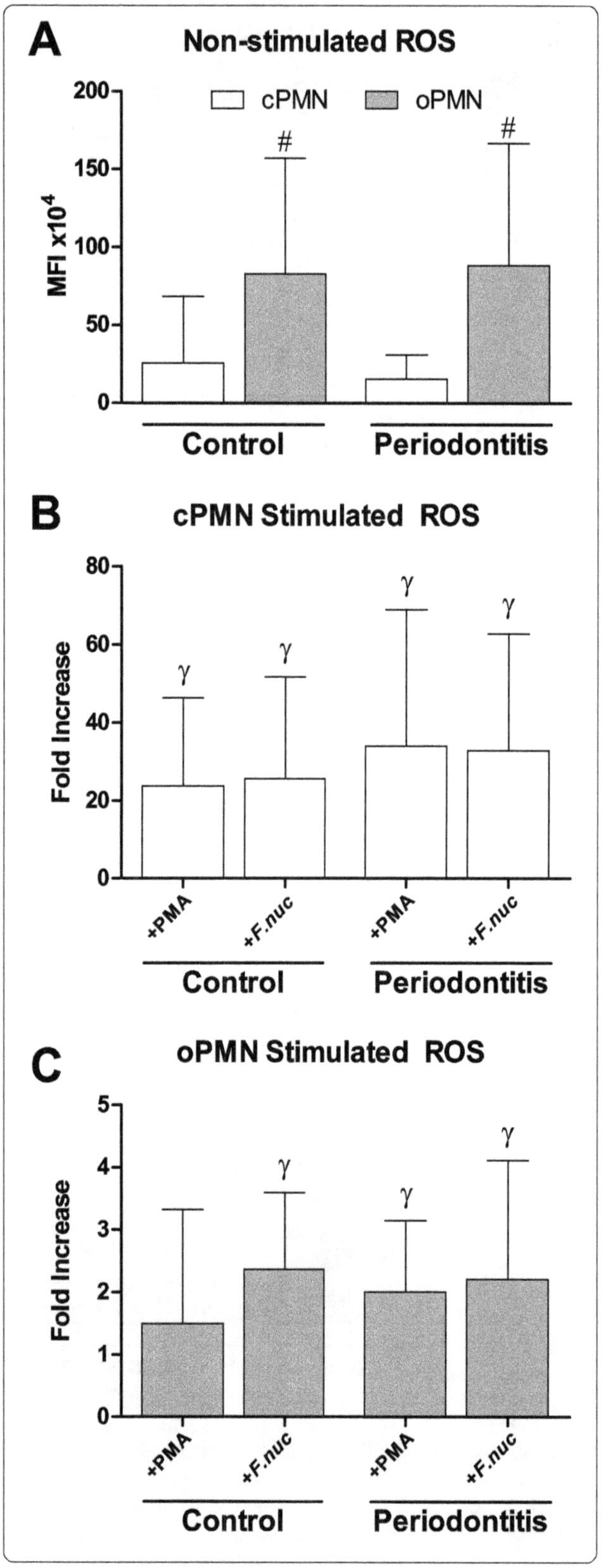

Fig. 3 Mean fluorescence intensity (MFI) of reactive oxygen species (ROS) produced by PMNs isolated from controls ($n = 16$) and periodontitis subjects ($n = 19$). **a** Non-stimulated ROS production was calculated and expressed as mean ± SD. **b** Stimulated ROS production produced by cPMNs when incubated with phorbol myristate acetate (+PMA) or *F. nucleatum* (+*F.nuc*). **c** Stimulated ROS production produced by oPMNs when incubated with phorbol myristate acetate (+PMA) or *F. nucleatum* (+*F.nuc*). Ratios were labeled as fold increase and were calculated for the stimulated ROS samples (MFI of the PMA-stimulated or *F.n.*-stimulated samples, divided by the MFI of the non-stimulated ROS samples). #*Comparisons oPMN* versus *cPMN within subjects*, Paired T-test, $^{\#}P < 0.001$. ᵞComparisons to corresponding non-stimulated samples (panel **a**), Student's T-test, all $^{\gamma}P < 0.05$

cells may be left with limited or depleted functional capabilities. The results of the present study showed a significant higher number of oPMNs in patients with untreated periodontitis compared to subjects without periodontitis. Confirming our previous results [11], the oPMNs showed increased expression of degranulation markers and unstimulated ROS release compared to the cPMNs; this was observed in both the periodontitis and control subjects. However, the periodontitis patients showed more apoptotic oPMNs and increased degranulation compared to the control group. Combined, these findings suggest that as the PMNs migrate through oral tissues and "travel" along the biofilms surrounding the teeth, these cells age, use their granule resources and lose ROS production capabilities; these traits are more pronounced in periodontitis.

On average, we found 4.5 times more oPMNs in the patient group. Our results confirm previous reports of increased PMN numbers in the presence of gingival inflammation and deepened pockets [4, 5, 7, 13, 18]. Higher numbers of oPMN in periodontitis is most likely explained by an increased periodontal inflamed surface area (PISA), which has been reported to reach 5–20 cm^2 [22, 23]. In response to the inflamed oral surroundings, PMNs leave the blood circulation, enter the periodontal space and mix in the oral fluid. Moreover, as the oral biofilm acquires pathogenic traits, more chemokines and cytokines are released into the periodontal tissues, resulting in increased recruitment of PMNs [24, 25].

We found more apoptotic oPMNs in periodontitis patients compared to controls. One explanation for this finding might be that there are more cPMNs being programmed for apoptosis in periodontitis and that these cells appear in patients' rinse samples. We suggest that more apoptotic cPMN could be a systemic characteristic of the periodontitis patients, and therefore also found in the oral cavity. More apoptotic oPMN in periodontitis is in contrast to the recent results of Lakschevitz and co-workers who suggested lower numbers of apoptotic oPMN in periodontitis compared to controls [8]. In our protocol, the participants repeated the oral rinsing 4

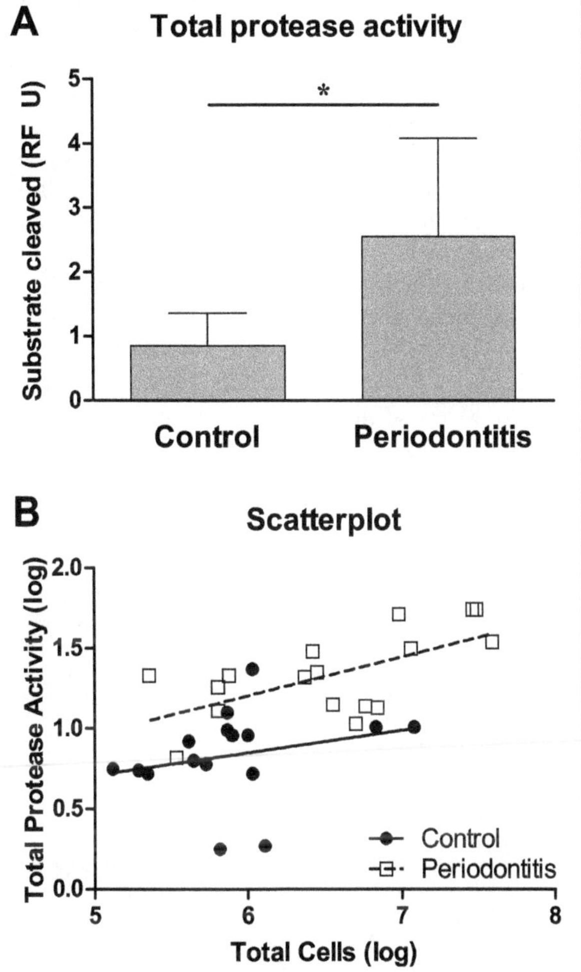

Fig. 4 Total protease activity measured from oral rinses originating from controls (n = 16) and periodontitis subjects (n = 16). **a** Total protease activity was measured as relative fluorescence per unit (RF U) and expressed as mean ± SD. *Comparisons periodontitis group versus control group, Student's T-test, $^{*}P < 0.001$. **b** Total protease activity was only predicted by oPMN counts in periodontitis patients (dashed line, $r^2 = 0.3989$, $P = 0.0065$) and not in the control group (straight line, $r^2 = 0.0629$, $P = 0.3486$)

times, while the subjects from Lakschevitz et al. rinsed 6 times consecutively [8]. In pilot experiments preceding the current study, we observed that the viability of oPMNs increased by 17.7% between the first rinse and the fourth successive rinse, suggesting that fresh, new PMNs are retrieved as the oral rinse is repeated (data not shown). Furthermore, Lakschevitz et al. based their conclusions about oPMN viability on a small sample subset ($N = 3$, for this sub-analysis) [8], whereas we analyzed nineteen periodontitis patients and observed inter-individual differences.

Upon PMN activation, the cytoplasmic granules fuse with the PMN cellular membrane and an upregulation of the granular markers (CD11b, CD63 and CD66b) becomes measurable. The increased expression of these CD markers in our study confirms that the oPMNs have undergone migration and degranulation relative to the cPMNs. Additionally, the upregulated expression of CD11b and the tendency for increased CD63 in periodontitis patients' oPMNs, suggest a higher release of granular content, possibly related to activation during the migration through the inflamed periodontal tissues and along the subgingival biofilm. Important to note is that periodontal inflammation can be present in various inflammatory states, ranging from a pre-inflammatory state within stressed tissues, to a full-fledged inflammatory state within damaged tissues. The results from this study corroborate the recent findings by Fine et al., who also found degranulated oPMNs in periodontitis [18].

Intrinsic increase of ROS production by cPMN has been proposed for patients with chronic periodontitis as a susceptibility trait [26–29]. In our study, we could not confirm this trait, since our results showed similar unstimulated and stimulated ROS levels originating from periodontitis patients and healthy controls. A plausible explanation for the discrepancy with the literature could be the application of different methods used to analyze ROS production. While most studies have used luminol enhanced chemi-luminescence for the measurement of total ROS generation (intra- and extracellular), our study has used flowcytometric analysis. In contrast to the chemi-luminescence method, which measures various ROS species in a multi-well assay, the flowcytometric analysis used in this study detects only hydrogen peroxide at a single cell level. However, the flowcytometric method is preferred because it is applicable in situations with low cell density, such as in our oral rinse samples.

Another possible reason may lie in the socio-demographic differences between study populations. Matthews et al. demonstrated that when periodontitis patients were compared with age-, and sex-matched controls, only the unstimulated cPMNs produced higher levels of ROS, while the stimulated levels were comparable between the measured groups [29]. In the present study, age and sex distribution were not different between the periodontitis and control subjects, however the ethnicity, BMI and smoking frequencies were different. Ethnic background can influence PMN numbers and ROS activity [30, 31]. Furthermore, it has been suggested that PMNs in obese subjects may be in a primed state compared to non-obese subjects, and can participate in the pathogenesis of obesity-related diseases, such as periodontitis [32]. Another study demonstrated that cigarette smoke extract could lower the PMN ROS production capabilities in response to *F. nucleatum* specifically [33].

Our group previously evaluated ROS levels of oPMNs and/or cPMNs in response to *F. nucleatum* [11, 12, 34]. Several PMN receptors are involved in active ROS production, like Toll-like receptors and protein kinase C agonists, from which Toll-like receptors are the most efficient in ROS generation [35, 36]. While PMA stimulation acts via protein kinase C, *F. nucleatum* is able to activate the PMNs' Toll-like receptors (TLR-2, TLR-4, TLR-9) [30]. *F. nucleatum* stimulation may therefore result in a different oPMN ROS response than PMA stimulation. The ROS levels that were recently reported in chronic periodontitis patients [18] were acquired using an extensive flowcytometric gating strategy in order to identify PMN sub-populations. Our study did not evaluate the PMNs to this extent. Fine and co-workers observed that PMA stimulation did not significantly induce ROS levels in chronic periodontitis patients and suggested that oPMNs from these subjects might have exhausted their ROS potential. Interestingly, the same results were observed in the control subjects in the current study, whereas we showed that ROS levels from the oPMNs isolated from periodontitis patients were significantly enhanced after stimulation. ROS production is known to show inter-individual variations and is stimulus dependent. In addition, the inflammatory state of the participants in our study may not be exactly identical to that of the participants from previous reports regarding ROS production in chronic periodontitis. We presume that the general inflammatory status of an individual (high – low) is reflected by the cPMNs, which does not necessarily reflect the oral inflammatory status. In this line, the oPMNs are a better reflection of the oral local environment than the cPMNs.

In addition to the biological processes within the periodontal environment, the high numbers of oPMNs in the oral cavity in periodontitis patients may also have consequences for the integrity of the oral mucosa. The increased protease levels that were observed in the periodontitis group were also positively correlated to the number of oPMNs. The combination of increased numbers, with unrestrained excessive ROS release and proteolytic enzymes, can negatively influence the balance of the healthy/normal oral ecology within an individual. As such, oxidative damage and degradative enzymes may contribute to the increasing vascular permeability [37, 38] and a continuous and excessive efflux of the PMNs into the oral cavity in untreated periodontal disease may contribute to collateral tissue damage not only within the periodontium, but also affect the integrity of the oral mucosa in these patients. Consequently these changes make the oral mucosa more vulnerable to environmental challenges including components of cigarette smoke, and metabolites of alcohol such as acetaldehyde and acetate.

Conclusions

In periodontitis, one can expect higher numbers of oral PMNs than in health. These cells are more degranulated and more often apoptotic than oPMNs from non-periodontitis individuals. We suggest that the primed cPMN is a systemic trait in periodontitis patients, showing an increased proportion of apoptotic cells compared to controls. This observed PMN characteristic could hamper their proper function in the periodontal tissues and their surveillance function in the oral cavity as a whole. Nevertheless, the oPMNs in periodontitis display sufficient functionality as shown by their responsiveness (ROS production) after ex vivo stimulation. We therefore suggest that the oPMNs in periodontitis participate in the maintenance of the oral ecosystem. However, the question remains whether in periodontitis, the increased oPMN counts, increased release of granule content, and excessive ROS and proteases can be detrimental to the oral mucosa integrity.

Abbreviations

BHI: Brain-heart infusion; BMI: Body mass index; CD: Clusters of differentiation; cPMN: Polymorphonuclear neutrophils isolated from the blood circulation; DHR: Dihydrorhodamine123; *F.n.*: *Fusobacterium nucleatum*; FITC: Fluorescein isothiocyanate; MFI: Mean fluorescence intensity; oPMN: Polymorphonuclear neutrophils isolated from the oral cavity; PBS: Phosphate-buffered saline; PE: Phycoerythrin; PI: Propidium iodide; PISA: Periodontal inflamed surface area; PMA: Phorbol myristate acetate; PMN: Polymorphonuclear neutrophils; ROS: Reactive oxygen species

Acknowledgements

The authors would like express their gratitude to S. Gunput, K. Hermes and W.J. Teeuw for their help in patient recruitment and collection of the samples.

Funding

Elena A. Nicu and P. Rijkschroeff were financially supported by the University of Amsterdam under the research priority area *'Oral Infections and Inflammation'*. The authors declare that the funding body played no role in the design of the study, the collection, analysis, and interpretation of the data and in writing the manuscript.

Authors' contributions

Substantial contributions to the design of the study: All authors. Substantial contributions to the acquisition of data: EAN, PR, EW and KN. Substantial contributions to the analysis of data: EAN, PR and KN. Substantial contributions to the interpretation of data: EAN, PR and BGL. Critically revising the manuscript: All authors. All authors read an approved the final manuscript.

Competing interests

The authors declare that they have no competing interest.

Author details

[1]Department of Periodontology, Academic Centre for Dentistry Amsterdam (ACTA), University of Amsterdam and VU University Amsterdam, Gustav Mahlerlaan 3004, 1081, LA, Amsterdam, The Netherlands. [2]Opris Dent SRL, Sibiu, Romania. [3]Department of Oral Biochemistry, Academic Centre for Dentistry Amsterdam (ACTA), University of Amsterdam and VU University, Amsterdam, The Netherlands.

References

1. Wade WG. The oral microbiome in health and disease. Pharmacol Res. 2013; 69:137–43.
2. Wu RQ, Zhang DF, Tu E, Chen QM, Chen W. The mucosal immune system in the oral cavity-an orchestra of T cell diversity. Int J Oral Sci. 2014;6:125–32.
3. Mayadas TN, Cullere X, Lowell CA. The multifaceted functions of neutrophils. Annu Rev Pathol. 2014;9:181–218.
4. Aps JKM, van den Maagdenberg K, Delanghe JR, Martens LC. Flow cytometry as a new method to quantify the cellular content of human saliva and its relation to gingivitis. Clin Chim Acta. 2002;321:35–41.
5. Bender JS, Thang H, Glogauer M. Novel rinse assay for the quantification of oral neutrophils and the monitoring of chronic periodontal disease. J Periodontol Res. 2006;41:214–20.
6. Aboodi GM, Goldberg MB, Glogauer M. Refractory periodontitis population characterized by a hyperactive oral neutrophil phenotype. J Periodontol. 2011;82:726–33.
7. Bhadbhade SJ, Acharya AB, Thakur S. Correlation between probing pocket depth and neutrophil counts in dental plaque, saliva, and gingival crevicular fluid. Quintessence Int. 2012;43:111–7.
8. Lakschevitz FS, Aboodi GM, Glogauer M. Oral neutrophil transcriptome changes result in a pro-survival phenotype in periodontal diseases. PLoS One. 2013;8 https://doi.org/10.1371/journal.pone.0068983.
9. Moosani A, Sigal MJ, Glogauer M, Lawrence HP, Goldberg M, Tenenbaum HC. Evaluation of periodontal disease and oral inflammatory load in adults with special needs using oral neutrophil quantification. Spec Care Dentist. 2014;34:303–12.
10. Wilcox ME, Charbonney E, d'Empaire PP, Duggal A, Pinto R, Javid A, Dos Santos C, Rubenfeld GD, Sutherland S, Liles WC, et al. Oral neutrophils are an independent marker of the systemic inflammatory response after cardiac bypass. J Inflamm. 2014;11:32.
11. Rijkschroeff P, Jansen ID, van der Weijden FA, Keijser BJ, Loos BG, Nicu EA. Oral polymorphonuclear neutrophil characteristics in relation to oral health: a cross-sectional, observational clinical study. Int J Oral Sci. 2016;8:191–8.
12. Rijkschroeff P, Loos BG, Nicu EA. Impaired polymorphonuclear neutrophils in the oral cavity of edentulous individuals. Eur J Oral Sci. 2017;125:371–8.
13. Klinkhamer JM, Zimmerman S. The function and reliability of the orogranulocytic migratory rate as a measure of oral health. J Dent Res. 1969; 48:709–15.
14. Dutzan N, Konkel JE, Greenwell-Wild T, Moutsopoulos NM. Characterization of the human immune cell network at the gingival barrier. Mucosal Immunol. 2016;9:1163–72.
15. Nussbaum G, Shapira L. How has neutrophil research improved our understanding of periodontal pathogenesis? J Clin Periodontol. 2011;38:49–59.
16. Calonius PE. The leukocyte count in saliva. Oral Surg Oral Med Oral Pathol. 1958;11:43–6.
17. Landzberg M, Doering H, Aboodi GM, Tenenbaum HC, Glogauer M. Quantifying oral inflammatory load: oral neutrophil counts in periodontal health and disease. J Periodontal Res. 2015;50:330–6.
18. Fine N, Hassanpour S, Borenstein A, Sima C, Oveisi M, Scholey J, Cherney D, Glogauer M. Distinct oral neutrophil subsets define health and periodontal disease states. J Dent Res. 2016;95:931–8.
19. World Medical A. World medical association declaration of Helsinki: ethical principles for medical research involving human subjects. JAMA. 2013;310: 2191–4.
20. van der Velden U. The Dutch periodontal screening index validation and its application in the Netherlands. J Clin Periodontol. 2009;36:1018–24.
21. Cummings RT, Salowe SP, Cunningham BR, Wiltsie J, Park YW, Sonatore LM, Wisniewski D, Douglas CM, Hermes JD, Scolnick EM. A peptide-based fluorescence resonance energy transfer assay for bacillus anthracis lethal factor protease. Proc Natl Acad Sci U S A. 2002;99:6603–6.
22. Loos BG. Systemic markers of inflammation in periodontitis. J Periodontol. 2005;76:2106–15.
23. Nesse W, Abbas F, van der Ploeg I, Spijkervet FKL, Dijkstra PU, Vissink A. Periodontal inflamed surface area: quantifying inflammatory burden. J Clin Periodontol. 2008;35:668–73.
24. Chin AC, Parkos CA. Pathobiology of neutrophil transepithelial migration: implications in mediating epithelial injury. Annu Rev Pathol. 2007;2:111–43.
25. Yin L, Chino T, Horst OV, Hacker BM, Clark EA, Dale BA, Chung WO. Differential and coordinated expression of defensins and cytokines by gingival epithelial cells and dendritic cells in response to oral bacteria. BMC Immunol. 2010;11:37.
26. Fredriksson M, Gustafsson A, Asman B, Bergstrom K. Hyper-reactive peripheral neutrophils in adult periodontitis: generation of chemiluminescence and intracellular hydrogen peroxide after in vitro priming and FcgammaR-stimulation. J Clin Periodontol. 1998;25:394–8.
27. Fredriksson MI, Gustafsson AK, Bergstrom KG, Asman BE. Constitutionally hyperreactive neutrophils in periodontitis. J Periodontol. 2003;74:219–24.
28. Matthews JB, Wright HJ, Roberts A, Cooper PR, Chapple IL. Hyperactivity and reactivity of peripheral blood neutrophils in chronic periodontitis. Clin Exp Immunol. 2007;147:255–64.
29. Matthews JB, Wright HJ, Roberts A, Ling-Mountford N, Cooper PR, Chapple IL. Neutrophil hyper-responsiveness in periodontitis. J Dent Res. 2007;86: 718–22.
30. Siddiqi M, Garcia ZC, Stein DS, Denny TN, Spolarics Z. Relationship between oxidative burst activity and CD11b expression in neutrophils and monocytes from healthy individuals: effects of race and gender. Cytometry. 2001;46:243–6.
31. Hsieh MM, Everhart JE, Byrd-Holt DD, Tisdale JF, Rodgers GP. Prevalence of neutropenia in the U.S. population: age, sex, smoking status, and ethnic differences. Ann Intern Med. 2007;146:486–92.
32. Brotfain E, Hadad N, Shapira Y, Avinoah E, Zlotnik A, Raichel L, Levy R. Neutrophil functions in morbidly obese subjects. Clin Exp Immunol. 2015; 181:156–63.
33. Matthews JB, Chen FM, Milward MR, Wright HJ, Carter K, McDonagh A, Chapple IL. Effect of nicotine, cotinine and cigarette smoke extract on the neutrophil respiratory burst. J Clin Periodontol. 2011;38:208–18.
34. Rijkschroeff P, Gunput STG, Ligtenberg AT, Veerman EC, Loos BG, Nicu EA. Polymorphonuclear neutrophil integrity and functionality are preserved when exposed to saliva. Arch Oral Biol. 2018;92:68–74.
35. Roberts A, Matthews JB, Socransky SS, Freestone PP, Williams PH, Chapple IL. Stress and the periodontal diseases: effects of catecholamines on the growth of periodontal bacteria in vitro. Oral Microbiol Immunol. 2002;17:296–303.
36. Chapple IL, Matthews JB. The role of reactive oxygen and antioxidant species in periodontal tissue destruction. Periodontol 2000. 2007;43:160–232.
37. Katakwar P, Metgud R, Naik S, Mittal R. Oxidative stress marker in oral cancer: a review. J Cancer Res Ther. 2016;12:438–46.
38. Nelson AR, Fingleton B, Rothenberg ML, Matrisian LM. Matrix metalloproteinases: biologic activity and clinical implications. J Clin Oncol. 2000;18:1135–49.

Effect of *TP53* rs1042522 on the susceptibility of patients to oral squamous cell carcinoma and oral leukoplakia

Zhen Sun[1†], Wei Gao[2†] and Jiang-Tao Cui[1*]

Abstract

Background: There are different and inconsistent conclusions regarding the genetic relationship between the human tumor suppressor p53 (*TP53*) rs1042522 polymorphism and the risk of oral squamous cell carcinoma (OSCC) and oral leukoplakia (OL). Therefore, the aim of the study was to comprehensively reassess this association through the performance of an updated meta-analysis.

Methods: After searching the available databases, we systematically screened and included the eligible case-control studies, which contain the full genotype frequency data of the *TP53* rs1042522 polymorphism for both OSCC/OL patients and the negative control groups. P_A (*P*-value of the association test) and ORs (odd ratios) with their corresponding 95% CIs (confidence intervals) were calculated to quantitatively evaluate the influence of *TP53* rs1042522 on the susceptibility of patients to OSCC or OL.

Results: In total, twenty eligible case-control articles were finally enrolled. Compared with the controls, no increased or decreased risk of OSCC was observed in the cases for six genetic models including allele C vs. G ($P_A = 0.741$), carrier C vs. G ($P_A = 0.853$), homozygote CC vs. GG ($P_A = 0.085$), heterozygote GC vs. GG ($P_A = 0.882$), dominant GC + CC vs. GG ($P_A = 0.969$), and recessive CC vs. GG + GC ($P_A = 0.980$). Furthermore, no statistically significant difference between the cases and controls was detected in most subgroup meta-analyses ($P_A > 0.05$). For the risk of OL, we did not observe the difference between the cases and controls for most genetic models in the overall meta-analysis and subsequent subgroup analysis ($P_A > 0.05$). Begg's test and Egger's test excluded the large risk of publication bias within the included studies in the meta-analysis of OSCC. The sensitivity analysis indicated the above relatively stable results.

Conclusions: Our updated meta-analysis (based on the current evidence) shows that *TP53* rs1042522 may not confer susceptibility to OSCC. In addition, for the first time, we provided evidence regarding the negative association between *TP53* rs1042522 and OL risk.

Keywords: TP53, OSCC, OL, Polymorphism, Meta-analysis

* Correspondence: cuijiangt@163.com
†Zhen Sun and Wei Gao contributed equally to this work.
[1]Department of Stomatology, Second Hospital of Tianjin Medical University, Ping-Jiang Road, He Xi District, 300211 Tianjin, People's Republic of China
Full list of author information is available at the end of the article

Background

The human tumor suppressor p53 *(TP53)* gene on chromosome 17p13, which is also known as *p53*, was reported to be involved in a group of cell biology events, such as the cell cycle, apoptosis and genomic stability [1, 2]. Some genetic variants of the *TP53* gene were reported to be linked to human carcinogenesis [2, 3]. The rs1042522 G/C, which is a very common polymorphism at exon 4 of the *TP53* gene, results in the alteration at codon 72 between arginine (Arg, R) and proline (Pro, P) and causes the TP53Arg72Pro mutation. This may affect the normal function of the TP53 protein and is implicated in susceptibility to several clinical diseases (e.g., colorectal cancer [4], endometriosis [5] or type 2 diabetes [6]).

Herein, we are interested in exploring the potential role of *TP53* rs1042522 in the risk of oral squamous cell carcinoma (OSCC) or oral leukoplakia (OL). OSCC, which is the main type of oral cancer, originates from squamous cells on the surface of the oral cavity or oropharynx [7, 8]. OL is considered the pre-cancerous lesion with white or gray keratosis on the oral mucosa [8, 9]. Life style (e.g., tobacco smoking, drinking, and chewing), human papillomavirus (HPV) infection, and other functional variants may be implicated in the etiology of OSCC and OL [7–9].

Currently, the association between rs1042522 of the *TP53* gene and OL/OSCC risks has been inconsistently reported among different populations. For instance, *TP53* rs1042522 was reported to be associated with the risk of oral potentially malignant disorders (OPMD), including OL, in Argentine patients [10]. However, the risk of OL was not found in Taiwanese patients [11]. *TP53* rs1042522 may have been linked to an increased risk of OSCC in an Indian population [12, 13]. However, the negative genetic conclusion between *TP53* rs1042522 and OSCC risk in India was also observed in another report [14]. Additionally, the GC genotype of *TP53* rs1042522 may be associated with a reduced risk of OSCC patients in Italy [15]. Therefore, the meta-analysis provides helpful insights into the genetic role of *TP53* rs1042522 in the susceptibility of the patient to OL or OSCC.

Currently, as far as we know, no meta-analysis has been previously published to investigate the relationship between rs1042522 of the *TP53* gene and the predisposition of OL. Regarding the association between *TP53* rs1042522 and OSCC risk, only two previous meta-analyses were published [16, 17]. Given the newly published case-control studies and the utilization of a strict screening strategy and quantitative synthesis, we performed an updated meta-analysis aiming to analyze the potential difference of *TP53* rs1042522 in the OSCC cases and the negative controls.

Materials and methods

Database searching

Our study was conducted in accordance with PRISMA (preferred reporting items for systematic reviews and meta-analyses) guidelines [18]. The PRISMA 2009 checklist is shown in the Additional file 1. Three online databases, including PUBMED, WOS (Web of Science), and EMBASE (Excerpta Medica Database), were searched up to June 2018 without any restrictions regarding language or the publication period. The principle of PICOS, namely, "population" (P), "intervention" (I), "comparator" (C), "outcomes" (O), and "study designs" (S), was considered. A series of terms regarding "population" (human patients with OSCC or OL disease) and "intervention" (polymorphism of the *TP53* gene) was utilized. To prevent the excessive filtering of articles, we checked the information of the "comparator" (negative control), "outcomes" (risk of OSCC or OL) and "study designs" (case-control study) by reading the text of the articles without a specific limitation in the electronic database search. The detailed search terms are shown in Additional file 2. Then, we removed the duplicates by using the "Find Duplicates" function of Endnote X7 software (Thomson Reuters, Philadelphia, PA, USA).

Inclusion and exclusion criteria

With reference to our inclusion and exclusion criteria, two authors (ZS and WG) independently screened and assessed the articles for eligibility based on the PICOS strategy. The inclusion criteria were as follows: (P) containing the patients with oral squamous cell carcinoma and oral leukoplakia; (I) focusing on the *TP53* rs1042522 polymorphism; (C) containing the negative controls; (O) the completed genotype distribution of GG, GC and CC and can be used for the assessment of OSCC or OL risk under the six genetic models, namely, C vs. G (allele), C vs. G (carrier), CC vs. GG (homozygote), GC vs. GG (heterozygote), GC + CC vs. GG (dominant), and CC vs. GG + GC (recessive); and (S) case-control studies.

The exclusion criteria were as follows: (P) animal or cell data, other disease or unconfirmed OSCC; (I) other genes, other variants or unconfirmed *TP53* mutation site; (C) lack of a control group or the genotype distributions of the control deviated from the HWE (Hardy--Weinberg Equilibrium) (*P*-value of HWE from χ^2 test < 0.05); (O) lack of full genotype frequency data in both the case and control group; and (S) a meta-analysis, review, and meeting abstracts.

Data collection and quality assessment

Then, we carefully extracted the data and listed the basic information (such as method, age, gender, smoking, alcohol, location, ethnicity, and disease type) and genotype frequency in the Tables. E-mails were sent for the missing data. We also evaluated the quality of each study using the NOS (Newcastle-Ottawa quality assessment Scale) system with the score of 1~ 9. The high quality was considered when the NOS score was larger than five. A full discussion was required for a conflicting or controversial issue during quality assessment.

Association and heterogeneity test

STATA 12.0 software (Stata Corporation, Texas, USA) was used for the quantitative synthesis and outcome measures. A two-sided *P*-value of association test, pooled ORs (odd ratios), and the 95% CI (confidence interval) were performed and used under the following six genetic models: C vs. G (allele); C vs. G (carrier); CC vs. GG (homozygote); GC vs. GG (heterozygote); GC + CC vs. GG (dominant); and CC vs. GG + GC (recessive). When $P < 0.05$ from the association test and the OR value > 1, the C minor allele of *TP53* rs1042522 will be considered the risk factor of OSCC or OL.

We performed the Q statistic and I^2 test to assess the between study heterogeneity. A random-effect model (DerSimonian and Laird method) for high heterogeneity will be used when *P*-values of the Q statistic are < 0.05 or the I^2 values are > 50%. Otherwise, a fixed-effect model (Mantel-Haenszel method) was used.

Additionally, we performed a group of subgroup analyses based on the control source (population-based or hospital-based), ethnicity (Caucasian or Asian), location (India, USA, China), and OSCC type (oral cavity, HPV16 −/+).

Publication bias

Taking into consideration that publication bias may exist, Begg's test and Egger's test were conducted when at least ten case-control studies were enrolled. Publication bias was indicated by a *P* value for Begg's test and Egger's test being less than 0.05.

Sensitivity analysis

We also conducted the sensitivity analyses under all of the genetic models. If there is no obvious change for the value of recalculated ORs (odd ratios), and the 95% CI (confidence interval) when the individual study was systematically omitted at a time, statistical stability of data was considered. The deleted case-control studies, which

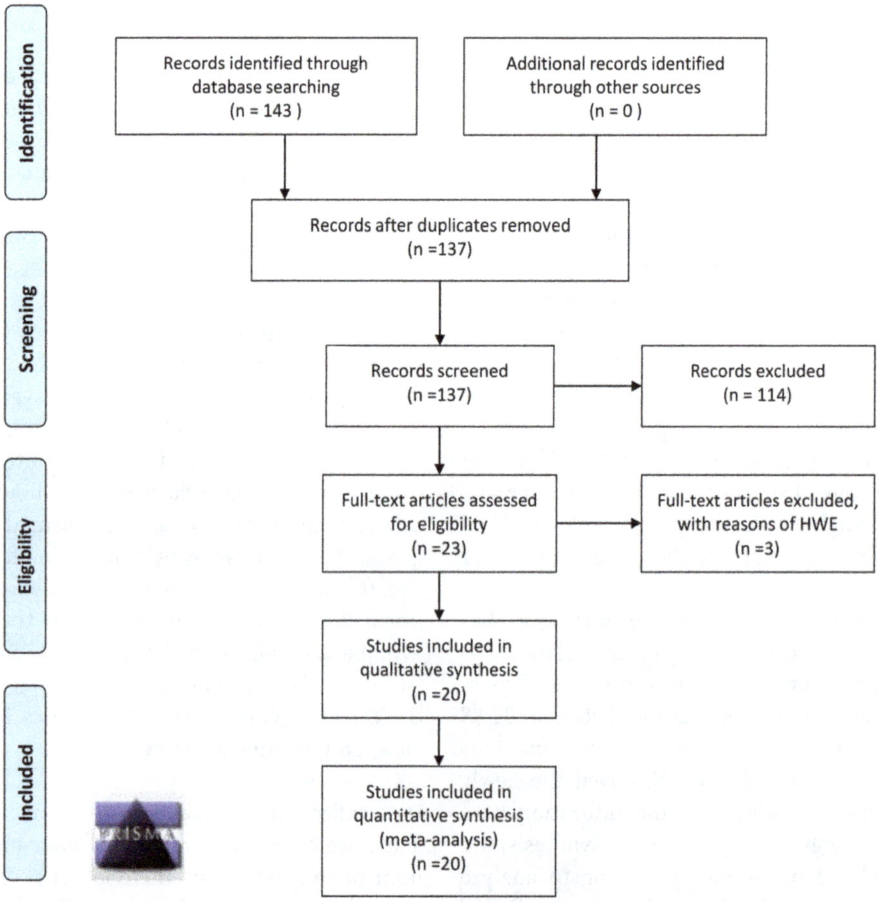

Fig. 1 The PRISMA 2009 flow diagram of our study

Table 1 Meta-analysis of *TP53* rs1042522 and OSCC risk

Genetic models	Overall/Subgroup		N	Case/control	ORs (95% CIs)	P_A	I^2 (%)	P_H	Statistical model
allele C vs. G	overall		17	3047/3305	1.02 (0.90, 1.15)	0.741	55.0	0.003	Random
	Control source	PB	13	2477/2485	1.01 (0.86, 1.18)	0.925	63.7	0.001	
		HB	3	381/704	1.01 (0.83, 1.22)	0.933	0.0	0.663	
	Location	India	4	577/498	1.29 (0.79, 2.08)	0.306	79.1	0.002	
		USA	4	942/1357	0.96 (0.84, 1.10)	0.560	0.0	0.768	
		China	3	1115/767	1.02 (0.79, 1.31)	0.886	68.5	0.042	
	Ethnicity	Asian	12	2028/1807	1.10 (0.93, 1.29)	0.253	58.4	0.006	
		Caucasian	4	817/1165	0.86 (0.70, 1.06)	0.158	46.0	0.135	
	Disease type	oral cavity	6	1295/1372	1.12 (0.92, 1.36)	0.244	59.5	0.030	
		HPV16(–)	4	208/255	1.06 (0.47, 2.40)	0.884	83.4	< 0.001	
		HPV16(+)	4	93/197	1.38 (0.88, 2.16)	0.157	0.0	0.865	
carrier C vs. G	overall		17	3047/3305	0.99 (0.91, 1.08)	0.853	0.0	0.460	Fixed
	Control source	PB	13	2477/2485	0.98 (0.89, 1.08)	0.685	20.0	0.242	
		HB	3	381/704	1.00 (0.80, 1.25)	0.990	0.0	0.878	
	Location	India	4	577/498	1.02 (0.84, 1.25)	0.820	40.6	0.168	
		USA	4	942/1357	0.97 (0.83, 1.12)	0.666	0.0	0.902	
		China	3	1115/767	1.01 (0.87, 1.18)	0.869	8.9	0.334	
	Ethnicity	Asian	12	2028/1807	1.03 (0.92, 1.15)	0.601	0.0	0.600	
		Caucasian	4	817/1165	0.89 (0.76, 1.05)	0.179	35.6	0.199	
	Disease type	oral cavity	6	1295/1372	1.06 (0.93, 1.20)	0.414	0.0	0.510	
		HPV16(–)	4	208/255	0.94 (0.66, 1.34)	0.729	69.4	0.020	
		HPV16(+)	4	93/197	1.20 (0.71, 2.01)	0.493	0.0	0.926	
homozygote CC vs. GG	overall		17	3047/3305	1.03 (0.88, 1.21)	0.085	33.9	0.733	Fixed
	Control source	PB	13	2477/2485	1.00 (0.83, 1.20)	0.989	45.0	0.040	
		HB	3	381/704	1.06 (0.69, 1.62)	0.799	0.0	0.587	
	Location	India	4	577/498	1.04 (0.74, 1.47)	0.812	75.6	0.006	
		USA	4	942/1357	0.97 (0.70, 1.34)	0.846	0.0	0.945	
		China	3	1115/767	1.00 (0.76, 1.32)	0.997	65.3	0.056	
	Ethnicity	Asian	12	2028/1807	1.06 (0.88, 1.28)	0.559	53.1	0.015	
		Caucasian	4	817/1165	0.91 (0.63, 1.31)	0.602	0.0	0.972	
	Disease type	oral cavity	6	1295/1372	1.16 (0.92, 1.46)	0.224	56.1	0.044	
		HPV16(–)	4	208/255	1.46 (0.79, 2.73)	0.230	51.4	0.103	
		HPV16(+)	4	93/197	2.40 (0.96, 5.99)	0.061	0.0	0.843	

Table 1 Meta-analysis of *TP53* rs1042522 and OSCC risk *(Continued)*

Genetic models	Overall/Subgroup		N	Case/control	ORs (95% CIs)	P_A	I^2 (%)	P_H	Statistical model
heterozygote GC vs. GG	overall		17	3047/3305	0.99 (0.89, 1.11)	0.882	37.4	0.061	Fixed
	Control source	PB	13	2477/2485	0.98 (0.86, 1.11)	0.706	50.1	0.020	
		HB	3	381/704	0.98 (0.75, 1.28)	0.861	0.0	0.969	
	Location	India	4	577/498	1.10 (0.82, 1.48)	0.541	0.0	0.402	
		USA	4	942/1357	0.94 (0.79, 1.12)	0.470	0.0	0.709	
		China	3	1115/767	1.10 (0.89, 1.35)	0.386	61.0	0.076	
	Ethnicity	Asian	12	2028/1807	1.10 (0.95, 1.28)	0.196	0.0	0.595	
		Caucasian	4	817/1165	0.81 (0.67, 0.98)	**0.030**	71.5	0.014	
	Disease type	oral cavity	6	1295/1372	1.15 (0.96, 1.38)	0.125	0.0	0.715	
		HPV16(−)	4	208/255	0.93 (0.30, 2.92)	0.904	80.6	0.001	
		HPV16(+)	4	93/197	0.96 (0.32, 2.86)	0.937	40.9	0.166	
dominant GC + CC vs. GG	overall		17	3047/3305	1.01 (0.86, 1.19)	0.969	47.6	0.015	Random
	Control source	PB	13	2477/2485	1.00 (0.81, 1.23)	0.936	57.5	0.005	
		HB	3	381/704	1.01 (0.86, 1.19)	0.181	0.0	0.877	
	Location	India	4	577/498	1.31 (0.77, 2.21)	0.321	57.8	0.068	
		USA	4	942/1357	0.94 (0.80, 1.11)	0.481	0.0	0.700	
		China	3	1115/767	1.07 (0.72, 1.58)	0.736	70.5	0.034	
	Ethnicity	Asian	12	2028/1807	1.13 (0.93, 1.36)	0.220	32.9	0.127	
		Caucasian	4	817/1165	0.78 (0.56, 1.07)	0.123	64.2	0.039	
	Disease type	oral cavity	6	1295/1372	1.15 (0.95, 1.40)	0.144	16.2	0.309	
		HPV16(−)	4	208/255	1.04 (0.32, 3.37)	0.942	83.9	< 0.001	
		HPV16(+)	4	93/197	1.21 (0.62, 2.37)	0.573	0.0	0.513	
recessive CC vs. GG + GC	overall		17	3047/3305	1.00 (0.87, 1.16)	0.980	22.8	0.189	Fixed
	Control source	PB	13	2477/2485	0.98 (0.84, 1.15)	0.794	36.4	0.092	
		HB	3	381/704	1.06 (0.71, 1.59)	0.765	0.0	0.560	
	Location	India	4	577/498	1.00 (0.75, 1.33)	0.997	75.6	0.006	
		USA	4	942/1357	0.99 (0.72, 1.36)	0.954	0.0	0.978	
		China	3	1115/767	0.95 (0.74, 1.21)	0.652	13.5	0.315	
	Ethnicity	Asian	12	2028/1807	1.00 (0.85, 1.18)	0.977	46.3	0.039	
		Caucasian	4	817/1165	0.98 (0.69, 1.40)	0.927	0.0	0.977	
	Disease type	oral cavity	6	1295/1372	1.00 (0.85, 1.18)	0.392	57.6	0.038	
		HPV16(−)	4	208/255	1.00 (0.85, 1.18)	0.353	16.3	0.310	
		HPV16(+)	4	93/197	1.00 (0.85, 1.18)	**0.031**	0.0	0.445	

OSCC, oral squamous cell carcinoma; *HPV*, Human papillomavirus; *N*, number of case-control studies; *PB*, population-based control; *HB*, hospital-based control; *HPV*, Human papillomavirus; *ORs*, odd ratios; *CIs*, confidence intervals; P_A, *P* value of association test; P_H, *P* values of heterogeneity test
P_A value <0.05, the number is in bold

lead to an obvious change, will be regarded as the source of heterogeneity and will be removed.

Results

Study selection and characteristics

Figure 1 shows the PRISMA 2009 flow diagram of our study. We obtained 143 records across three databases, including PUBMED ($n = 31$), WOS ($n = 84$) and EMBASE ($n = 28$). Then, a total of 137 records were screened after the duplicates were removed. After screening the titles and abstracts, 114 records were excluded for various reasons: animal or cell data, other disease or unconfirmed OSCC (n = 31); other genes, other variants or an unconfirmed *TP53* mutation site ($n = 35$); lack of a control group or full genotype frequency data in both the case and the control group ($n = 21$); meta-analysis, review, and meeting abstracts ($n = 27$). Next, the eligibility of 23 full-text articles was evaluated. From these articles, the genotype distributions of three articles did not adhere to HWE. Finally, a total of twenty articles were rigorously included in our quantitative synthesis. Of these twenty articles, sixteen studies [11–15, 19–29] examined oral squamous cell carcinoma (OSCC), and five studies [10, 11, 30–32] examined oral leukoplakia (OL). The basic information and genotype frequency of the included studies are listed in Additional file 3 and Additional file 4. NOS assessment system data (Additional file 5) showed that all of the enrolled case-control studies are high quality because all NOS quality scores were larger than five.

TP53 rs1042522 and OSCC risk

First, a total of 17 case-control studies from 16 articles with 3047 cases and 3305 controls were recruited for the meta-analysis of *TP53* rs1042522 and OSCC risk. Table 1 shows the heterogeneity for the three genetic models: allele C vs. G [$I^2 = 55.0\%$, P_H (*P*-value of heterogeneity = 0.003) and dominant GC + CC vs. GG ($I^2 = 47.6\%$, $P_H = 0.015$), which led to the use of a random-effects model (DerSimonian and Laird method). A fixed-effects model (Mantel-Haenszel method) was utilized for others. The summary data in Table 1 show that compared with the controls, no increased or decreased risk of OSCC was observed in the cases for the six genetic models including allele C vs. G [P_A (*P*-value of association test) =0.741], carrier C vs. G ($P_A = 0.853$), homozygote CC vs. GG ($P_A = 0.085$), heterozygote GC vs. GG ($P_A = 0.882$), dominant GC + CC vs. GG ($P_A = 0.969$), and recessive CC vs. GG + GC ($P_A = 0.980$). Forest plot data of the allele C vs. G model are depicted in Fig. 2.

Subgroup meta-analyses were also performed by PB (population-based)/HB (hospital-based), Caucasian/Asian, India/USA/China, and oral cavity/HPV16 (–)/HPV16(+).

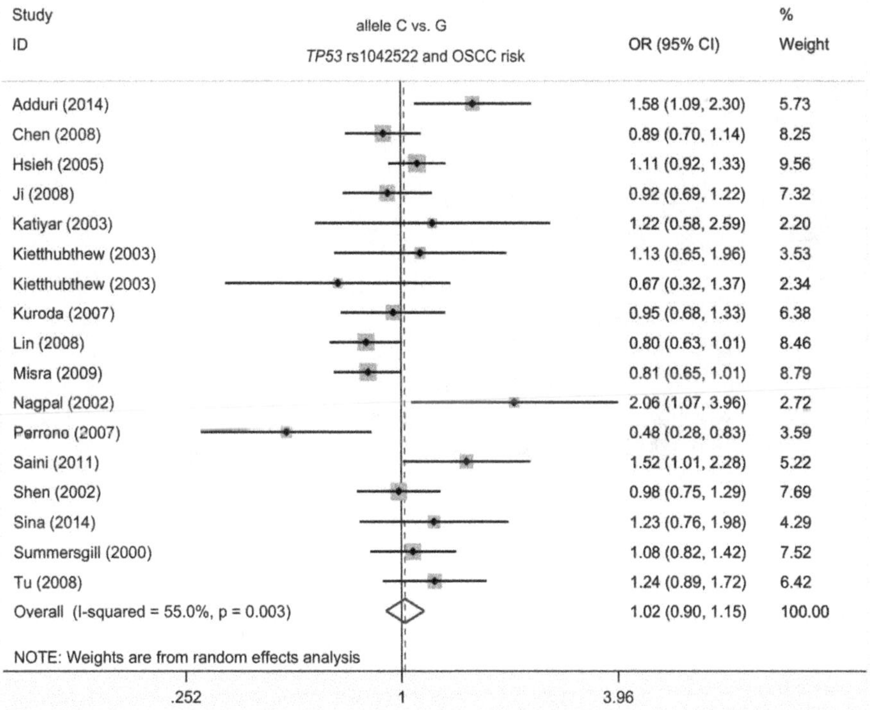
Study
ID
allele C vs. G
TP53 rs1042522 and OSCC risk
OR (95% CI)
%
Weight
Adduri (2014) 1.58 (1.09, 2.30) 5.73
Chen (2008) 0.89 (0.70, 1.14) 8.25
Hsieh (2005) 1.11 (0.92, 1.33) 9.56
Ji (2008) 0.92 (0.69, 1.22) 7.32
Katiyar (2003) 1.22 (0.58, 2.59) 2.20
Kietthubthew (2003) 1.13 (0.65, 1.96) 3.53
Kietthubthew (2003) 0.67 (0.32, 1.37) 2.34
Kuroda (2007) 0.95 (0.68, 1.33) 6.38
Lin (2008) 0.80 (0.63, 1.01) 8.46
Misra (2009) 0.81 (0.65, 1.01) 8.79
Nagpal (2002) 2.06 (1.07, 3.96) 2.72
Perrono (2007) 0.48 (0.28, 0.83) 3.59
Saini (2011) 1.52 (1.01, 2.28) 5.22
Shen (2002) 0.98 (0.75, 1.29) 7.69
Sina (2014) 1.23 (0.76, 1.98) 4.29
Summersgill (2000) 1.08 (0.82, 1.42) 7.52
Tu (2008) 1.24 (0.89, 1.72) 6.42
Overall (I-squared = 55.0%, p = 0.003) 1.02 (0.90, 1.15) 100.00
NOTE: Weights are from random effects analysis
.252
1
3.96

Fig. 2 Meta-analysis (allele C vs. G) of *TP53* rs1042522 and OSCC risk

Table 2 Meta-analysis of *TP53* rs1042522 and OL risk

Genetic models	Overall/Subgroup		N	Case/control	ORs (95% CIs)	P_A	I^2 (%)	P_H	Statistical model
allele C vs. G	Overall		6	391/763	1.16 (0.73, 1.84)	0.525	77.1	0.001	Random
	Control source	PB	4	291/647	0.77 (0.59, 1.01)	0.055	21.7	0.280	
	Location	India	4	307/465	1.05 (0.57, 1.92)	0.879	78.7	0.003	
	Ethnicity	Asian	5	377/745	0.99 (0.65, 1.49)	0.952	71.8	0.007	
carrier C vs. G	overall		6	391/763	0.93 (0.76, 1.15)	0.510	41.0	0.132	Fixed
	Control source	PB	4	291/647	0.82 (0.65, 1.03)	0.090	0.0	0.713	
	Location	India	4	307/465	0.89 (0.70, 1.13)	0.353	39.1	0.177	
	Ethnicity	Asian	5	377/745	0.90 (0.73, 1.11)	0.334	19.3	0.292	
homozygote CC vs. GG	overall		6	391/763	1.14 (0.49, 2.62)	0.764	69.2	0.006	Random
	Control source	PB	4	291/647	0.52 (0.34, 0.80)	**0.003**	1.0	0.387	
	Location	India	4	307/465	1.06 (0.33, 3.37)	0.920	75.6	0.006	
	Ethnicity	Asian	5	377/745	0.93 (0.41, 2.08)	0.854	67.5	0.015	
heterozygote GC vs. GG	overall		6	391/763	0.95 (0.71, 1.29)	0.760	45.2	0.104	Fixed
	Control source	PB	4	291/647	0.85 (0.61, 1.18)	0.330	0.0	0.700	
	Location	India	4	307/465	0.81 (0.57, 1.15)	0.239	0.0	0.827	
	Ethnicity	Asian	5	377/745	0.87 (0.64, 1.19)	0.388	0.0	0.803	
dominant GC + CC vs. GG	overall		6	391/763	1.20 (0.66, 2.18)	0.557	63.1	0.019	Random
	Control source	PB	4	291/647	0.73 (0.53, 1.00)	0.050	0.0	0.460	
	Location	India	4	307/465	0.88 (0.51, 1.50)	0.629	32.0	0.220	
	Ethnicity	Asian	5	377/745	0.87 (0.60, 1.25)	0.446	21.0	0.281	
recessive CC vs. GG + GC	overall		6	391/763	1.04 (0.53, 2.05)	0.907	68.9	0.007	Random
	Control source	PB	4	291/647	0.59 (0.41, 0.85)	**0.004**	0.0	0.505	
	Location	India	4	307/465	1.11 (0.42, 2.98)	0.829	79.7	0.002	
	Ethnicity	Asian	5	377/745	0.97 (0.47, 2.01)	0.943	73.6	0.004	

OL, oral leukoplakia; N, number of case-control studies; PB: population-based control; ORs, odd ratios; CIs, confidence intervals; P_A, *P* value of association test; P_H, *P* values of heterogeneity test
P_A value <0.05, the number is in bold

As shown in Table 1 and Additional file 6, Additional file 7, Additional file 8, Additional file 9, there is no statistically significant difference between the cases and the controls in all of the subgroup analyses (all $P_A > 0.05$) except for the Caucasian subgroup for the heterozygote model (P_A=0.030) and the HPV16(+) subgroup for the recessive model ($P_A = 0.031$). These results indicate that *TP53* rs1042522 may have no significant influence on the risk of oral squamous cell carcinoma.

TP53 rs1042522 and OL risk

Six case-control studies with 391 cases and 763 controls were included from five articles for the meta-analysis of *TP53* rs1042522 and OL risk. As shown in Table 2, a fixed-effects model (Mantel-Haenszel method) was used for the carrier (I^2 = 41.0%, $P_H = 0.132$) and heterozygote (I^2 = 45.2%, $P_H = 0.104$) models, whereas a random-effects model (DerSimonian and Laird method) was used for the other alleles (I^2 > 50.0%). We did not detect a difference between the cases and the controls for all of the genetic models in the overall meta-analysis (Table 2, $P_A > 0.05$). After stratification by PB, India and Asia, similar negative results were detected (Table 2, $P_A > 0.05$) and only separate from the homozygote ($P_A = 0.003$) and recessive ($P_A = 0.004$) model of PB subgroup. The forest plots are illustrated in Fig. 3 and in Additional file 10, Additional file 11, Additional file 12. These findings suggest that *TP53* rs1042522 may not be associated with the susceptibility to oral leukoplakia.

Publication bias and sensitivity analysis

We performed both the Begg's test and Egger's test to qualitatively assess the presence of publication bias. Because no more than ten case-control studies in this meta-analysis examined OL, we only analyzed the publication bias in the meta-analysis of OSCC. As shown in Table 3, the *P*-value of Begg's test and Egger's test was larger than 0.05 for all the above genetic models [P_B (*P*-value of Begg's test) > 0.05; P_E (*P*-value of Egger's test) > 0.05]. The Begg's funnel plot (Fig. 4A) and Egger's publication bias plot (Fig. 4B) of the allele model are shown as an example. Thus, there was no large publication bias in our study.

Moreover, we observed a similar summarized OR value in our sensitivity analysis (Fig. 5 for the allele model of OSCC; Additional file 13 for the allele model of OL; and other data not shown), which indicated the reliability of our results.

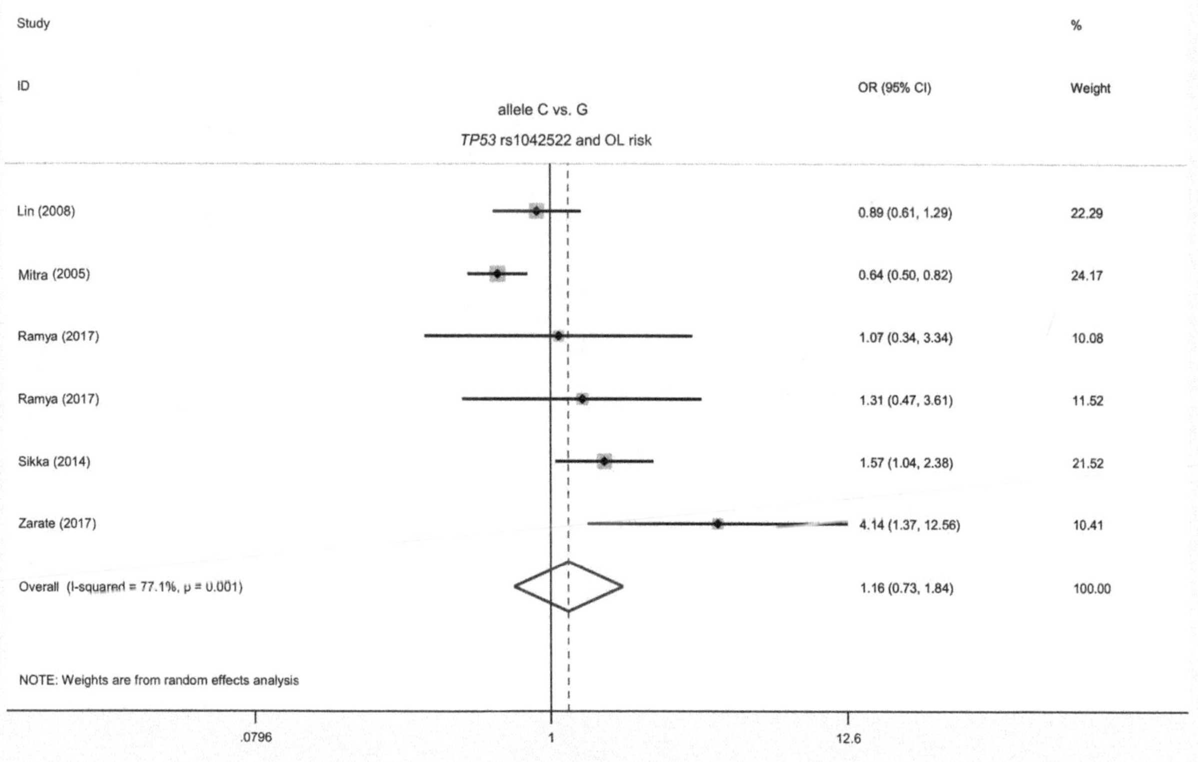

Fig. 3 Meta-analysis (allele C vs. G) of *TP53* rs1042522 and OL risk

Table 3 Publication bias evaluation

Genetic models	Begg's test*		Egger's test	
	z	P_B	t	P_E
allele C vs. G	1.03	0.303	0.88	0.393
carrier C vs. G	0.78	0.434	0.52	0.609
homozygote CC vs. GG	0.78	0.434	1.51	0.152
heterozygote GC vs. GG	0.95	0.343	0.19	0.856
dominant GC + CC vs. GG	0.78	0.434	0.69	0.504
recessive CC vs. GG + GC	0.87	0.387	1.63	0.124

*continuity corrected; *OSCC*, oral squamous cell carcinoma; *OL*, oral leukoplakia; P_B, P value of Begg's test; P_E, P value of Egger's test

Discussion

In this study, we focused on the potential role of *TP53* rs1042522 in the risk of oral squamous cell carcinoma through a meta-analysis of sixteen case-control studies. Overall, the results of the present meta-analysis failed to find any significant association (*P*-value of the association test> 0.05) between *TP53* rs1042522 and the risk of OSCC in either the Asian or Caucasian population. Additionally, the current meta-analysis investigated the potential role of *TP53* rs1042522 in oral leukoplakia risk based on all the published articles that were available. The results showed that *TP53* rs1042522 may not be a susceptible factor for oral leukoplakia disease.

Our meta-analysis data of OSCC coincides with the results reported earlier [16, 17]. In 2009, Zhou et al. performed the first meta-analysis of nine studies [11, 13, 14, 19–21, 23, 25, 28] and found that *TP53* rs1042522 does not seem to be associated with the risk of OSCC [16]. In 2014, Zeng et al. selected eleven case-control studies [11, 13, 19, 22, 23, 26, 28, 29, 33–35] for a meta-analysis regarding the role of *TP53* rs1042522 in the risk of OSCC risk among the Asian population and reported that *TP53* rs1042522 is not linked to the risk of an HPV-negative OSCC patient among Asians [17]. In the present meta-analysis, we worked toward identifying the effect *TP53* rs1042522 on the risk of OSCC in not only the Asian population but also the Caucasian

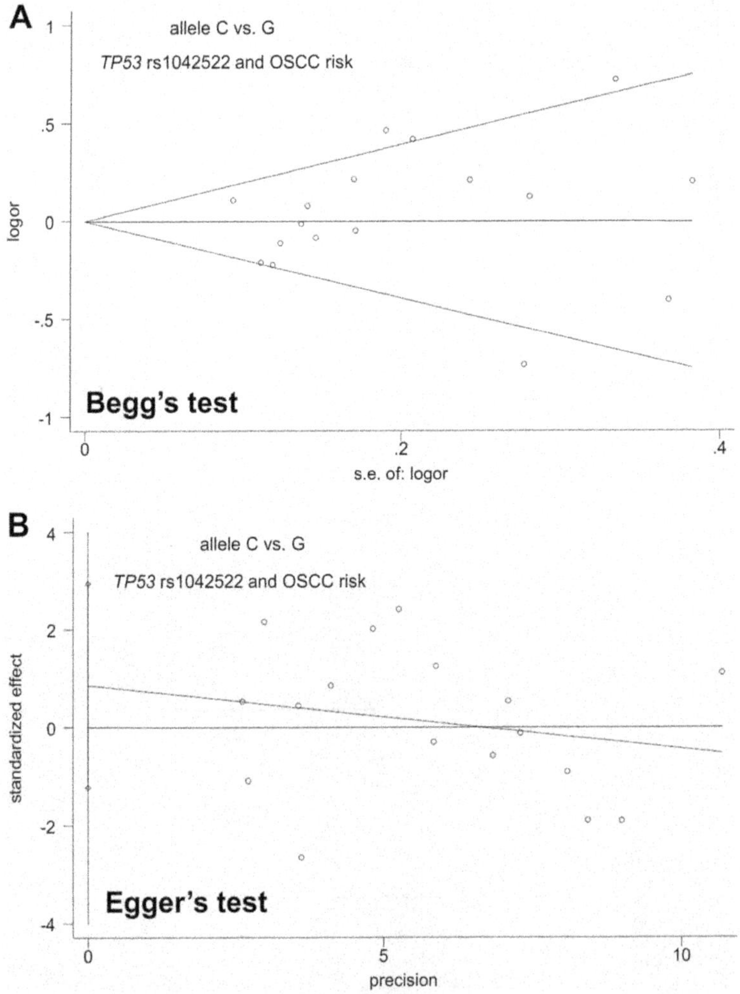

Fig. 4 Publication bias evaluation (allele C vs. G) of *TP53* rs1042522 and OSCC risk. (**a**) Begg's test; (**b**) Egger's test

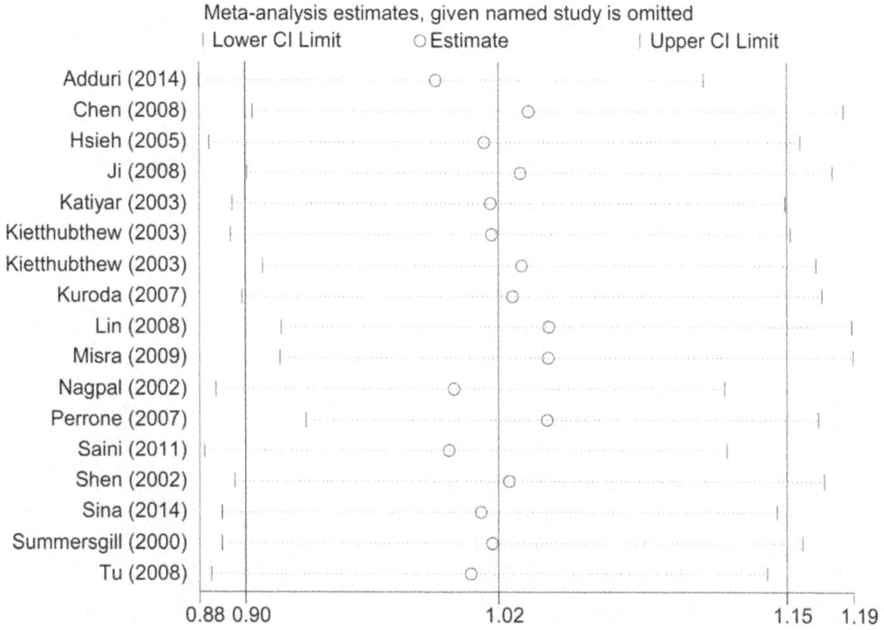

Fig. 5 Sensitivity analysis (allele C vs. G) of *TP53* rs1042522 and OSCC risk

population. We removed one study [33], in which oral cancer was not histopathologically confirmed as SCC, and two other studies [34, 35] for deviation from the Hardy-Weinberg equilibrium. More importantly, we added another eight new case-control studies [12, 14, 15, 20, 21, 24, 25, 27] in our updated meta-analysis.

Despite the above negative association between *TP53* rs1042522 and OSCC risk, different conclusions were observed in meta-analyses regarding the genetic relationship between *TP53* rs1042522 and oral cancer risk [36, 37]. In 2013, Jiang et al. identified 17 case-control studies [11, 13, 14, 19–23, 25, 26, 28, 29, 33, 35, 38–40] for a meta-analysis and reported a lack of a genetic link between *TP53* rs1042522 and oral cancer risk [36]. However, In 2015, Hou et al. statistically pooled 13 studies [11, 19, 20, 22–24, 26, 39, 41–45] for another meta-analysis of the association between *TP53* rs1042522 and oral cancer and revealed that *TP53* rs1042522 may be linked to the pathogenesis of oral cancer [37]. Among these included studies, we noted that several case-control studies [33, 39, 40] do not provide the pathological typing information of oral cancer; however, OSCC accounts for most of oral cancer cases. In addition, the genotype distributions of the control group in two studies [35, 38] were not in line with Hardy-Weinberg Equilibrium.

Our updated meta-analysis enrolled as much articles as possible. Strict inclusion and exclusion criteria were utilized to select the eligible case-control studies. The reliability of our results was also observed in our sensitivity analysis. However, the limitations still exist in our study. The following concerns should be addressed. (1) Our statistical conclusion should be further verified by more case-control studies with a larger number of subjects. Only six case-control studies from five articles [10, 11, 30–32] were included for the meta-analysis of oral leukoplakia, and only four case-control studies [13–15, 26] were enrolled in the HPV 16 +/− subgroup meta-analysis of OSCC. We only detected the role of HPV 16 but not any other type of HPV. In addition, we only enrolled four case-control studies [15, 20, 21, 24] for the "non-Asian, Caucasian" subgroup analysis of *TP53* rs1042522 and OSCC risk. Furthermore, no case-control study population was obtained for the "Caucasian" subgroup analysis of *TP53* rs1042522 and OL risk. (2) The existence of between-study heterogeneity was observed in some comparisons. For example, the high heterogeneity among the case-control studies in the overall meta-analysis of *TP53* rs1042522 and OSCC risk under allele and dominant genetic models disappears in the hospital-based, USA and HPV16(+) subgroups. The complexity of OSCC/OL pathogenesis, the source of control, location and ethnicity may be involved in this dynamic. (3) We did not perform the meta-analysis regarding the role of the other loci of the *TP53* gene or the variant combination between the *TP53* gene and other genes. (4) No case-control study in the Caucasian population was enrolled in the meta-analysis of *TP53* rs1042522 and OL risk. In addition, we did not perform Begg's test and Egger's test to assess the risk of publication bias in meta-analysis of OL because the number of included case-control studies was less than ten. Even though our data from Begg's test and Egger's test show no proof of publication bias for the meta-analysis of

OSCC, we still cannot ignore the impact of publication language, time, and regional variation on the presence of selection bias. (5) Even though the basic information of gender, age, smoking and alcohol consumption was gathered, the relevant stratification analyses by adjusted factors were not performed due to the lack of original genotype frequency data in both the case and control groups.

Conclusions

In conclusion, according to the currently available case-control studies, our updated meta-analysis data together with previous reports fail to statistically support the genetic relationship between *TP53* rs1042522 and the risk of oral squamous cell carcinoma. Additionally, our meta-analysis is the first study to report that the *TP53* rs1042522 polymorphism does not appear to confer susceptibility to oral leukoplakia patients. Additional high-quality case-control studies will help us to scientifically assess the significance of the *TP53* rs1042522 polymorphism on the risk of oral leukoplakia and oral squamous cell carcinoma.

Abbreviations

CI: confidence interval; Embase: Excerpta Medica Database; HPV: papillomavirus; HWE: Hardy-Weinberg Equilibrium; OL: oral leukoplakia; OPMD: oral potentially malignant disorders; ORs: odd ratios; OSCC: oral squamous cell carcinoma; PRISMA: preferred reporting items for systematic reviews and meta-analyses; TP53: tumor suppressor p53; WOS: Web of Science

Funding

Not applicable.

Authors' contributions

ZS designed the study. ZS, WG and JTC extracted, analyzed, and interpreted the data. ZS and JTC drafted the manuscript. All authors read and approved the final version of the manuscript.

Competing interests

The authors declare that they have no competing interests.

Author details

[1]Department of Stomatology, Second Hospital of Tianjin Medical University, Ping-Jiang Road, He Xi District, 300211 Tianjin, People's Republic of China. [2]Department of Interventional Therapy, Tianjin Medical University Cancer Institute and Hospital, National Clinical Research Center for Cancer, Key Laboratory of Cancer Prevention and Therapy, Tianjin's Clinical Research Center for Cancer, Huan Hu West Road, 300060 Tianjin, People's Republic of China.

References

1. Isobe M, Emanuel BS, Givol D, Oren M, Croce CM. Localization of gene for human p53 tumour antigen to band 17p13. Nature. 1986;320(6057):84–5.
2. Hanel W, Moll UM. Links between mutant p53 and genomic instability. J Cell Biochem. 2012;113(2):433–9.
3. Merino D, Malkin D. p53 and hereditary cancer. Subcell Biochem. 2014;85:1–16.
4. Tian X, Dai S, Sun J, Jiang S, Jiang Y. The association between the TP53 Arg72Pro polymorphism and colorectal cancer: an updated meta-analysis based on 32 studies. Oncotarget. 2017;8(1):1156–65.
5. Yan Y, Wu R, Li S, He J. Meta-analysis of association between the TP53 Arg72Pro polymorphism and risk of endometriosis based on case-control studies. Eur J Obstet Gynecol Reprod Biol. 2015;189:1–7.
6. Burgdorf KS, Grarup N, Justesen JM, Harder MN, Witte DR, Jorgensen T, et al. Studies of the association of Arg72Pro of tumor suppressor protein p53 with type 2 diabetes in a combined analysis of 55,521 Europeans. PLoS One. 2011;6(1):e15813.
7. Sathiyasekar AC, Chandrasekar P, Pakash A, Kumar KU, Jaishlal MS. Overview of immunology of oral squamous cell carcinoma. J Pharm Bioallied Sci. 2016;8(Suppl 1):S8–s12.
8. Yu CH, Lin HP, Cheng SJ, Sun A, Chen HM. Cryotherapy for oral precancers and cancers. J Formos Med Assoc. 2014;113(5):272–7.
9. Arduino PG, Bagan J, El-Naggar AK, Carrozzo M. Urban legends series: oral leukoplakia. Oral Dis. 2013;19(7):642–59.
10. Zarate AM, Don J, Secchi D, Carrica A, Galindez Costa F, Panico R, et al. Study of the TP53 codon 72 polymorphism in oral cancer and oral potentially malignant disorders in argentine patients. Tumour Biol. 2017; 39(5):1010428317699113.
11. Lin YC, Huang HI, Wang LH, Tsai CC, Lung O, Dai CY, et al. Polymorphisms of COX-2 -765G>C and p53 codon 72 and risks of oral squamous cell carcinoma in a Taiwan population. Oral Oncol. 2008;44(8):798–804.
12. Adduri RSR, Katamoni R, Pandilla R, Madana SN, Paripati AK, Kotapalli V, et al. TP53 Pro72 Allele Is Enriched in Oral Tongue Cancer and Frequently Mutated in Esophageal Cancer in India. PLoS One. 2014:9(12).
13. Nagpal JK, Patnaik S, Das BR. Prevalence of high-risk human papilloma virus types and its association with P53 codon 72 polymorphism in tobacco addicted oral squamous cell carcinoma (OSCC) patients of eastern India. Int J Cancer. 2002;97(5):649–53.
14. Katiyar S, Thelma BK, Murthy NS, Hedau S, Jain N, Gopalkrishna V, et al. Polymorphism of the p53 codon 72 Arg/pro and the risk of HPV type 16/ 18-associated cervical and oral cancer in India. Mol Cell Biochem. 2003; 252(1–2):117–24.
15. Perrone F, Mariani L, Pastore E, Orsenigo M, Suardi S, Marcomini B, et al. p53 codon 72 polymorphisms in human papillomavirus-negative and human papillomavirus-positive squamous cell carcinomas of the oropharynx. Cancer. 2007;109(12):2461–5.
16. Zhuo XL, Li Q, Zhou Y, Cai L, Xiang ZL, Yuan W, et al. Study on TP53 codon 72 polymorphisms with oral carcinoma susceptibility. Arch Med Res. 2009; 40(7):625–34.
17. Zeng XT, Luo W, Geng PL, Guo Y, Niu YM, Leng WD. Association between the TP53 codon 72 polymorphism and risk of oral squamous cell carcinoma in Asians: a meta-analysis. BMC Cancer. 2014;14:469.
18. Moher D, Liberati A, Tetzlaff J, Altman DG. Preferred reporting items for systematic reviews and meta-analyses: the PRISMA statement. PLoS Med. 2009;6(7):e1000097.
19. Kuroda Y, Nakao H, Ikemura K, Katoh T. Association between the TP53 codon72 polymorphism and oral cancer risk and prognosis. Oral Oncol. 2007;43(10):1043–8.
20. Chen X, Sturgis EM, El-Naggar AK, Wei Q, Li G. Combined effects of the p53 codon 72 and p73 G4C14-to-A4T14 polymorphisms on the risk of HPV16-associated oral cancer in never-smokers. Carcinogenesis. 2008;29(11):2120–5.
21. Shen H, Zheng Y, Sturgis EM, Spitz MR, Wei Q. P53 codon 72 polymorphism and risk of squamous cell carcinoma of the head and neck: a case-control study. Cancer Lett. 2002;183(2):123–30.
22. Misra C, Majumder M, Bajaj S, Ghosh S, Roy B, Roychoudhury S. Polymorphisms at p53, p73, and MDM2 loci modulate the risk of tobacco associated leukoplakia and oral cancer. Mol Carcinog. 2009;48(9):790–800.
23. Tu HF, Chen HW, Kao SY, Lin SC, Liu CJ, Chang KW. MDM2 SNP 309 and p53 codon 72 polymorphisms are associated with the outcome of oral carcinoma patients receiving postoperative irradiation. Radiother Oncol. 2008;87(2):243–52.

24. Ji X, Neumann AS, Sturgis EM, Adler-Storthz K, Dahlstrom KR, Schiller JT, et al. p53 codon 72 polymorphism associated with risk of human papillomavirus-associated squamous cell carcinoma of the oropharynx in never-smokers. Carcinogenesis. 2008;29(4):875–9.
25. Summersgill KF, Smith EM, Kirchner HL, Haugen TH, Turek LP. p53 polymorphism, human papillomavirus infection in the oral cavity, and oral cancer. Oral Surg Oral Med Oral Pathol Oral Radiol Endod. 2000;90(3):334–9.
26. Saini R, Tang TH, Zain RB, Cheong SC, Musa KI, Saini D, et al. Significant association of high-risk human papillomavirus (HPV) but not of p53 polymorphisms with oral squamous cell carcinomas in Malaysia. J Cancer Res Clin Oncol. 2011;137(2):311–20.
27. Sina M, Pedram M, Ghojazadeh M, Kochaki A, Aghbali A. P53 gene codon 72 polymorphism in patients with oral squamous cell carcinoma in the population of northern Iran. Med Oral Patol Oral Cir Bucal. 2014;19(6):e550–5.
28. Hsieh LL, Huang TH, Chen IH, Liao CT, Wang HM, Lai CH, et al. p53 polymorphisms associated with mutations in and loss of heterozygosity of the p53 gene in male oral squamous cell carcinomas in Taiwan. Br J Cancer. 2005;92(1):30–5.
29. Kietthubthew S, Sriplung H, Au WW, Ishida T. The p53 codon 72 polymorphism and risk of oral cancer in southern Thailand. Asian Pac J Cancer Prev. 2003;4(3):209–14.
30. Mitra S, Sikdar N, Misra C, Gupta S, Paul RR, Roy B, et al. Risk assessment of p53 genotypes and haplotypes in tobacco-associated leukoplakia and oral cancer patients from eastern Idia. Int J Cancer. 2005;117(5):786–93.
31. Ramya AS, Majumdar S, Babu TM, Uppala D, Srinivas B, Rao AK. Expression of human papillomavirus DNA and p53 polymorphisms through polymerase chain reaction in normal mucosa and oral leukoplakia individuals with deleterious oral habits. Int J Appl Basic Med Res. 2017;7(2):134–8.
32. Sikka S, Sikka P. Association of Human Papilloma Virus 16 infection and p53 polymorphism among tobacco using oral leukoplakia patients: a Clinicopathologic and genotypic study. Int J Prev Med. 2014;5(4):430–8.
33. Bau DT, Tsai MH, Lo YL, Hsu CM, Tsai Y, Lee CC, et al. Association of p53 and p21(CDKN1A/WAF1/CIP1) polymorphisms with oral cancer in Taiwan patients. Anticancer Res. 2007;27(3b):1559–64.
34. Saleem S, Azhar A, Hameed A, Khan MA, Abbasi ZA, Qureshi NR, et al. P53 (Pro72Arg) polymorphism associated with the risk of oral squamous cell carcinoma in gutka, niswar and manpuri addicted patients of Pakistan. Oral Oncol. 2013;49(8):818–23.
35. Tandle AT, Sanghvi V, Saranath D. Determination of p53 genotypes in oral cancer patients from India. Br J Cancer. 2001;84(6):739–42.
36. Jiang N, Pan J, Wang L, Duan YZ. No significant association between p53 codon 72 Arg/pro polymorphism and risk of oral cancer. Tumour Biol. 2013;34(1):587–96.
37. Hou J, Gu Y, Hou W, Wu S, Lou Y, Yang W, et al. P53 codon 72 polymorphism, human papillomavirus infection, and their interaction to oral carcinoma susceptibility. BMC Genet. 2015;16:72.
38. Drummond SN, De Marco L, Pordeus Ide A, Barbosa AA, Gomez RS. TP53 codon 72 polymorphism in oral squamous cell carcinoma. Anticancer Res. 2002;22(6a):3379–81.
39. Ihsan R, Devi TR, Yadav DS, Mishra AK, Sharma J, Zomawia E, et al. Investigation on the role of p53 codon 72 polymorphism and interactions with tobacco, betel quid, and alcohol in susceptibility to cancers in a high-risk population from north East India. DNA Cell Biol. 2011;30(3):163–71.
40. Jing G, Lv K, Jiao X. The p53 codon 72 polymorphism and the risk of oral Cancer in a Chinese Han population. Genetic Testing and Molecular Biomarkers. 2012;16(9):1149–52.
41. Kitkumthorn N, Yanatatsaneejit P, Rabalert J, Dhammawipark C, Mutirangura A. Association of P53 codon 72 polymorphism and ameloblastoma. Oral Dis. 2010;16(7):631–5.
42. Patel KR, Vajaria BN, Begum R, Shah FD, Patel JB, Shukla SN, et al. Association between p53 gene variants and oral cancer susceptibility in population from Gujarat, West India. Asian Pac J Cancer Prev. 2013;14(2):1093–100.
43. Storey A, Thomas M, Kalita A, Harwood C, Gardiol D, Mantovani F, et al. Role of a p53 polymorphism in the development of human papillomavirus-associated cancer. Nature. 1998;393(6682):229–34.
44. Wang Z, Sturgis EM, Zhang Y, Huang Z, Zhou Q, Wei Q, et al. Combined p53-related genetic variants together with HPV infection increase oral cancer risk. Int J Cancer. 2012;131(3):E251–8.
45. Zemleduch T, Lianeri M, Rydzanicz M, Gajecka M, Szyfter K, Jagodzinski PP. Contribution of polymorphism in codon 72 of TP53 gene to laryngeal cancer in polish patients. Oral Oncol. 2009;45(8):683–6.

31

Socioeconomic status, oral health and dental disease in Australia, Canada, New Zealand and the United States

Gloria C. Mejia[1*], Hawazin W. Elani[2], Sam Harper[3], W. Murray Thomson[4], Xiangqun Ju[1], Ichiro Kawachi[5], Jay S. Kaufman[3] and Lisa M. Jamieson[1]

Abstract

Background: Socioeconomic inequalities are associated with oral health status, either subjectively (self-rated oral health) or objectively (clinically-diagnosed dental diseases). The aim of this study is to compare the magnitude of socioeconomic inequality in oral health and dental disease among adults in Australia, Canada, New Zealand and the United States (US).

Methods: Nationally-representative survey examination data were used to calculate adjusted absolute differences (AD) in prevalence of untreated decay and fair/poor self-rated oral health (SROH) in income and education. We pooled age- and gender-adjusted inequality estimates using random effects meta-analysis.

Results: New Zealand demonstrated the highest adjusted estimate for untreated decay; the US showed the highest adjusted prevalence of fair/poor SROH. The meta-analysis showed little heterogeneity across countries for the prevalence of decayed teeth; the pooled ADs were 19.7 (95% CI = 16.7–22.7) and 12.0 (95% CI = 8.4–15.7) between highest and lowest education and income groups, respectively. There was heterogeneity in the mean number of decayed teeth and in fair/poor SROH. New Zealand had the widest inequality in decay (education AD = 0.8; 95% CI = 0.4–1.2; income AD = 1.0; 95% CI = 0.5–1.5) and the US the widest inequality in fair/poor SROH (education AD = 40.4; 95% CI = 35.2–45.5; income AD = 20.5; 95% CI = 13.0–27.9).

Conclusions: The differences in estimates, and variation in the magnitude of inequality, suggest the need for further examining socio-cultural and contextual determinants of oral health and dental disease in both the included and other countries.

Keywords: Socioeconomic factors, Dental caries, Self-report, Oral health

Background

Socioeconomic status has long held interest for its effect on general and oral health. Most evidence indicates that socioeconomic inequalities are associated with oral health status, whether subjectively (self-rated oral health) or objectively (clinically-diagnosed dental diseases) determined [1–4]. Monitoring social inequalities in oral health is important to provide information on population differences in oral health care needs, preventive practices and oral health system priorities.

* Correspondence: gloria.mejia@adelaide.edu.au
[1]Australian Research Centre for Population Oral Health, Adelaide Dental School, The University of Adelaide, Adelaide, SA 5005, Australia
Full list of author information is available at the end of the article

Previous studies have demonstrated that socioeconomic position is negatively associated with oral health and dental disease [3, 5], which means the higher the socioeconomic position, the better the perception of oral health and the less experience of clinically-diagnosed dental diseases. Education and income are the most common and relevant indicators used in epidemiology for socioeconomic status measurement [3–7]. Oral health, as a significant constituent of general health, relies on subjective perceptions, whereas disease measurement uses objective clinical indicators [1, 2].

Most previous studies estimated the association between socioeconomic and oral health status based on national surveys or on a specific population [5, 7–10].

Population determinants of health and disease are more likely to vary across countries than within countries, but it is impossible to generalize the strength and direction of associations across populations and time [11]. Therefore, a global approach is considered fundamental to 'public health epidemiology' because it allows identification of international patterns that lead to hypothesis generation, essential to scientific progress [11]. In addition, these studies generally estimated the association by using only one socioeconomic factor with clinical indicators of dental disease. Few studies have tackled both subjective (health) and objective or normative (disease) aspects [12]. Some have focused on low to middle income countries, with few cross-national comparisons [13–18]. Hence, the aim of this paper is to compare the magnitude of socioeconomic inequality in oral health and dental disease using representative datasets of adults in Australia, Canada, New Zealand and the United States.

Methods

Comparable high-income countries with dental health care delivery for the adult population based largely on fee-for-service [19, 20] were selected on the availability of nationally-representative survey examination data within a 5 year timeframe. The sources of data were: (1) Australia's National Survey of Adult Oral Health (NSAOH), conducted between 2004 and 2006 [21]; (2) the Canadian Health Measures Survey (CHMS) that was conducted between 2007 and 2009 [22]; (3) the New Zealand Oral Health Survey (NZOHS) that was conducted from February to December 2009 [23] and; (4) the 2003–2004 module of the US National Health and Nutrition Examination Survey (NHANES) [24]. All surveys included a comprehensive oral examination and detailed demographic and socioeconomic position data.

The NSAOH used a three-stage, stratified clustered design, with 14,123 adults aged 15 years and older taking part in a telephone interview. Of these, 5,505 respondents were invited for, and accepted, a dental examination [21]. The CHMS used a multi-stage stratified sampling design to interview and examine a total of 5,586 participants, including both children and adults [22]. The NZOHS examined 3,196 children and adults. The study base were participants in the previous New Zealand 2006/2007 health survey who agreed to be contacted for future surveys; this second survey was still found to be representative [23]. NHANES, a stratified multistage probability sample of the civilian non-institutionalized population of the US, examined 7,072 people [24].

The response rates for each survey were 49.0% (the interview participation rate) and 43.7% (the examination rate) (NSAOH) [21]; 69.9% of the selected households and among households, 88.3% and 84.9% of individuals (questionnaire and clinic component, respectively) (CHMS) [22], 41.0% (NZOHS) and 79% (interview) and 76% (examination) (NHANES) [25].

In this study, health was captured through the variable self-rated oral health, an indicator of subjective oral health status. In the NSAOH, the self-rated question read: "How would you rate your own dental health?" In the CHMS, the question used was "In general, would you say the health of your mouth is..." The NZOHS asked "How would you describe the health of your teeth or mouth?" In NHANES, the question was "How would you describe the condition of your teeth?" All surveys used the following ordinal response options: 'Excellent', 'Very good', 'Good', 'Fair' or 'Poor'. The responses were dichotomized into 'excellent, very good or good' and 'fair or poor'. Disease was assessed through clinical examination by registered and calibrated dental examiners by using a standard oral epidemiological method /the examination protocol - the U.S. National Institute of Dental Research (National Institute of Dental Research 1987) [26], as untreated tooth decay (% DT > 0) and the mean number of decayed teeth (mean DT). All analyses were based on 28 teeth, excluding third molars.

We used education and income as measures of socioeconomic position. Education was grouped into 4 comparable categories across the surveys (primary, secondary, post-secondary and University). We grouped income categories for each country by quantiles into equal thirds (low, medium, high). However, when converting the categories of income from the survey into tertiles, the resulting proportions were not exactly equal because of prior categorization in the original data collected in each survey.

We limited the analysis to adults aged 25 years and older in order to have a more stable measure of final educational attainment. We calculated absolute differences in prevalence (AD) to examine socioeconomic inequalities and we estimated pooled measures of inequality estimates using random effects meta-analysis.

All analyses were age and gender adjusted to the average covariate distribution of the four surveys combined. In addition, to make population inferences, we utilized survey weights to account for individual probabilities of selection and complex survey designs [21–24]. We used Stata statistical software (version 13.1) for all analyses [27].

Results

The combined study sample included 14,960 participants, of whom 33.9% were from Australia, 21.9% from Canada, 13.6% from New Zealand and 30.5% from the United States. Table 1 indicates that, across all countries, a slightly higher proportion of females were represented, with the mean population age ranging between 47.9 years for Canada and 49.5 years for Australia. In Australia, a greater proportion of individuals had a University educational

Table 1 Socio-demographic and outcome characteristics

Variables	Australia	Canada	New Zealand	United States
	National Survey of Adult Oral Health	Canadian Health Measures Survey[a]	New Zealand Oral Health Survey	National Health and Nutrition Examination Survey
	2004–2006	2007–2009	2009	2003–2004
	N = 5,073	*N* = 3,278	*N* = 2,041	*N* = 4,568
	N (%)[b]	N (%)[b]	N (%)[b]	N (%)[b]
Gender				
Male	2,016 (49.8)	(49.1)	793 (48.2)	2,200 (48.0)
Female	3,057 (50.2)	(50.9)	1,248 (51.9)	2,368 (52.0)
Education				
Primary	1,196 (22.8)	(12.8)	467 (19.8)	1,366 (18.6)
Secondary	478 (10.9)	(17.6)	307 (16.4)	1,134 (26.9)
Post-Secondary	1,521 (32.0)	(42.1)	800 (40.0)	1,189 (30.4)
Tertiary	1,634 (34.4)	(27.5)	444 (23.3)	865 (24.2)
Income				
Low	2,189 (37.4)	(6.3)	776 (24.7)	2,075 (36.1)
Medium	1,590 (35.0)	(36.0)	592 (29.0)	1,157 (30.2)
High	1,069 (27.6)	(57.7)	728 (46.4)	1,060 (33.8)
Mean age (years)	49.5 ± 14.7	47.9 ± 12.4	48.9 ± 13.0	48.9 ± 13.0

NB: all numbers are based on individuals aged 25 years or older
[a]Due to reasons of confidentiality, the only estimates available for Canada are weighted proportions (i.e. not N)
[b]Weighted proportions

level; in Canada, New Zealand and the United States, there was a greater proportion with post-secondary education. Australia also had the highest proportion of individuals with only primary education, and Canada the lowest.

Table 2 shows differences in prevalence and mean estimates among countries; for example, the prevalence of decayed teeth for highly educated New Zealanders was equal to that of the lowest educated group in the United States. The same was observed in the mean number of teeth with untreated decay. Downward gradients by educational level and income within countries favored the more socially advantaged socioeconomic groups. Australia showed a clear gradient in the adjusted estimate for the two disease measures (% DT > 0 and Mean DT) but it is less obvious for fair/poor self-rated oral health. Canada presents a gradient in the proportion of individuals with at least one untreated decayed tooth. New Zealand shows educational gradients in the proportion with untreated decay and fair/poor self-rated oral health. The apparent inconsistency in educational gradients for Canada and New Zealand in disease severity (mean DT) was minor and is likely explained by sampling variability. The United States consistently showed gradients that favor the most highly educated. By income, all countries present gradients for all measures in which lower income groups are more heavily burdened with poorer oral health.

As indicated by the adjusted absolute differences in Table 2, the greatest absolute inequalities between the extreme levels of education (Primary versus University) were in Canada for the proportion of individuals with untreated decay (AD = 22.1), in New Zealand for the mean number of untreated decayed teeth (AD = 0.8), and in the United States for fair/poor self-rated oral health (AD = 40.4). Also, shown in Table 2, the greatest absolute inequality in outcomes between extreme levels of income (Low versus High) is in New Zealand for the proportion with untreated decay (AD = 17.5) and the mean number of untreated decayed teeth (AD = 0.99), whereas, for fair or poor self-rated oral health, the greatest gap is in the United States (AD = 20.5).

Figure 1 presents meta-analysis estimates for educational inequality. The findings on educational inequality for the proportion of individuals with at least one tooth with untreated decay indicate that all variability in the effect sizes is attributable to sampling error ($I^2 = 0.0\%$); results for this measure may be considered to be essentially homogenous, with a pooled adjusted AD of 19.7. There was moderate heterogeneity ($I^2 = 57.5\%$) for the mean number of untreated decayed teeth; that is, roughly half of the variability was among countries and half of the variability was within

Table 2 Adjusted estimates and adjusted absolute difference (AD) for multiple oral health outcomes

	% DT > 0		Mean DT		% Fair/poor self-rated oral health	
	Adjusted estimate (95% CI)	AD (95% CI)	Adjusted estimate (95% CI)	AD (95% CI)	Adjusted estimate (95% CI)	AD (95% CI)
Australia[a]						
Education						
Primary	32.7 (28.1, 37.2)	18.4 (13.1, 23.7)	0.8 (0.7, 1.0)	0.6 (0.4, 0.8)	24.5 (22.4, 26.6)	10.9 (8.4, 13.3)
Secondary	28.6 (22.7, 34.6)	14.4 (7.7, 21.0)	0.5 (0.4, 0.7)	0.3 (0.2, 0.5)	16.3 (13.4, 19.1)	2.7 (−0.4, 5.7)
Post-secondary	23.3 (19.9, 26.6)	9.0 (4.9, 13.1)	0.5 (0.4, 0.6)	0.3 (0.2, 0.4)	17.7 (16.1, 19.4)	4.1 (2.0, 6.3)
University	14.3 (11.8, 16.8)	Ref	0.2 (0.2, 0.3)	Ref	13.6 (12.1, 15.1)	Ref
Income						
Low	27.7 (24.3, 31.0)	11.9 (6.8, 17.0)	0.6 (0.5, 0.7)	0.4 (0.2, 0.5)	25.3 (23.2, 27.4)	13.9 (11.1, 16.8)
Medium	22.5 (19.5, 25.5)	6.8 (2.1, 11.4)	0.4 (0.4, 0.5)	0.2 (0.1, 0.3)	14.4 (13.0, 15.9)	3.1 (0.9, 5.2)
High	15.8 (12.3, 19.3)	Ref	0.3 (0.2, 0.3)	Ref	11.4 (9.6, 13.1)	Ref
Canada[b]						
Education						
Primary	32.3 (25.2, 39.5)	22.1 (14.2, 30.0)	0.9 (0.6, 1.1)	0.7 (0.4, 0.9)	23.7 (17.7, 29.6)	13.0 (6.2, 19.7)
Secondary	25.4 (19.9, 31.0)	15.2 (8.8, 21.6)	0.9 (0.6, 1.3)	0.7 (0.4, 1.1)	24.5 (18.7, 30.3)	13.8 (7.3, 20.4)
Post-secondary	18.0 (15.0, 21.1)	7.8 (3.7, 12.0)	0.4 (0.4, 0.5)	0.2 (0.1, 0.3)	13.1 (10.6, 15.5)	2.4 (−1.3, 6.1)
University	10.2 (7.3, 13.2)	Ref	0.2 (0.1, 0.3)	Ref	10.7 (7.9,13.5)	Ref
Income						
Low	31.1 (22.5, 39.8)	16.7 (7.5, 25.9)	0.9 (0.6, 1.2)	0.6 (0.3, 1.0)	28.4 (20.7, 36.0)	16.9 (8.9, 24.9)
Medium	22.4 (18.5, 26.4)	8.0 (3.0, 12.9)	0.7 (0.5, 0.8)	0.4 (0.2, 0.5)	19.7 (16.3, 23.1)	8.3 (4.1, 12.5)
High	14.5 (11.9, 17.1)	Ref	0.3 (0.2, 0.4)	Ref	11.4 (9.2, 13.7)	Ref
New Zealand[c]						
Education						
Primary	46.5 (37.6, 55.5)	17.7 (6.6, 28.7)	1.4 (1.0, 1.7)	0.8 (0.4, 1.2)	41.0 (32.0, 49.9)	17.6 (7.1, 28.1)
Secondary	42.9 (36.8, 49.0)	14.1 (5.1, 23.1)	0.9 (0.8, 1.1)	0.4 (0.1, 0.6)	30.1 (24.4, 35.8)	6.7 (−1.3, 14.7)
Post-secondary	35.6 (30.9, 40.3)	6.8 (−1.3, 14.8)	1.1 (0.9, 1.3)	0.5 (0.2, 0.8)	27.5 (23.3, 31.8)	4.2 (−2.9, 11.2)
University	28.8 (22.4, 35.3)	Ref	0.6 (0.4, 0.7)	Ref	23.4 (17.9, 28.9)	Ref
Income						
Low	43.4 (36.0, 50.8)	17.5 (8.0, 26.9)	1.5 (1.1, 2.0)	1.0 (0.5, 1.5)	38.3 (31.1, 45.5)	18.8 (9.8, 27.8)
Medium	40.3 (33.2, 47.4)	14.3 (5.4, 23.3)	0.9 (0.7, 1.1)	0.4 (0.2, 0.6)	31.4 (24.6, 38.2)	11.9 (3.7, 20.1)
High	26.0 (20.5, 31.4)	Ref	0.5 (0.4, 0.7)	Ref	19.6 (14.8, 24.3)	Ref
United States[d]						
Education						
Primary	28.7 (24.1, 33.3)	20.1 (15.8, 24.5)	0.6 (0.5, 0.7)	0.4 (0.3, 0.5)	64.5 (61.1 67.9)	40.4 (35.2, 45.5)
Secondary	19.0 (13.8, 24.2)	10.4 (4.7, 16.2)	0.4 (0.3, 0.5)	0.3 (0.1, 0.4)	51.7 (47.4, 56.0)	27.5 (22.6, 32.5)
Post-secondary	16.3 (12.7, 19.9)	7.7 (3.6, 11.8)	0.3 (0.2, 0.4)	0.2 (0.1, 0.2)	45.0 (41.1, 48.9)	20.8 (16.3, 25.4)
University	8.6 (5.5, 11.7)	Ref	0.2 (0.1, 0.2)	Ref	24.1 (20.1, 28.2)	Ref
Income						
Low	21.1 (17.4, 24.8)	8.9 (4.8, 13.1)	0.4 (0.3, 0.5)	0.2 (0.1, 0.4)	54.0 (50.0, 58.1)	20.5 (13.0, 28.0)
Medium	15.6 (11.3, 20.0)	3.4 (−2.2, 9.0)	0.3 (0.2, 0.4)	0.1 (−0.1, 0.2)	43.5 (38.6, 48.4)	10.0 (3.8, 16.2)
High	12.2 (8.3, 16.2)	Ref	0.2 (0.1, 0.3)	Ref	33.5 (28.7, 38.4)	Ref

NB: Data based on ages 25 years and older. Education adjusted for age and gender and Income adjusted for age, gender and education
[a]National Survey of Adult Oral Health, 2004–2006
[b]Canadian Health Measures Survey, 2007–2009
[c]New Zealand Oral Health Survey, 2009
[d]National Health and Nutrition Examination Survey, 2003–2004

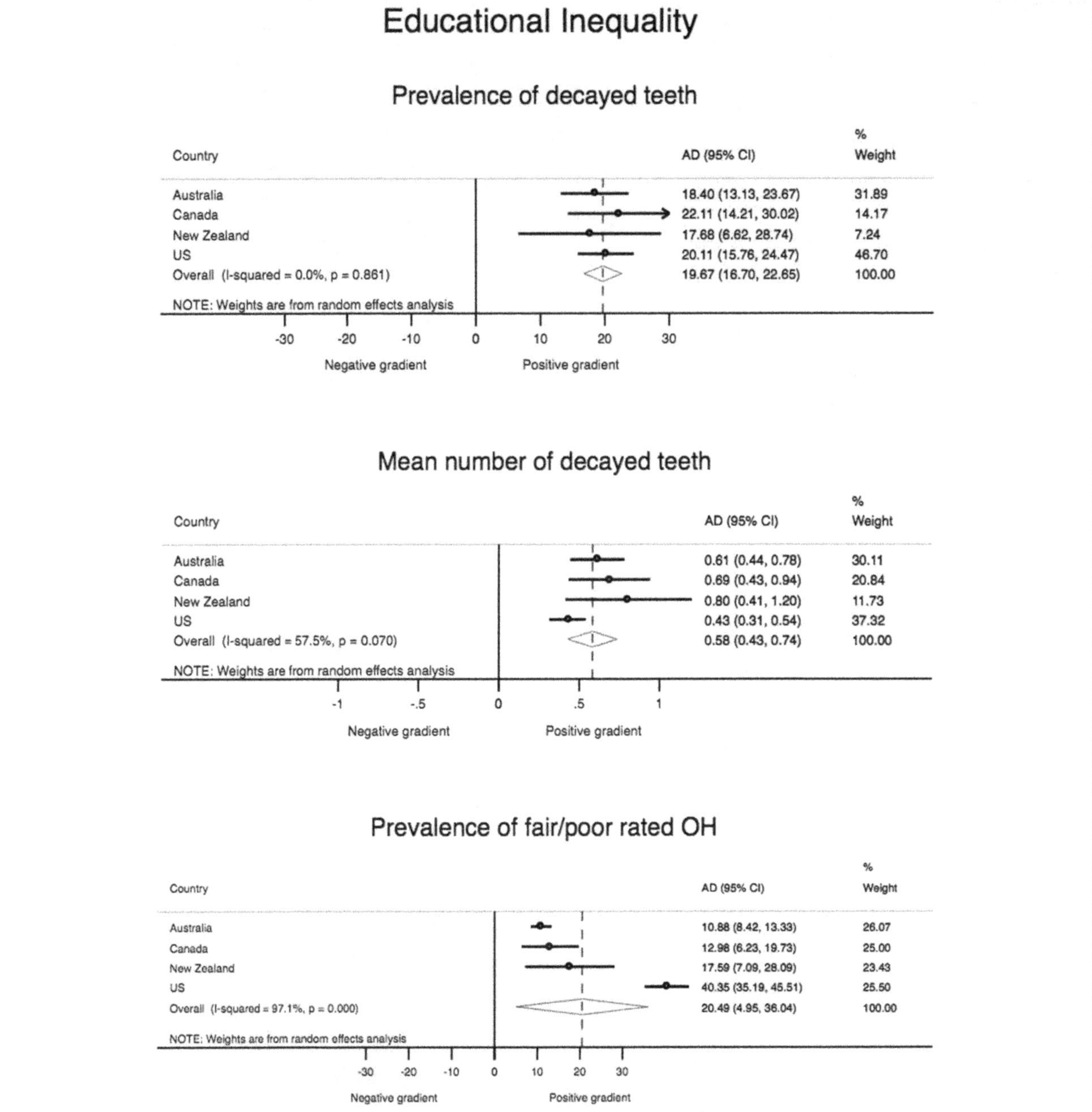

Fig. 1 Meta-analysis estimates for educational inequality

countries. New Zealand had the widest absolute socioeconomic inequality (AD = 0.8) and the United States had the narrowest (AD = 0.4). For fair or poor self-rated oral health, the United States had the widest inequality gap (AD = 40.4) and Australia the narrowest (AD = 10.9) with almost all of the variation occurring across countries ($I^2 = 97.1\%$).

The meta-analysis for income inequality (Fig. 2) indicates modest heterogeneity across countries in the pooled estimate for the prevalence of untreated decayed teeth ($I^2 = 29.3\%$), with New Zealand having the widest gap and the United States the narrowest (AD = 17.5 and 8.9, respectively). The other measure of dental disease — the mean number of teeth with untreated decay — showed more profound heterogeneity of effect estimates ($I^2 = 76.4\%$). Again, New Zealand presented the greatest magnitude of absolute inequality (AD = 0.99), translating into a clinical difference of one tooth, and the United States presented the lowest magnitude of effect (AD = 0.22). There was low heterogeneity in the measure of fair/poor self-rated oral health, with a pooled adjusted absolute difference of 15.8 percentage points, ranging from 13.9 for Australia to 20.5 for the United States.

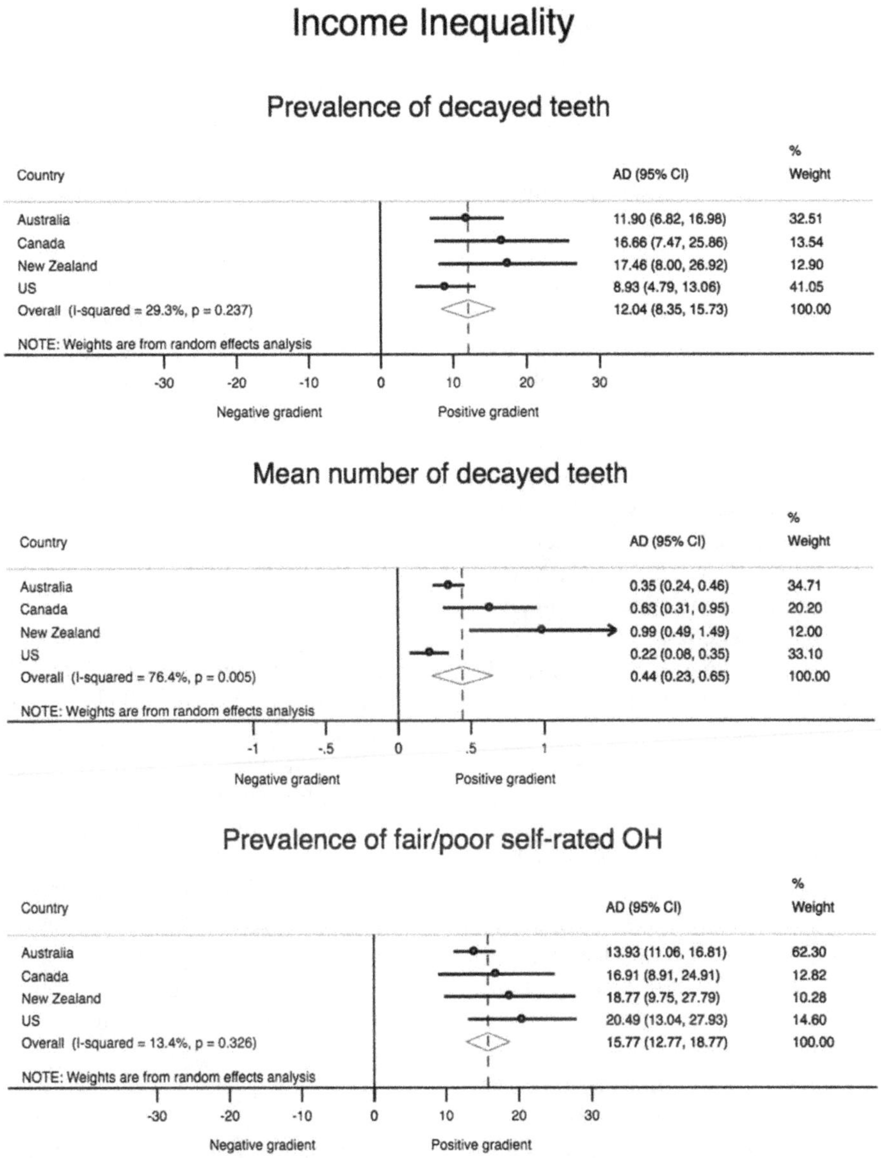

Fig. 2 Meta-analysis for income inequality

Discussion

The findings demonstrate socioeconomic inequality in self-rated oral health and untreated dental caries among adults in Australia, Canada, New Zealand and the United States, yet they also highlight some important differences across countries. While New Zealand had the highest absolute inequality in measures of disease, the United States had the highest gaps in perceptions of oral health.

Measures of health status based solely on the objective assessment of pathological abnormality do not include non-biological aspects of health such as the mental and social wellbeing of individuals. We represented disease through normative clinical measures of untreated tooth decay and the magnitude or extent of the disease through the mean number of decayed teeth. To measure oral health, we used self-rated health, considered as "the most feasible, most inclusive and most informative measure of health status" [28].

Interestingly, our findings indicate that New Zealand had greater disease and wider socioeconomic gaps in the proportion and mean number of untreated decay than the other countries, despite having arguably the most comprehensive, wide ranging and free public dental service in the world, that is available to all aged below 18 years (through the School Dental Service). A possible explanation may lie in New Zealand not having a means-tested public dental service for low-income adults (those aged 18+ years), whereas such services are available in Canada, Australia and, to some extent, the United States.

Our study did not examine the effects of other contributing factors such as water fluoridation. It is estimated that 79% of the Australian population, 53% of the New Zealand population, 42% of Canadian population and 60% of the US population is supplied with artificially fluoridated water [29]. Water fluoridation has been regarded as the most effective way to reduce the prevalence and severity of caries, as well as socioeconomic disparities in its occurrence [30]. Although a side-effect of water fluoridation is mild fluorosis of enamel, manifesting a slightly more opaque enamel that is generally perceived by lay people as being aesthetically better, with concomitant effects on their self-rated oral health [31].

The United States had the most unfavorable indicators of oral health, in terms of self-ratings, which is in sharp contrast with self-ratings of general health, in which Americans perform relatively well [32]. In global health measures, the intrinsic value individuals assign to health is driven by a multitude of factors including socio-cultural environments and personal experiences [33].

Dissatisfaction with dental appearance is associated with tooth alignment and crowding, fractures in anterior teeth, and discrepancies in tooth shade [34–36]. It relates respectively to orthodontic treatment, aesthetic restorations and tooth bleaching [34, 35, 37]. Oro-facial aesthetics and appearance have been shown to be associated with self-ratings of oral health in diverse population samples [36, 38–41]. It is possible that the contemporary emphasis on dental aesthetics (such as tooth whitening) contributes to a general dissatisfaction in dental appearance and hence poorer self-rated oral health, whereas the same does not occur for general health.

Differences in reporting may arise from cultural perceptions of health, differences in health expectations and adaptability to ill-health, but also from the way in which the ordinal scale is understood by different individuals and how they weigh the different factors involved in the global measure [42, 43]. In this study, the wording of the SROH question varied slightly among the countries, with NSAOH and NHANES asking specifically about dental health/teeth, Canada framed the question in terms of health of the mouth and New Zealand asked for the health of both the teeth and mouth. Also noteworthy is that the United States asked about the 'condition' of the teeth, whereas all other countries framed the question around 'health', which could influence how the question is interpreted and may aid in explaining the large difference between the United States and the other countries. A limitation of the study was the inability to measure the extent to which the differences in terminology influenced the findings.

Differences in self-reports may be explained in terms of optimism, such as the ability among older people to adapt to slow declining health, and higher expectations when more socially advantaged groups, for example, report poorer health states [44]. Rousseau and colleagues [45] reported as such, arguing that the complete loss of all teeth is considered by middle-class people to be far more catastrophic than it is by working-class people, because of differing social norms. It is also possible that the frame of reference through which societies in a given country view disease differs; for example, Australians had the lowest levels of self-rated fair or poor health yet their levels of disease were as high as or higher than disease in the United States. Even subtle differences in subjective ratings point towards cultural, social and psychosocial influences on oral health [46]. Given the cultural and context-specific nature of self-rated health, our findings cannot necessarily be generalized to countries beyond those included in the analysis, and caution needs to be taken when making international comparisons [28, 33].

The study explored two socioeconomic indicators to draw a clear picture of social inequalities. Education has the potential to translate into employment opportunities, receptiveness to health messages and the ability to navigate health care systems, as well as representing values, beliefs, and attitudes. It captures the long-term effects of early life conditions and adult resources on health [47]. Income, which measures material resources and living standards, has a cumulative effect over the life course yet is dynamic in the short-term and may be prone to reverse causality if deteriorating health contributes to changes in income [47].

Whereas educational gradients in oral health and disease show some inconsistencies among countries, income shows consistently clear gradients across all countries. In terms of dental disease, this reflects the ability to access oral health care, favoring populations with higher income. In terms of perceived oral health, those with lower incomes reported lower self-ratings. If this general dissatisfaction were to lead to lower self-ratings than warranted by 'objective' health, and higher social groups were to systematically report better health than justified, such differences could lead to overestimates of health inequities [43]. Our study did not explore such possibilities at the individual level, but, on average, socially advantaged groups had better oral health, indicating that such overestimation is unlikely.

The limitations of the study were:

(1) there was no overlap of time period for all four surveys, although it is unlikely inequality estimates would differ systematically as major changes in chronic dental diseases are not expected within short time frames; and (2) Missing data for each survey could affect the findings; however, analyses of bias due to survey non-response was carried out independently, at least in the NSAOH, [21] indicating estimates are unlikely to be affected by systematic error. In addition we used weighted data to

account for sampling probabilities and adjusted for age and gender.

An important next step is to compare socio-cultural and health system characteristics that shape disease and health status measures among different countries in order to have a better understanding of the roles these factors and other social determinants play in population oral health.

Conclusion

Our findings demonstrate differences in oral health and dental disease experience across income and education groups, with socioeconomic gradients for both clinically determined and self-reported indicators. Individuals from lower income and education groups consistently experienced higher burdens of untreated dental decay and poorer self-rated oral health. Differences in outcome estimates within countries also indicate conceptual differences between health and disease. The variation in the magnitude of inequality across countries suggests the need for further understanding socio-cultural and contextual determinants of oral health and dental disease.

Abbreviations

AD: Absolute differences; CHMS: The Canadian Health Measures Survey; DT: Decayed teeth; NHANES: The US National Health and Nutrition Examination Survey; NSAOH: Australia's National Survey of Adult Oral Health; NZOHS: The New Zealand Oral Health Survey; SROH: Self-rated oral health; US: The United States

Funding

JSK was supported by the Canada Research Chairs program. SH was partially supported by a Chercheur-boursier Junior 2 grant from the Fonds de recherche du Québec—Santé. NSAOH was supported by Australian Government health agencies, including National Health and Medical Research Council (NHMRC) grants #299060, #349514, and #349537. The Australian Dental Association and state and territory health departments and dental services are also acknowledged. Colgate Oral Care provided gifts for participants.

Authors' contributions

GM contributed to the conception and design of the study, data acquisition, analysis and interpretation, drafting of the manuscript, critical revisions and approval of the final version. HE contributed to conception and design, acquisition, analysis and interpretation of data, critical review of manuscript drafts and approval of version to be published. SH and JK contributed to the conception and design of the study, interpretation of data, critical review of manuscript and approval of final version. MT contributed to the conception and study design, acquisition of data, analysis and interpretation, critically reviewed the manuscript and approved the final version. XJ contributed to the analysis and interpretation of the data, was involved in drafting and reviewing the manuscript and approved the final version. IK critically revised the manuscript for important intellectual content and provided final approval. LJ contributed to the conception and design of the study, acquisition of the data, interpretation of results, critical review of manuscript drafts and provided final approval. All authors read and approved the final manuscript

Competing interests

The authors declare that they have no competing interests.

Author details

[1]Australian Research Centre for Population Oral Health, Adelaide Dental School, The University of Adelaide, Adelaide, SA 5005, Australia. [2]Harvard School of Dental Medicine, Harvard University, Boston, MA, USA. [3]Department of Epidemiology, Biostatistics & Occupational Health, McGill University, Montreal, Quebec H3A 1A2, Canada. [4]Sir John Walsh Research Institute, Faculty of Dentistry, The University of Otago, Dunedin, New Zealand. [5]Social and Behavioral Sciences, Harvard T.H. Chan School of Public Health, Boston, MA 02115, USA.

References

1. Locker D, Slade G. Association between clinical and subjective indicators of oral health status in an older adult population. Gerontology. 1994;11:108–14.
2. Bowling A. Concepts of functioning, health, well-being and quality of life. In: Measuring health. A review of quality of life measurement scales. 3rd ed. Maidenhead: Open University Press; 2005. p. 1–9.
3. Tsakos G, Demakakos P, Breeze E, Watt RG. Social gradients in oral health in older adults: findings from the English longitudinal survey of aging. Am J Public Health. 2011;101:1892–9.
4. Watson CA, Nilam S. Educational level as a social determinant of health and its relationship to periodontal disease as a health outcome. J Dent Sci Ther. 2017;1:8–11.
5. Mejia G, Jamieson LM, Ha D, Spencer AJ. Greater inequalities in dental treatment than in disease experience. J Dent Res. 2014;93:966–71.
6. Steele J, Shen J, Tsakos G, Fuller E, Morris S, Watt R, et al. The Interplay between socioeconomic inequalities and clinical oral health. J Dent Res. 2015;94:19–26.
7. Borrell LN, Burt BA, Neighbors HW, Taylor GW. Social factors and periodontitis in an older population. Am J Public Health. 2004;94:748–54.
8. Tsakos G, Sheiham A, Iliffe S, Kharicha K, Harari D, Swift CG, et al. The impact of educational level on oral health-related quality of life in older people in London. Eur J Oral Sci. 2009;117:286–92.
9. Sabbah W, Tsakos G, Sheiham A, Watt RG. The role of health-related behaviors in the socioeconomic disparities in oral health. Soc Sci Med. 2009; 68:298–303.
10. Moradi G, Moinafshar A, Adabi H, Sharafi M, Mostafavi F, Bolbanabad AM. Socioeconomic inequalities in the oral health of people aged 15-40 years in Kurdistan, Iran in 2015: a cross-sectional study. J Prev Med Public Health. 2017;50:303–10.
11. Pearce N. Global epidemiology: the importance of international comparisons and collaborations. OA Epidemiology. 2013;1:15.
12. Takagi D, Watanabe Y, Edahiro A, Ohara Y, Murakami M, Murakami K, et al. Factors affecting masticatory function of community-dwelling older people: investigation of the differences in the relevant factors for subjective and objective assessment. Gerodontology. 2017;34:357–64.
13. Bhandari B, Newton JT, Bernabé E. Social inequalities in adult oral health in 40 low- and middle-income countries. Int Dent J. 2016;66:295–303.
14. Shen J, Listl S. Investigating social inequalities in older adults' dentition and the role of dental service use in 14 European countries. Eur J Health Econ. 2016. https://doi.org/10.1007/s10198-016-0866-2.
15. Elani HW, Harper S, Allison PJ, Bedos C, Kaufman JS. Socio-economic inequalities and Oral health in Canada and the United States. J Dent Res. 2012;91:865–70.
16. Peres MA, Luzzi L, Peres KG, Sabbah W, Antunes JL, Do LG. Income-related inequalities in inadequate dentition over time in Australia, Brazil and USA adults. Community Dent Oral Epidemiol. 2015;43:217–25.
17. Sanders AE, Slade GD, John MT, Steele JG, Suominen-Taipale AL, Lahti S, et al. A cross-national comparison of income gradients in oral health quality of life in four welfare states: application of the Korpi and Palme typology. J Epidemiol Community Health. 2009;63:569–74.
18. He S, Thomson WM. An oral epidemiological comparison of Chinese and New Zealand adults in 2 key age groups. Community Dent Oral Epidemiol. 2018;46:154–60.
19. Downer MC, Drugan CS, Blinkhorn AS. Salaried services in the delivery of dental care in Western industrialised countries: implications for the National Health Service in England. Int Dent J. 2006;56:7–16.
20. Ju X, Brennan DS, Spencer AJ, Teusner DN. Longitudinal change in dental visits provided by Australian dentists. J Public Health Dent. 2016;76:30–7.
21. Slade GD, Spencer AJ, Roberts-Thomson KD. Australia's dental generations. the National Survey of Adult Oral Health 2004–06. AIHW cat. No. DEN 165. Canberra: Australian Institute of Health and Welfare (Dental Statistics and Research Series No. 34); 2007. https://www.adelaide.edu.au/arcpoh/downloads/publications/reports/dental-statistics-research-series/nsaoh-report.pdf

22. Health Canada. Report on the findings of the oral health component of the Canadian Health Measures Survey 2007–2009. HC Pub.:100183. Ottawa: Publications Health Canada; 2010. http://publications.gc.ca/collections/collection_2010/sc-hc/H34-221-2010-eng.pdf Accessed 26 June 2017
23. New Zealand Ministry of Health. Our oral health: Key findings of the 2009 New Zealand oral health survey (NZOHS). Ministry of Health. 2010. http://www.health.govt.nz/publication/our-oral-health-key-findings-2009-new-zealand-oral-health-survey. Accessed 26 June 2017.
24. Centers for Disease Control and Prevention. National Center for Health Statistics. National Health and nutrition examination survey. 2005. https://wwwn.cdc.gov/nchs/nhanes/Default.aspx. Accessed 26 June 2017.
25. Centers for Disease Control and Prevention. National Center for Health Statistics. National Health and Nutrition Examination Survey. https://wwwn.cdc.gov/nchs/data/nhanes3/ResponseRates/RRT0304MF.pdf. Accessed 16 February 2018.
26. National Institute of Dental Research. Oral Health of United States adult. National finding. NIH Publication. 87–2868. US Department of Health and Human Services, Public Service, National Institutes of Health, 1987.
27. StataCorp. Stata Statistical Software. Release 13. College Station: StataCorp LP; 2013.
28. Jylhä M. What is self-rated health and why does it predict mortality? Towards a unified conceptual model. Soc Sci Med. 2009;69:307–16.
29. O'Mullane DM, Baez RJ, Jones S, Lennon MA, Petersen PE, RuggGunn AJ, et al. Fluoride and oral health. Comm Dent Health. 2016;33:69–99.
30. Burt BA. Fluoridation and social equity. J Public Health Dent. 2002;62:195–200.
31. Do LG, Spencer AJ. Oral health-related quality of life of children by dental caries and fluorosis experience. J Public Health Dent. 2007;67(3):132–9.
32. Office of Disease Prevention and Health Promotion (ODPHP). Healthy People 2020. Washington: US Dept of health and human services; 2007. https://www.healthypeople.gov/2020/prevention-portal-508/office/office-of-disease-prevention-and-health-promotion. Accessed 26 June 2017
33. Hardy MA, Acciai F, Reyes AM. How health conditions translate into self-ratings: a comparative study of older adults across Europe. J Health Soc Behav. 2014;55:320–41.
34. Al-Zarea BK. Satisfaction with appearance and the desired treatment to improve aesthetics. Int J Dent. 2013;912368:7. https://doi.org/10.1155/2013/912368. Epub 2013 Feb 20.
35. Maghaireh GA, Alzaraikat H, Taha NA. Satisfaction with dental appearance and attitude toward improving dental esthetics among patients attending a dental teaching center. J Contemp Dent Pract. 2016;17:16–21.
36. Larsson P, John MT, Nilner K, List T. Normative values for the oro-facial esthetic scale in Sweden. J Oral Rehab. 2014;41:148–54.
37. Silva FBD, Chisini LA, Demarco FF, Horta BL, Correa MB. Desire for tooth bleaching and treatment performed in Brazilian adults: findings from a birth cohort. Braz Oral Res. 2018;32:e12.
38. Matthias RE, Atchison KA, Lubben JE, De Jong F, Schweitzer SO. Factors affecting self-ratings of oral health. J Public Health Dent. 1995;55:197–204.
39. Pattussi MP, Olinto MTA, Hardy R, Sheiham A. Clinical, social and psychosocial factors associated with self-rated oral health in Brazilian adolescents. Comm Dent Oral Epidemiol. 2007;35:377–86.
40. Pattussi MP, Peres KG, Boing AF, Peres MA, da Costa JSD. Self-rated oral health and associated factors in Brazilian elders. Comm Dent Oral Epidemiol. 2010;38:348–59.
41. Carlsson V, Hakeberg M, Blomkvist K, Boman UW. Orofacial esthetics and dental anxiety: associations with oral and psychological health. Acta Odontol Scand. 2014;78:703–13.
42. Allison P, Locker D, Jokovic A, Slade G. A cross-cultural study of oral health values. J Dent Res. 1999;78:643–9.
43. Dowd JB. Whiners, deniers, and self-rated health: what are the implications for measuring health inequalities? A commentary on Layes, et al. Soc Sci Med 2012;75:10–13.
44. Layes A, Adada Y, Kephart G. Whiners and deniers – what does self-rated health measure? Soc Sci Med. 2012;75:1–9.
45. Rousseau N, Steele J, May C, Exley C. Your whole life is lived through your teeth: biographical disruption and experiences of tooth loss and replacement. Sociol Health Illn. 2014;36:462–76.
46. Slade GD, Nuttall N, Sanders AE, Steele JG, Allen PF, Lahti S. Impacts of oral disorders in the United Kingdom and Australia. British Dent J. 2005;198:489–93.
47. Shaw M, Galobardes B, Lawlor D, Lynch J, Wheeler B, Davey-Smith G. The handbook of inequality and socioeconomic position: concepts and measures. Chicago: The Policy Press; 2007.

Permissions

All chapters in this book were first published in OH, by BioMed Central; hereby published with permission under the Creative Commons Attribution License or equivalent. Every chapter published in this book has been scrutinized by our experts. Their significance has been extensively debated. The topics covered herein carry significant findings which will fuel the growth of the discipline. They may even be implemented as practical applications or may be referred to as a beginning point for another development.

The contributors of this book come from diverse backgrounds, making this book a truly international effort. This book will bring forth new frontiers with its revolutionizing research information and detailed analysis of the nascent developments around the world.

We would like to thank all the contributing authors for lending their expertise to make the book truly unique. They have played a crucial role in the development of this book. Without their invaluable contributions this book wouldn't have been possible. They have made vital efforts to compile up to date information on the varied aspects of this subject to make this book a valuable addition to the collection of many professionals and students.

This book was conceptualized with the vision of imparting up-to-date information and advanced data in this field. To ensure the same, a matchless editorial board was set up. Every individual on the board went through rigorous rounds of assessment to prove their worth. After which they invested a large part of their time researching and compiling the most relevant data for our readers.

The editorial board has been involved in producing this book since its inception. They have spent rigorous hours researching and exploring the diverse topics which have resulted in the successful publishing of this book. They have passed on their knowledge of decades through this book. To expedite this challenging task, the publisher supported the team at every step. A small team of assistant editors was also appointed to further simplify the editing procedure and attain best results for the readers.

Apart from the editorial board, the designing team has also invested a significant amount of their time in understanding the subject and creating the most relevant covers. They scrutinized every image to scout for the most suitable representation of the subject and create an appropriate cover for the book.

The publishing team has been an ardent support to the editorial, designing and production team. Their endless efforts to recruit the best for this project, has resulted in the accomplishment of this book. They are a veteran in the field of academics and their pool of knowledge is as vast as their experience in printing. Their expertise and guidance has proved useful at every step. Their uncompromising quality standards have made this book an exceptional effort. Their encouragement from time to time has been an inspiration for everyone.

The publisher and the editorial board hope that this book will prove to be a valuable piece of knowledge for researchers, students, practitioners and scholars across the globe.

List of Contributors

Eijiro Yamaga, Yusuke Sato and Shunsuke Minakuchi
Gerodontology and Oral Rehabilitation, Department of Gerontology and Gerodontology, Graduate School of Medical and Dental Sciences, Tokyo Medical and Dental University, Yushima Bunkyo-ku, Tokyo 113-8549, Japan

Nicola Schmidt, Michael Schauseil, Steffen Stein and Heike Maria Korbmacher-Steiner
Department of Orthodontics, University Hospital Giessen and Marburg, Campus Marburg, Georg-Voigt-Strasse 3, 35039 Marburg, Germany

Andreas Hellak
Department of Orthodontics, University Hospital Giessen and Marburg, Campus Marburg, Georg-Voigt-Strasse 3, 35039 Marburg, Germany
Abt. für Kieferorthopädie, UKGM Standort Marburg, Georg-Voigt-Strasse 3, 35039 Marburg, Germany

Thomas Drechsler
Private practice, Wiesbaden, Germany

Yu-Hsuan Hu, Aileen Tsai, Li-Wei Ou-Yang, Li-Chuan Chuang and Pei-Ching Chang
Department of Pediatric Dentistry, Chang Gung Memorial Hospital, Linkou, Taiwan, Republic of China
Department of Pediatric Dentistry, Chang Gung Memorial Hospital, No. 5 Fu-Hsing Street. Kuei Shan Hsiang, Taoyuan, Taiwan, Republic of China

Manika Govil and Nandita Mukhopadhyay
Center for Craniofacial and Dental Genetics, Department of Oral Biology, School of Dental Medicine, University of Pittsburgh, Suite 500 Bridgeside Point, 100 Technology Drive, Pittsburgh, PA 15219, USA

John R. Shaffer and Alexandre R. Vieira
Center for Craniofacial and Dental Genetics, Department of Oral Biology, School of Dental Medicine, University of Pittsburgh, Suite 500 Bridgeside Point, 100 Technology Drive, Pittsburgh, PA 15219, USA
Department of Human Genetics, Graduate School of Public Health, University of Pittsburgh, Pittsburgh, PA, USA

Eleanor Feingold
Center for Craniofacial and Dental Genetics, Department of Oral Biology, School of Dental Medicine, University of Pittsburgh, Suite 500 Bridgeside Point, 100 Technology Drive, Pittsburgh, PA 15219, USA
Department of Human Genetics, Graduate School of Public Health, University of Pittsburgh, Pittsburgh, PA, USA
Department of Biostatistics, Graduate School of Public Health, University of Pittsburgh, Pittsburgh, PA, USA

Mary L. Marazita
Center for Craniofacial and Dental Genetics, Department of Oral Biology, School of Dental Medicine, University of Pittsburgh, Suite 500 Bridgeside Point, 100 Technology Drive, Pittsburgh, PA 15219, USA
Department of Human Genetics, Graduate School of Public Health, University of Pittsburgh, Pittsburgh, PA, USA
Clinical and Translational Science Institute, and Department of Psychiatry, School of Medicine, University of Pittsburgh, Pittsburgh, PA, USA

Daniel E. Weeks
Department of Human Genetics, Graduate School of Public Health, University of Pittsburgh, Pittsburgh, PA, USA
Department of Biostatistics, Graduate School of Public Health, University of Pittsburgh, Pittsburgh, PA, USA

Steven M. Levy
Department of Preventive and Community Dentistry, University of Iowa College of Dentistry, Iowa City, IA, USA
Department of Epidemiology, University of Iowa College of Public Health, Iowa City, IA, USA

Rebecca L. Slayton
Department of Pediatric Dentistry, School of Dentistry, University of Washington, Seattle, WA, USA

Daniel W. McNeil
Dental Practice and Rural Health, West Virginia University School of Dentistry, Morgantown, WV, USA

Department of Psychology, Eberly College of Arts and Sciences, West Virginia University, Morgantown, WV, USA

Robert J. Weyant
Department of Dental Public Health and Information Management, School of Dental Medicine, University of Pittsburgh, Pittsburgh, PA, USA

Richard J. Crout
Department of Periodontics, West Virginia University School of Dentistry, Morgantown, WV, USA

Hongru Su and Wenhao Qian
Xuhui District Dental Centre, Shanghai, China

Renren Yang, Qinglong Deng and Jinming Yu
Collaborative Innovation Centre of Social Risks Governance in Health, School of Public Health, Fudan University, Shanghai, China

Felice Amoo-Achampong, David E. Vitunac and Kathleen Deeley
Departments of Oral Biology, University of Pittsburgh School of Dental, Medicine, 412 Salk Pavilion, Pittsburgh, PA 15261, USA

Adriana Modesto and Alexandre R. Vieira
Departments of Oral Biology, University of Pittsburgh School of Dental, Medicine, 412 Salk Pavilion, Pittsburgh, PA 15261, USA
Pediatric Dentistry, University of Pittsburgh School of Dental Medicine, 412 Salk Pavilion, Pittsburgh, PA 15261, USA

Minmin Tan, Zhaowu Chai, Chengjun Sun, Bo Hu, Xiang Gao and Yunjia Chen
College of Stomatology, Chongqing Medical University, Chongqing, China
Chongqing Key Laboratory of Oral Diseases and Biomedical Sciences, College of Stomatology, Chongqing Medical University, Chongqing, China
Chongqing Municipal Key Laboratory of Oral Biomedical Engineering of Higher Education, College of Stomatology, Chongqing Medical University, Chongqing, China

Jinlin Song
College of Stomatology, Chongqing Medical University, Chongqing, China
Chongqing Key Laboratory of Oral Diseases and Biomedical Sciences, College of Stomatology, Chongqing Medical University, Chongqing, China
Chongqing Municipal Key Laboratory of Oral Biomedical Engineering of Higher Education, College of Stomatology, Chongqing Medical University, Chongqing, China
Stomatological Hospital affiliated to Chongqing Medical University, No. 426, N. Songshi Rd, Chongqing 401147, China

A. J. Lubon, D. J. Erchick, J. Katz and L. C. Mullany
Department of International Health, Johns Hopkins Bloomberg School of Public Health, 615 N. Wolfe Street W5009, Baltimore, MD 21205, USA

S. C. Le Clerq
Department of International Health, Johns Hopkins Bloomberg School of Public Health, 615 N. Wolfe Street W5009, Baltimore, MD 21205, USA
Nepal Nutrition Intervention Project - Sarlahi (NNIPS), Krishna Galli, Lalitpur, Kathmandu, Nepal

S. K. Khatry
Nepal Nutrition Intervention Project - Sarlahi (NNIPS), Krishna Galli, Lalitpur, Kathmandu, Nepal

N. K. Agrawal
Department of Dentistry, Institute of Medicine, Tribhuhvan University, Kathmandu, Nepal

M. A. Reynolds
Department of Periodontics, University of Maryland School of Dentistry, Baltimore, MD, USA

Ahmad A. Madarati
Restorative Dental Sciences Department, College of Dentistry, Taibah University, , Madina 43353, Saudi Arabia
Faculty of Dentistry, Aleppo University, Aleppo, Syria

Ezi A. Akaji, Nkolika P. Uguru, Sam N. Maduakor and Etisiobi M. Ndiokwelu
Department of Preventive Dentistry, Faculty of Dentistry, College of Medicine, University of Nigeria, UNTH, Enugu, Nigeria

Tamanna Tiwari and Anne Wilson
Department of Community Dentistry and Population Health, School of Dental Medicine, University of Colorado Anschutz Medical Campus, Aurora, Colorado, USA

Matthew Mulvahill
School of Medicine, University of Colorado Anschutz Medical Campus, Aurora, Colorado, USA.

Nayanjot Rai
Colorado School of Public Health, University of Colorado Anschutz Medical Campus, Aurora, Colorado, USA

Judith Albino
Center for Native Oral Health Research, University of Colorado Anschutz Medical Campus, Aurora, Colorado, USA

Yilkal Tafere
Department of Public health, College of Health Sciences, Debre Tabor University, Debre Tabor, Ethiopia

Selam Chanie
Department of Nursing, Debre Tabor General hospital, Debre Tabor, Ethiopia

Tigabu Dessie
Department of Nursing, College of Health Sciences, Debre Tabor University, Debre Tabor, Ethiopia

Haileyesus Gedamu
Department of Nursing, College of Medicine and Health Sciences, Bahirdar University, Bahirdar, Ethiopia

Wentian Sun, Kai Xia, Xinqi Huang, Qing Liu and Jun Liu
State Key Laboratory of Oral Diseases, National Clinical Research Center for Oral Diseases, Department of Orthodontics, West China Hospital of Stomatology, Sichuan University, Chengdu 610041, China

Xiao Cen
State Key Laboratory of Oral Diseases, National Clinical Research Center for Oral Diseases, Department of Oral and Maxillofacial Surgery, West China Hospital of Stomatology, Sichuan University, Chengdu 610041, China

Neel Shimpi and Ingrid Glurich
Center for Oral and Systemic Health, Marshfield Clinic Research Institute, 1000 North Oak Avenue, Marshfield 54449, WI, United States of America

Amit Acharya
Center for Oral and Systemic Health, Marshfield Clinic Research Institute, 1000 North Oak Avenue, Marshfield 54449, WI, United States of America
Family Health Center of Marshfield Inc., 1307 N St Joseph Ave, Marshfield 54449, WI, United States of America
Office of Research Computing and Analytics, Marshfield Clinic Research Institute, 1000 North Oak Avenue, Marshfield 54449, WI, United States of America

Monica Jethwani and Aditi Bharatkumar
Center for Oral and Systemic Health, Marshfield Clinic Research Institute, 1000 North Oak Avenue, Marshfield 54449, WI, United States of America
Family Health Center of Marshfield Inc., 1307 N St Joseph Ave, Marshfield 54449, WI, United States of America

Po-Huang Chyou
Office of Research Computing and Analytics, Marshfield Clinic Research Institute, 1000 North Oak Avenue, Marshfield 54449, WI, United States of America

Hyemin Lee and Jooly Cha
Graduate School of Clinical Dentistry, Ewha Womans University, Seoul, South Korea

Youn-Sic Chun and Minji Kim
Department of Orthodontics, College of Medicine, Ewha Womans University, Seoul, South Korea

Keisuke Matsumura, Yuji Sato, Noboru Kitagawa, Toshiharu Shichita, Daisuke Kawata and Mariko Ishikawa
Department of Geriatric Dentistry, Showa University, School of Dentistry, 2-1-1 kitasenzoku Ota Ward, Tokyo 145-8515, Japan

Alessandra Giuliani and SerenaMazzoni
Sezione di Biochimica, Biologia e Fisica Applicata, Department of Clinical Sciences, Università Politecnica delle Marche, Via Brecce Bianche 1, 60131 Ancona, Italy

Carlo Mangano and Francesco Mangano
Private Practice, Gravedona, CO, Italy

Piero Antonio Zecca, Alberto Caprioglio, Nicolò Vercellini and Mario Raspanti
Department of Medicine and Surgery, University of Insubria, Via Guicciardini 9, Varese, Italy

Adriano Piattelli and Giovanna Iezzi
Department of Medical, Oral and Biotechnological Sciences, University of Chieti-Pescara, Via dei Vestini 31, 66100 Chieti Scalo, CH, Italy

Rosamaria Fastuca
Department of Biomedical Sciences, Dentistry and Morphological and Functional Imaging, University of Messina, Messina, Italy

Arthur Kemoli
Department of Paediatric Dentistry, University of Nairobi, Nairobi, Kenya

Hans Gjørup
Center for Oral Health in Rare Diseases, Department of Maxillofacial Surgery, Aarhus University Hospital, Aarhus C, Denmark

Marie-Louise Milvang Nørregaard and Dorte Haubek
Section for Pediatric Dentistry, Department of Dentistry and Oral Health, Health, Aarhus University, Aarhus C, Denmark

Mark Lindholm
Division for Oral Microbiology, Odontology, Umeå University, Umeå, Sweden

Tonnie Mulli
Department of Periodontology, University of Nairobi, Nairobi, Kenya

Anders Johansson
Molecular Periodontology, Odontology, Umeå University, Umeå, Sweden

Z. H. Zhou, X. Z. Chen, X. W. Chen, Y. X. Wang and J. Z. Zhen
Department of Oral and Maxillofacial Surgery, School of Medicine, Ninth People's Hospital, Shanghai Jiao Tong University, 639 Zhi Zao Ju Road, Shanghai 200011, People's Republic of China

S. F. Sun
Department of Stomatology, Tongren Hospital Affiliated to Shanghai Jiao Tong University School of Medicine, Shanghai 200336, People's Republic of China

S. Y. Zhang
Department of Oral and Maxillofacial Surgery, School of Medicine, Ninth People's Hospital, Shanghai Jiao Tong University, 639 Zhi Zao Ju Road, Shanghai 200011, People's Republic of China
Department of Oral Surgery, Shanghai Key Laboratory of Stomatology and Shanghai Research Institute of Stomatology, College of Stomatology, Ninth People's Hospital, Shanghai Jiao Tong University School of Medicine, No. 639, Zhi-Zao-Ju Road, 200011 Shanghai, People's Republic of China

Işıl Sarıkaya and Yeliz Hayran
Department of Prosthodontics, Tokat Gaziosmanpasa University Faculty of Dentistry, 60100 Tokat, Turkey

Cande V. Ananth
Department of Obstetrics and Gynecology, College of Physicians and Surgeons, Columbia University, New York, NY 10032, USA
Department of Epidemiology, Joseph L. Mailman School of Public Health, Columbia University, New York, NY 10032, USA

Emilie Bruzelius
Department of Epidemiology, Joseph L. Mailman School of Public Health, Columbia University, New York, NY 10032, USA
Section of Population Oral Health, College of Dental Medicine, Columbia University, New York, NY 10032, USA

Howard F. Andrews
Department of Biostatistics, Joseph L. Mailman School of Public Health, Columbia University, New York, NY 10032, USA
New York State Psychiatric Institute, New York, NY 10032, USA.

Panos N. Papapanou
Division of Periodontics, Section of Oral, Diagnostic and Rehabilitation Sciences, College of Dental Medicine, Columbia University, New York, NY 10032, USA

Angela M. Ward and David A. Albert
Section of Population Oral Health, College of Dental Medicine, Columbia University, New York, NY 10032, USA

Mary Lee Conicella
Aetna Inc., Pittsburgh, PA 15220, USA

Hongbing Lv, Yuemin Chen, Lishan Lei, Ming Zhang, Ronghui Zhou and Xiaojing Huang
School and Hospital of Stomatology, Fujian Medical University, Fuzhou 350002, China

Zhiyu Cai
Department of Stomatology, Fujian Medical University Union Hospital, Fuzhou 350001, China

Sun-Hyun Kim
Department of Clinical Oral Health Science, Graduate School of Clinical Dentistry, Ewha Womans University, Seoul, Korea

Jong-Bin Lee
Department of Periodontology, Mokdong Hospital, Ewha Womans University, Seoul, Korea

Min-Ji Kim
Department of Orthodontics, School of Medicine, Ewha Womans University, Seoul, Korea

Eun-Kyoung Pang
Department of Periodontology, School of Medicine, Ewha Womans University, 1071 Anyangcheon-ro, Yangcheon-gu, Seoul 07985, Republic of Korea

Dada Oluwaseyi Temilola
Department of Child Dental Health, Obafemi Awolowo University, Ile-Ife, Nigeria

Morenike Oluwatoyin Folayan
Department of Child Dental Health, Obafemi Awolowo University, Ile-Ife, Nigeria
Department of Child Dental Health, Obafemi Awolowo University Teaching Hospitals' Complex, Ile-Ife, Nigeria

Nneka Maureen Chukwumah
University of Benin Teaching Hospital, Benin City, Edo State, Nigeria

Bamidele Olubukola Popoola and Folake Barakat Lawal
University of Ibadan, Ibadan, Nigeria

Nneka Kate Onyejaka
University of Nigeria, Enugu, Nigeria

Titus Ayo Oyedele
Department of Surgery, Benjamin Carson, Snr, School of Medicine, Babcock University, Ilisan-Remo, Ogun State, Nigeria
Dental Department, Babcock University Teaching Hospial, Ilisan-Remo, Ogun State, Nigeria

Rim Hmaidouch and Paul Weigl
Department of Postgraduate Education, Master of Oral Implantology, Oral and Dental Medicine at Johann Wolfgang Goethe-University, Theodor-Stern-Kai 7 / building 29, 60596 Frankfurt am Main, Germany

Louise Sidenö
Department of Postgraduate Education, Master of Oral Implantology, Oral and Dental Medicine at Johann Wolfgang Goethe-University, Theodor-Stern-Kai 7 / building 29, 60596 Frankfurt am Main, Germany
Stockholm, Sweden

Jan Brandt
Department of Dental Prosthodontics, Faculty of Oral and Dental Medicine at Johann Wolfgang Goethe-University, Theodor-Stern-Kai 7 / building 29, 60596 Frankfurt am Main, Germany

Nadine von Krockow
Department of Oral Surgery, Faculty of Oral and Dental Medicine at Johann Wolfgang Goethe-University, Theodor-Stern-Kai 7 / building 29, 60596 Frankfurt am Main, Germany

Hiu Tung Bonnie Ling, Fung Hou Kumoi Mineaki Howard Sum, Hai Ming Wong and Yanqi Yang
Department of Paediatric Dentistry and Orthodontics, Faculty of Dentistry, Prince Philip Dental Hospital, The University of Hong Kong, 2/F, 34 Hospital Road, Sai Ying Pun, Hong Kong SAR, China

Linkun Zhang
Department of Orthodontics, Tianjin Stomatological Hospital of Nankai University, 75 Dagu Road, Tianjin, China

Cindy Po Wan Yeungm and Kar Yan Li
Translational Research Laboratory, Faculty of Dentistry, Prince Philip Dental Hospital, The University of Hong Kong, Room 7A26, 7/F, 34 Hospital Road, Sai Ying Pun, Hong Kong SAR, China

L. A. Foster Page
Department of Oral Sciences, Faculty of Dentistry, University of Otago, Dunedin 9054, New Zealand

D. Boyd and W. M. Thomson
Department of Oral Sciences, University of Otago, Dunedin, New Zealand

A. Stevenson
Hutt Valley District Health Board, Wellington, New Zealand

K. Goad
Waikato District Health Board, Hamilton, New Zealand

K. Fuge
Community Oral Health Service, Hutt Valley Hospital, Wellington, New Zealand

D. Sim
Southern District Health Board, Dunedin, New Zealand

Najlaa M. Alamoudi
Pediatric Dentistry Department, Faculty of Dentistry, King Abdulaziz University, Jeddah 21589, Saudi Arabia

Azza A. El-Housseiny
Pediatric Dentistry Department, Faculty of Dentistry, King Abdulaziz University, Jeddah 21589, Saudi Arabia
Pediatric Dentistry Department, Faculty of Dentistry, Alexandria University, mAlexandria, Egypt

Alaa M. Baik
Pediatric Dentistry Department, King Abdulaziz University Dental Hospital, Jeddah, Saudi Arabia

Tariq S.Abu Haimed
Biomaterial Department, Faculty of Dentistry, King Abdulaziz University, Jeddah, Saudi Arabia

Ahmed S. Bakry
Operative Dentistry Department, Faculty of Dentistry, King Abdulaziz University, Jeddah, Saudi Arabia
Conservative Dentistry Department, Faculty of Dentistry, Alexandria University, Alexandria, Egypt

Patrick Rijkschroeff, Eva Wartewig and Bruno G. Loos
Department of Periodontology, Academic Centre for Dentistry Amsterdam (ACTA), University of Amsterdam and VU University Amsterdam, Gustav Mahlerlaan 3004, 1081, LA, Amsterdam, The Netherlands

Elena A. Nicu
Department of Periodontology, Academic Centre for Dentistry Amsterdam (ACTA), University of Amsterdam and VU University Amsterdam, Gustav Mahlerlaan 3004, 1081, LA, Amsterdam, The Netherlands
Opris Dent SRL, Sibiu, Romania

Kamran Nazmi
Department of Oral Biochemistry, Academic Centre for Dentistry Amsterdam (ACTA), University of Amsterdam and VU University, Amsterdam, The Netherlands

Zhen Sun and Jiang-Tao Cui
Department of Stomatology, Second Hospital of Tianjin Medical University, Ping-Jiang Road, He Xi District, 300211 Tianjin, People's Republic of China

Wei Gao
Department of Interventional Therapy, Tianjin Medical University Cancer Institute and Hospital, National Clinical Research Center for Cancer, Key Laboratory of Cancer Prevention and Therapy, Tianjin's Clinical Research Center for Cancer, Huan Hu West Road, 300060 Tianjin, People's Republic of China

Gloria C. Mejia, Xiangqun Ju and Lisa M. Jamieson
Australian Research Centre for Population Oral Health, Adelaide Dental School, The University of Adelaide, Adelaide, SA 5005, Australia

Hawazin W. Elani
Harvard School of Dental Medicine, Harvard University, Boston, MA, USA

Sam Harper and Jay S. Kaufman
Department of Epidemiology, Biostatistics and Occupational Health, McGill University, Montreal, Quebec H3A 1A2, Canada

W. Murray Thomson
Sir John Walsh Research Institute, Faculty of Dentistry, The University of Otago, Dunedin, New Zealand

Ichiro Kawachi
Social and Behavioral Sciences, Harvard T.H. Chan School of Public Health, Boston, MA 02115, USA

Index

www.ingramcontent.com/pod-product-compliance
Lightning Source LLC
Chambersburg PA
CBHW061315190326
41458CB00011B/3813
* 9 7 8 1 6 3 2 4 1 5 7 0 7 *